W9-BFZ-229

MOLECULAR
BASIS
of
AGING

Edited by
Alvaro Macieira-Coelho, M.D., D.Sc., D.h.c.
Research Director
INSERM
Versailles, France

CRC Press
Boca Raton   New York   London   Tokyo

Library of Congress Cataloging-in-Publication Data

Molecular basis of aging/edited by Alvaro Macieira-Coelho.
     p. cm.
    Includes bibliographical references and index.
    ISBN 0-8493-4786-6
      1. Aging–Molecular aspects. 2. Aging–Genetic aspects.
    I. Macieira–Coelho, Alvaro, 1932-
     [DNLM: 1. Aging–genetics. 2. Mammals–genetics. 3. Evolution.
    WT 104 M7174 1995]
    QP863.M683 1995
    599′ .0372--dc20
    DNLM/DLC
    for Library of Congress
                                       95-15170
                                          CIP

© 1995 by CRC Press, Inc.

No claim to original U.S. Government works
International Standard Book Number 0-8493-4786-6
Library of Congress Card Number 95-15170
Printed in the United States of America 1 2 3 4 5 6 7 8 9 0
Printed on acid-free paper

THE EDITOR

Alvaro Macieira-Coelho, M.D., D.Sc., D.h.c., is Research Director at the French National Institute of Health (INSERM), Department of Immunology, Medical School Pitié-Salpetrière, University of Paris VI.

Dr. Macieira-Coelho obtained his M.D. at the University of Lisbon, Portugal and his D.Sc. from the University of Uppsala, Sweden. From 1958–1961 he was an intern at the Lisbon University Hospital and a research associate at the Wistar Institute of the University of Pennsylvania (1961–1964) and in the Department of Pathology of the University of Uppsala (1964–1967). He was head of the Department of Cell Pathology at the Institute of Cancerology and Immunogenetics, Villejuif, France (1967–1986) and visiting professor at the Department of Cell Biology at the University of Linköping, Sweden (1987–1989).

Dr. Macieira-Coelho currently teaches at the University of Paris. He has given over 100 invited lectures at international meetings and at various institutes and universities, has published more than 100 research papers, and is the author of one book. He was the editor of one book on aging and is on the editorial board of four international gerontology journals.

Dr. Macieira-Coelho received the Johananoff International Visiting Professorship from the Mario Negri Institute (Milan) in 1982, the Fritz-Verzaàr Prize for Gerontology from the University of Vienna in 1988, and a Dr. Honoris Causa from the University of Linköping, Sweden, in 1991.

He is a member of the New York Academy of Sciences, American Society for Cell Biology, American Association for Cancer Research, and the Gerontological Society of America.

His current research interests concern the role of cell replication in aging of the human organism, for which he received support from a grant from the Sandoz Foundation for Gerontological Research.

CONTRIBUTORS

Paul S. Agutter, Ph.D.
Department of Biological Sciences
Napier University
Edinburgh, Scotland

Hervé Allain, M.D., Ph.D.
Pharmacology Laboratory
Faculty of Medicine
University of Rennes I
Rennes, France

Fiorenzo Battaini, Ph.D.
Department of Experimental Medicine and
Biochemical Sciences
University of Rome Tor Vergata
Rome, Italy

Danièle Bentue-Ferrer, Ph.D.
Pharmacology Laboratory
Faculty of Medicine
University of Rennes I
Rennes, France

Philippe van den Bosch de Aguilar,
Ph.D.
Laboratory of Cell Biology
Catholic University of Louvain
Louvain-la-Neuve, Belgium

Ulf Brunk, Ph.D.
Department of Pathology
University of Linköping
Linköping, Sweden

James W. Gaubatz, Ph.D.
Department of Biochemistry and Molecular
Biology
College of Medicine
University of South Alabama
Mobile, Alabama

Stefano Govoni, Ph.D.
Institute of Pharmacological Sciences
University of Milan
Milan, Italy

Siegfried Hoyer, M.D.
Department of Pathochemistry and General
Neurochemistry
University of Heidelberg
Heidelberg, Germany

Kenneth H. Johnson, M.D.
Department of Veterinary PathoBiology
College of Veterinary Medicine
University of Minnesota
St. Paul, Minnesota

M. S. Kanungo, Ph.D.
Molecular Biology Laboratory
Department of Zoology
Banaras Hindu University
Varanasi, India
and
Institute of Life Sciences
Bhaneswar, India

Paul J. M. Klosen, Ph.D.
Laboratory of Cell Biology
Catholic University of Louvain
Louvain-la-Neuve, Belgium

J. Labat-Robert, Ph.D.
Department of Cell Biology
University of Paris VII
Paris, France

Hans U. Lutz, Ph.D.
Laboratory for Biochemistry
Swiss Federal Institute of Technology
Zurich, Switzerland

Alvaro Macieira-Coelho, M.D., D.Sc.,
D.hc.
Research Director, INSERM
Versailles, France

Jaime Miquel, Ph.D.
Chief, Division of Applied Neuroscience
Institute of Neurosciences
University School of Medicine
Alicante, Spain
and
Institute of Molecular Medical Sciences
Palo Alto, California

Werner E. G. Müller, Ph.D.
Department of Applied Molecular Biology
Institute of Physiological Chemistry
Mainz, Germany

Atsushi Miyamoto, M.S., Ph.D.
Department of Pharmacology
Sapporo Medical University School of
Medicine
Sapporo, Japan

Hans Niedermüller, Ph.D.
Austrian Society for Geriatrics and
Gerontology
Institute of Physiology
and
The Ludwig Boltzmann Institute of
Experimental Gerontology
Veterinary Medical University
Vienna, Austria

Suresh I. S. Rattan, Ph.D., D.Sc.
Laboratory of Cellular Aging
Department of Chemistry
Aarhus University
Aarhus, Denmark

Ladislas Robert, M.D., Ph.D.
Department of Cell Biology
University of Paris VII
Paris, France

George S. Roth, Ph.D.
Molecular Physiology and Genetics Section
Laboratory of Cellular and Molecular Biology
Gerontology Research Center
NIH, National Institute on Aging
Baltimore, Maryland

Heinz C. Schröder, M.D., Ph.D.
Department of Applied Molecular Biology
Institute of Physiological Chemistry
Mainz, Germany

D. F. Swaab, M.D., Ph.D.
Director, Graduate School Neurosciences
Netherlands Institute for Brain Research
Amsterdam, The Netherlands

Marco Trabucchi, M.D.
Department of Experimental Medicine and
Biochemical Sciences
University of Rome Tor Vergata
Rome, Italy

Per Westermark, M.D., Ph.D.
Department of Pathology
Linköping University
Linköping, Sweden

Dazhong Yin, Ph.D.
Department of Pathology
Linköping University
Linköping, Sweden

J. N. Zhou, M.D.
Graduate School Neurosciences
Netherlands Institute for Brain Research
Amsterdam, The Netherlands
and
Ningxia Medical College
Ningxia, China

TABLE OF CONTENTS

INTRODUCTION

Those without expertise in gerontology, but interested in understanding the investigations carried out to elucidate the mechanisms of aging, face many difficulties.

PROBLEMS ARISING FROM COMPARATIVE BIOLOGY AND PHYSIOPATHOLOGY

One difficulty comes from the tendency that many gerontologists have of looking for a global view of the mechanisms of aging along the evolutionary scale, extrapolating data, and then seeking for universal explanations. Comparative biology has shown that the mechanisms of aging cannot be universal.[1] This does not mean, however, that studies performed on lower organisms along the evolutionary scale are useless in understanding human aging. Some mechanisms may be conserved, but as an organism becomes more complex other regulatory mechanisms come into the picture, and as a result the homeostatic regulation of the life span also increases in complexity. Moreover, along the evolutionary road some mechanisms have remained preponderant in some species, while becoming secondary in others.

It is obvious that the mechanisms controlling the life span in *Drosophila*, for instance, where there is no cell turnover in the mature organism, cannot be the same as those in a mammal, where permanent renewal occurs throughout the life span in many cell compartments, and whose genome is more complex than that of a fly. Initial mortality rates are also extremely high in flies; as compared with humans, they are 1000 times higher.[1] This illustrates fundamental developmental differences, showing that the mechanisms regulating the life span in *Drosophila* cannot be extrapolated to vertebrates.

A disregard for comparative biology and physiopathology has led to shortcuts and misinterpretations that have retarded the advancement of gerontology and handicapped communications between gerontologists.

We have limited this volume to experimental approaches performed with mammals but even among mammals striking differences appear, indicating that extrapolations should be carried out with restraint.

Among mammals, rodents are the laboratory animals most often used in gerontology studies, and the data obtained are often extrapolated to humans in spite of fundamental biologic differences. It has been considered that "molecular genetics and cell biology reinforce the evidence that rats and men are basically similar, so that many of the laboratory findings on aging in rats are substantially valid for our own species."[2] However, at the molecular and cellular levels, specificities exist which have obvious implications for survival. For instance, human cells are capable of removing *Micrococcus luteus* UV-endonuclease-susceptible sites, as opposed to rat cells which almost completely lack this type of DNA repair.[3] It has been suggested that this characteristic may render rat cells more dependent on postreplication repair systems which are error prone.[3] This may lead to an increased frequency of genetic changes in rat cells.

Another difference between the genetic material of rodents and humans became apparent in transfection experiments, which showed that a significantly lower number of sequences become stably incorporated by human cells as compared to hamster cells.[4] This shows that human cells are less prone to be modified by new information integrated from external sources.

Many experimental results on the biology of aging of mice have been thought to be applicable to humans. However, this is hardly conceivable when one considers the profound differences in the molecular and cellular biology of these two species. The DNA repair abilities of mouse cells differ from human cells and may be implicated in the cellular instability that characterizes this rodent group, expressed by the predisposition to malignant transformation. Mouse cells have a reduced capacity for excision repair as revealed by the low host-cell reactivation of UV-irradiated herpes simplex virus.[5,6] Single-strand break repair also differs; the relative increased efficiency of this type of repair is higher in human than in mouse fibroblasts.[7] Moreover, contrary to the situation in human cells, telomere shortening does not occur in mouse cells during aging.[8]

Furthermore, hybridization experiments between human and mouse cells revealed an incompatibility between the two genomes, making genetic interpretation of the transmission of interspecies phenotypic markers impossible.[9] These experiments showed that expression of the marker in the hybrid does not obey any law, even that of Mendelian genetics. These results have implications for certain experiments that are supposed to determine the presence of putative genes responsible for cell senescence.

Even the morphological comparison of mice and human chromosomes (Figure 1) highlights the fundamental differences existing in the organization of the two genomes. One can assume a different hierarchy within the centromere-telomere segment, implying specific regulatory constraints for each species.[10]

In addition to their particular morphology, mouse chromosomes display interesting features that could be responsible for some aspects of the

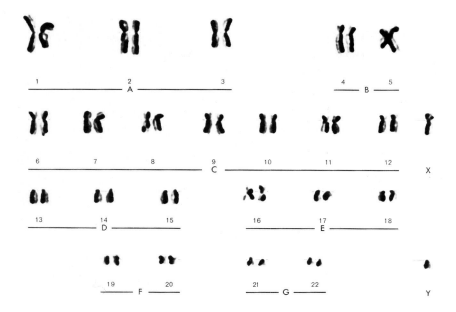

Human

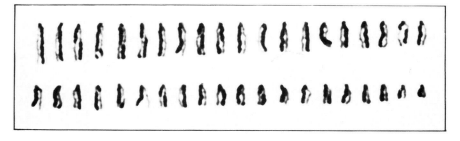

Mouse

Figure 1

Human (top) and mouse (bottom) chromosomes. The cells were labeled with bromodeoxyuridine during two rounds of replication, then prepared for visualization of the karyotype. After fixation they were stained with Giemsa. The chromatid which incorporated the precursor in both DNA strands is stained dark, the one that incorporated only in one strand is lightly stained. A few exchanges between sister chromatids can be seen, although more frequently in the mouse chromosomes.

physiopathology of this rodent's life span; this is reviewed in detail in Chapter 1, dealing with the reorganization of the genome. Mouse chromosomes display a pronounced instability which is manifested as a high probability of recombinational events.[11] This must be due to some yet-unknown structural organization of the mouse genome, and to the presence of molecules that regulate recombination. The efficiency of converting nicks into crossovers due to the transient appearance of a protein called R-protein, which facilitates DNA reannealing, seems to be greater in the mouse.[10]

This characteristic of the mouse genetic material seems to be responsible, at least in part, for the particularly high transformation frequency of mouse cells; it must also be responsible for the high frequency of mutable events of this species. This might be useful for the group's survival as it provides a greater capacity to adapt and evolve with environmental changes, but is deleterious to the individual because of the instability it creates at the molecular and cellular levels.

The "plasticity" of the genome, i.e., the potential for rearrangements, seems to play an essential role in development, aging, and disease; this is a feature that has been neglected in gerontology. A suitable potential for genome rearrangements must be important for differentiation to progress through development. Plasticity of the genome diminishes through development, maturity, and aging (see Chapter 1); this could be a control mechanism to avoid deviations from normal development that could lead to disease. Indeed, unregulated genome plasticity, such as the expansion of small repeats, can lead to disease. An increased potential for chromosomal recombinational events is also related to a predisposition for neoplastic transformation.[12]

The lack of plasticity seems to lead to deviations from normal development as is the case with Werner's syndrome patients. The cytogenetic studies of this disease have shown that it is characterized by rearrangements which become fixed.[13]

A puzzling feature, seemingly correlated to the plasticity of the genome and one that distinguishes the cells of mammalian species, has been observed during the *in vitro* cultivation of their fibroblasts. This feature is their relative propensity to overcome proliferative senescence and acquire the potential for unlimited proliferation. This has been one of the interesting windfalls of the aging of proliferative cells concept and of its opposite, cell immortalization;[14] it has implications for evolutionary differences between species that also have a bearing on cancer and aging *in vivo*.

Swim and Parker[15] had obtained data suggesting that cells from some species might be endowed with a limited number of doublings, while others were able to divide indefinitely. Later, it became apparent that the probability of escaping proliferative senescence, and of becoming immortalized, has a bearing on the susceptibility to be transformed by all types of carcinogens and oncogenes.[12,16] The failure to grasp this important conclusion led to the indiscriminate use of cells in the study of the effects

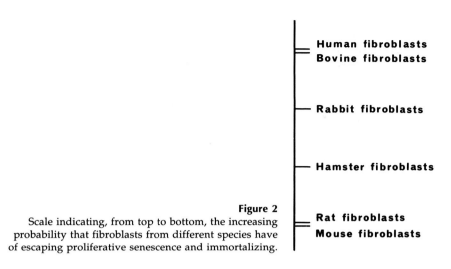

Human fibroblasts
Bovine fibroblasts

Rabbit fibroblasts

Hamster fibroblasts

Figure 2
Scale indicating, from top to bottom, the increasing
probability that fibroblasts from different species have
of escaping proliferative senescence and immortalizing.

Rat fibroblasts
Mouse fibroblasts

of carcinogens, and to incorrect interpretations of the action of oncogenes due to misunderstandings of the target cell biology. Indeed, when comparing fibroblasts from different species based on the probability of spontaneously yielding a population with unlimited growth potential, the resulting scale goes from very low to 100% probability (Figure 2). The latter occurs with rat and mouse fibroblasts regardless of the animal strain.[17] In general, murine fibroblasts tend to have a higher probability of yielding permanent cell lines than, for instance, their human and bovine counterparts. This led to the claim that one or two genes were necessary for the transformation of murine cells. In fact, these cells evolve spontaneously through the different transformation steps, and the introduction of those genes simply accelerates a latent potential.[12,16]

It is also easier to induce cancers in those species whose fibroblasts have a higher probability of escaping *in vitro* senescence. The species whose fibroblasts immortalize easily also seem to be more short lived. Is there a possible causality relationship between cell instability and a short life span? The question remains open but the relationship seems reasonable, especially with the realization that cellular instability seems to be related to the instability of the genome.[12,16] These fundamental molecular and cellular interspecies differences, expressed in their respective physiopathologies, have not been considered by gerontologists.

Other aspects of comparative physiopathology also illustrate the difficulty in extrapolating data from one species to another. Women, for instance, have a unique propensity for breast cancer (25% of all malignant tumors) as compared to other mammals. Breast cancer in dogs constitutes approximately 13%, in cats 5%, and in cattle and horses 1% of all cancers.[18] There are also marked differences in the pathology of atherosclerosis.

CONCLUSIONS FROM EXPERIMENTAL SYSTEMS SHOULD FIT THE PHYSIOLOGY OF ORGANISM AGING

Another difficulty for gerontology students comes from the incorrect utilization of certain experimental systems. This is particularly true for experiments attempting to elucidate the mechanisms that alter the proliferative potential of some cell compartments during aging of the organism. This has created a wall between cytogerontologists and the other gerontologists, through which communication is barely possible.

Both the investigators studying the proliferative potential of cells and the gerontologists working in other fields were misdirected, following claims that the decline of the proliferative potential of some somatic cells is due to an increase in the fraction of nondividing cells. Cloning of cells was first used to determine the cell fraction capable of division during the proliferative history of human fibroblast populations.[19] It concluded that "the increase in the fraction of nondividing cells is approximately exponential, as is the increase in the probability of death for certain privileged human populations." Other investigations, where ^{3}H-thymidine labeling of cells was used for the same purpose, claimed that "the data showed a continual decrease in the fraction of cells synthesizing DNA during aging."[20]

Both of these works reached a conclusion incompatible with the physiology of a mammalian organism, i.e., that cellular senescence is due to the increase of nondividing cells during serial population doublings. Surprisingly, this conclusion was accepted by most investigators using this experimental system; it led to the almost obsessive search for an evaluation of the number of nondividing cells, and for the stage of the division cycle where cell growth is arrested. Cells that had lost their division potential were called senescent cells, and cellular senescence was defined as the reproductive failure after a period of replication. Most works claiming to study cellular senescence still attempt to identify the events that occur when a cell population enters the final nondividing phase. Some investigations, claiming to have discovered inductors of cell senescence, were simply reporting on the way to make cells enter the postmitotic stage.

These types of interpretations also led to an association between the limited proliferation potential and apoptosis, for which there is no experimental evidence. In regard to senescence of proliferative cells, chromatin studies have shown that the terminal postmitotic cell is not in apoptosis.[21] At this time, apoptosis appears as a homeostatic mechanism of cell elimination and renewal, which might in fact protect the organism from cells that have completed their life span and from disorderly proliferations. When uncontrolled, it is also implicated in pathological states.

It is obvious that aging of the mammalian organism is not due to the loss of the division potential of proliferative cell compartments. The transition to a postmitotic phase is an interesting and important problem of

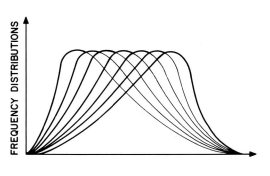

Figure 3
Shift to the right of the heterogeneity of generation times of human mesenchymal cells, summarized from the data obtained on the kinetics of proliferation during proliferative aging.[23-30] The shift in generation times is the expression of the functional drift.

FREQUENCY DISTRIBUTIONS

GENERATION TIMES AT DIFFERENT PASSAGES

cell biology, but there is no evidence whatsoever of its relevance to aging of the organism. Therefore, many gerontologists that used other experimental systems dismissed the one proposed by Hayflick,[22] claiming that it is irrelevant to the study of aging.

Meanwhile, other works gave a different view of aging of proliferative cells — one compatible with the physiology of aging of the organism. They showed that long before a cell population enters the final nondividing phase, progressive changes can be detected in the response to growth stimuli and in the way the cells transit through the cycle.[23-30] These works demonstrated the uncertainty and heterogeneity that are implicated in the probability of cycling, in contrast to the other data that assume an all-or-none event, obviously incompatible with the physiology of the organism.

Most investigators missed the point that the significance for aging of the experimental system proposed by Hayflick[22] is to have revealed how serial replication affects the coordination of the response to growth factors, and the way cells progress through the divison cycle rather than how cells are arrested when they become postmitotic. Furthermore, the ability to divide is just one function among others; if the response to growth stimuli and the way the cells transit through the cycle are progressively modified by serial divisions, then other functions are modified as well.

The commitment to divide depends on several factors such as the substratum for cell attachment, concentration of nutrients, growth factors and inhibitors, cooperation between cells, intracellular modifications, etc. As for aging of the organism, the relevance of modifications occurring through serial proliferation is the increased heterogeneity in the response of proliferative cell compartments to those different parameters; this shows the functional evolution of a cell compartment.

During the course of proliferation, cells progress through different functional stages so that their distribution among those stages is modified (Figure 3). This implicates new cell interactions and regulations and is an important component of the permanent evolution suffered by a mammalian organism through its life span. This occurs not only in several mitotic cell systems,[31] but also in conditionally mitotic compartments such as hepatocytes.[32]

The implications that cellular changes occurring during proliferation have on aging of the organism are presented in detail in Chapter 1 concerning these cell compartments.

It should be stressed that the cellular changes taking place in mitotic cell populations can also be created by events independent from those occurring during the division cycle, such as pathological conditions or external events (e.g., action of the sun on the skin).[33]

There is growing evidence that favors the proposal in which the evolution of a fibroblast population through proliferation is a differentiation process.[34] The mesenchyme is known for its inductive properties on neighboring cells; however, the specific functions of the different phases traversed by its cells have not been ascertained. The function of the terminal fibroblastic cell has yet to be determined; until this is elucidated, the terminal differentiation hypothesis shall remain a hypothesis. In any case, one has to distinguish the life cycle of a cell population that is part of homeostasis from those changes due to and contributing to aging of the organism.

The terminal postmitotic fibroblast is present in the normal adult organism,[21] but its eventual role in the aging process has not been found. However, the terminal cell was found in increased amounts in aging-related pathological states;[21,35] the interesting possibilities this finding offers to distinguish between physiological and pathological aging are discussed in Chapter 1. Since this volume deals mainly with aging per se, and not with the problem of terminal differentiation or the pathology of aging, the extensive work done on the mechanisms intervening in the switch to the terminal postmitotic fibroblast is not discussed herein.

THE UNITY AND INTERDEPENDENCE OF PHENOMENA IN THE ORGANISM

Additional problems have plagued the field of gerontology. The insatiable quest for a Holy Grail, rooted in our culture, has led to attempts to explain aging with regard to a keystone — an initial trigger, followed by a chain reaction leading to senescence. There have been several fads, some at the molecular level such as DNA mutations, cross-links, protein errors, free radicals, etc., and others of a more general nature, such as the influence of stress. This does not fit the physiology of complex organisms regulated by infinite interactions between the different hierarchical orders of organization that constitute them. Hence, it is not surprising that the hypotheses proposed to explain aging, whether of a general nature or focalized at the molecular level, are actually all connected; it illustrates the unity and interdependence of all phenomena in an organism.

Stress as a cause of aging has been proposed by Selye, who postulated that individuals are born with a fixed quantity of adaptive energy which is progressively consumed during the increased exposure to hormones secreted during stress.[36] Selye was able to induce a progeria-like syndrome in rats using dihydrotachysterol, and to prevent it using spironolactone which he termed a catatoxic hormone, i.e., capable of canceling the toxic effects of other hormones.

The stress of reproduction is a major hormone-releasing event in some species — one that triggers a chain of reactions leading to rapid senescence and death. In humans, it was found that castration prolonged the life of inmates in a mental hospital;[37] this could be an example of a mechanism that obviously plays an important role in limiting the life span in some species but became relatively unimportant in others.

It is unquestionable that stress can accelerate aging, not only through the triggering of diseases, but also by hastening changes at the molecular and cellular levels that lead to senescence. An interesting study showed that arterial smooth muscle cells from hypothalamus-stimulated animals grow faster when explanted *in vitro* than do those of the control donors.[38] This work demonstrates the repercussions of a broad reaction in the organism at the molecular, cellular, and tissue levels. It is also representative of the influence external events can have on the proliferative history of a cell compartment.

In addition to or because of its accelerating effect on senescence, stress plays a role in mortality which becomes increasingly significant with aging, since the amplitude of the insult needed to kill diminishes as the organism ages.[39]

The stress hypothesis is a variant, although more specific, of the "rate of living" theory. This theory claimed that the duration of life varies in inverse proportion to the rate of energy expended, as a result of a finite, total amount of "vitality" being used. This proposal eventually acquired a scientific basis when a correlation was ascertained between life span and metabolic rate and temperature.[2]

The way energy expenditure is regulated is a crucial problem in cell biology and one which unfortunately is almost completely unknown to us. The problem of the control of energy transduction and its role in aging is related, at the molecular level, to the proposal that the fundamental cause of aging resides in the mitochondria, the power house of the cell. It postulates that dysfunction of the mitochondria would be due to alterations of the mitochondrial genome, leading to disorganization of free radical production on the mitochondrial membrane.

Free radicals are molecules with an impaired electron. They are generated along the electron transport chain, when electromagnetic energy is transformed into chemical energy. The ultimate electron acceptor along the chain is oxygen, which then becomes a superoxide radical. The goal of this electron transport is to create chemical energy with the production of a high-phosphate donor, i.e., ATP. This transformation of energy is obviously a crucial process in the life of a cell, therefore anything that takes place in the cell must be influenced by, or influences, this transport chain.

Thanks to oxidative metabolism, molecules are modified — in this way constituting signals for homeostatic molecular and cellular elimination and renewal (see Chapter 6).

The free radical theory of aging has been one of the most popular. It demonstrates how arguments proposed to explain both maximal life span and organism aging can be used indiscriminately to find a single explanation for everything. This has been one of the problems for those interested in learning the methods used to identify the mechanisms of aging: the combination of conceptual contributions made to explain maximum life span with the theories and experiments attempting to explain aging of an organism. Although the two phenomena may overlap in some respects, some mechanisms are proper to each. The correlation between oxidative damage and species life span[40] could provide a mechanism to explain the former rather than the latter.

The role of free radicals in aging-related pathologies is well documented; their influence on the mechanisms of aging, though, has a less firm basis and is difficult to fit into many of the features involved in longevity. The prolongation of the life span, measured as a function of the survival curve of a population of individuals, is usually used to ascertain the causal relationship between aging and a given parameter. However, prolonged survival can be due to the elimination of pathologies that curtail the life span without having an effect on the process of senescence. This has been shown to be the case in the improved survival of calorie-restricted animals.[41] The same could hold true for life span manipulations through the action of free radical metabolism. There are other pitfalls in using survival curves to identify phenomena influencing aging, but they will not be discussed in this volume.

The free radical theory of aging does not explain many features, inter alia the clock-type behavior of the mammalian life span and the parental genetic influence on aging.

Inherited longevity cannot be due to genes either, since accelerated physiologic aging has never been reported. Individuals die before reaching their maximal life span potential because of accidents or disease. Furthermore, all the known so-called syndromes of premature aging actually involve a variety of pathologies and only have a vague similitude with physiologic aging. The Werner's syndrome of so-called premature aging has a very complex genetic picture that has no analogy to physiological aging. All progeroid syndromes seem to be more a deviation from normal development associated with several pathologies than accelerated aging.

The parental influence on longevity could be due to the genetically determined probability of developing or not developing diseases that curtail the life span, rather than to modifications of the process of aging per se. In that case genes would naturally be involved, since a correlation between the presence of certain genes and the probability of developing specific diseases is well documented.

The inherited genetic determinants of longevity could also influence aging through the heritable character of time, as proposed by Gedda and Brenci.[42] These two investigators suggested that there are two properties for every gene, one consisting of the informational potential which they called the ergon, and the other corresponding to its informational activity period which they called the chronon. They reported an interesting correlation in monozygotic twins as to when different developmental and senescent processes were manifested such as first word, first pubic hair, onset of menarch, first gray hair, use of eyeglasses, or onset of menopause.

Aging is determined from the embryonic stage onward, and the events that occur during development can be critical for the pattern of aging.[43] Longevity could be influenced by the periodicity of the different developmental stages; genetic determinants of this periodicity could, in part, be parentally transmitted. This way, the hereditary determinants of longevity could be related to the phenomenon of hereditary biological time, the chronon.[42]

The constant desire to find a rationale in evolution led to the proposal that specific genes and specific genomic modifications are responsible for species life span, aging of the organism, as well as cell aging. This does not make sense in the face of the complexity of the genome and of its interactions with other levels of information storage.

Genes must be involved in the determination of a species life span, but theories that propose sets of genes as the main determinants of life span seem simple-minded. It is more likely that the whole genome is involved in the determination of a species life span, with the coding and noncoding regions as well as the folding of DNA. The examples mentioned earlier concerning differences between the genomes of humans and rodents support this view. It is becoming increasingly obvious that regions occupied by repetitive sequences are equally important. They have been found to play a role in recombinational events; this may be due to a preferential nicking of DNA in regions of moderate repeats.[10] On the other hand, an increase in the number of certain repeats can destabilize genomic regions and lead to disease.

The genome though, cannot be the sole determinant of the life span in such complex systems as mammalian organisms. As pointed out by Sacher,[44] "the length of life is the expression of the total capability of a set of physiological, biochemical and behavioral performances directed towards stabilizing the organism and maintaining life." The good correlation between brain size and life span led him to the stochastic theory of mortality, according to which an increase in brain size during hominid evolution initiated an increase in the encephalization index, and consequently in the precision of homeostatic regulation of the life span. It also led to increased intelligence, and thus to the possibility of avoiding environmental hazards. This view seems to be more realistic than any other focalized proposals of the mechanisms responsible for the life span.

Another very popular cascade-type theory is the protein error theory; its basis is more cultural than scientific. It focuses on a concept common to several cultures, i.e., that the human organism is basically perfect but perishes because of errors committed. However, none of the numerous experimental attempts to test for the presence of proteins with errors could provide any support to the theory.

Another problem encountered with many reviews of works describing the organism's changes over time, is that the reader is faced with a description of the phenomenon of aging at the molecular level that sounds more like a catalogue of findings, rather than an integrative explanation of the physiology of a mammalian organism.

These are some of the complexities facing those attempting to describe the state of the art of molecular gerontology.

THE FOCUS OF THE PRESENT VOLUME

To avoid a labyrinthine review of age-related molecular events in which the reader would get lost, we have focused this volume on a fundamental aspect of mammalian physiology that is of primary importance to understanding development, maturity and aging, and which has not been presented so far.

Functioning of an organism basically depends upon the capacity of its cells to maintain their genetic information and to work cooperatively; in other words, it fundamentally depends upon the storage and the flow of information. It has become apparent that these two requisites evolve permanently from the beginning to the end of the mammalian life span, and that functioning of the organism evolves accordingly.

Countless modifications occur in the information stored in the genome — some are programmed, which is obvious from the cyclical evolution of the functions of the organism through its life span, others are stochastic. Stochastic modifications of the information stored are partly due to the reorganization taking place in the nuclear and mitochondrial DNA. As described in this volume, one of the sources of this reorganization is the inevitable modifications that occur in the genome through the division cycle, within proliferative cell compartments. It has become apparent that after each division, a daughter cell is not exactly identical to the mother cell and its sister cell. Quantitative and qualitative changes create a drift that progressively becomes expressed in cell functioning. Cell division is a necessary renewal mechanism, but has its price. It creates a drift in a cell compartment that modifies its function and its subsequent interactions with other compartments.

Genomic DNA of nondividing cells also undergoes modifications. Changes can occur by the introduction of new genetic information carried by viruses, or through damage, repair, and metabolic activity. The molecule can be modified through methylation, and genes can be modified through amplification, conversion, transposition, or deletion. Loss of genes and DNA conformational changes have been reported in postmitotic tissues of old animals.[45,46] On the other hand, exchanges were found to take place between genomic and mitochondrial DNA.[47] Examples of the modifications that occur in nuclear and mitochondrial DNA are described in the respective chapters.

In this volume we focused mainly on the storage of information in the genome. Information, however, is not stored only in DNA. Some gene products, such as the extracellular molecules of connective tissue, can also be considered as information sites which feed back on the genome. Changes in the information stored results in new coordinations of the information flowing between the different hierarchical orders of organization.

The flow of information depends on short- and long-range molecular intermediates responsible for the transmission of signals, and also on structure. Structure is both a source of storage and of the transmission of information. The organism is constituted of different hierarchical structural orders of organization. From DNA to the cell membrane and to the extracellular matrix, a structural continuum extends to the whole tissue or organ. The structure-dependent flow of information evolves during the organism's life span, making it an interesting aspect of mammalian physiology. The organism is permanently remodeled at the molecular, cellular, tissue, and organ levels, and the modifications occurring at one level of structure are transmitted to other levels of organization. The organism evolves from the beginning to the end through a complex interaction of its constituents, their structural changes reflecting on each of the other's structure and function.

This integrative view of the organism was well expressed by Schrödinger's statement: "the fundamental characteristic of life is the production of order from order, and the only source of biological order is biological order." Development, maturity, and aging, in part, are the result of the continuous evolution of biological order taking place through the organism's life span. Since structure and function are closely coupled at all levels of organization, the structural modifications are translated into functional modifications and vice versa.

For molecules, cells, and tissues, the flow of information depends on structural flexibility; this is what Valery Ivanov has coined as the "biology of conformation." One of the characteristics of aging of the mammalian organism is the loss of flexibility partly caused by structural remodeling.

At the molecular and cellular levels, flexibility is achieved through energy mobilization and transduction. This is regulated through phosphorylation and dephosphorylation, one of the tools developed by nature to switch a molecule between configurations with different responses to substrates and regulator molecules. When a ligand binds with a receptor, it can become a kinase through steric modification, this way initiating the transmission of signals through energy barriers.

Molecular conformation is also regulated through gradients of electric potential created through currents of electrons, protons, and ions which activate energy barriers such as membranes. On the other hand, a change in the conformation of a molecule is in itself a generator of a current by charged elements. Examples of how these mechanisms evolve over time in the organism, and the repercussions they have on cell function, are given in this volume.

Tissue flexibility also depends on the secretion of molecules such as hyaluronan, which seem to play a crucial role in the elasticity of different tissues. During aging, a decline in the secretion of this molecule by connective tissue cells has been reported. All the large molecules of the extracellular matrix in connective tissue (collagen, elastine, and proteoglycans) also play a role in local flexibility.

The flexibility of tissues and organs also depends on the relative proportion of their molecular and cellular components and on their structural integrity. Modifications in the skin, for instance, are visible externally and result from a progressive variation in the relative proportion of molecular and cellular components;[48,49] this remodeling is expressed on the skin surface. In the bone, continuous remodeling due to an evolution of the interaction between osteoblasts and osteoclasts leads to a structure unsuitable for adequate function.

In summary, fusion of the gametes triggers a molecular and cellular remodeling that creates an organism made up of different levels of organization connected by structural continuity, and by the molecular information flowing between them. The remodeling process is continuous, although the pace evolves. It causes changes in the information stored — changes that are partly stochastic and partly programmed. The restructuring undertaken at the different levels of organization is the result of events intrinsic to a living organism and of its interaction with the external milieu. This reorganization creates new coordinations in the flow of information. Function evolves accordingly.

Development, maturity, and aging correspond to different stages of this progression which tends to reach a limit; its pace differs and assumes characteristics inherent to each mammalian species. This book is meant to present the reader with experiments illustrating some aspects of this complex evolution of the mammalian organism: one that starts with the fusion of the gametes, progresses until its extinction, changes its function, and is eventually accompanied by a decreased probability of survival.

REFERENCES

1. Finch, C. E., *Longevity, Senescence and the Genome*, University of Chicago Press, Chicago, 1990, 657.
2. Sacher, G. A., Longevity, aging, and death: an evolutionary perspective, *The Gerontologist*, 18, 110, 1978.
3. Vijg, J., Mullaart, E. P., VanderSchans, G., Lohman, P. H., and Knook, D. L., Kinetics of ultraviolet induced DNA excision repair in rat and human fibroblasts, *Mutat. Res.*, 132, 129, 1984.
4. Hoeijmakers, J. H., Hanny, O., and Westerweld, A., Differences between rodent and human cell lines in the amount of integrated DNA after transfection, *Exp. Cell Res.*, 169, 111, 1987.
5. Yagi, T., DNA repair ability of cultured cells derived from mouse embryos in comparison with human cells, *Mutat. Res.*, 96, 89, 1982.
6. Elliot, G. C. and Johnson, R. I., DNA repair in mouse embryo fibroblasts. II. Responses of nontransformed preneoplastic and tumorigenic cells to ultraviolet irradiation, *Mutat. Res.*, 145, 185, 1985.
7. Diatloff-Zito, C., Deschavanne, P. J., Loria, E., Malaise, E., and Macieira-Coelho, A., Comparison between the radiosensitivity of human, mouse and chicken fibroblast-like cells using short-term endpoints, *Int. J. Rad. Biol.*, 39, 419, 1981.
8. Kipling, D. and Cook, H. J., Hypervariable ultra-long telomeres in mice, *Nature*, 347, 400, 1990.
9. LeBorgne de Kaouel, C., Billard, C., and Macieira-Coelho, A., Analysis of the growth in vitro of hybrids between normal and transformed cell lines, *Int. J. Cancer*, 21, 338, 1978.
10. Lima de Faria, A., *Molecular Evolution and Organization of the Genome*, Elsevier, Amsterdam, 1983, 210.
11. Macieira-Coelho, A., Implications of the reorganization of the cell genome for aging or immortalization of dividing cells in vitro, *Gerontology*, 26, 276, 1980.
12. Macieira-Coelho, A., Cancer and aging, *Exp. Geront.*, 21, 483, 1986.
13. Salk, D., Au, K., Hoehn, H., and Martin, G. M., Cytogenetics of Werner's syndrome cultures skin: variegated translocation mosaicism, *Cytogenet. Cell Genet.*, 30, 92, 1981.
14. Hayflick, L., Oncogenesis in vitro, *J. Natl. Cancer Inst.*, 26, 355, 1967.
15. Swim, H. E. and Parker, R. F., Culture characteristics of human fibroblasts propagated serially, *Am. J. Hyg.*, 66, 235, 1957.
16. Macieira-Coelho, A., Cancer and aging at the cellular level, in *Cancer and Aging*, Macieira-Coelho, A. and Nordenskjöld, B., Eds., CRC Press, Boca Raton, FL, 1990, 11.

17. Macieira-Coelho, A. and Azzarone, B., The transition from primary culture to spontaneous immortalization in mouse fibroblast populations, *Anticancer Res.*, 8, 165, 1989.
18. Glimelius, B., Hodgkin's disease, in *Cancer and Aging*, Macieira-Coelho, A. and Nordenskjöld, B., Eds., CRC Press, Boca Raton, FL, 1990, 227.
19. Merz, G. S. and Ross, J. D., Viability of human diploid cells as a function of in vitro age, *J. Cell. Physiol.*, 74, 219, 1969.
20. Cristofalo, V. J. and Sharf, B. B., Cellular senescence and DNA synthesis. Thymidine incorporation as a measure of population age in human diploid cells, *Exp. Cell Res.*, 76, 419, 1973.
21. Macieira-Coelho, A., Chromatin reorganization during senescence of proliferating cells, *Mutat. Res.*, 256, 81, 1991.
22. Hayflick, L., The limited in vitro lifetime of human diploid cell strains, *Exp. Cell Res.*, 37, 614, 1965.
23. Macieira-Coelho, A., Pontén, J., and Philipson, L., The division cycle and RNA synthesis in diploid human cells at different passage levels in vitro, *Exp. Cell Res.*, 42, 153, 1966.
24. Macieira-Coelho, A., Pontén, J., and Philipson, L., Inhibition of division cycle in confluent cultures of human fibroblasts in vitro, *Exp. Cell Res.*, 43, 20, 1966.
25. Macieira-Coelho, A., Influence of cell density on growth inhibition of human fibroblasts in vitro, *Proc. Soc. Exp. Biol. Med.*, 125, 548, 1967.
26. Macieira-Coelho, A. and Berumen, L., The cell cycle during growth inhibition of human embryonic fibroblasts in vitro, *Proc. Soc. Exp. Biol. Med.*, 144, 43, 1973.
27. Macieira-Coelho, A., Are non-dividing cells present in ageing populations of human fibroblasts in vitro?, *Nature*, 248, 421, 1974.
28. Macieira-Coelho, A. and Taboury, F., A re-evaluation of the changes in proliferation in human fibroblasts during ageing in vitro, *Cell Tiss. Kinet.*, 15, 213, 1982.
29. Macieira-Coelho, A. and Azzarone, B., Aging of human fibroblasts is a succession of subtle changes in the cell cycle and has a final stage with abrupt events, *Exp. Cell Res.*, 141, 325, 1982.
30. Macieira-Coelho, A., Contributions made by the studies of cells in vitro for understanding of the mechanisms of aging, *Exp. Gerontol.*, 28, 1, 1993.
31. Macieira-Coelho, A., Biology of normal proliferating cells in vitro. Relevance for in vivo aging, in *Interdisciplinary Topics in Gerontology*, von Hahn, H. P., Ed., Karger, Basel, 1988, 1.
32. Ishigami, A., Reed, T.A., and Roth, G., Effect of aging on EGF stimulated DNA synthesis and EGF receptor levels in primary cultured rat hepatocytes, *Biochem. Biophys. Res. Commun.*, 196, 181, 1993.
33. Gilchrest, B. A., Prior chronic sun exposure decreases the lifespan of human skin fibroblasts in vitro, *J. Gerontol.*, 35, 537, 1980.
34. Martin, G. M., Sprague, C. A., Norwood, T. H., and Pendergrass, W. R., Clonal selection, attenuation and differentiation in an in vitro model of hyperplasia, *Am. J. Pathol.*, 74, 137, 1974.
35. Macieira-Coelho, A., Genome reorganization through cell division. Implications for aging of the organism and cancer development, in *The Aging Clock*, Pierpaoli, W., Regelson, W., and Fabris, N., Eds.; *Ann. N.Y. Acad. Sci.*, 719, 108, 1994.
36. Selye, H., Stress and aging, *J. Am. Geriatr. Soc.*, 18, 669, 1970.
37. Hamilton, J. B. and Mestler, G. E., Mortality and survival. Comparison of eunuchs with intact men and women in a mentally retarded population, *J. Gerontol.*, 24, 395, 1969.
38. Gutstein, W. H., Wang, C. H., Wu, J. M., Ore, J., Cui, Y. N., and Lee, M. K., Growth retardation in senescent arterial smooth muscle cells and its reversal following brain stimulation. Implications for atherogenesis, *Mech. Ageing Dev.*, 60, 89, 1991.

39. Fries, J. F., The compression of morbidity: miscellaneous comments about a theme, *The Gerontologist*, 24, 354, 1984.

40. Cutler, R., Peroxide-producing potential of tissues. Inverse correlation with longevity of mammalian species, *Proc. Natl. Acad. Sci. U.S.A.*, 82, 4798, 1985.

41. Turturro, A., Duffy, P. H., and Hart, R. W., Modulation of toxicity by diet and dietary macronutrient restriction, *Mutat. Res.*, 295, 151, 1993.

42. Gedda, L. and Brenci, G., *Chronogenetics. The Inheritance of Biological Time*, Charles C Thomas, Springfield, IL, 1978, 95.

43. Muggleton-Harris, A. L., Hardy, K., and Higbee, N., Rescue of developmental lens abnormalities in chimaeras of noncataractous and congenital cataractous mice, *Development*, 99, 473, 1987.

44. Sacher, G. A., Maturation and longevity in relation to cranial capacity in hominid evolution, in *Primate Functional Morphology and Evolution*, Tuttle, R., Ed., Mouton, The Hague, 1975, 417.

45. Johnson, R. and Strehler, B. L., Loss of genes coding for ribosomal RNA in ageing brain cells, *Nature*, 240, 412, 1972.

46. Kanungo, M. S., *Biochemistry of Ageing*, Academic Press, London, 1980, 35.

47. Tsuzuki, T., Nomiyama, H., Setoyama, C., Maeda, S., and Shimada, K., Presence of mitochondrial-DNA-like sequences in the human nuclear DNA, *Gene*, 25, 223, 1983.

48. Boyer, B., Kern, P., Fourtanier, A., and Labat-Robert, J., Age-dependent variations of the biosynthesis of fibronectin and fibrous collagens in mouse skin, *Exp. Gerontol.*, 26, 375, 1991.

49. Pieraggi, M. T., Julian, M., and Bouissou, H., Fibroblast changes in cutaneous ageing, *Virchows Arch. [Pathol. Anat.]*, 402, 275, 1984.

I
THE STORAGE OF INFORMATION

Chapter 1

REORGANIZATION OF THE GENOME DURING AGING OF PROLIFERATIVE CELL COMPARTMENTS

A. Macieira-Coelho

CONTENTS

0-8493-4786-6/95/$0.00+$.50

I. RATIONALE OF THE SEARCH FOR A MOLECULAR REORGANIZATION OF THE GENOME DURING CELL PROLIFERATION

A. Chromosomal Rearrangements During Serial Cell Divisions

Studies of the kinetics of proliferation during senescence of mitotic cell compartments with a finite division potential[1-7] led to the conclusion that the decline of the growth potential is due mainly to an increased heterogeneity in the initiation and transit through the division cycle. This is summarized in Figure 1.

This conclusion was contrary to the main trend in the field, which favored the idea that at each doubling of the cell population there was an increase in the number of nondividing cells — an idea that was obviously incompatible with *in vivo* aging, since an accumulation of nondividing cells is not a characteristic of the aged organism.

The conclusion illustrated in Figure 1, which is compatible with what is known to take place with *in vivo* aging, was seminal for the understanding of the mechanisms leading to the decline of the growth potential through proliferation. As a matter of fact, it implied that at each division events that occur during the cell cycle must change the cells cumulatively, creating a drift that increases the heterogeneity to growth stimuli. The relevance for aging of the organism and of the data obtained with mitotic cell systems *in vitro* lies not in the fact that the end point to proliferation is reached, but rather in the finding that cells are progressively modified through division.[1-7]

What could be the events that modify the cells continuously through proliferation? It was proposed[8,9] that the events that create the cellular drift during proliferation are the result of the genome reorganization that takes place through the division cycle, causing cumulative quantitative and qualitative changes in DNA.

Several data indicate that a genome reorganization does indeed take place during the division cycle. The well-known exchanges between sister chromatids constitute one example;[10] another is the asymmetry in sister chromatids after DNA replication that can be observed with chromosome banding.[11]

Direct evidence for chromosomal recombination taking place during serial divisions comes from cytogenetic analyses performed on human

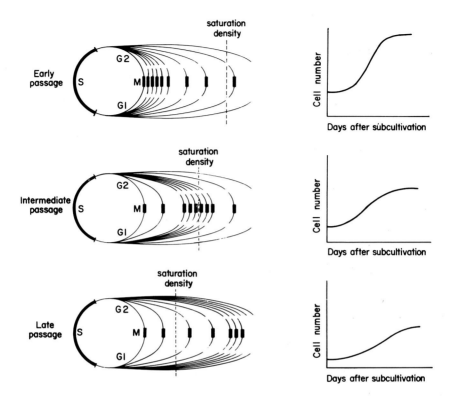

Figure 1
Schematic representation of the distribution of cell cycles through the life span of a human fibroblast population. Each circle or ellipse represents the generation time of a cell. There is a progressive shift to long cycles at the expense of the G1 and G2 periods, with increasing population doubling levels. The vertical dashed lines correspond to the maximal cell density reached, which declines. On the right-hand side are represented the growth curves obtained at the corresponding passage levels.

fibroblasts where chromosomal markers were used to detect somatic segregation in cells obtained from subjects heterozygous for chromosomal variants.[12] Somatic segregation (chromosomal recombination) for three different autosomes could be observed. Recombinant diploid cells appeared within cultures of tetraploid clones, and tetraploid cells regularly occurred within clones of diploid cells, with a parasexual cycle 2n→4n→2n.

Additional evidence for genome reorganizations occurring during the cell cycle comes from cytogenetic experiments showing that several rearrangements can be observed during serial divisions of cells. Human fibroblasts have been well-studied in this respect; translocations, inversions, dicentrics, breaks, and deletions have all been described, and increase through the cell population's life span.[13-15]

A pertinent observation was the one reported by Chen and Ruddle[16] who found that during the proliferation of normal human embryonic fibroblasts there are minor stem cell populations which compete, but none that dominate. The cells are not uniformly diploid; rather, several recurring chromosomal rearrangements can be detected at sufficiently high frequencies to insure their generation by minor stem cell populations.

It seemed reasonable to assume that reorganizations at the molecular level underlie the chromosomal rearrangements observed cytogenetically in proliferative cell compartments.

B. Relationship Between the Potential for Chromosome Recombination and the Long-Term Division Potential

On the other hand, there is evidence that the potential for chromosome rearrangements has a direct relationship with the long-term potential for proliferation of mitotic cells.

Human embryonic fibroblasts when cultivated *in vitro* go through continuous chromosomal rearrangements without any definite pattern becoming predominant.[16,17] The data suggested that multiple clones arise continuously, and compete among each other without one overgrowing the others. These cells have a longer division potential than postnatal fibroblasts, which go through more stable clonal-type chromosomal rearrangements during serial divisions *in vitro*.[17,18]

Moreover, fibroblasts from Werner's syndrome patients, which have a reduced doubling potential when compared with cells from age-matched donors, present chromosomal rearrangements (variegated translocation mosaicism) which become predominant and fixed during the cell population *in vitro* life span.[19]

These findings at the cytogenetic level suggest that a "rigidity" of the genome is associated with a shorter doubling potential, as opposite to a higher "plasticity" which would lead to a prolonged proliferative life span.

Another pertinent finding is the one showing that sister chromatid exchanges in human fibroblasts which have used most of their doubling capacity are less stimulated by drugs known to induce them.[20] These results suggest that in this cell system the loss of the division potential is associated with a loss of the "plasticity" of the genome.

It has also become apparent that a higher "plasticity" of the genome is related to the propensity to overcome proliferative senescence and to engage into the path of malignant transformation through the action of carcinogens. The study of the response of fibroblasts from different origins to ionizing radiation buttressed this view.

Human embryonic fibroblasts irradiated with low-dose-rate radiation at low population doubling levels (PDLs) when they have a higher poten-

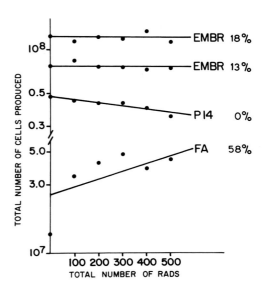

Figure 2
Total amount of cells produced in nonirradiated (ordinate) human fibroblast cultures and in the same cells irradiated with the different doses of ionizing radiation during their proliferative history *in vitro*. EMBR = embryonic lung fibroblasts; P14 = postnatal lung fibroblasts; FA = skin fibroblasts from a Fanconi's anemia patient. The % indicates the frequency of chromosome rearrangements observed in the respective nonirradiated cells through their *in vitro* life span.

tial for chromosome recombination are more resistant to radiation, and their life span can be prolonged.[21] If irradiated late during their life span, however, when they are less prone to rearrangements, their doubling potential is shortened. On the other hand, irradiation shortens the division potential of early passage postnatal fibroblasts which have a lower potential for chromosome recombination than the embryonic ones,[18] but can prolong the life span of human postnatal fibroblasts from donors with genetic diseases with a high rate of chromosome recombinations that are at high risk of cancer.[22] These findings are illustrated in Figure 2 which compares the effect of different doses of ionizing radiation on the doubling potential of human fibroblast populations, with the frequency (%) of chromosome rearrangements observed in the respective nonirradiated cells through their proliferative history. No chromosome rearrangements were observed in postnatal cells whose life spans were shortened by radiation. By contrast, a high frequency of rearrangements was observed in the cell population whose doubling potential was prolonged by radiation (skin fibroblasts from a Fanconi's anemia patient). Finally, the cells whose life spans were unaffected or slightly prolonged by radiation (human embryonic lung fibroblasts)[21] had an intermediate number of chromosome rearrangements. These results suggest that the effect of this carcinogen depends upon the potential of the cell population for chromosome rearrangements and that ionizing radiation under the experimental conditions used accentuates the intrinsic long-term growth potential of fibroblasts, maybe by accelerating changes in the genome which take place anyway during cell replication.

Another pertinent observation was the finding[18] that in the irradiated cells most of the breaks involved in exchanges (53 out of 62) concerned the centromeric and telomeric regions (Figure 3). Thus, the intrachromosomal break distribution where exchanges took place was preferentially located at regions rich in repetitive DNA, which have been implicated in recombinational events.[23]

We also found that the prolongation of the doubling potential of skin fibroblasts from retinoblastoma patients by low-dose-rate ionizing radiation showed a correlation with the potential for sister chromatid exchanges of the cells of the respective patients (Table 1). Hence, the presence of the deletion was not enough to confer susceptibility of the cells to this carcinogen; other genetic factors responsible for the high probability of chromosome recombination confer the proneness to transformation of these cells *in vitro* by radiation.

These results fit the hypothesis proposed at the start of the century by Boveri, establishing a relationship between malignant transformation and chromosomal rearrangements; they also agree with the proposal by Duesberg[25] that malignant transformation results from recombinations in cellular genes rather than mutations in latent cancer genes ("protooncogenes").

Low-dose-rate ionizing radiation can also accelerate the acquisition of an infinite growth potential in mouse fibroblasts *in vitro*,[26] a cell whose genome seems to be endowed with a high degree of "plasticity" and a high probability of spontaneous immortalization. Indeed, additional evidence in favor of an association between genome plasticity and prolonged division potential comes from observations on some characteristics of the mouse genome. The chromosomes of mouse fibroblasts cultivated *in vitro* show a very unusual capacity of recombination; images of crossing-overs and bridges between chromosomes (Figure 4), suggestive of interchromosomal exchanges, can be observed with a high frequency. Another difference between the mouse and the human genomes is the higher rate of sister chromatid exchanges in the former (Table 2) and the rapidity with which mouse cells can switch from the diploid to the tetraploid state.[27] Furthermore, the chromatin lability which accumulates during cellular aging disappears in the case of mouse cells during the chromosomal rearrangements that occur during the transition from senescence to immortalization.[28] We have also observed an interesting phenomenon of DNA elimination in mouse fibroblasts during the period preceding immortalization,[29] which could be germane to the disappearance of the fragile chromatin sites.

The potential for chromosomal recombinational events expressed by mouse fibroblasts *in vitro* also has a counterpart *in vivo*. Although 40 acrocentric chromosomes is the usual diploid number of the mouse species, localized races with 38 to 22 chromosomes resulting from Robertsonian fusions have been found in the wild.[30] This property of the mouse genome could be responsible for the high probability of mouse cells to escape

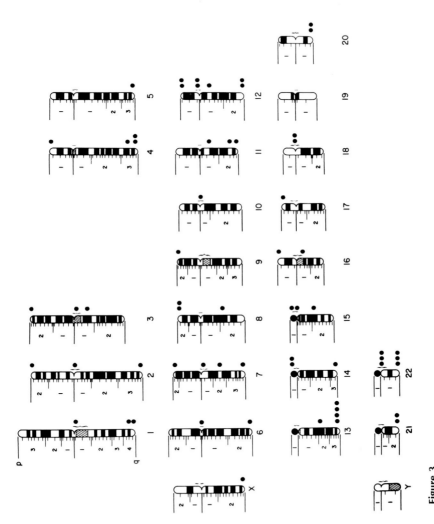

Figure 3
Distribution of breaks involved in exchanges in irradiated embryonic and postnatal human lung fibroblasts.

TABLE 1.

Percent Changes in Cell Population Doublings (CPD) in Skin Fibroblast Cultures from Retinoblastoma Patients that Received 2 ×1 Gy and Frequency of Sister Chromatid Exchanges in the Respective Nonirradiated Cell Populations

Donor	%Change in CPD	Mean SCE/cell[a]
1	+89	19.6(11–30)
2	+47	11.0(4–20)
3	−36	9.4(1–16)

[a] Mean of 20 cells; values within parentheses indicate the maximal and minimal number of SCE found in a cell.

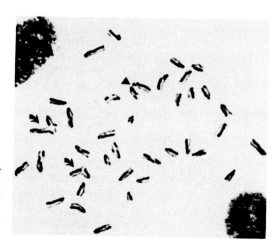

Figure 4
Radial figures (arrows) and bridge between chromosomes (triangle) found in karyotypes of mouse fibroblastic cultures before immortalization.

senescence and to immortalize, for the high frequency of spontaneous malignant transformations, the high susceptibility to viral, chemical, and physical carcinogens and oncogenes, and the facility with which one can induce tumors in mice.[24]

Thus it is not the chromosome constitution that is important for cell longevity, but rather the capacity of the genetic material to recombine. The data described above show that the problem of the growth potential of cells is not an artifact of *in vitro* cultivation, and that it has important correlations with evolutionary, developmental, and physiopathological characteristics of the organism from which the cells are derived.

The observations on the relationship between the capacity of cells to proliferate and the potential for recombinational events of their genome led to a new paradigm for the explanation of the mechanisms determining the long-term growth potential of certain mitotic cell compartments.[8,9]

TABLE 2.

Number of SCE/Cell[a] in Human and Mouse Fibroblasts at Different PDL After Two Division Cycles in the Presence of BRDU

Human		Mouse	
PDL	SCE	PDL	SCE
33	7	1	11
37	5	3	11
41	8	4	17
46	6	12	12

[a] Mean of 100 cells.

According to the paradigm, the trigger for a progressive shift in cell behavior leading to senescence of these cell compartments is the genome reorganization that inevitably accompanies cell division and modifies DNA at different levels of its structure. This is due *inter alia* to chromosomal rearrangements, sister chromatid exchanges, DNA strand switching, DNA loss, displacement of transposable elements, gene amplification, recombinations, deletions, and other events that occur during the cell cycle. This reorganization is the inevitable event which, although providing the cell with a way to evolve, adapt, and survive, will also determine its permanent drift and lead to the loss of the division potential. In some cells, however, for yet-unknown reasons, there is a higher probability to overcome this reorganization, to escape from proliferative senescence, and to engage in the path of malignant transformation. The reasons may lie in the organization of the coding and noncoding regions of the genome, which create different relationships and regulations.

The paradigm led to the search of a genome reorganization at the molecular and supramolecular levels developing during serial cell proliferation.

II. GENOME REORGANIZATION DURING SENESCENCE OF PROLIFERATIVE CELLS

A. Asymmetric Partition of DNA During Cell Division

The problem of quantitative changes in DNA originating during cell division was approached with cytofluorometric and cytophotometric measurements, and autoradiography.[31] The amount of DNA was measured on cells in interphase, prophase, metaphase, and anaphase; it was found that the scatter of DNA contents of cells in these different phases is

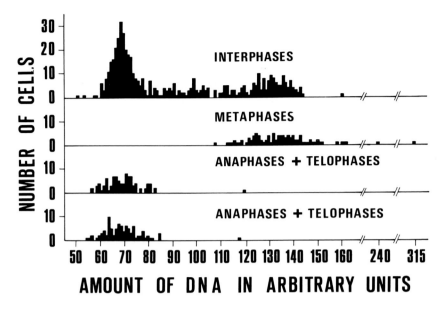

Figure 5
Distribution of DNA content in arbitrary units, found on interphases, metaphases, and on anaphases and telophases of human embryonic lung fibroblasts stained with ethidium bromide.

the same regardless of the stages of the cell cycle (Figure 5). It suggested that the scatter of values is due to real differences in DNA contents and not to methodological flaws.

To see if the scatter of DNA contents between cells varied with cell divisions, the distribution of DNA contents of each half of the anaphases and telophases, and that of the metaphases was plotted on probit paper in such a way that the scale of the abscissa for metaphases was twice that of the anaphases plus telophases (Figure 6). The values corresponding to each half of the anaphases and telophases and metaphases were linear, i.e., had a normal distribution, had identical slopes, and overlapped.

The data collected from cells close to the end of their proliferative life span (Phase IV), however, showed that the plot of DNA contents was an S-shaped curve, both for the anaphases and metaphases (Figure 7). Furthermore, the DNA contents of the metaphases and anaphases diverged. The cells' DNA content also reached significantly higher figures during this final phase of the fibroblast population proliferative life span. These results suggest a final chaos-type synthesis and partition of DNA during cell division, leading to an irreversible postmitotic state.

Staining with Feulgen also showed that the same DNA contents are obtained regardless of the stage of the cell cycle (Figure 8). These data reinforced the idea that the variation of DNA content between cells is due

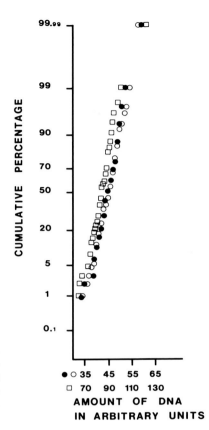

Figure 6

Plot on probit paper of the distribution of the amount of DNA found on human embryonic lung fibroblasts, measured on metaphases (□) and on each half of anaphases and telophases (●○). Ethidium bromide staining.

to quantitative differences and not to within-sample variation caused *inter alia* by changes in the binding of the dye to DNA at different stages of the division cycle, or to a different geometry of the cell. It takes place at a constant rate during the proliferative life span of the cells and assumes a chaos-type pattern during the last mitoses.

The differences in the DNA content of each half of the anaphases and telophases were expressed as the percentage of the mean value of each pair. The distribution of differences in DNA content between daughter cells was constant throughout the life span of the fibroblast population and increased only during the last two or three doublings (Figure 9).

Repeated measurements were made on the same samples stained with Feulgen-pararosaniline to evaluate the differences attributable to methodology. The white area in Figure 10 represents the differences, with three standard deviations, found with repeated measurements of the same cells. The data showed that differences in DNA content larger than 4% of the mean of the pair of daughter cells are significant.

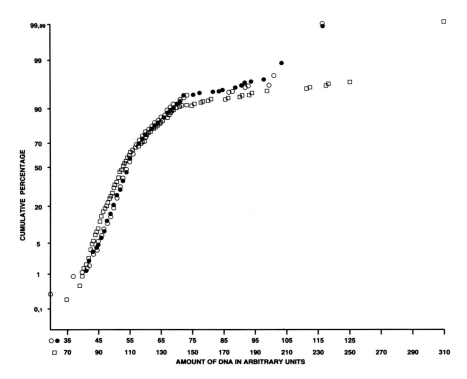

Figure 7
Plot on probit paper of the distribution of the amount of DNA found on human
embryonic lung fibroblasts in Phase IV, measured on metaphases (□) and on each
half of anaphases-telophases (○●). Ethidium bromide staining.

The spread of the distribution of DNA contents did not vary through
the cell population life span (Figure 11) although in cells close to the
terminal phase there were two modes; this is in agreement with the
deviation from parallelism of the plot presented in Figure 7, and with the
increase in the number of sister cells with large differences in DNA content
(Figure 9) for the cultures approaching the end of their proliferative history.

To determine if the DNA synthesized during the preceding S period
is unequally distributed, the number of grains on each half of the anaphases
and telophases was measured after labeling the DNA with ^{3}H-thymidine
during a whole S period. To choose the amount of the precursor that does
not interfere with cell division, cells were labeled with different concentrations of ^{3}H-thymidine and the distribution of the differences in DNA
contents between anaphases and telophases found in the different groups
of cultures was plotted. It was found that 0.5 μCi/ml increased the number of pairs with differences larger than 4% of the mean (Figure 12,
compare with Figure 9A). Thus, radioactivity increased the fraction of
cells with significant differences in DNA contents. This was considered as

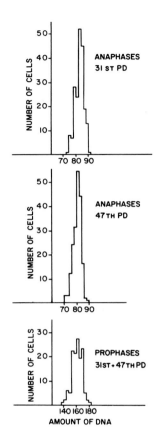

Figure 8
Distribution of DNA content in arbitrary units
(Feulgen-pararosaniline staining) found on anaphases
and prophases of human embryonic lung fibroblasts at
the 31st and 47th population doubling.

further proof that beyond 4% of the mean of the pair the differences in DNA contents between sister cells are significant.

Nontoxic concentrations of ^{3}H-thymidine were then used to measure the distribution of grains on each half of the anaphases and telophases on autoradiographs of cells labeled during a whole S period. The plot obtained with this experiment was compared with a computer simulation (Figures 13A and B) which showed that, in a significant fraction of cells, newly synthesized DNA was not distributed evenly between daughter cells. The fraction of cells with significant differences was smaller than that found when measuring the DNA contents, which was to be expected since the precursor is incorporated in a limited number of sites while cytophotometry, on the contrary, evaluates the whole DNA content.

The quantitative changes in DNA could originate during semiconservative DNA synthesis, chromosome assembly, or chromosome segregation. It was concluded that the three mechanisms are implicated.[31] Screening of mitoses could indeed detect disturbances in chromosome segregation.

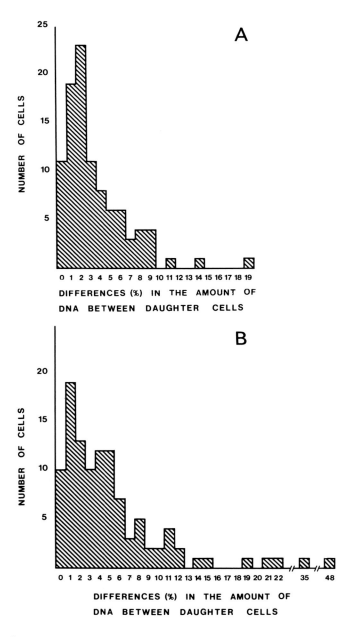

Figure 9
Distribution of the differences in the amount of DNA (ethidium bromide staining, expressed as a percentage of the mean of the pair) found between daughter cells (anaphase-telophase) in Phase II (A) and Phase IV (B) human embryonic lung fibroblasts.

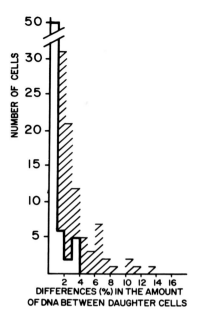

Figure 10
Distribution of the differences in the amount
of DNA (Feulgen-pararosaniline staining)
expressed as percentage of the mean of
the pair, found between daughter cells
(anaphase-telophase) in human embryonic
lung fibroblast cultures at the 31st population
doubling. The white area corresponds to the
differences, with three standard deviations,
found between repeated measurements
of the same samples.

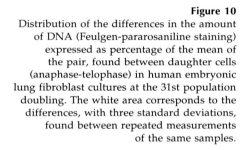

The results showed that this process of uneven distribution of DNA goes on at a constant rate in serially dividing cells and becomes amplified at the very end of the proliferative life span with a chaos-type event. It must be a source of genetic drift and of progressive cell heterogeneity. Results obtained with lymphocytes from human donors of different ages, showing an increased variance with age in the DNA content between cells,[32] are germane to the results described above.

One can now say, in regard to the dogma of the semiconservative partition of DNA during cell division, that it holds only when the phenomenon is analyzed at the level of the cell population; when analyzed at the level of each cell, however, a much more complicated picture becomes apparent. In fact, the genetic information received by the daughter cell after division is different from that of the mother cell and of the other daughter cell. The problem of DNA distribution between the daughter cells after a division cycle could constitute an interesting biological model for the study of chaos.

An event that can give rise to an uneven distribution of DNA during cell division concerns the telomeric region of chromosomes. It originates from the inability of DNA polymerase to fully replicate the ends of the discontinuously synthesized DNA strand. This was proposed to be a source of cell senescence.[33] The first experimental evidence favoring Olovnikov's proposal[33] was obtained by Harley et al.[34,35] who hybridized with the appropriate probe the terminal restriction fragments (TRF) of the

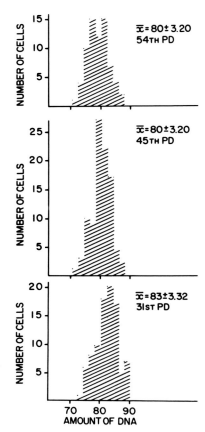

Figure 11
Distribution of the DNA content in arbitrary units, found on anaphases-telophases of human embryonic lung fibroblasts at the indicated population doubling levels (stained with Feulgen-pararosaniline). The mean DNA content with 95% confidence limits is indicated.

DNA from fibroblasts from postnatal donors of different ages; the cell populations were cultivated *in vitro* up to the end of their growth potential. The mean length of the TRF decreased in all fibroblast populations, with a mean loss of 48+21 bp/population doubling. The loss of the hybridization signal intensity was compatible with the loss of TTAGGG repeats, without the decrease of other internal repetitive sequences. Cells kept in a resting phase during long periods of time did not display a decrease in the lengths of TRFs. A significant direct correlation was also found between TRF length and donor age, with a loss of 14±6 bp of telomeric DNA per year.[34,35] A higher loss of telomeric DNA (33 bp/year) was reported for human peripheral leukocytes.[36] A significantly higher rate of telomere loss with donor age (133±15 bp/year) was found in lymphocytes from Down's syndrome (DS) patients, which display premature aging.[37] Telomere loss during aging *in vitro* of lymphocytes from normal individuals was approximately 120 bp/cell population doubling. Telomere lengths of lymphocytes from centenarians and from older DS patients were similar to those of terminal lymphocytes *in vitro*.[37]

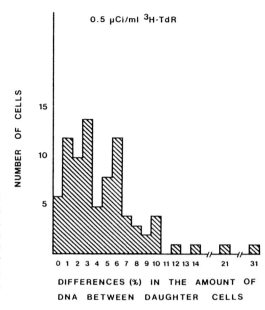

0.5 µCi/ml ³H-TdR

DIFFERENCES (%) IN THE AMOUNT OF DNA BETWEEN DAUGHTER CELLS

Figure 12
Distribution of the differences in the amount of DNA (ethidium bromide staining) expressed as percentage of the mean of the pair, found between daughter cells (anaphase-telophase) in cultures labeled during 10 h with 0.5 µCi/ml ³H-TdR.

Since telomeres apparently function in the attachment of chromosome ends to the nuclear envelope,[38] the alterations of the organization of chromatin fibers at DNA synthesis-initiating sites close to the lamina densa, described below, could be germane to the shortening of telomeres during serial division. Telomeres also seem to prevent aberrant recombinations;[39] hence, modifications at the chromosome ends may explain the increased frequency of ring chromosomes and of dicentric chromosomes known to occur during cell aging.[13,18,40]

Some immortal cell lines express the enzyme telomerase and thus develop the capacity to reconstitute telomeres after each replication.[41] This, though, does not seem to be universal since B lymphocytes immortalized by Epstein-Barr virus display a loss of subtelomeric and telomeric sequences.[42] Moreover, in mice, telomere repeats are longer than in humans and no shortage could be detected over the life cycle of the donor.[43]

These works concerning telomere shortening have to be viewed under the general scope of the loss of the hybridization signal described for different probes during cellular senescence (see section below). The loss of the hybridization signal can be due to loss of sequences, but can also be attributed to recombinations in the region, which will decrease the efficiency of hybridization. Indeed, telomere-promoted recombination can lead to degeneration of the telomeric sequence and subsequent loss of the hybridization ability.[44] Apparent terminal deletions, in fact, can be subtelomeric translocations which are not detected by conventional methods.[45] Hence, although there seems to be a relationship in the human species between cell aging and modifications in the telomere regions, the

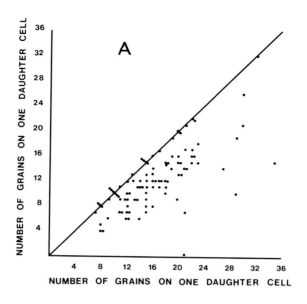

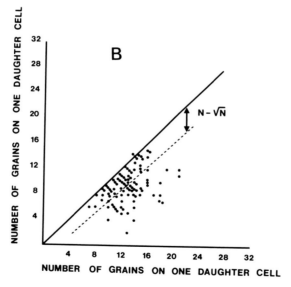

Figure 13
(A) Number of grains found on each daughter cell in human embryonic lung fibroblasts when the grain count saturated after proliferating in the presence of ^{3}H-TdR; daughter cells with the smallest number of grains were represented on the ordinate. The diagonal corresponds to the ideal line where the number of grains should fall if each daughter cell would have had the same grain count. (B) Number of grains on each daughter cell computed with a Monte Carlo simulation. The dashed line corresponds to the deviation expected from a Poisson distribution.

exact nature of these modifications has yet to be determined. They could be part of the reorganization taking place in the genome through proliferation, to which TTAGGG repeats seem particularly prone.

B. Reorganization in the Different Hierarchical Structures of DNA During Cell Proliferation

1. Reorganization of the 30-nm Chromatin Fiber

The first hierarchical order of DNA organization that was analyzed was the 30-nm solenoid chromatin fiber.[28] Observation with electron microscopy, after treatment of cells with a loosening procedure, revealed that at early PDLs the nucleolar region contained highly contrasted filamentous masses organized in a fine, regular network (Figure 14a). In the rest of the nucleus the chromatin fibers were evenly distributed, forming a continuity with the lamina densa at the periphery (Figure 14c). On the other hand, in cells at the end of their proliferative potential (Phase IV), the nucleolar filamentous masses displayed a granular appearance due to the knobby configuration of their entangled filaments (Figure 14b). The fibrils which constituted the nucleolar masses of young nuclei were 6 to 7 nm thick, whereas they reached 10 to 15 nm in old nuclei. In the rest of the nucleus of the terminal cells the chromatin threads were rarer, especially at the nuclear periphery, where the threads were shorter and unusually spaced along the lamina densa which sometimes was entirely devoid of chromatin threads (Figure 14d). The frequency of the nuclei with these changes is indicated in Table 3. They were absent during Phase II (up to the 40th doubling), then increased to 5% during Phase III (41st to 49th doublings), and finally increased rapidly during Phase IV (50th to 56th doublings). This showed that the rapid fall in the fraction of cells capable of entering DNA synthesis within a 24-h period is accompanied by dramatic changes in the nucleus simultaneous with an increase in cell size.

Postnatal skin fibroblasts were also analyzed in this regard and compared at an early *in vitro* PDL with embryonic cells. The results, presented in Table 4, show that cells with old-type chromatin are absent in early passage embryonic cells, as expected from the results presented in Table 3. In the cells of two normal donors, 30 and 59 years old, a fraction of cells presented old-type chromatin although the nucleoli in these cells displayed a normal pattern of organization. A significant increase of the percent of cells with old-type chromatin was observed in the cultures obtained from a 96-year-old normal donor; these cells also displayed abnormal nucleoli. In the cell population obtained from a 60-year-old donor with Werner's syndrome, 89% had old-type chromatin with abnormal nucleoli. These results suggest that a small fraction of cells from young and middle-aged normal adults have old-type chromatin with

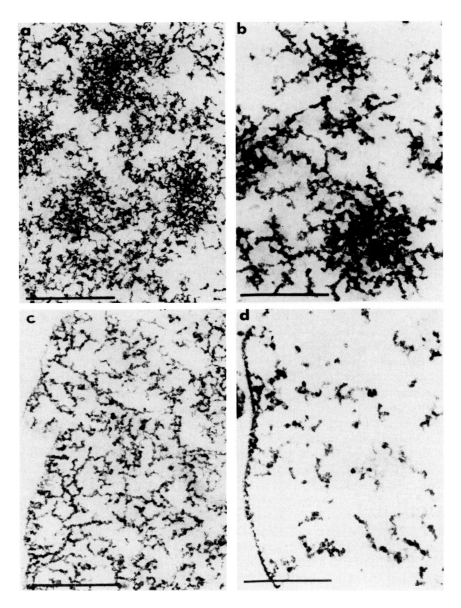

Figure 14
30-nm chromatin fibers following mild loosening of early population doubling human embryonic lung fibroblasts (a and c) and of the same cells at the end of their proliferative history (b and d). Nucleolar (a and b) and peripheral nuclear (c and d) regions. Bar = 0.5 μm.

TABLE 3.

Percent Nuclei With Altered Nucleoli
and Chromatin Found at Different
PDL During the Serial Subcultivation
of the Human Embryonic Lung
Fibroblast Line ICIG-7

PDL	%
10th to 40th	0
41st to 49th	5
50th to 56th	98

TABLE 4.

Percent Nuclei With Altered Nucleoli and Chromatin Found in Low PDL
Cultures of Human Skin Fiborblasts

	Cell Line	Age (Years)	PDL/Maximal Number of Doublings	Nucleoli	Chromatin
Fetal	ICIG-9		4/~50		
	AG 4525		6/~50		
Postnatal	MVL	30	12/30	—	17
	AG 4353	59	6/40	—	7
	AG 4059	96	5/29	63	63
	AG 780 (Werner's Syndrome)	60	6/19	89	89

normal nucleoli. A pronounced increase of cells with old-type chromatin
and old-type nucleoli are present only late during the human life span at
a time where, inevitably, underlying pathologies are present; these cells
seem to have additional functional deficiency because of their defective
nucleoli. In Werner's syndrome the majority of the cells are of the defective type. Hence the data suggest that an increase in the number of cells
with ultrastructural features identical to those of terminal cells may be
associated with pathological conditions.

Since we have found that changes in cell cycling can be detected long
before the terminal Phase IV (Figure 1),[1,2,6,7] attempts were also made to
detect more subtle modifications in the organization of the chromatin
fibers. This was done by screening with an image analyzer[46] the periphery
of nuclear preparations from human embryonic fibroblasts at different
PDL during *in vitro* proliferation. Experiments with ^{3}H-thymidine labeling
suggested that the peripheral nuclear area close to the lamina densa is the
zone where DNA synthesis-initiating sites are located.[47] Indeed, whatever
the duration of labeling with ^{3}H-TdR and the presence or absence of

a long chase period, silver grains were mainly located at the periphery of nuclei of human fibroblasts at different PDLs (Figure 15) and at a short distance from the lamina densa. The few grains scattered through the nucleus probably correspond to peripheral sites seen through the nuclear layers.

Hence, the peripheral areas were chosen to try to detect more subtle modifications in the arrangement of the chromatin fibers by screening those areas on electron microscope pictures with an image analyzer.[46] Two measurements were made. One expressed the ratio between the dark and light areas and was called the density of the fibers; the other, which was called the spacing, was obtained with a sieve-like computerized procedure that calculated the areas between the fibers. The density of the fibers, mainly at the level of their anchorage close to the lamina densa, was found to decrease progressively during proliferation. On the other hand, the spacing of the fibers was found to follow a two-step pattern; it varied very little during most of the cell population's life span and increased abruptly at the end when the cells entered the terminal postmitotic stage.

These modifications in the organization of the 30-nm solenoid fibers have functional implications, since the fall in the density correlated with the decline in the rate of DNA synthesis initiation after cell attachment and spreading; whereas the evolution of the spacing correlated with the terminal fall in the maximal number of cells capable of initiating DNA synthesis during a 24-h period. Hence, density and spacing must correspond to two different parameters within the high-order structure of chromatin, the pronounced changes in the spacing corresponding to more profound chromatin reorganizations.

Electron microscopy, after glutaraldehyde fixation of nuclei from cells at different stages of their proliferative history, has shown that the heterochromatin of terminal Phase IV cells is decondensed (Figure 16); this indicates that the more profound changes in chromatin structure concern the organization of heterochromatin. These observations show that Phase IV cells are not in apoptose, since in the latter chromatin appears condensed and fragmented. It is pertinent to remember that at high PDL there is also a change in the timing of DNA replication in the centromere of chromosome 9, a region rich in heterochromatin.[48]

Measurements with the image analyzer were also made on fibroblasts cultivated from skin biopsies of normal donors of different ages and of two patients with Werner's syndrome (Figure 17). It was found that the density decreased in an inverse relationship with the age of the donor and that the values found for the cells of the Werner patients did not differ from the aged-matched controls. However, the spacing increased in a direct relationship with the age of the donor and the values found for the

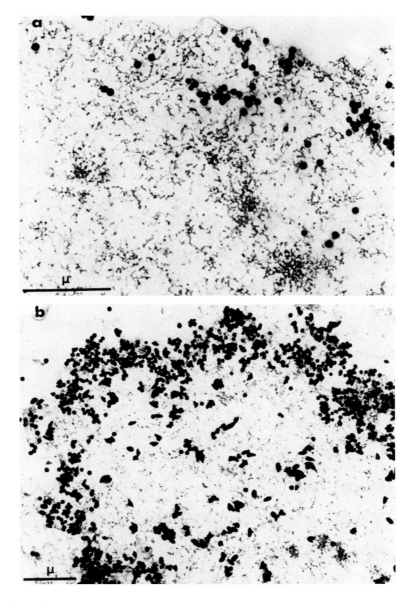

Figure 15
Autoradiograms of human embryonic lung fibroblasts at the end of their proliferative history, incubated with ^{3}H-TdR during (a) 10 min and (b) 66 h, and prepared with the loosening procedure for electron microscopy.

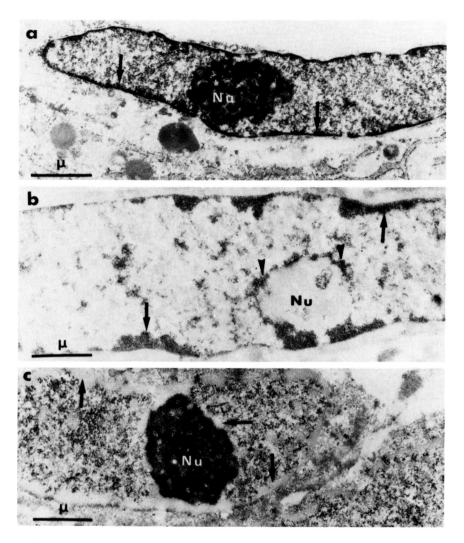

Figure 16
Nucleoprotein organization following conventional fixation with glutaraldehyde
alone of Phase II (A) and Phase IV (B) cells. Bar = 1 μm; (a) uranyl and lead staining;
chromatin is condensed at the nuclear periphery (arrows) in Phase II cells and is
more dispersed in the nucleoplasm of Phase IV cells, which appear clearer than in
young cells. The nucleolus (Nu) is prominent and presents a bud (arrow) in the
Phase IV cell. (b) Specific DNA staining; dense chromatin is accumulated at the
nuclear (arrows) and nucleolar (arrow heads) peripheries of young cells, but not old

cells from the Werner patients were significantly higher than those of the
age-matched controls. The values found for the cells of the 60-year-old
patient were identical to those of the 96-year-old donor. This again suggests

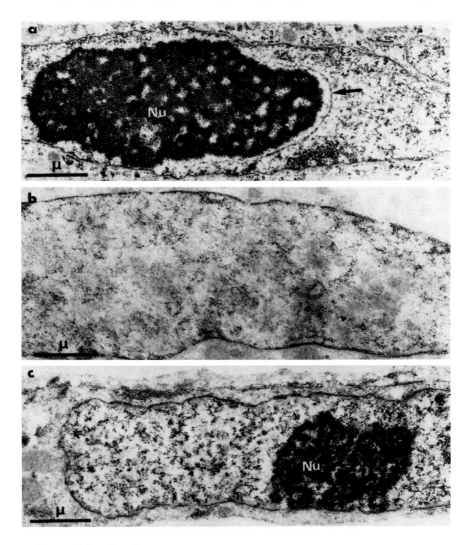

Figure 16 (continued)
ones. In addition, the reaction shows chromatin to be less dispersed in the nucleoplasm of young than of Phase IV cells. (c) Preferential RNP staining; in young cells the bleached chromatin is mainly located at the nuclear periphery and around the nucleolus (arrows). The latter (Nu), and the nucleoplasm which contains RNP structures, remain heavily contrasted. In Phase IV cells the nucleolus is well contrasted, whereas nonnucleolar RNP structures are more dispersed than in early PDL cultures, consequently the nucleoplasm appears clear.

that density and spacing express different parameters of the high-order organization of chromatin, with only the spacing being prematurely disturbed in the cases of pathological aging. These results reiterate the

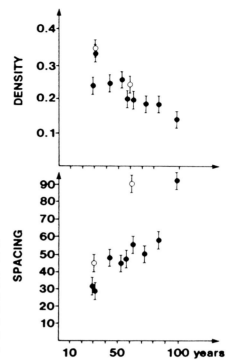

Figure 17
Plot of the values of the density and spacing of the 30-nm chromatin fibers, obtained with an image analyzer, found in human postnatal skin fibroblasts before the fourth PDL, from normal donors (●) and from two patients with Werner's syndrome (○) of different ages. The bars represent the 95% confidence limits.

idea that an increasing fraction of cells with structural changes identical to those of terminal cultures are associated with a pathological condition.

We have performed further studies on human fibroblasts from normal donors of different ages, using the cells from the Baltimore Longitudinal Study of Aging, maintained by the Institute for Medical Research in New Jersey. The cells from a 39-year-old supposedly normal donor yielded values for the density and spacing of chromatin fibers that corresponded to those found at a much later age in the rest of the samples, with the presence of an increased fraction of cells with old-type chromatin. We asked the investigators responsible for the Cell Repository for further information concerning this donor; it turned out that he had diabetes and hypertension. This interesting finding, which deserves further investigation with a larger number of samples, buttresses the conclusion that an increased presence of terminal-type cells may be correlated with pathological aging.

Overall, the results reported above show that the changes in the organization of chromatin fit the pattern of evolution of the proliferation kinetics of human fibroblast populations and of the partition of DNA during mitosis, i.e., aging of these cells is characterized by a succession of subtle changes in the cell cycle and a final short stage with abrupt events.[7]

2. Reorganization of the 10-nm Chromatin Fiber

The next level of organization of DNA was approached through study of the 10-nm beaded chromatin fiber at the ultrastructural level with electron microscopy[28] and by digestion with micrococcal nuclease.[49]

The ultrastructural studies revealed that 10-nm chromatin fibers from young cells (early PDL) displayed a typical nucleosomal organization (Figure 18a), whereas in terminal cells most of the DNA fibers were punctuated by highly spaced nucleosomes or were entirely extended. The latter was observed in Phase IV of the *in vitro* life span of human embryonic fibroblasts (Figure 18b) and in an increased fraction of cells obtained from a skin biopsy from a 60-year-old patient with Werner's syndrome (Figure 18c). These results reiterate the conclusion reported above: that changes occurring in the chromatin of terminal postmitotic fibroblasts are also observed in a pathological situation having the characteristics of premature aging.

These changes, observed with Miller spreads, could be due to shear forces acting on a more fragile structure as a result of the ionic detergent, the alkaline pH, and the hypotonic solution used during preparation of the sample for electronic microscopy. They also may be secondary to alterations of the synthesis of histone H1,[50] which plays a crucial role in stabilizing the 10 additional base pairs at both ends of the 140-bp core particle. A confirmation of these structural changes in the 10-nm fiber was later reported.[51] In addition, in spreads of Werner's syndrome nuclei, short pieces of unbeaded DNA fibers with lengths distributed between 0.1 and 0.2 μm were frequently seen, occasionally forming a circle (Figure 18).

Positioning of nucleosomes may be important to maintain the condensed nature of heterochromatin;[52] it would create a spatial arrangement of DNA favorable for chromosome positioning. Hence, our findings suggesting a change in nucleosomal spacing could be related to the decondensation of heterochromatin found in postmitotic cells (Figure 16), and be part of the explanation for the sudden difficulty in the progression through the division cycle.

We have also tried to see if one can detect changes at this level of DNA organization, before the terminal stage. This was done by digesting chromatin with micrococcal nuclease, which cuts the 10-nm fiber at the linker region.[49] The data showed that the initial velocity of the reaction and the final plateau were unchanged when young cells were compared with older cells (Figure 19); at intermediate times, however, the velocity was higher in older cells. These results are compatible either with an increased heterogeneity of DNA repeat lengths or with conformational changes of the substrate. The possibility that the increased digestion velocity was due to nucleosome sliding in older cells during the incubation was ruled out by running the reaction at 4°C to inhibit the exonuclease activity of

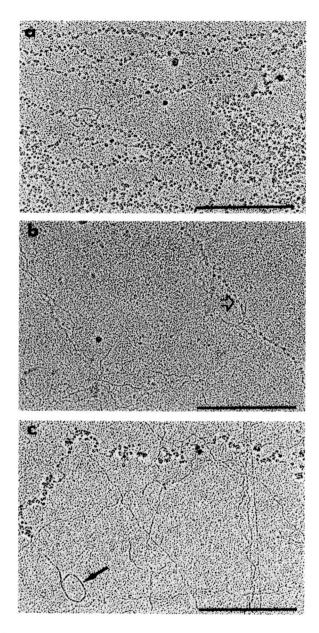

Figure 18
Studies of 10-nm chromatin fibers. Beaded chromatin fibers are abundant in early
PDL human embryonic lung fibroblasts. (a). Most of the fibers are extended in the
same cells in Phase IV; however, chromatin fibers with a "bead-on-a-string" configuration (empty arrow) can be found. (b). Most DNA fibers are fully extended in
Werner's cells; (c) short pieces of unbeaded DNA fibers are dispersed, sometimes
forming a circle (arrow). Bars = 0.5 μm.

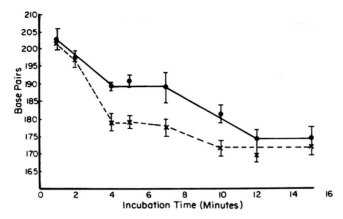

Figure 19
Digestion velocity with micrococcal nuclease of DNA from low PDL (six experiments 13–23 PDL) (●) and from high PDL (seven experiments 51–70 PDL) (x) postnatal human skin fibroblasts. Each value corresponds to the mean, and the standard errors of the mean are indicated. (From Dell'Orco, R.T., Whittle, W.L., and Macieira-Coelho, A., *Mech. Ageing Dev.*, 35, 199, 1986. With permission.)

micrococcal nuclease and fixing the nuclei prior to digestion with formaldehyde to induce reversible DNA-protein cross links.

When the size of the monosome fragment was analyzed for all digestion times with the cells of different PDL, the size of the fragment declined with longer digestion times to a constant value of about 146 bp after 7 min of digestion, and was identical for low and high PDL cells (Figure 20). These results indicate that the structural changes detected with the micrococcal nuclease (Figure 19) are located in the linker region.

A proliferation-related inhibition of DNA digestion by DNAase I is also suggestive of chromatin conformational changes developing through cell divisions.[53]

3. Gene Reorganization

Attempts to detect changes at the gene level were made by hybridizing genomic DNA from cells at different PDLs with the cDNA probes for two genes that are expressed (beta-actin and beta-interferon) and one that is not expressed (alpha-globin) in human mesenchymal cells.[54] The intensity of the band corresponding to the two alpha-globin genes decreased at high PDL during proliferative aging *in vitro* (Figure 21A). The autoradiogram of the hybridization with the cloned cDNA probe for the actin gene showed multiple bands whose intensity diminished with the DNAs extracted from cells at higher PDLs (Figure 21B). The ethidium bromide fluorescence of DNA in the gel used for the blots showed that the decline in the hybridization signal is not due to variations in the amount of DNA

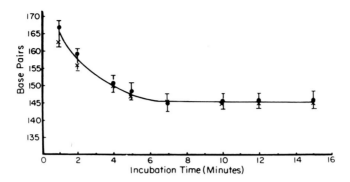

Figure 20
Size of the monosome fragment from low (●) and high (x) PDL cells determined
from the same experiments illustrated in Figure 19. (From Dell'Orco, R.T., Whittle,
W.L., and Macieira-Coelho, A., *Mech. Ageing Dev.*, 35, 199, 1986. With permission.)

loaded on the gel. Filters used with these probes were dehybridized and
rehybridized with the interferon probe. The human beta-interferon DNA
of 1.8 kb hybridized with identical intensity to the DNA extracted from
cells at different PDLs (Figure 21C). These results suggested structural
changes in some, though not all, genes during cell proliferation, some
regions being better conserved than others. Skin fibroblasts from postnatal
donors with Werner's syndrome and Hutchinson-Gilford progeria had a
decreased hybridization signal with the globin probe even at early PDL
(Figure 22).

DNA from young and terminal human fibroblasts was extracted with
the Hirt method, centrifuged to equilibrium in CsCl gradients containing
ethidium bromide, and collected in four different fractions. DNA from
these fractions, undigested or cleaved with Bam H1 restriction enzyme,
was hybridized to the alpha-globin and beta-actin probes (Figure 23). For
DNA isolated from cells at the 16th doubling, the alpha-globin and beta-
actin probes hybridized as a very faint band at 5 kb (fraction 2) (Figures
23A′ and B′). In old cells the autoradiogram of the undigested DNA
sample from fraction 2° (density 1.62) showed several bands of hybridization with the alpha-globin and beta-actin probes (Figures 23A′ and B′). The
fastest running band (I) corresponds to covalently closed circular extrachromosomal DNA, the second band (II) contains nicked circular molecules,
and the other bands are dimers and multimers of the form I. The Bam H1-
digested material ran as 5 and 14 kb (doubling 59, fraction 2) (Figures 24A′
and B′). The interferon probe had no homology with the DNA extracted
according to Hirt. In preparations from both young and terminal cells,
DNA was visible by UV fluorescence after ethidium bromide staining in
fraction 3 (density 1.59) (Figure 23A and B). It probably corresponded to
mitochondrial DNA since it could be cleaved by Bam H1 in a single

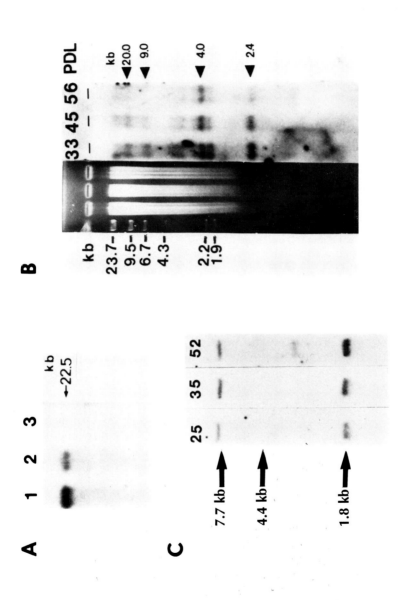

Figure 21
Hybridization of ^{32}P-labeled alpha-globin (A), beta-actin (B), and beta-interferon (C) probes with Eco R1-digested DNA from human embryonic lung fibroblasts at doublings 33 (1), 45 (2), and 56 (3). The numbers to the right and left of the blots indicate lengths in kilobases.

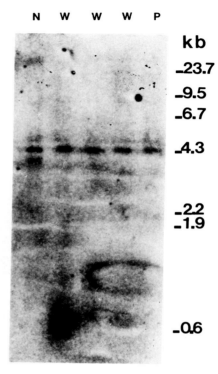

Figure 22
Hybridization of the ^{32}P-labeled alpha-globin probe with Eco R1-digested DNA from postnatal human skin fibroblasts before the sixth population doubling: from a normal donor (N) and from patients with Werner's syndrome (W), and with progeria (P). The band corresponding to the hybridization can be seen on the top of the gel column N. The band at 4.3 kb which does not vary and is unknown; serves as an internal control.

fragment of 17 kb. This DNA did not hybridize to the globin and actin cDNA probes (Figure 23). The Alu human highly repeated sequence probe, BLUR-8, hybridized to the circular DNA present in fractions 2°, 2, 3°, and 3 (Figure 24).

To see if circular DNA molecules could hybridize to specific bands on a genomic DNA blot, the extrachromosomal DNA from terminal cells (fraction 2) was purified by migration on a 0.7% agarose gel and electroelution. This yielded a pure population of circular molecules with a modal size of 5 kb, free of 17-kb mitochondrial molecules. This small size DNA, used as a probe, was hybridized to Eco R1-digested genomic DNA from human fibroblasts (Figure 25). Three main bands could be detected on the autoradiogram at 22, 9, and 8.5 kb. Identical results were obtained using genomic DNA from earlier passage cultures.

DNAs from fractions 2 and 3 were prepared for electron microscopy.[54] Covalently closed circular molecules could be seen in undigested DNA of fraction 2 from terminal cells with sizes of around 5 kb (Figures 26A and 27C) and between 8 and 14 kb (Figure 27C). In the third fraction of the CsCl gradient, molecules of 17 kb were found in DNA preparations from cells at doubling 16 as well as at doubling 59 (Figures 26C, 27B, and 27D). Most of the mitochondrial DNA molecules seemed to be nicked into form

II, probably due to the formamid present in the spreading buffer (50%). A few additional circular molecules ranging between 0.8 and 2.7 kb could be seen at the same density (1.59) in preparations from terminal cells (Figure 27D). Small linear fragments of DNA, heterogeneous in size, were also abundant in the fractions examined.

Undigested DNA from young (early PDL) and terminal cells were laid on a 10 to 40% sucrose gradient and centrifuged.[54] Each fraction collected was electrophoresed in a 0.5% agarose gel, transferred to a nitrocellulose filter, and hybridized with the alpha-globin probe as described above. Hybridization of the alpha-globin probe occurred with fractions from the lower 2/3 of the gradient obtained with DNA from cells of both PDLs, although this hybridization was weaker with DNA from old cells. Hybridization of the probe with the fractions from the upper 1/3 of the gradient, i.e., small molecular weight DNA, occurred only with DNA from terminal cells.

These results show that the decreased hybridization of the probes of the alpha-globin and beta-actin genes are due, in part, to loss of sequences into extrachromosomal circular DNA. This, however, cannot be the sole explanation since the decline in the hybridization signals occurs well before the increase of DNA in an extrachromosomal form — an event that seems to occur only during the transition to the postmitotic state. The faint band detected in young cells could be due to a small fraction of terminal cells that are present at early PDLs. A decreased hybridizability of the DNA coding for ribosomal RNA has been previously reported *in vivo* during aging of mammals.[55-57] Other mechanisms could be implicated in the decreased hybridizability, such as chromosome deletion or mispairing deletions,[58] an age-related increase in tightly bound proteins to DNA,[59] or increased cross links due to oxidized SH groups.[60] A decreased hybridization signal can also be due to rearrangements within these multigene families. This could be germane to the loss of the hybridization signal with the probe for the telomere region. It is interesting that the alpha-globin genes are among the most terminal genes known, i.e., located close to telomeres.

The lack of loss of the hybridization signal with the interferon probe shows that some regions are better conserved than others. The interferon gene does not have introns, a feature that may limit the probability of recombinations for this gene. In this respect, it is pertinent to remember that the beta-interferon gene product remains unchanged up to the end of the life span of human fibroblasts.[54]

It is believed that during the division cycle circular DNA detaches and reintegrates again in the genome. It is possible that in the postmitotic cells the circles do not reintegrate into the chromosomes because of the profound chromatin structural reorganization. The presence of highly repeated sequences near the two alpha-globin genes, as well as in the

A

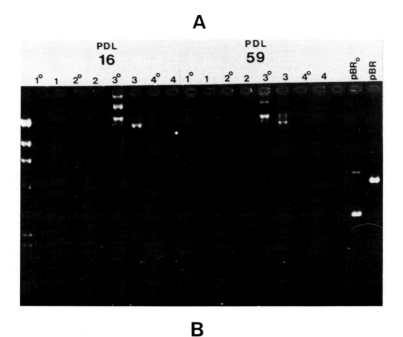

B

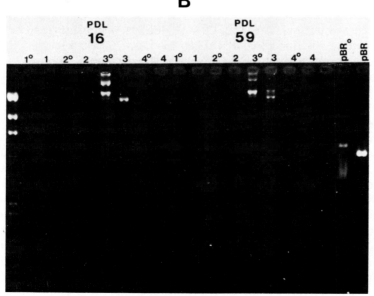

Figure 23
Identification of alpha-globin and beta-actin probes in extrachromosomal sequences.
(A and B) UV fluorogram of DNA banded in CsCl-isopycnic gradient. (A' and B')
DNA blot hybridization with alpha-globin and beta-actin ³²P-labeled probes to

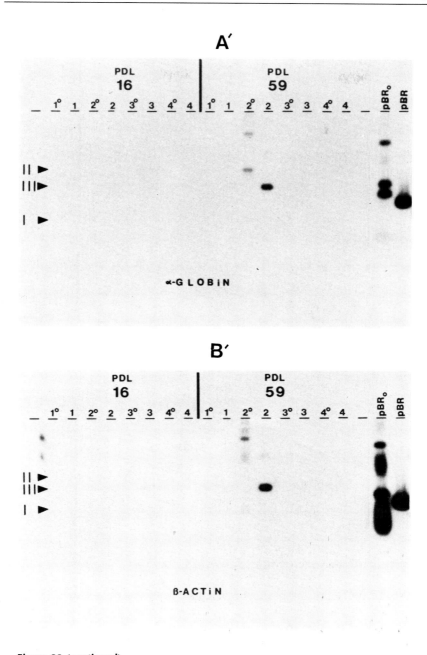

Figure 23 (continued)
fractions from the CsCl gradient. Undigested DNA (1°–4°) and Bam H1-digested
DNA (1–4) from cells at the 16th and 59th doubling. (I) Covalently closed circular
DNA; (II) nicked circular DNA; (III) linear DNA.

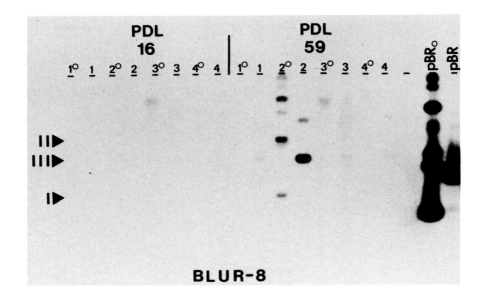

Figure 24
Identification of BLUR-8 probe in extrachromosomal sequences. See legend to Figure 23 for explanation.

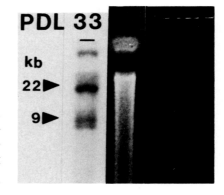

Figure 25
Hybridization of ^{32}P-labeled extrachromosomal DNA probe with Eco R1-digested chromosomal DNA isolated from human embryonic fibroblasts at the 33rd DPL (UV fluorogram shown on the right).

vicinity of the actin genes and in circular molecules detected in terminal cells,[54] suggests a mechanism by which these circles could be recovered in an extrachromosomal form, i.e., this repeated sequence may work as a transposable element. On the other hand, extrachromosomal DNA can replicate in cells that differentiate from G2. It has been suggested that this is due to the failure of nascent replicons to join when cells reach G2, leaving gaps that serve as recognition sites for the initiation of DNA

A   B   C

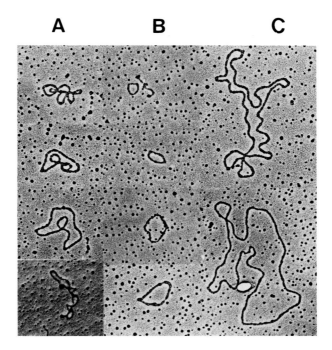

Figure 26
Electron micrograph of circular DNA from human embryonic fibroblasts at doubling 59. DNA preparations of 4.91+1.1 kb (A), 1.5+0.4 kb (B), and 17.2+2.4 kb (C) were obtained with the Hirt method. Length measurements were made relative to the plasmid pBR322 (4361 bp). Magnification ×51,000.

amplification.[61] Hence, the presence of extrachromosomal circular DNA in the terminal cells could support the terminal differentiation hypothesis of the evolution of these cell populations.

A defect in the gap-filling step could indeed be detected by following the sedimentation velocity of newly synthesized DNA after heating the cells during lysis. Resting phase cells were stimulated with a medium change and labeled with ^{3}H-thymidine; they were harvested at different times thereafter and centrifuged in alkaline sucrose gradients. In both Phase II and Phase IV cells, 45 min after labeling the radioactivity was distributed in small peaks through the gradients (Figure 28). Then DNA progressively sedimented in young cells as a single peak which was completed 10 h after labeling, i.e., after covering the time of a S period. In terminal cells, however, even at the 16th hour after addition of the labeled precursor, DNA sedimented in several peaks with different sedimentation velocities although most of the cells had gone through the S period. This suggests an increased thermolability of the gap-filling step, caused by a

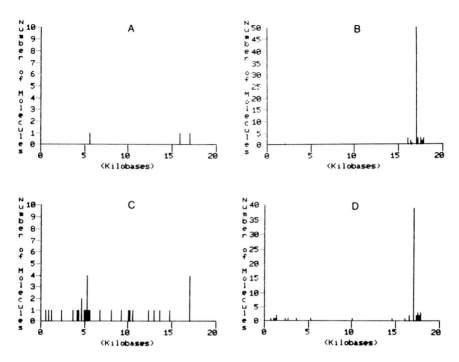

Figure 27
Computer printout of the size distribution of extrachromosomal circular DNA present in young and old cells. (A) Circular DNA from cells at doubling 16 (density 1.62) present in fraction 2 of the CsCl gradient; (B) circular DNA from cells at doubling 16 (density 1.59) present in fraction 3; (C) circular DNA from cells at doubling 59 (density 1.62); (D) circular DNA from cells at doubling 59 (density 1.59). Data from the same experiment shown in Figure 26.

defect of the ligation step. This data could explain the prolongation of the G2 period that accompanies the decline of the growth potential of these proliferative cell compartments (Figure 1).

Amplification of extrachromsomal circular DNA was also found to increase in human lymphocytes during aging of the organism; the amplification of restricted size classes of circular DNAs occurs only in the latter part of the human life span.[62] Circular DNA was also found to be present in the lymphocytes of Werner syndrome patients, although not amplified when compared with the cells from age-matched normal donors; in a murine model of accelerated senescence, it was found to be increased.[62]

The findings reported above buttress the view that the terminal Phase IV is characterized by drastic new characteristics at the molecular and supramolecular levels. Hence, it is not surprising that a multitude of changes occur in gene expression during Phase IV. Indeed, screening of Go subtractive cDNA libraries from young and terminal cells in the resting

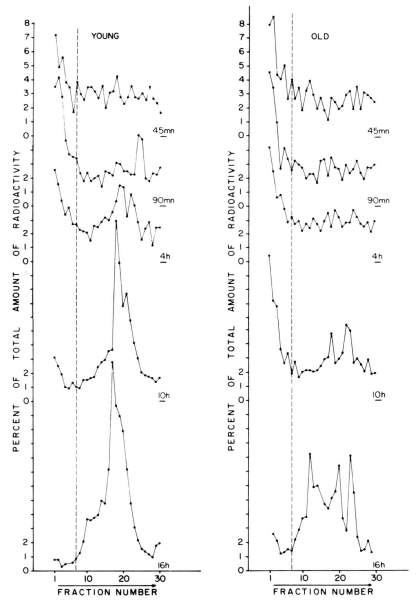

Figure 28
Radioactivity collected from the different fractions after alkaline sucrose gradient centrifugation of DNA from resting cells taken at the indicated times after stimulation. The dashed line indicates the fraction where denatured lambda phage DNA (40.5S) sedimented. Young cells were at the 27th PDL and old cells at the 52nd PDL. The sedimentation direction was from left to right.

phase has uncovered at least 17 differentially expressed genes.[63] The extensive work done to identify the transition to the terminal postmitotic cell will not be reviewed, since we believe that it does not have any relevance for the physiology of aging of the organism; it does have, though, implications for the pathology of aging as shown above. This aspect is further discussed below.

A progressive diminished capacity of serially proliferating fibroblasts to express the transcript of the EPC-1 (early PDL cDNA-1) gene has been reported,[64] as well as an age-related diminished capacity of skin fibroblasts from postnatal donors to express the transcript. This gene is a Go-specific marker in young fibroblasts, identical to the pigmented epithelial-derived differentiation factor, and bears a sequence similarity with a family of serine protease inhibitors. The EPC-1 gene is expressed in young quiescent cells, but not in terminal cells. The full implications of the regulatory properties of the product of this gene are not yet elucidated.

An interesting system that has been studied in regard to the progressive changes occurring during aging *in vitro* is the bovine adrenocortical cell.[65-67] There is a change in the conditions for reinduction of 11-beta-hydroxylase by agents that raise intracellular cyclic AMP. This is preceded at a much earlier time by changes in methylation in the gene flanking region. Satellite I DNA shows a slow and apparently random loss of methylation that extends over the entire replicative life span. There is also a loss of the synthesis of the normal final product of steroidogenesis, i.e., cortisol.

4. *Other Reorganizations*

Age-related conformational rearrangements of DNA were also reported in human peripheral blood lymphocytes.[68] Between 20 and 90 years of age the content of negative superhelical turns increases. These data were considered suggestive of an immature lymphoid cell state arising with aging.

The molecular weight of DNA from human peripheral lymphocytes was also measured on alkaline sucrose density gradients.[69] The average molecular weight of DNA decreased as the age of the donor increased.

A reduction of the methylation level of the c-myc gene, was described in T cells during aging. The relation of this alteration with the age-related reduced proliferation response, however, could not be established.[70]

In summary, one can say that different molecular biology approaches have ascertained that a reorganization of the genome takes place in the different hierarchical structures of DNA of proliferative cell compartments. It underlies the functional, structural, and morphological drifts that accompany cell divisions.

III. IMPLICATIONS FOR AGING OF THE ORGANISM OF THE GENOME REORGANIZATION OCCURRING DURING CELL PROLIFERATION

The problem of the growth potential of cells is crucial for aging; it concerns phenomena such as the regeneration of tissues, wound healing, the immune response, and stem cell renewal. The fibroblast, for instance, plays an important role during wound healing;[71] it migrates and invades the wound on a fibrin layer, followed by the deposition of collagen which immobilizes the fibroblasts, so that the epithelial cells can move in to fill the wound. Many of the changes occurring in fibroblasts during aging can explain the disturbances in wound healing observed with senescence.[72] But there are other aspects of the changes taking place in proliferative cell compartments that are relevant for understanding the manifestations of aging and which are often overlooked by those who ignore the physiology of a mammalian organism.

The changes that occur in fibroblasts through proliferation have led some investigators to suggest that the different stages of the fibroblast life span is a differentiation process.[73] This suggestion was buttressed by the claim that four main morphologically distinguishable cell types, corresponding to the phases illustrated in Figure 29, can be identified in cloned fibroblast populations. In other words, the cells would progress via a process of clonal attenuation to a terminal postmitotic differentiated cell, fulfilling a role in homeostasis.[74]

A biochemical marker has been described during proliferative senescence of human fibroblasts.[75] It consists in the linear decrease of the ratio of the histone variants H2A.1/H2A.2 as a function of cumulative population doublings of human fibroblasts. This decrease was found during differentiation of other cell systems and was considered as proof that the evolution of fibroblast cell compartments is a differentiation process.

The studies reported above show that the terminal postmitotic cells are indeed in a different state and are present in human postnatal tissues. The differentiation hypothesis, however, will remain speculative until a definite role for that cell *in vivo* is found, such as is the case for erythrocytes or keratinocytes.

On the other hand, evidence is accumulating that the terminal cell may have implications for pathologic conditions with a bearing on aging. As mentioned above, there is the presence of an increased number of terminal fibroblasts in the skin of patients with Werner's syndrome, in a patient with diabetes and hypertension, and in a 96-year-old donor — an age when different pathologies are inevitably present. Moreover, atypical fibroblast-like cells have been observed in the articular cartilage of older animals;[77,78] the aged cells seemed to be atypical in function as well as in

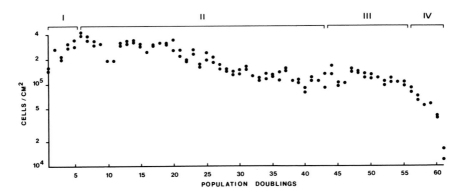

Figure 29

Maximal cell densities recorded before each subcultivation during the entire life span of a human embryonic lung fibroblast population. Each dot corresponds to a cell count from a different culture vessel. Phase I concerns the first five doublings, when the cell densities increase due to selection of the fibroblast population and elimination of other cell types. Phase II lasts from the 5th to approximately the 43rd doubling, when close to 100% of the cells enter DNA synthesis during a 24-h period and the population doubling time is stable. Phase III lasts from the 43rd to around the 55th doubling, when close to 100% of the cells still synthesize DNA during a 24-h period but the population doubling time increases. Phase IV corresponds to the last three to five doublings, when the number of cells capable of synthesizing DNA during a 24-h period declines rapidly and the doubling time increases pronouncedly.

structure. Since it is presumed that an interaction between synovial cells and cartilage is of importance in the pathogenesis of arthritis,[78] "old" fibroblasts must be directly implicated in the latter.

Another pathological situation related to aging, where the final stage of the cells' growth potential could constitute an important aspect of the pathogenesis of the disease at the local tissue level, is atherosclerosis. It has been reported[79] that smooth muscle cells from the fibrous plaques of arteries have a decreased growth response to whole-blood serum, analogous to that observed in senescent cells in culture at the end of their life span.

This leads us to a fundamental question at the core of gerontology research: is it possible to establish a breaking point at the cellular level where one can distinguish an imbalance in the evolution of cell populations that signals a switch from physiological to pathological aging? A given fraction of cells with structural characteristics of terminal phase IV cells are normally present in the tissues of postnatal donors. The end point, though, if reached in excess, could be related to pathological states. The breaking point between physiological and pathological aging would be an excess production of terminal cells that would disturb the homeostasis of the tissue. This could constitute an interesting biomarker to investigate the border between physiological and pathological aging at the cellular level.

It should be stressed, contrary to the view of most investigators in the field, that the relevance for the physiological aging of the organism is not the final step of the proliferative history of a mitotic cell compartment. What is relevant for organism aging is the evolution of a cell population through different functional stages, whether through a stochastic or a programmed process. The following examples illustrate this point.

In the case of the fibroblast, at any time a differentiated cell, its specific functions evolve due to the modifications accumulated in the genome through cell divisions. Many of these functions are known; the fibroblast is an ubiquitous cell in the organism, and in this respect it is responsible for the creation of a microenvironment either through the synthesis of macromolecules (collagen, proteoglycans, elastin, structural glycoproteins)[80] or of small diffusible molecules that act as regulators of homeostasis.

Fibroblasts differ in their properties depending on the organ or tissue they come from; during development the fibroblast evolves into different metabolic pathways acquiring tissue specificity adequate for the local homeostasis. Fibroblasts can also evolve to fulfill certain roles; they can, for instance, acquire the expression of alpha smooth-muscle actin which is required during wound healing.[82]

The need for the interactions between fibroblasts and other cell types during development is well known. Indeed, mouse embryo mammary rudiments fail to develop in the absence of mesenchyme,[83] and the response to sex hormones of the epithelia from the genital tract is mediated via the connective tissue.[84] The need of these cell interactions for organ function prevails through the organism's life span; it is obvious that if there is a drift in cell functions, then cell-to-cell interactions must also evolve, thereby continuously creating new constraints in the organism.

It has been shown[85] that the mesenchymal feeder layer is fundamental for the maturation of thymocytes. Early during development, the site where the thymus will be located is invaded by an intensive proliferation of mesenchymal cells that will constitute the feeder layer. The early involution of the organ could be due in part to the changes of the mesenchymal cells through division at the initial stages of the development of the gland, modifying their feeder properties.

Some aspects of the aging syndrome can be attributed to disturbances in these cell-to-cell interactions. In the developing prostate, the mesenchyme is the actual target and mediator of androgenic effects upon the epithelium.[84] Prostatic hypertrophy, a typical entity of the aging syndrome where the prostate resumes growth late in life, is thought to be due to a change in the inductive activity of the stroma.[86]

Vice versa, fibroblasts also respond to other cell compartments. Epithelial cells of the growing mammary ducts have a stimulatory effect on stromal DNA synthesis.[87] This activity changes during senescence so that an aged epithelium fails to elicit this response.

The drift that takes place through cell division was found to occur in several cell systems; the permanent restructuring that occurs in bone is an example of the evolution in the balance between osteoblasts and osteo-clasts that follows the change in the growth potential of the former cells, and eventually leads to a functionally deficient architecture. The changes that take place in bone through the organism's life span are obviously not due only to changes in osteoblasts through division, but the latter is an important contributing factor.

The finding[88] that the loss of human bone marrow fibroblast-like progenitor cells during aging is compensated for by an increase in the number of epithelial-like cells is another example of this new balance between cell systems that evolves during the life span of the organism.

The physiology of the brain constitutes an example of the relevance of the interactions between dividing and nondividing cells that evolve during the organism's life span. Glial cells are fundamental for the survival of neurons *inter alia*, through their action on myelination and neuron mem-brane recycling,[89] creation of the blood-brain barrier,[90] and regulation of the neuron's ionic environment.[91] Therefore, modifications in the glial cell metabolism through division will alter its multiple interactions with the neuron and must be responsible for many aspects of aging of the brain. Indeed, the changes occurring with aging in the kinetics of proliferative compartments, which were identified *in vitro* in fibroblast cultures,[6] were also found to be displayed *in vivo* by astrocytes.[92]

Another aspect of the influence of dividing cells on the function of nondividing cell compartments concerns the muscle. Myotubes regener-ate through the injection of the nucleus of satellite cells into the myotube; the progressive loss of the satellite cells' division potential[93] limits their capacity to fulfill this role. The replication of satellite cells is also under the control of fibroblasts and, thus, the changes of the latter will also influence muscle senescence.

The tissue modifications that progress through the organism's life span are not due only to cell-cell interactions. Because of the alterations in cell metabolism, the relative proportions of the molecules secreted by the cells into the extracellular space change. Indeed, an evolution with age in the hydroxylation of collagen and in the proportion of collagen type III in relation to type II, as well as an increase in the synthesis of fibronectin, have been observed.[94,95]

In brief, the main contribution of the data obtained from the studies of mitotic cells is to have shown that successive divisions originate a drift in cell function. It is created by the evolution in the storage and the flow of information, and is one of the mechanisms responsible for the continuous physiological changes progressing through development, maturity, and aging of the mammalian organism.

REFERENCES

1. Macieira-Coelho, A., Pontén, J., and Philipson, L., The division cycle and RNA synthesis in diploid human cells at different passage levels in vitro, *Exp. Cell Res.*, 42, 153, 1966.
2. Macieira-Coelho, A., Pontén, J., and Philipson, L., Inhibition of the division cycle in confluent cultures of human fibroblasts in vitro, *Exp. Cell Res.*, 43, 20, 1966.
3. Macieira-Coelho, A., Influence of cell density on growth inhibition of human fibroblasts in vitro, *Proc. Soc. Exp. Biol. Med.*, 125, 548, 1967.
4. Macieira-Coelho, A. and Berumen, L., The cell cycle during growth inhibition of human embryonic fibroblasts in vitro, *Proc. Soc. Exp. Biol. Med.*, 144, 43, 1973.
5. Macieira-Coelho, A., Are non-dividing cells present in ageing populations of human fibroblasts in vitro?, *Nature*, 248, 421, 1974.
6. Macieira-Coelho, A. and Taboury, F., A re-evaluation of the changes in proliferation in human fibroblasts during ageing in vitro, *Cell Tiss. Kinet.*, 15, 213, 1982.
7. Macieira-Coelho, A. and Azzarone, B., Aging of human fibroblasts is a succession of subtle changes in the cell cycle and has a final stage with abrupt events, *Exp. Cell Res.*, 141, 325, 1982.
8. Macieira-Coelho, A., Reorganization of the cell genome as the basis of aging in dividing cells, in *Recent Advances in Gerontology*, Orimo, H., Shimada, K., Iriki, M., and Maeda, D., Eds., Excerpta Medica, Amsterdam, 1979, 111.
9. Macieira-Coelho, A., Implications of the reorganization of the cell genome for aging or immortalization of dividing cells in vitro, *Gerontology*, 26, 276, 1980.
10. Taylor, J.H., Sister chromatid exchanges in tritium-labelled chromosomes, *Genetics*, 43, 515, 18.
11. Goradia, R.Y. and Davis, B.K., Asymmetry in sister chromatids of human chromosomes, *J. Hered.*, 69, 369, 1978.
12. Martin, G.M. and Sprague, C.A., Parasexual cycle in cultivated human somatic cells, *Science*, 166, 761, 1969.
13. Saksela, E. and Moorhead, P.S., Aneuploidy in the degenerative phase of serial cultivation of human cell strains, *Proc. Natl. Acad. Sci. U.S.A.*, 50, 390, 1963.
14. Benn, P.A., Specific chromosome aberrations in senescent fibroblast cell lines derived from human embryos, *Am. J. Hum. Genet.*, 28, 465, 1976.
15. Miller, R.C., Nichols, W.W., Pottash, J., and Aronson, M.M., Cytogenetic comparison of diploid human fibroblast and epithelioid cell lines, *Exp. Cell Res.*, 110, 63, 1977.
16. Chen, T.R. and Ruddle, F.H., Chromosome changes revealed by the Q-Band staining method during cell senescence of WI-38, *Proc. Soc. Exp. Biol. Med.*, 147, 533, 1974.
17. Harnden, D.G., Benn, D.A., Oxford, J.M., Taylor, A.M.R., and Webb, T.P., Cytogenetically marked clones in human fibroblasts cultured from normal subjects, *Somatic Cell Genet.*, 2, 55, 1976.
18. Bourgeois, C.A., Raynaud, N., Diatloff-Zito, C., and Macieira-Coelho, A., Effect of low dose rate ionizing radiation on the division potential of cells in vitro. VIII. Cytogenetic analysis of human fibroblasts, *Mech. Ageing Dev.*, 17, 225, 1981.
19. Salk, D., Werner's Syndrome: A review of recent research with an analysis of connective tissue metabolism, growth control of cultured cells and chromosomal aberrations, *Hum. Genet.*, 62, 1, 1982.
20. Schneider, E.L. and Gilman, B., Sister chromatid exchanges and aging. III. The effect of donor age on mutagen-induced sister chromatid exchange in human diploid fibroblasts, *Hum. Genet.*, 46, 57, 1979.

21. Macieira-Coelho, A., Diatloff, C., Billardon, C., and Bourgeois, C.A., Effect of low dose rate ionizing radiation on the division potential of cells in vitro. III. Human lung fibroblasts, *Exp. Cell Res.*, 104, 215, 1977.
22. Diatloff, C. and Macieira-Coelho, A., Effect of low-dose-rate irradiation on the division potential of cells in vitro. V. Human skin fibroblasts from donors with a high risk of cancer, *J. Natl. Cancer Inst.*, 63, 55, 1979.
23. Schmid, C.W. and Jelinek, W.R., The Alu family of dispersed repetitive sequences, *Science*, 216, 1065, 1982.
24. Macieira-Coelho, A., Cancer and aging at the cellular level, in *Cancer and Aging*, Macieira-Coelho, A. and Nordenskjöld, B., Eds., CRC Press, Boca Raton, FL, 1990, 11.
25. Duesberg, P., Cancer genes: rare recombinants instead of activated oncogenes. A review, *Proc. Natl. Acad. Sci. U.S.A.*, 84, 2117, 1987.
26. Macieira-Coelho, A. and Diatloff, C., Doubling potential of fibroblasts from different species after ionizing radiation, *Nature*, 261, 586, 1976.
27. Macieira-Coelho, A., Implications of the reorganization of the cell genome for aging or immortalization of dividing cells in vitro, *Gerontology*, 26, 276, 1980.
28. Macieira-Coelho, A., Chromatin reorganization during senescence of proliferating cells, *Mutat. Res.*, 256, 81, 1991.
29. Macieira-Coelho, A. and Azzarone, B., The transition from primary culture to spontaneous immortalization in mouse fibroblast populations, *Anticancer Res.*, 8, 669, 1988.
30. Capanna, E., *Cytotaxonomy and Vertebrate Evolution*, Academic Press, London, 1973, 783.
31. Macieira-Coelho, A., Bengtsson, A., and VanderPloeg, M., Distribution of DNA between sister cells during serial subcultivation of human fibroblasts, *Histochemistry*, 75, 11, 1982.
32. Staiano-Coico, L., Darzynkiewicz, Z., Melamed, M.R., and Weksler, M., Changes in DNA content of human blood mononuclear cells with senescence, *Cytometry*, 3, 79, 1982.
33. Olovnikov, A.M., A theory of marginotomy, *J. Theor. Biol.*, 41, 181, 1973.
34. Harley, C.B., Futcher, A.B., and Greider, C.W., Telomeres shorten during aging of human fibroblasts, *Nature*, 345, 458, 1990.
35. Allsop, R.C., Vaziri, H., Patterson, C., Goldstein, S., Younglai, E.V., Futcher, A.B., Greider, C.W., and Harley, C.B., Telomere length predicts replicative capacity of human fibroblasts, *Proc. Natl. Acad. Sci. U.S.A.*, 89, 10114, 1992.
36. Hastie, N.D., Dempster, M., Dunlop, M.G., Thompson, A.M., Green, D.K., and Allshire, R.C., Telomere reduction in human colorectal carcinoma and with aging, *Nature*, 346, 866, 1990.
37. Vaziri, H., Schächter, F., Uchida, I., Wei, L., Zhu, X., Effros, R., Cohen, D., and Harley, C., Loss of telomeric DNA during aging of normal and trisomy 21 human lymphocytes, *Am. J. Hum. Genet.*, 52, 661, 1993.
38. Agard, D.A., and Sedat, J.W., The three dimensional architecture of the nucleus, *Nature*, 302, 676, 1983.
39. Orr-Weaver, T.L., Szostak, T.L., and Rothstein, R.J., Yeast transformation: a model system for the study of recombination, *Proc. Natl. Acad. Sci. U.S.A.*, 78, 6354, 1981.
40. Pezzolo, A., Gimelli, G., Cohen, A., Lavagetto, A., Romano, C., Fogu, G., and Zuffardi, O., Presence of telomeric and subtelomeric sequences at the fusion points of ring chromosomes indicates that the ring syndrome is caused by ring instability, *Hum. Genet.*, 92, 23, 1993.
41. Harley, C.B., Telomere loss: mitotic clock or genetic time bomb?, *Mutat. Res.*, 256, 271, 1991.

42. Guerrini, A.M., Camponeschi, B., Ascenzioni, F., Piccolella, E., and Donini, P., Subtelomeric as well as telomeric sequences are lost from chromosomes in proliferating B lymphocytes, *Hum. Mol. Genet.*, 2, 455, 1993.
43. Kipling, D. and Cooke, H.J., Hypervariable ultra-long telomeres in mice, *Nature*, 347, 400, 1990.
44. Ashley, T. and Ward, D.C., A "hot spot" of recombination coincides with an interstitial telomeric sequence in the armenian hamster, *Cytogenet. Cell Genet.*, 62, 169, 1993.
45. Meltzer, P.S., Guan, X.Y., and Trent, J.M., Telomere capture stabilizes chromosome breakage, *Nature Genetics*, 4, 252, 1993.
46. Macieira-Coelho, A. and Puvion-Dutilleul, F., Evaluation of the reorganization in the high order structure of DNA during aging of human fibroblasts, *Mutat. Res.*, 219, 165, 1989.
47. Puvion-Dutilleul, F., Puvion, E., Icard-Liepkalns, C., and Macieira-Coelho, A., Chromatin structure, DNA synthesis and transcription through the lifespan of human embryonic fibroblasts, *Exp. Cell Res.*, 151, 283, 1984.
48. Lindgren, U. and Farber, J.R.A., Chromosome replication in aging human diploid fibroblasts, *Exp. Cell Res.*, 142, 301, 1982.
49. Dell'Orco, R.T., Whittle, W.L., and Macieira-Coelho, A., Changes in the higher order organization of DNA during aging of human fibroblast-like cells, *Mech. Ageing Dev.*, 35, 199, 1986.
50. Mitsui, Y., Sakagami, H., Murota, S.I., and Yamada, M.A., Age-related decline in histone H1 fraction in human diploid fibroblast cultures, *Exp. Cell Res.*, 126, 289, 1980.
51. Ishimi, Y., Kojima, M., Takeuchi, F., Miyamato, T., Yamada, M.A., and Hanaoka, F., Changes in chromatin structure during aging of human skin fibroblasts, *Exp. Cell Res.*, 169, 458, 1987.
52. Igo-Kemenes, T., The structure of satellite-containing chromatin of the rat, in *Structure and Function of the Genetic Apparatus*, Nicoline, C. and Ts'o, P.O.P., Eds., Plenum Press, New York, 1985, 55.
53. Dell'Orco, R.T. and Whittle, V.L., Microccocal nuclease and DNAase I digestion of DNA from aging human diploid cells, *Biochem. Biophys. Res. Commun.*, 107, 117, 1982.
54. Icard-Liepkalns, C., Doly, J., and Macieira-Coelho, A., Gene reorganization during serial divisions of normal human cells, *Biochem. Biophys. Res. Commun.*, 141, 112, 1986.
55. Johnson, R. and Strehler, B.L., Loss of genes coding for ribosomal RNA in aging brain cells, *Nature*, 240, 412, 1979.
56. Strehler, B.L., Chang, M.P., and Johnson, L.K., Loss of hybridizable ribosomal DNA from human postmitotic tissues during aging. I. Age-dependent loss in human myocardium, *Mech. Ageing Dev.*, 11, 371, 1977.
57. Strehler, B. and Chang, M.P., Loss of hybridizable ribosomal DNA from human postmitotic tissues during aging. II. Age dependent loss in human cerebral cortex-hypocampal and somato sensory cortex comparison, *Mech. Ageing Dev.*, 11, 375, 1979.
58. Strehler, B.L., Roles and mechanisms of rDNA changes during aging, in *Genetic Defects of Aging*, National Foundation March of Dimes Birth Defects, Bergsma, D. and Harrison, G., Eds., 1978, 445.
59. Gaubatz, J.W. and Cutler, R.G., Age-related differences in the number of ribosomal RNA genes of mouse tissues, *Gerontology*, 24, 179, 1978.
60. Tas, S., Tam, C.F., and Walford, R.L., Disulfide bonds and the structure of the chromatin complex in relation to aging, *Mech. Ageing Dev.*, 12, 65, 1980.

61. Van't Hof, J. and Bjerknes, C.A., Cells of pea (Pisum sativum) that differentiate from G2 phase have extrachromosomal DNA, *Mol. Cell. Biol.*, 2, 339, 1982.

62. Kunisada, T., Yamagishi, H., Ogita, Z.I., Kirakawa, T., and Mitsui, Y., Appearance of extrachromosomal circular DNAs during in vivo and in vitro ageing of mammalian cells, *Mech. Ageing Dev.*, 29, 89, 1985.

63. Hara, E., Yamaguchi, T., Tahara, H., Tsuyama, N., Tsurui, H., Ide, T., and Oda, K., DNA-DNA subtractive cDNA cloning using oligo(dT)-latex and PCR. Identification of cellular genes which are overexpressed in senescent human diploid fibroblasts, *Anal. Biochem.*, 214, 58, 1993.

64. Pignolo, R.J., Cristofalo, V.J., and Rotenberg, M.O., Senescent WI-38 cells fail to express EPC-1, a gene induced in young cells upon entry into the Go state, *J. Biol. Chem.*, 268, 8949, 1993.

65. Hornsby, P.J., Simonian, M.H., and Gill, G.N., Aging of adrenocortical cells in culture, *Int. Rev. Cytol.*, Suppl. 10, 131, 1979.

66. Hornsby, P.J., Aldern, K.A., and Harris, S.E., Adrenocortical cultures as model systems for investigating cellular aging, in *Free Radicals in Molecular Biology, Aging and Disease*, Armstrong, D., Sohal, R., Cutler, R., and Slater, B., Eds., Raven Press, New York, 1984, 203.

67. Hornsby, P.J., Yang, L., Raju, S.J., and Cheng, C.Y., Changes in gene expression and DNA methylation in adrenocortical cells senescing in culture, *Mutat. Res.*, 256, 331, 1991.

68. Hartwig, M. and Körner, I.J., Age-related changes of DNA winding and repair in human peripheral lymphocytes, *Mech. Ageing Dev.*, 38, 73, 1987.

69. Turner, D.R., Morley, A.A., Seshadri, R.S., and Sorrell, J.R., Age-related variations in human lymphocyte DNA, *Mech. Ageing Dev.*, 17, 305, 1981.

70. Deguchi, Y., Negoro, S., Hara, H., Nishio, S., and Kishimoto, S., Age-related changes of proliferative response, kinetics of expression of protooncogenes after the mitogenic stimulation, and methylation level of the protooncogene in purified human lymphocytic subsets, *Mech. Ageing Dev.*, 44, 153, 1988.

71. Gabbiani, J., The role of contractile proteins in normal healing and fibrocontractive diseases, in *Methods and Achievements in Experimental Pathology*, Vol. 9, Jasmin, D. and Cantin, P., Eds., Karger, Basel, 1979, 187.

72. Holm-Pedersen, P., Fenstad, A.M., and Folke, E.A., DNA, RNA and protein synthesis in healing wounds in young and old mice, *Mech. Ageing Dev.*, 3, 173, 1974.

73. Martin, G.M., Sprague, C.A., Norwood, T.H., and Pendergrass, W.R., Clonal selection, attenuation and differentiation in an in vitro model of hyperplasia, *Am. J. Pathol.*, 74, 137, 1974.

74. Bayreuther, K., Aging in the human dermal fibroblast stem cell system *in vivo* and in vitro, in *Molecular Biology of Aging*, Finch, C.E. and Johnson, T.E., Eds., Alan R. Liss, New York, 1990, 205.

75. Rogakou, E.P. and Sekeri-Pataryas, K.E., A biochemical marker for differentiation is present in an in vitro aging cell system, *Biochem. Biophys. Res. Commun.*, 196, 1274, 1993.

76. Silberberg, R., Silberberg, M., and Feir, D., Life cycle of articular cartilage cells. An electron microscopic study of the hip joint of the mouse, *Am. J. Anat.*, 114, 17, 1964.

77. Weiss, C., Ultrastructural characteristics of osteoarthritis, *Fed. Proc.*, 32, 1459, 1975.

78. Peeter-Joris, C. and Vaes, G., Degradation of cartilage proteoglycan and collagen by synovial cells, lymphocyte factors, bacterial products or other inflammatory stimuli, *Biochem. Biophys. Acta*, 804, 474, 1984.

79. Ross, R., The pathogenesis of atherosclerosis. An update, *New Engl. J. Med.*, 314, 488, 1986.
80. Robert, B. and Robert, L., Aging of connective tissues, in *Frontiers in Matrix Biology*, Vol. 1, Karger, Basel, 1973, 1.
81. Macieira-Coelho, A., Biology of normal proliferating cells in vitro. Relevance for in vivo aging, in *Interdisciplinary Topics in Gerontology*, Vol. 23, von Hahn, H.P., Ed., Karger, Basel, 1988, 168.
82. Desmoulières, A., Rubbia-Brandt, L., Abdiu, A., Walz, T., Macieira-Coelho, A., and Gabbiani, J., Alpha-smooth muscle actin is expressed in a subpopulation of cultured and cloned fibroblasts and is modulated by gamma-interferon, *Exp. Cell Res.*, 201, 64, 1992.
83. Kratochwill, K., Organ specificity in mesenchymal induction demonstrated in the embryonic development of the mammary gland of the mouse, *Develop. Biol.*, 20, 46, 1969.
84. Cunha, G.R, Donjacour, A.A., Cooke, P.S., Mee, S., Bigsby, R.M., Higgins, S.S., and Sugimura, Y., The endocrinology and developmental biology of the prostate, *Endocrinol. Rev.*, 8, 338, 1987.
85. Auerbach, R., Morphogenetic interactions in the development of the mouse thymus gland, *Develop. Biol.*, 2, 217, 1961.
86. McNeal, J.E., The prostate gland morphology and pathobiology, *Monogr. Urol.*, 4, 3, 1983.
87. Berger, J.J. and Daniel, C.W., Stromal DNA synthesis is stimulated by young, but not serially aged mouse mammary epithelium, *Mech. Ageing Dev.*, 23, 277, 1983.
88. Mets, T. and Verdonk, G., Variations in the stromal cell population of human bone marrow during aging, *Mech. Ageing Dev.*, 15, 41, 1981.
89. Cuadras, J., Are glial cells involved in neuron membrane recycling?, *J. Electron Microsc.*, 34, 419, 1985.
90. Janzer, R.C. and Raff, M.C., Astrocytes induce blood-brain barrier properties in endothelial cells, *Nature*, 325, 253, 1987.
91. Walz, W. and Herz, L., Functional interactions between neurons and astrocytes. Potassium homoeostasis at the cellular level, *Progr. Neurobiol.*, 20, 133, 1983.
92. Fedoroff, S., Ahmed, I., and Wang, E., The relationship of expression of statin, the nuclear protein of nonproliferating cells, to the differentiation and cell cycle of astroglia in cultures and in situ, *J. Neurosci. Res.*, 26, 1, 1990.
93. Mezzorgiono, A., Coletta, M., Zani, B.M., Cossu, G., and Molinaro, M., Paracrine stimulation of senescent satellite cell proliferation by factors released by muscle or myotubes from young mice, *Mech. Ageing Dev.*, 70, 35, 1993.
94. Boyer, B., Kern, P., Fourtanier, A., and Labat-Robert, J., Age-dependent variations of the synthesis of fibronectin and fibrous collagens in mouse skin, *Exp. Gerontol.*, 26, 375, 1991.
95. Pieraggi, M.T., Julian, M., and Bouissou, H., Fibroblast changes in cutaneous ageing, *Virchows Archiv (Pathol. Anat.)*, 402, 275, 1984.

Chapter 2

GENOMIC INSTABILITY DURING AGING OF POSTMITOTIC MAMMALIAN CELLS

James W. Gaubatz

CONTENTS

0-8493-4786-6/95/$0.00+$.50
71

I. INTRODUCTION

A. Genome-Based Theories of Aging

To provide a conceptual framework for the experimental results presented in this chapter, some of the more prominent genome-based theories of aging will be briefly covered first. In metazoans, biological instability as manifested by biological changes over time is exceedingly complex and likely to have multiple causes. Nevertheless, some biological changes may be more fundamental to the aging process in that they are capable of producing secondary, tertiary, and more long-range effects to generate a complex physical and functional appearance. Genomic instability has the power to account for complex, pleiotropic changes which occur in all systems of all living organisms at virtually every level of organization.[1] The central idea common to most genome-based theories of aging is the proposal that alterations which take place in the genome with time produce physiological decrements characteristic of natural aging.[1-3]

With the dawn of the atomic age, there was considerable interest in the effects of radiation on living organisms. Various experiments using X-rays or γ-rays were conducted, leading to the concepts (among others) of radiation-induced cell death, mutation, and transformation. It was noted that the death rate of chronically irradiated rodents exceeded that of controls and that irradiated rats seemed to age more quickly than nonirradiated rats.[4] These observations led to the hypothesis that radiation-induced life shortening is mechanistically related to natural senescence, and stimulated Failla[5] to propose that the aging process was due to a random accumulation of somatic mutations which he regarded as dominant. Subsequently, Szilard[6] considered the hypothetical hits of genetic targets to be recessive and culminate in cell death. The latter proposal meant that both alleles of a diploid genome must become inactivated, i.e., mutated, to observe an effect. Maynard Smith[7] and Kirkwood[8-10] have evaluated and discussed these early somatic mutation theories of aging. Their critiques have focused on comparative and evolutionary aspects of aging, and in some cases analyzed the quantitative aspects of some theories.[7,11]

The somatic mutation theory of aging was later championed by Curtis,[12,13] who was the first to provide interspecies and intraspecies evidence which supported a role for mutations in aging of somatic cells (see below). However, there is evidence both for and against the hypothesis that radiation-induced life shortening and pathology are related to accelerated or premature aging, and a thoughtful discussion of the data can be found in Walburg's article[14] on radiation and aging. Alexander[15] argued that if somatic mutations are responsible for causing aging, then the administration of mutagens to animals should accelerate aging, but the experimental data, including much of Curtis's work,[12,13] do not agree with the notion of somatic mutations per se being a major determinant of longevity. Alexander[15] went on to reason that DNA lesions, not mutations, were likely to exert their most profound effects in nondividing cells. DNA acts as a template to duplicate itself, and deleterious mutations would disrupt the flow of information through progeny cells, many of which might die or be lost by selection to be replaced by wild-type cells. Therefore, there may not be any observable physiological loss to the animal as a whole. Alternatively, the other major function of DNA is to guide the formation of RNA molecules which continually turn over and need to be replaced. Lesions involving DNA which interfere with RNA synthesis might be lethal to postmitotic cells if new proteins cannot be made, or might reduce physiological functions if reduced or altered proteins are made. Thus in regard to senescence, Alexander[15] switched the emphasis from an accumulation of sequence changes in dividing cells to an accumulation of damages in nondividing cells. A more extended version of somatic damage theories is the disposable soma hypothesis of aging[8-11] which predicts that an accumulation of unrepaired somatic defects leads to aging, and rates of aging are thus regulated by altering levels of maintenance and repair processes. More recently, Gensler and Berstein[16,17] have stressed the importance of the DNA damage hypothesis of aging in relationship to the effects of damage on gene expression in nonrenewing somatic mammalian cells.

As basic knowledge concerning eukaryotic cell and molecular biology emerged, new variants of genome-based theories of the aging process were spawned. Yielding[18] reworked the somatic mutational theory of aging to accommodate differential DNA repair. A previous difficulty of somatic mutation theories was to rationalize how single hits at random loci in different cells could lead to the cumulative expression of uniformly depressed function seen at the macroscopic level. His model viewed DNA as a nonuniform substrate for somatic mutational damage. There are active chromosomal sectors that are responsible for cell-specific functions, and these sectors are physically accessible for transcription and other enzyme processes. In addition, there are inactive chromosomal sectors which are functionally not transcribed, physically masked, and inaccessible to repair enzymes. Due to variations in the availability of sequences to repair enzymes, damage to DNA of somatic cells accumulates preferentially in the chromosomal sectors which are not actively transcribed. Yielding[18] viewed the major effect of DNA alterations, accumulating in the quiescent fraction of the genome, as interfering with the normal replenishing of cells and, in a quantitative sense, cells with equal damage but at different loci would be equally impaired in their replicative ability. Research on gene-specific repair over the past decade has shown that differential repair (with transcriptionally active sequences generally being repaired preferentially) is indeed a basic mechanism of cell survival.[19-21] Little thought was initially given to postmitotic cells, except to state that cells which rarely divide would be relatively immune from the accumulation of damage to inactive chromosomal sectors since they are not subjected to the same selective pressures as proliferating cells.[18] Although it is obvious that replicative pressures would not exist, it is not at all clear that postmitotic cells would escape such damage unscathed.

The error catastrophe theory[22] is another variant of the somatic mutation theory of aging. Error theory considers the effects of mutations generating more mutations. For example, a random mutation in a DNA polymerase that increases copying mistakes will contribute to a higher mutation frequency. This type of feedback loop is predicted to give rise to an exponential type of increase in somatic mutations with age. Obviously, this theory is not easily tested in postmitotic mammalian cells *in vivo*. It would be difficult to determine if a few cells out of many are in some phase of a nonlinear increase of mutations, particularly if such cells were rather rapidly eliminated from the population by the accumulation of deleterious mutations.

The accumulation of epigenetic modifications has been suggested to contribute to genomic instability during aging.[23] The modification to DNA that has received the most attention is methylation of cytosine. 5-Methylcytosine is the only known covalent modification that occurs normally to mammalian DNA as part of cellular differentiation.[24-26] These epigenetic modifications are clonally propagated in replicating cells by maintenance *trans*-methylases that recognize half-methylated CpG substrates following replication.[23-26] Therefore, different cell types exhibit sequence-specific methylation patterns characteristic of one cell type. In animal cells there is a fairly strong inverse correlation between gene expression and the methylation status of CpG clusters in regulatory regions of a gene.[27] Since 5-methylcytosine can undergo spontaneous deamination to thymine, there may be a relationship between a time-dependent accumulation of undermethylated genes and an age-related accumulation of DNA damage (G-T mismatches) in the same genomes.[23,28]

Many theories of aging consider DNA as a primary target for damage but stress the source of damage induction, such as oxygen radicals,[29,30] while others point to possible sources of genetic instability such as transposon-mediated sequence rearrangements,[31] chromosomal deletions of tandemly repeated genes,[32] or selective loss of telomeric repetitive sequences.[33] In contrast, other theories focus on the types of damage such as a single class of lesions, e.g., cross-linkages.[34] In conjunction with underscoring the genome as a target of aging, some theories have featured genes and genetic mechanisms that counteract stochastic aging processes;[2,3,35] these have included gene redundancy,[36] DNA replication[2,3,37,38] and repair machinery,[2,3,39,40] and antioxidant defenses.[41] The possibility that biological aging is genetically programmed has received some attention, too.[9]

Lastly, there is the more recent presumption that the mitochondrial genome might be the primary pace-setter of aging for postmitotic mammalian cells.[42,43] The genome-bases theories that were developed regarding the nuclear genome will need to be redefined considering mitochondrial DNA as the foremost target of genetic instability and, thus, a regulator of senescence. There have been a rather high number of review articles discussing age-related aspects of genomic instability, such as DNA damage and repair, published from 1990 to the present, and the reader is referred to these commentaries for additional information and perspectives.[44-54]

B. Objectives and Viewpoints

The objective of this review is to examine critically the evidence for genomic instability in postmitotic mammalian cells during their life span. The analysis will concentrate on aging characteristics that have stood the tests of time and confirmation, as supplemented by more recent data generated with newer techniques/methods that will need to withstand future scrutiny. Most of the studies discussed in this article were carried out with the aim of identifying types of genomic instability and quantifying levels of lesions in a particular tissue as a function of age. Thus, the data are largely descriptive and not mechanistic in that the origins and operations behind the instability were not investigated. Furthermore, the coverage will be selective in representing a personal viewpoint or bias.

To lay a basis for eventually understanding the role of genomic instability in the deterioration of biological performance with age, it will be assumed that the accumulation of somatic mutations and pernicious DNA damage, due to nonrepaired or incorrectly repaired lesions, are causes of mammalian aging. The ability of cells to sustain both performance and viability in the face of continued genomic insults with time is therefore a critical factor in longevity, and the degenerative changes associated with senescence are ultimately the consequences of an individual's inability to preserve the function and viability of its cellular components.

We start with the premise that DNA damage is going to be continuously introduced into the genomes of all cells. Many forms of DNA damage occur naturally as a consequence of metabolic processes, reactions involving normal cellular constituents, and the intrinsic chemical instability of DNA.[44,45,55-60] Additional DNA lesions arise from environmental and dietary components.[61-64] UV irradiation, ionizing radiation, viruses, dietary mutagens, and xenobiotics are exogenous DNA damaging agents, whereas oxygen radicals, body heat, endogenous alkylating agents, and Mallard products of sugars are examples of normal mammalian metabolism that illustrate unavoidable DNA damaging agents.[44,45,55-64] This damage is an attack on the integrity of the cellular information. Some types of damage are normally efficiently removed.[65-71] Other types of damage can persist for long times. Various DNA adducts can block transcription and replication.[66-68,70,72] Other alterations cause miscoding during replication and thus lead to mutations.[58,66-72] Still different alterations separate and rearrange genetic codes. Modifications to DNA might have a transient local effect such as a base mismatch, or a long-range permanent effect, e.g., double-strand breaks.

The end points of unrepaired DNA damage can be different between replicating cells and nonreplicating cells. Cell death or mutations can be an outcome for both cell types. However, mutations in the proliferating cell will give rise to a population of progeny cells, whereas the nonproliferating cell will not expand its genome and remain unique. For replicating cells, amplification from stem or blast cells will either result in selection for wild-type cells or mutant cells which can compete effectively, for a variety of reasons, with a concurrent selection against mutant cells that are defective in some aspect of competition *in vivo*. Therefore, what one measures in a proliferating cell compartment in an organism is skewed due to selective pressure.

The vast majority of mammalian cell *in vivo* are postmitotic and exist in a state of terminal differentiation.[73] We can ask if a specific type of damage can be detected or measured in these cells. Indeed, many attempts have been made to measure changes in DNA as organisms grow old. The problem is again complicated by the fact that there are dividing cells and nondividing cells in the same organ or tissue. Cellular division does not allow analysis of certain aspects of aging information. For example, the original elements with resident damages that constitute a genome will be rapidly diluted out to vanishingly small proportions in mitotic cells. The emphasis here will be on those cells that, for the most part, are not dividing in the adult animal and the term postmitotic, meaning cells that are through dividing at birth or shortly thereafter, will be used. The discussion will also be restricted to mammalian studies.

Since there are a large number of diverse lesions, is there a class of modifications that will be more informative than others? The opinion that will be stressed here is that single-strand breaks in DNA will give a more comprehensive picture of the damaged state of a genome than any other single lesion. The rationale for this argument stems from the knowledge that single-strand breaks arise spontaneously,[74] other abundant lesions (such as abasic sites) lead to DNA strand breaks,[75,76] and processing of most DNA adducts involves enzymic single-strand incisions.[65-71] Hence, damage-induction and damage-processing pathways intersect at a single measurable parameter. Table 1 lists direct and indirect sources for single-strand DNA breaks originating *in vivo* and predicts proximal biological effects for postmitotic mammalian cells.

Genetic instability, genomic instability, and chromosomal instability are terms that have been used somewhat interchangeably, although they tend to have different connotations. In this review, chromosomal instability will be used to describe visible changes in the nucleoprotein complexes that constitute the characteristic structure of individual mitotic chromosomes, i.e., a change in the individual cell's normal karyotype. Genetic instability will be used to discuss changes in the primary structure of DNA, including covalent modifications (damage) and replication-dependent events (mutations). Lastly, genomic instability will be used to describe all changes that affect DNA-based information in a cell, encompassing both chromosomal and genetic instability, in addition to epigenetic changes. In a final section, the effects of aging on the stability of mitochondrial genomes will be examined. To conclude, there will be an attempt to summarize the evidence that genomic instability is a primary aging process, to determine if sets of data define age-related patterns, to see if predictions can be made from such patterns, and to outline attractive candidates for future study or experimental strategies that might yield more meaningful results.

TABLE 1.

Sources of Single Strand Breaks in Postmitotic Mammalian Genomes[a]

Sources	Intermediates	Outcomes[b]
Direct Sources		
1. Spontaneous strand scission	None	Loss of template capacity;
2. Oxygen radical induced breakage		diminished propagation of long-range regulatory signals;
3. Nonspecific endonucleases		disruption of chromatin
4. Topoisomerases		organization in nucleus
5. Recombination endonucleases		
6. Retroviruses/retroposons		
Indirect Sources		
1. Base loss	Abasic sites	Single-strand breaks
a. Spontaneous release		
b. Base adducts		
i. Accelerated spontaneous loss		
ii. N-glycosylase action		
2. Nucleotide modifications[c]	Mismatched bases,	Repair endonuclease action
a. Base alterations	helical distortions,	(single-strand cleavages)
b. Sugar alterations	structural	
c. Phosphate alterations	abnormalities	
d. Complex alterations		

[a] References for sources of single-strand breaks can be found in the text.
[b] Only the most proximal effects are listed for single-strand DNA breaks from direct and indirect sources.
[c] Complex alterations are those involving more than one nucleotide component.

II. GENOMIC INSTABILITY

A. Chromosomal Instability

1. *Spontaneous Chromosomal Aberrations*

The presence of abnormal chromosomes in dividing cells is a classical cytological index of genomic instability. Howard Curtis[12,13] considered chromosomal aberrations to be a manifestation of somatic mutations. This supposition evolved from mutation studies with plants, wherein somatic cells can differentiate in the next mitosis to germinal cells whose mutations can be scored via phenotypic markers. In this system, it was found that the numbers of mutations were proportional to the numbers of chromosome aberrations under a wide variety of experimental conditions.[77] This supposition was bolstered by correlations between radiation-induced pathologies and chromosomal instability.[77-80] Hence, by extrapolation to animal cells, scoring somatic chromosome abnormalities was an indirect measure of mutation frequency. Mammalian liver cells rarely divide in the adult animal, but can be induced to divide *in vivo* by partial hepatectomy.[81]

Therefore, regenerating liver tissue was used to test the somatic theory of aging by scoring chromosomal aberrations as a function of age. The cytological methods used by Curtis and co-workers[81-85] consisted of injecting rodents with carbon tetrachloride to destroy part of the liver. At the height of liver regeneration, the animals were killed, the tissue was fixed and stained, and cell squash preparation were examined microscopically. All cells in anaphase or early telophase were scored as either normal or abnormal. Although other types of abnormalities were noted, the most common aberrations consisted of either bridges (dicentrics) or fragments (acentrics).[81,82] In an effort to avoid incorrect interpretations, only bridges and fragments were counted to measure somatic cell DNA damage and mutations.[81-85]

In a study of the late somatic effects of radiomimetic compounds that induce chromosomal abnormalities, Stevenson and Curtis[81] discovered that liver cells of normal, untreated CF_1 mice exhibited steadily increasing numbers of chromosomal aberrations with age, reaching 22% by 10 months of age. Subsequent work verified that the frequency of chromosomal aberrations in regenerating liver cells increased steadily with age and can reach as high as 75% in some very old animals.[82] These results also showed that, at least in some strains of mice, the rate at which aberrations increase with age is inversely related to the life expectancy of the particular strain.[82,83] In addition, it was shown that dogs, which age much more slowly than mice, also develop aberrations in their liver cells at a much slower rate than mice.[84] The dog data are limited, however, because only seven dogs were used in the study, and there were much fewer scorable figures in the dog study than in the rodent studies.[84] Even though the dog data were scanty, the overall conclusion was that the accumulation of aberrations in postmitotic cells of dogs and mice proceeded at a rate roughly inversely proportional to the life expectancy of the species, and it was suggested that the frequency of chromosomal aberrations may be influenced by the rate of cellular metabolism.[84]

To further examine the relationship between longevity and chromosomal aberrations, Curtis and Miller[85] repeated the experiments using guinea pigs, which have a median life span between those for mice and dogs. It was found that the spontaneous chromosome aberration rate for guinea pigs lies between the rates for mice and dogs. With the inclusion of the guinea pig results to give a three-species comparison, the data indicated that the rate at which animals accumulate spontaneous chromosomal aberrations in hepatocytes is inversely proportional to their life span, and these data strongly supported the concept that senescence in mammals occurs because somatic cells develop mutations, i.e., chromosomal aberrations.[85]

Brooks et al.[86] studied the effects of aging in the Chinese hamster liver, scoring chromosomal aberrations in metaphase plates. Using surgical partial-hepatectomy to first stimulate cell division, colchicine was then injected to arrest mitosis in metaphase. Their results supported the hypothesis that the frequency of chromosome aberrations in liver cells increases with age.[86] The percentage of cells with aberrant chromosomes increased almost linearly with age. An algebraic equation describing the regression line that fit the chromosomal aberration frequency vs. age data revealed a slope of 0.016, expressed as percentage of abnormal cells per day. The Y intercept (zero days) was less than 1%. By 1000 days of age, the percentage of abnormal cells per total cells scored was 16% in Chinese hamsters. The most abundant types of metaphase aberrations observed were isochromatid deletions and dicentric chromosomes.[86] Compared to the results of Curtis' laboratory,[81-85] the slope of the Chinese hamster age-response curve was less than that observed for mice (0.04 to 0.12%/day), greater than that for dogs (0.0014%/day), and about equal to that seen for guinea pigs. The earlier studies,[81-85] however, had reported initial frequencies (zero days) ranging from 9 to 15%; so there is a large discrepancy in the chromosomal aberration frequency at the beginning ages. Brooks et al.[86] attributed the differences to the two experimental methods used to score aberrations. Curtis and others[81-85] did not arrest cells at metaphase, but analyzed anaphase-telophase cells instead. In anaphase-telophase cells, the chromosomes are grouped together and are not viewed separately. The results are therefore subject to a much higher background count of aberrations which, in turn, contributes to the high frequency baseline of the former studies.[81-85] It was noted that if the rate of aging and life span directly correlated with chromosome damage, then the slopes of chromosomal aberration lines would decrease in the following order: mice, Chinese hamsters, guinea pigs, and dogs. This order was indeed followed with the single exception of the relationship of Chinese hamster to guinea pig.[86] Guinea pigs have a life span that is approximately twice that of the hamster, but the two slopes were essentially the same. Given the differences in methodology and the somewhat uncertain maximum life span values of these two species, this one discordance is probably understandable. Therefore, in general, the results of Brooks et al.[86] provided independent confirmation that there is a positive correlation between the frequency of chromosomal lesions and chronological age, and the rate of accumulation is roughly inversely proportional to longevity.

The investigation of Martin et al.[87] broadened the analysis of chromosomal stability to include kidney cells. Chromosomal aberrations were determined in the first metaphases of cells isolated from the kidneys of 8-month-old and 40-month-old CB6F1 hybrid (BALB.cNNia x C57BL/6NNia) mice. Colcemid was added to arrest cells in metaphase and 11 different types of aberrations were scored, including chromatid and chromosome gaps, chromatid breaks, double minutes, acentric fragments, pulverization (extreme fragmentation), Robertsonian (whole-arm) translocations, complex exchanges, and chromosomes with three or four arms. The results showed that old kidney cells had a sixfold higher percentage of cells containing chromosome aberrations. The frequency of cells with aberrations was 4.6% for 8-month-old animals, whereas the percentage of cells with one or more aberrations was 27.1% in 40-month-old mice. The age-specific increase in abnormal chromosomes was greatest for the acentric and pulverized types. Martin et al.[87] suggested that a single mechanism appears to be insufficient to generate all the atypical chromosomes, but many of the lesions that are produced in the senescent kidney cells could originate from one or more double-strand breaks, e.g., gaps, pulverization, translocations, acentric fragments, etc. These data generalize to a limited extent the findings of Curtis' laboratory,[81-85] but they are more in agreement with the values of Brooks et al.[86] who also examined metaphase plates instead of early anaphase-telophase chromosomes. Whereas the previous studies analyzed liver parenchymal cells, it is not clear what types of cells displayed abnormal chromosomes in the kidney studies.[87]

Similar findings have been made in many studies with proliferating cells, such as lymphocytes, including those of humans.[88,89] An age-related increase in chromosomal instability is indicated for dividing cells of aged normal human diploid fibroblasts.[91] Furthermore, the frequency of aberrations in peripheral lymphocytes of healthy humans is related to donors age.[90] Recent results of somatic mutations in proliferating cells have been summarized by others.[48,49,50,91,92] Of greater interest here is the study on the frequency of metaphase chromosome aberrations in the small intestine of aged rats by Ellsworth and Schimke.[93] A cytogenetic analysis of jejunal crypt cells from young (3 to 7 months) and old (24 to 26 months) rats revealed an age-dependent increase in metaphase aberrations. The magnitude of the change observed in crypt cells (twofold increase) was not as great as that previously noted for liver and kidney cells (sixfold to sevenfold increases),[81-87] but importantly, these investigators were able to correlate the frequency of chromosomal aberrations with histological evidence of cell death in the small intestine of senescent rats.[93] Therefore, chromosomal aberrations seem to be a general feature of natural senescence in both dividing and nondividing mammalian cells, and may signal the approach of death for dividing cells.

Genetic factors play an important role in determining life expectancy. It is possible to postulate that chromosomal stability is genetically controlled, and this control contributes importantly to a species longevity. The genetic control can be found in multiple biochemical processes that protect the flow of genetic information from injuries on the one hand, and repair damages on the other hand. Curtis et al.[94] undertook experiments to clarify the genetic components of chromosomal stability by scoring aberrations between inbred strains of mice. Mice of the C58/J strain, which spontaneously develop tumors at 10 to 12 months of age, were compared with the long-lived 129/J and C57BL/6J strains. There was no significant difference in the rate at which the C58/J strain and the C57BL/6J and 129/J strains produced aberrations. While there are many possible interpretations of why the leukemia-prone strain did not have a higher frequency of aberrations, it is likely that chromosomal instability in white blood cells may result from causes different than those in liver cells.

To further examine the influence of genetic factors in the aging process, Curtis et al.[94] scored chromosomal aberrations in regenerating liver cells of the long-lived C57BL/6J mouse strain, the short-lived A/HeJ strain, and hybrids from the two inbred strains (C57BL/6J males X A/HeJ females). It had previously been shown that the short-lived A/HeJ strain accumulated higher levels of aberrations in liver cells than the C57BL/6J strain.[82,83] Female hybrid mice developed chromosomal aberration at a rate between the two parental strains. Male offspring displayed aberration frequencies that were essentially the same as the short-lived A/HeJ strain.[95] The frequency of aberrations were then compared to mortality data. At variance with the chromosomal damage results, the survival rate of male hybrid mice was not significantly different from that of the long-lived C57BL/6J strain.[94] (No survival data were reported for female hybrids.) Superficially, the results imply that genetic elements of chromosomal stability can segregate independently from elements of longevity. One conclusion to be drawn from this experiment is that the rate of formation of chromosomal aberrations is not the sole determinant responsible for longevity. Therefore, chromosomal instability as an index of aging is not a dominant characteristic, but may be one of multiple mechanisms involved in the genesis of senescence.

The senescence-accelerated mouse (SAM) was developed as a murine model of aging.[95] The senescence-prone (SAM-P) strains, derived from AKR/J mice, were founded by repeated selection of less robust littermates. The SAM-P mice are characterized by a shorter life span and an advancement in time of the senescent phenotype, including age-related pathologies. In contrast with the genetic studies of Curtis et al.,[94] senescence-prone mice show an enhanced rate of chromosomal instability over senescent-resistant (SAM-R) strains of mice derived from normal littermates of the same parental strain.[96] The rate of increase of chromosomal aberration frequency in bone marrow cells paralleled the advancement of senescence in both strains, and is approximately proportional to the aging rate of the animal. In old SAM-P mice, the percentage of bone marrow cells having chromosome aberrations was nearly twice that observed for age-matched SAM-R mice. However, the average number of aberrations per cell was roughly three- to four-fold higher in SAM-P mice.[96] The qualitative aspects of this study are consistent with the results from liver regeneration studies,[81-86] whereas the quantitative aspects of the work are more in agreement with the data on proliferating cells *in vivo*.[93] Direct analogy to the genetic studies cited above[94] cannot be made because the SAM mice have a single genetic background in contrast to F1 hybrids produced by crosses of two inbred strains.

Since chromosomal aberrations appear to be associated with normal *in vivo* aging of nondividing and dividing mammalian cells, it is obvious to look at naturally occurring diseases that exhibit greater instability than normal. Human genetic disorders, such as ataxia telangiectasia and Werner's syndrome, show increased chromosomal instability.[48,97-100] These disorders have certain aspects that might be interpreted as evidence for the premature onset of senescence or accelerated aging processes, and are therefore referred to as segmental progeroid syndromes.[99] Segmental progeroid syndromes are defined as those genetic disorders in which multiple major features of the senescent phenotype appear much earlier than clinically normal age-matched subjects.[100] A marked increase in the predisposition to cancers is part of the syndrome phenotype. Both disorders are rare autosomal recessive alleles. Werner's syndrome patients present clinically with a number of geriatric symptoms beginning about the time of puberty and culminating at death with a median age of 47 years.[99] The replicative life span of cultured Werner's syndrome cells is significantly less than controls.[101] Cytogenetic analysis of cultured somatic cells from patients with Werner's syndrome have revealed a high frequency of translocations, deletions, and inversions.[102-105] This instability was also observed at the level of the gene. Spontaneous mutations in the hypoxanthine-guanine phosphoribosyl transferase (HPRT) gene, mostly relatively large deletions, were eightfold higher than those of control subjects.[106] These observations have been interpreted as a coupling of chromosomal instability, cancer, and aging.[48]

The use of data from human genetic disorders to support the genomic instability hypotheses of aging, however, is a double-edged sword. If chromosomal instability is a direct index of aging rate, then all disorders that have higher than normal frequencies of aberrations would be expected to age at an accelerated rate, and there are many different inherited disorders that do not demonstrate precocious or accelerated aging.[100,107] However, some have rationalized this discrepancy by postulating that it is the distribution and type of damage in the genome and in the cells of tissues, i.e., the genes and cell types that are affected, that determines aging vs. pathology phenotypes.[17]

To summarize the data in this section, it can be stated that the spontaneous frequency of chromosomal aberrations of a normally nonreplicating differentiated mammalian cell, that is, the hepatocyte, increases as a function of chronological age. Furthermore, this increase seems to progress in a linear fashion with time. Similar results have been obtained for other cell types, including replicating cells of different lineages. The fact that the rate of development of chromosomal aberrations is roughly inversely proportional to an animal's life span for several mammalian species, suggests that the lesions responsible for chromosomal aberrations are related to basic processes of aging. However, there is evidence to indicate that chromosomal aberrations per se are not an invariant biomarker for the rate of aging because there are examples of enhanced rates and frequencies of aberrations that do not correlate simply with longevity.

2. Induced Chromosomal Aberrations

Curtis[12,13,81-85] suggested that there was a relationship between somatic mutations (chromosomal aberrations), γ-irradiation, and shortening of the life span. It can be argued that if somatic mutations are related to aging, agents that increase the frequency of chromosomal aberrations should also accelerate the rate of aging. Indeed, mice given a very large dose of radiation have greatly increased frequencies of chromosomal aberrations and do not live as long as nonirradiated controls.[12,80,108] The fraction of liver cells containing radiation-induced chromosomal aberrations decreases with time from some initial level toward the spontaneous level, but never appears to reach the uninduced levels for age-matched controls.[81,83]

The idea that radiation-induced life shortening is comparable to premature aging was based on a number of criteria. The single most important criterion was that irradiation increased the death rate from all causes, and appeared to advance in time the occurrence of all diseases.[14] This is in contrast to accelerated aging, in which the rate of development is increased for all manifestations of aging.[4] Early investigations into the late-somatic effects of radiation, wherein rodents were given enormous doses of radiation, seemed to support the arguments that irradiation produces premature aging.[4,12-15,80,108] In particular, radiation preserved the normal-shaped survival curve, but decreased the mean survival of the experimental group. However, these early studies suffered from some inadequacies of pathological analysis. More vigorous analyses in later studies, and a critical reassessment of the original work, showed that the dominant effect of radiation was an increase in the death rate from cancers and nephrosclerosis.[4,14,15] While some types of cancer were advanced in time, very few degenerative diseases were brought on sooner in rodents exposed to high doses of radiation. Furthermore, moderate to low multiple doses of radiation shorten the life span principally by induction of neoplastic diseases.[15] Other classical events associated with aging, such as changes in neuromuscular function and collagen cross linking, appear to be somewhat refractory to radiation.[14] Therefore, the hypothesis that irradiation causes premature aging does not seem to be valid based on the total weight of the evidence.

If chromosomal aberrations are the basis for radiation shortening the life span, then any agent capable of inducing chromosomal aberrations should cause the same effect. The ability of nitrogen mustard and other radiomimetic compounds to bring on chromosomal abnormalities, such as breaks and rearrangements, is just one of a number of properties that they share in common with radiation.[14] Some radiomimetic agents, when given in fractional doses, were reported to shorten the life span,[108-110] but many experiments demonstrated that nitrogen mustard did not decrease life span when given either as massive single doses or as multiple smaller doses split over the first half of the animals' life span.[12,81,83] Likewise, ethyl methane sulfonate, a known mutagen, did not decrease life span, but greatly increased tumor incidence at death.[15] However, the rate of accumulation of chromosomal aberrations of the nitrogen mustard-treated mice was only slightly higher than control mice.[12] This result suggests that significant repair of nitrogen mustard-induced lesions took place in the interphase liver cells.

There are data on chromosomal aberration frequency that are simply inconsistent with direct correlations between chromosomal aberrations and aging. For example, if a moderate, nonfatal dose of neutron radiation is administered to a group of mice, chromosomal aberrations in liver cells approach 100% and persist through the life span of the mice.[12,81] However, this dosage produces no measurable life-shortening effects, and liver function appears to be normal in spite of the various lesions in the hepatocyte genomes. Such results suggest that the bulk of these lesions are in DNA sequences which are not essential for function. These results also indicate that aberrations are not a quantitative marker of senescence. What is missing from an evaluation of the data is knowledge about the types of lesions associated with spontaneous, γ-radiation-induced, and neutron radiation-induced chromosomal aberrations. It is possible that some types of damages correlate with aging whereas other types of damages do not.

3. Nature of the Lesions in Chromosome Aberrations

Aberrant chromosomes include dicentric chromosomes, acentric chromosomes, centric ring fusions, chromosomal deletions, inversions, breakage and translocations, and chromatid gaps or breaks. What do these chromosomal aberrations represent at the molecular level? It is reasonable to propose that single-strand breaks, double-strand breaks, interstrand and intrastrand cross-linkages, inappropriate or abnormal recombination, inaccurately processed covalent DNA damages (adducts), and replication errors (perhaps associated with fragile sites or unstable nucleotide repeats[111,112]) are some of the mechanisms giving rise to abnormal chromosomes. It is interesting to note that liver cells seldom divide, if at all, yet their frequency of chromosomal aberrations increase steadily during aging. This indicates that these lesions are made by some mechanism independent of cell division and are not due to an accumulation of replication errors. The nature of DNA lesions that lead to chromosomal aberrations induced by ionizing radiation has been studied by Natarajan et al.[113] and others.[114-118] Ionizing radiation efficiently induces chromosomal aberrations *in vivo*. There are four types of abundant DNA damage produced by ionizing radiation: (1) single-strand breaks, (2) double-strand breaks, (3) base modification, and (4) DNA-protein cross-links.[113] Of these damages, double-stand breaks are thought to be most responsible for causing chromosomal instability. Some of the data supporting this premise include: (1) there is an increase in chromosomal aberrations when X-irradiated cells are treated with single-strand-specific nucleases which convert single-strand lesions to double-strand breaks;[116] (2) the repair kinetics of double-strand breaks is similar to the kinetics of aberration disappearance induced by split radiation doses;[116] (3) radiation that produces proportionately more double-strand breaks also induces more aberrant chromosomes,[113] and; (4) double-strand breaks created by restriction endonucleases induce chromosomal aberrations in treated cells.[117,118] The contribution of single-strand breaks to the frequency of aberrations is difficult to ascertain since a fraction of these lesions will lead to excision repair, and base modification can lead to single-strand breaks via repair endonucleases. Nonetheless, some experimental evidence[113] has been interpreted as single-strand breaks potentiating the frequency of chromosomal aberrations.

Other studies have suggested that an increase in chromosomal aberrations does not necessarily mean increased strand breaks. Gille et al.[119] analyzed chromosomal stability in oxygen-tolerant Chinese hamster ovary cells under an atmosphere of 99% O_2. Hyperoxic stress contributed to a 20-fold higher frequency of chromosome aberrations. Surprisingly, no increased levels of DNA breaks in the same cells were measured by the alkaline elution technique.[119] Since sister chromatid exchanges under hyperoxic conditions were barely twice the control values, it was thought that oxygen stress either affected replication and repair or resulted in DNA damages that were resistant to alkaline elution from filters.

One possible source of genetic instability in chromosomes is trinucleotide repeats, such as the $(CCG)_n$ sequence of the Fragile X gene.[111] When these repeats become amplified from a normal level of 2 to 60 copies to more than 200 copies, the defect presents as a segmental gap of poorly staining chromatin that predisposes the marker chromosome to breaks.[111,120,121] Other unstable trinucleotide repeats include those associated with Huntington's disease chromosomes[122] and monotonic dystrophy.[123] The mechanisms behind trinucleotide expansion and contraction and the production of fragile sites are not known. Simple repetitive sequences may adopt structures[123] or accumulate modifications[111] that make completely accurate replication difficult, if not impossible.

B. Genetic Instability

1. DNA Damage: Base Alterations and Adducts

There are a number of different types of covalent modifications that can alter the bases in DNA. These consist of base deaminations, covalent additions (adducts) of small aliphatic groups, large bulky adducts, oxygen radical modifications, interstrand cross-links, intrastrand cross-links, and cross-links to other macromolecules such as proteins. There is now solid experimental data that show these alterations, e.g., alkyl-, aromatic-, and oxygen-adducts, can be measured at uninduced background levels in somatic cells and in most cases these levels change with age. There is circumstantial evidence that some of the other types of lesions, i.e., cross-linkages, exist *in vivo* and may change with age. Lastly, there are either no data or negative data for age-related changes in base deaminations.

a. Alkyl Adducts

Gaubatz[124] used ^{32}P-postlabeling methods to discover DNA damage during aging of mouse heart cells. This postlabeling analysis showed that a modified nucleotide increased in an age-dependent manner. The modified nucleotide appeared to be 7-methyl-deoxyguanosine-5'-monophosphate, the most abundant alkylation product formed in DNA,[125] based on its mobility in two-dimensional, thin-layer chromatography systems. The adduct was observed to increase about ninefold in heart DNA in mice between 2 and 39 months of age.[124] This increase with age seemed to be more of an exponential change rather than a linear increase. Park and Ames[126] subsequently observed indigenous 7-methylguanine adducts in DNA of rat liver, using HPLC separation with electrochemical detection. A contaminating unidentified adduct that coeluted with 7-methylguanine prevented quantifying this adduct in rat liver, however.[127]

Using two independent HPLC systems and two different methods of detection, Tan et al.[128] showed that low levels of 7-methylguanine are present in nuclear DNA of normal postmitotic mouse tissues. The structural identity of the adduct was confirmed by fast atom bombardment mass spectrometry. The results demonstrated that the steady-state levels of 7-methylguanine increased approximately twofold between mature (11 months) and old (28 months) brain, liver, and kidney tissues of C57BL/6NNia male mice.[128] Figure 1 shows the number of 7-methylguanine adducts in postmitotic mouse tissues as a function of age. For the ages and tissues studied, adduct levels reached their highest point in 28-month-old kidney, where 1 out of every 30,000 guanine bases was methylated. These data suggest that indigenous alkyl adducts are present at biologically meaningful levels in postmitotic mammalian genomes and increase with age. Furthermore, 7-methylguanine levels have been measured in white

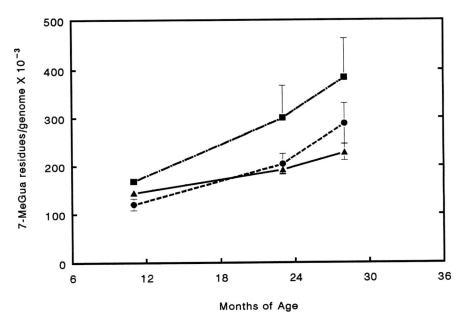

Figure 1
Content of 7-methylguanine adducts (7-MeGua) in postmitotic mouse genomes as
a function of age. The data are taken from Tan et al.[128] and are calculated on a diploid
genome basis. Error bars show standard errors of the mean for multiple determinations. Where error bars are not evident, the standard errors are less than the symbol
representing the mean. Brain data are shown as triangles, liver data as circles, and
kidney data as squares. Alkylation damage ranged from a low of 120,000 residues/
genome for 11-month-old liver to a high of 384,000 residues/genome for 28-month-
old kidney.

blood cell DNA of humans, using the ^{32}P-postlabeling approach.[129] The
range of adduct levels for this replicating cell were 600 to 4,200 residues
per diploid genome. DNA methylation of this type is thought to arise in
untreated genomes as a consequence of endogenous processes, perhaps as
a consequence of nonenzymatic reactions involving endogenous
S-adenosylmethionine as a methyl donor.[59, 130] Recent *in vivo* studies suggest a role for endogenous DNA alkylation damage, including 7-
methylguanine, as a source of spontaneous mutations in eukaryotic cells.[131]

b. Oxygen Radical Modifications

Adelman et al.[132] have measured thymine glycol and thymidine glycol
adducts, removed from DNA by repair enzymes, in urine samples of four
different mammalian species. This biomarker of oxidative DNA damage
correlated highly with the specific metabolic rates of mice, rats, monkeys,
and humans, consistent with the idea that free radicals are a major source
of indigenous DNA damage. Thus, mice excrete 18 times more glycol

adducts than do humans, and monkeys excrete 4 times more glycol adducts than do humans on a normalized-weight basis; so the rate of oxidative DNA damage excretion is inversely related to the life span.[132] To distinguish between oxidative damage to nuclear DNA and to mitochondrial DNA, methods were developed to measure the oxidized nucleoside 8-hydroxydeoxyguanosine.[133] It was found that 8-hydroxydeoxyguanosine residues were 16 times higher in mitochondrial DNA than in nuclear DNA from rat liver;[134] a result in keeping with the former molecule's closer proximity to the sites of oxidative metabolism. Further experiments demonstrated that oxidative damage to somatic cell chromosomes was extensive. Steady-state levels of 8-hydroxydeoxyguanosine ranged from 8 to 73 modifications per million normal deoxyguanosines. The amounts of oxidized nucleoside increased with age in Fischer 344 rat liver, kidney, and intestine.[135] On the other hand, data indicated that the levels of 8-hydroxydeoxyguanosine did not change with age in brain tissue and testes. Figure 2 shows the content of 8-hydroxydeoxyguanosine in DNA from different rat tissues as a function of age. The lines were obtained by linear regression analysis of the data. It can be seen that kidney cells had higher levels of oxidized nucleoside than the other tissues, and the slopes (indicating rates of change) are similar for liver and kidney tissues, but are lower in the brain.

It is of interest to compare the results from the indigenous 7-methylguanine studies in mice with those of oxidation damage to nuclear DNA of rat tissues. The total number of lesions per diploid genome (or per somatic cell) are of the same order of magnitude for liver and kidney tissues of the two species. For example, calculations indicate that there are 67,000 residues of 8-hydroxydeoxyguanosine per kidney cell in 4-month-old rats and 120,000 molecules of 7-methylguanine per kidney cell in 11-month-old mice. The higher levels of methyl adducts in mouse cells probably reflect the differences in rates of damage accumulation between the two species. For kidney tissue, it can be estimated that rats accumulate 8-hydroxydeoxyguanosine at 80 residues per day,[135] whereas mice increase their steady-state levels of 7-methylguanine by 440 residues per day,[128] or 5.5 times more rapidly than the oxidation damage. Whether these differences are due to species differences or to the nature of the lesions and their respective removal from DNA is not known. It is known that there are 12 sites of alkylation on DNA, but modification at N[7]-guanine occurs with the greatest frequency.[72,125] In fact, 7-methylguanine represents roughly 70% of all lesions produced by simple direct-acting methylating agents *in vivo* and *in vitro*.[125] Relatively speaking, 7-methylguanine is not removed as actively from DNA as some other methyl adducts and can persist for long times *in vivo*.[72,125,128,179] By contrast, 8-hydroxydeoxyguanosine is only one of 20 known oxidative damages incurred by DNA *in vivo*.[132,135] Its relative proportion to all other indigenous oxidative-DNA lesions in normal cells

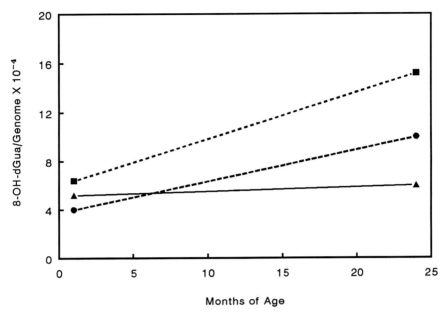

Figure 2
Levels of 8-hydroxydeoxyguanosine (8-OH-dGua) in postmitotic rat tissues at different ages. The data are taken from Fraga et al.,[135] and individual results are not shown. The lines represent a molecular conversion of linear regression analyses of femtomoles of adduct per microgram of DNA obtained with all data points, but only adduct levels calculated for the ages of 1 month and 24 months are presented. The data were calculated for diploid genomes. Triangles, circles, and squares represent brain, liver, and kidney cells, respectively.

is not known, but the available data indicate that this modified nucleoside is very actively removed from DNA.[68-71] Perhaps the most interesting difference in damage accumulation between the two rodents is the absence of an increase with age of 8-hydroxydeoxyguanosine in rat brain. Brain tissue is very active metabolically and consumes large amounts of oxygen[136] which would seem to put brain genomes at risk for higher levels of oxidative damage, yet initial levels of 8-hydroxydeoxyguanosine are roughly the same as in other tissues, and moreover, did not change significantly with aging.[135] Methyl adducts in brain DNA were fewer than in liver or kidney DNA for age-matched younger animals,[128] and of the three tissues, brain adducts increased at the slowest rate of 150 adducts per cell per day, which gives the overall impression that brain DNA is more resistant to damage accumulation than many other cell types.

c.   Bulky Adducts

Do postmitotic genomes accumulate bulky hydrophobic types of DNA adducts as a function of age? The evidence for a positive answer is not clear. Randerath and colleagues[137,138] first described covalent modifications in untreated rats using postlabeling assays. Tissue-specific patterns of ^{32}P-labeled spots were observed following autoradiography of thin-layer chromatograms. These spots were first termed I-spots, then were later renamed as I-compounds based on the assumption that they are nonpolar, covalent DNA modifications that arise indigenously.[137] In addition, polar types of I-compounds have been described.[144] The numbers and quantities of I-compounds vary with tissue, sex, age, species, diet, individual nutrients and minerals, and physiological and pathological processes.[137-146] It was postulated that I-compounds were derived from endogenous DNA-reactive compounds generated during normal metabolism.[137] In the context of aging, I-compounds associated with DNA isolated from tissues of rats appeared to increase early in the life span then level off after maturity, although there seemed to be a jump in levels in kidney and liver DNAs from the oldest animals.[137,138,143,144] Age-dependent increases in a selected group of I-compound spots in human brain DNA have been reported and appear to accumulate in a nonlinear fashion.[144]

The original notion that I-compounds represent covalent modifications to DNA, and are therefore DNA-adducts, was built on the facts that (1) polynucleotide kinase catalyzed the transfer of γ-^{32}P-phosphate to the compounds, (2) the association of the labeled phosphate to its receptor molecule is chemically stabile, and (3) their chromatographic properties resemble nucleotides containing bulky, hydrophobic moieties.[137-142] However, the chemical structure of a single I-compound has yet to be determined. Given the observations that so many factors modulate I-compounds, qualitatively and quantitatively, including the evidence that treatment of rats with various carcinogens and toxins depressed the age-related increases of I-compounds in liver tissue[140,145,146] and the findings that calorically restricted rats have higher levels of I-compounds than controls,[143] it is difficult to view I-compounds as DNA damage. This issue will need to be resolved before any type of definitive statement regarding the effects of I-compounds can be made.

Another postlabeling analysis of indigenous aromatic-like DNA adducts accumulating during aging was performed with mouse myocardium.[147] Unlike the other studies that measured low levels of adducts,[137] nonpolar constituents of deoxynucleotide digests were first isolated by phase transfer to 1-butanol, prior to labeling. The results showed that several adducts were more abundant in ^{32}P-maps of senescent heart DNA. One adduct showed a striking 10-fold higher content in 39-month-old mice, compared to 17-month-old mice.[147] The relationship between these "aromatic DNA adducts" and I-compounds is not known.

d.   Cross-Links

Over the years there has been circumstantial evidence related to the possible accumulation of cross-linkages in DNA of nondividing mammalian cells.[34,55] The indirect signs that cross-links increase in somatic cell DNA with time involve age-related changes in the melting temperature or other physical-chemical properties of DNA and chromatin, the degree of difficulty in removing proteins bound to DNA, and in nuclear template activity for exogenous RNA polymerases. The results from various investigations have been reviewed by Tice and Setlow[55] and by Cutler.[34] A different approach has been to purify DNA from a tissue, hydrolyze DNA in 6 N HCl to release the bases, then separate the individual bases from larger products using molecular exclusion chromatography.[148] It was shown by this approach that age-related modifications of DNA in the liver of mice and rats exhibit an unusually high fluorescence, indicative of DNA-DNA or DNA-protein cross-links in which covalent bonds between ring systems produce larger fluorescent effects. Similar compounds are formed when solutions of DNA are irradiated with γ-photons.[149] Yamamoto et al.[150] examined fluorescent modifications to DNA in liver tissue of the New Zealand white rabbit. Chromatographically separated modified bases, which were obtained in relatively large yields from old animals, were highly fluorescent, and mass spectrometry using the secondary ion mass method indicated the compounds were cross-linked base products.[150] The yield of highly fluorescent products from rabbit liver DNA increased with age (after 6 months of age) in a way that data could be fitted with an exponential function. Livers from 10-year-old rabbits had four times the amount of modified bases found for young rabbit livers.[150] Thus, these data give some direct evidence for an age-dependent accumulation of DNA cross-linkages in mammalian liver tissue.

e. Deaminations

Hydroxymethyluracil is an oxidation product of thymine, and uracil is the deamination product of cytosine. It has been suggested that deamination of deoxycytidine is a common event in the genome of a mammalian cell at 37°C.[44,55,63] The work of Ames and others,[132-135] moreover, has shown that oxidation damage to mammalian DNA can be extensive for some cells. Therefore, it is surprising that Kirsh et al.[151] failed to detect deoxyuridine or 5-hydroxymethyldeoxyuridine in DNAs from various tissues of mice ranging in age from 7 to 31 months. The absence of altered deoxynucleosides in somatic cell DNA implies exceedingly efficient repair of these lesions. This investigation employed reversed-phase HPLC separation of deoxynucleosides, coupled with UV-detection/quantification.[151] The limits of detection corresponded to approximately 10 pmol of modified deoxynucleosides per micromole of normal deoxynucleosides, or 1 modification per 10^5 residues. To compare this method with those that were used to measure indigenous methyl adducts[128] and oxidative damage,[133,135] one can estimate that UV detection is 10- to 20-fold lower than electrochemical detection, depending on the electrochemical activity of the individual base or deoxynucleoside. Therefore if background, steady-state levels of deoxyuridine and 5-hydroxymethyldeoxyuridine in DNA are similar to those for 7-methylguanine or 8-hydroxdeoxyguanosine, minimum detection limits of 1×10^{-6} will be required to measure them.

The results discussed in this section lead to the conclusion that a variety of altered bases and nucleotide adducts can be found in somatic cell genomes, and there is convincing evidence that the levels of most forms of indigenous damage that have been measured to date increase in nondividing cells as a function of age. However, there are exceptions, such as the intriguing example of 8-hydroxydeoxyguanosine in rat brain.[135] In view of the number of diverse methods that now exist to detect and quantify minute amounts of DNA damage, it seems reasonable to expect more reports concerning relationships between DNA modifications and aging in the future.

2. DNA Damage: Strand Breaks and Alkaline-Sensitive Sites

DNA single-strand breaks have been the most widely examined form of DNA damage in age-related studies. There are several reason for this: (1) sensitive methods to directly measure single-strand breaks have been around for many years; (2) other methods, such as DNA polymerase template activity give indirect evidence for single-strand breaks; and (3) as discussed earlier, single-strand breaks are likely to be a more informative marker of the damaged state of a genome, since they arise from multiple routes — spontaneously, as a consequence of modifying enzymes, and as a result of repair enzyme processing of many diverse lesions. Table 2 lists the results of experiments that have searched for single-strand breaks or gaps during aging of postmitotic mammalian organ systems.

Three categories of assays have been used to analyze somatic cells for single-strand breaks — alkaline assays, enzyme assays, and miscellaneous assays. Alkaline sucrose gradients,[152] alkaline elution from membrane filters,[153] and alkaline-induced DNA unwinding[154] are three denaturing assays that investigators have exploited in gerontological research. Abasic sites (apurinic or apyrimidinic sites) and phosphotriesters will appear as single-strand breaks when alkaline assays are used since these lesions have alkali-labile bonds.[65] Therefore, it is not clear what contribution each type of lesion makes toward the total number measured by alkaline assays.

Detection of single-strand breaks by alkaline sucrose gradient sedimentation is sensitive and quantitative. It is estimated that 1 break per 10^8 Da (20,000 breaks/cell) can be detected via alkaline sucrose gradients.[65] Since relatively little DNA can be loaded on gradients, fluorescence spectroscopy is a commonly employed means to quantify DNA in these gradients. Alkaline elution assays are judged to be about 20 times more

TABLE 2.

Results of Studies Examining Single-Strand Breaks in Postmitotic
Mammalian Tissues at Different Ages.[a]

Tissue	Animal	Age (months)	Method[b]	Result	Ref.
Brain	Mouse	3–35	Template activity	Increase	158
	Mouse	3–35	Template activity	Increase	159
	Mouse	6–30	ASGS	Increase	165
	Mouse	1–22	ASGS	No change	169
	Mouse	1–12	Immunofluorescence	Increase	167
	Mouse	0–20	ASGS	No change	170
	Peromyscus	0–60	ASGS	No change	170
	Rat	0–36	Alkaline elution	No change	155
	Dogs	2–156	ASGS	Increase	171
Liver	Mouse	3–35	Template activity	Increase	158
	Mouse	2–22	ASGS	Increase	169
	Mouse	1–12	Immunofluorescence	Increase	167
	Mouse	0–20	ASGS	Increase	170
	Mouse	6–24	Alkaline elution	Increase	172
	Peromyscus	0–60	ASGS	Increase	170
	Rat	6–36	Alkaline elution	Increase	155,173
	Rat	1–35	ASGS and viscosity	Increase	168
Heart	Mouse	3–35	Template activity	Increase	158
	Mouse	6–30	ASGS/CsCl-ES	Increase	164
Muscle	Human	12–1092	SS-nuclease/EM	Increase	166
Kidney	Mouse	0–20	ASGS	Increase	170
	Peromyscus	0–60	ASGS	No change	170
Spleen	Mouse	1–22	ASGS	No change	169
Retina	Rabbit	1–93	Zonal-ASGS	Increase	174

[a]   This table originated from similar tables in the reviews of Tice and Setlow, and
      Holmes et al.
[b]   Template activity was measured with calf thymus DNA polymerase; ASGS, alkaline
      sucrose gradient sedimentation; immunofluorescence with anti-cytidine antibodies;
      CsCl-ES, cesium chloride equilibrium sedimentation; SS-nuclease/EM, electron
      microscopy of single-strand-specific nuclease-digested DNA molecules.

sensitive than alkaline sucrose gradients, with sensitivity limits of 1,000
breaks/cell.[155] The newer method of alkaline-induced DNA unwinding
has not been used as much as the other two assays. In the unwinding
assay, nuclear suspensions are treated with solutions of urea-sodium
dodecyl sulfate (SDS), then treated with urea-SDS in alkali for 30 min at
0°C to allow for equilibration.[156] To initiate the unwinding, nuclear lysates
are shifted to 15°C for varying times and reactions are stopped by neutralization and chilling. Mixtures are next briefly sonicated and ethidium
bromide is added to fluorometrically detect DNA unwinding. Experimental samples are compared to those which were not treated with alkali (total
double-stranded DNA) and to those which were sheared by sonication

prior to alkali addition (background).[156] No age-related accumulation of single-strand breaks has been noted thus far with the unwinding assay.[156,157] In fact, the rate of DNA unwinding decreased as a function of age for rat brain, liver, and intestinal epithelium, which implies that there are less strand breaks or alkaline-sensitive sites in senescent mammalian cells.[156] It was noted in the study just cited, however, that DNA preparations from older animals contained less double-stranded DNA at the beginning of these experiments, suggesting that considerable unwinding had occurred *in situ* or during sample preparation.[156] Therefore, until this assay has been shown to accurately measure single-strand breaks *in situ*, perhaps by calibration of the same samples with one or both of the other alkaline assays, the unwinding data are equivocal and are not included in Table 2.

Polymerase template activities have been used to probe for single-strand breaks or gaps in nuclear chromatin and DNA isolated at different ages.[158] The rationale for studying strand breaks with DNA-dependent DNA polymerases comes from the knowledge that the initial rates of deoxynucleotide incorporation by *E. coli* DNA polymerase I and mammalian α-DNA polymerase, e.g., calf thymus DNA polymerase, are directly proportional to the number of 3'-OH template primer sites, i.e., strand nicks or gaps.[159] Synthesis is usually determined by autoradiography, in conjunction with radiolabeled precursors, as grains over the nucleus. Results from polymerase template activity experiments are more descriptive than those from alkaline assays in the sense that values are only indirectly related to primary lesions, and there are alternative interpretations to explain incorporation differences.[65]

Chetsanga et al.[160] were the first to use single-strand-specific nucleases to probe age-related changes in DNA structure. DNAs isolated from liver tissue of CBF1 mice of different ages were subsequently treated with S1 nuclease. It was reported that S1 nuclease digestion of liver DNAs to acid-soluble, $A_{260 \text{ nm}}$-absorbing material showed an increase from background levels at 15 months of age to approximately 25% at 30 months of age. Several different labs have not been able to reproduce these results,[161-163] and it is probably unrealistic to think that there are such large differences in the primary structure of senescent somatic cell DNA that they can be detected by this approach. On the other hand, the use of single-strand-specific nucleases to convert DNA nicks into double-strand breaks, which can then be measured by sedimentation,[164,165] electron microscopy,[166] or other techniques, appears to be a valid approach for looking at these lesions.

Under miscellaneous assay, one study has employed antibodies directed against cytosine nucleosides to examine DNA single-strandedness in cell preparations derived from mouse brain and liver tissues.[167] Control experiments indicated that the antibodies could bind their epitopes only in single-stranded regions of DNA as determined by immunofluorescence, and cells obtained from older animals exhibited qualitatively more immunofluorescence than cells from younger animals. In one of the earliest studies on single-strand breaks, Massie et al.[168] used hydrodynamic methods such as viscosity, sucrose gradient sedimentation, and buoyant density, in addition to alkaline sucrose gradients, to analyze rat liver DNA for intactness. Their results were generally consistent in that alkaline sucrose gradients, viscosity, and neutral sucrose gradients all indicated an increase in strand breaks.[168] There was no change in buoyant densities, which was not surprising since a decrease in DNA molecular weight would not be revealed in density differences but in the peak width-to-height ratios. One interesting conclusion from this investigation was that the greatest changes in liver DNA strand breaks occurred between 1 and 12 months of age, with relatively small changes thereafter.[168]

An inspection of the results in Table 2 shows that liver and brain tissue have been the systems studied most frequently. If results from alkaline unwinding and single-strand-specific nuclease digestion experiments per se are excluded, all the results with rodent liver cells are in agreement. Eight independent studies, employing five different assays, have demonstrated that DNA single-strand breaks (or alkali-labile bonds) increased in rodent liver tissue as a function of age.[155,158,167-170,172,173] The results with brain tissue are not so straightforward. About half of the studies indicate no age-related differences in single-strand lesions.[155,158,159,167, 169-171] In fact, three out of the five experiments using the more analytical methods of alkaline assays gave negative results.[155,165,169-171] These latter results were from comparative studies in which more than one tissue was examined. For example, Ono et al.[169] observed an age-dependent increase of DNA strand breakage in mouse liver, but not mouse brain or spleen, with the alkaline sucrose gradient assay. Likewise, Su et al.[170] found DNA strand breaks associated with aging in mouse and *Peromyscus* liver cells but not in brain cells of the same animals, which makes these results all the more meaningful.

Mullaart and others[155] measured spontaneous DNA strand breaks in rat brain during development and aging using the alkaline elution technique. They found a constant low level of DNA breaks in nuclei isolated from the cerebral cortex and cerebellum of rat embryos. The level of DNA strand breaks remained the same in 6- and 36-month-old rodents.[155] In contrast to these static results, DNA strand breaks increased twofold in rat liver DNA between the same ages.[155] The results[155,169,170] show that, as signified by levels of DNA strand breaks, aging affects different tissues variably. It was also noted in the study by Mullaart et al. that rat brain DNA rather quickly accumulated strand breaks after death. The relevance of this latter observation should be considered in all studies measuring *in vivo* DNA strand breaks. In 6-month-old rats, the level of liver DNA breaks was twice as high as brain strand breaks, i.e., 1.1×10^3 breaks per brain cell compared to 2.2×10^3 breaks per liver cell.[155] Earlier work by this same group demonstrated that an age-related increase in liver DNA breaks took place exclusively in the postmitotic parenchymal cells, and no increase in breaks was observed for the proliferative nonparenchymal cells,[173] a result that suggested the accumulation of strand breaks was a property of postmitotic cells, not mitotic cells. With this latter result in mind, it does not seem unreasonable to suggest that the genomes of senescent hepatocytes have fourfold more strand breaks than neurons at the same age. One conclusion gained from this analysis is that the aging processes associated with increased DNA alterations is not uniform across postmitotic cells in different tissues of one animal. In this regard, the effects of aging on the accumulation of single-strand breaks or alkaline-sensitive sites in DNA of postmitotic mammalian cells are consistent with the data on base alterations and adducts discussed above, i.e., senescent brain genomes have lower levels of lesions than liver and kidney genomes in the same animals.

In addition to results already discussed in this section, there are several studies that deserve special mention; one is the work of Zahn et al.[166] The only data regarding humans listed in Table 2 is from the research of Zahn et al.[166] This investigation represented a massive study on muscle tissues, covering 470 subjects in age-groups from 1 to 91 years old. The experimental approach was to isolate DNA from individual subjects, treat the DNA with single-strand-specific nucleases (S1, BAL31, and pea endonuclease were compared), then measure the contour lengths of double-stranded DNA molecules from electron micrographs (20 to 200 molecules analyzed for each individual.). The results showed that the average molecular weight of DNA strands decreased in a highly significant fashion with the age of the donor.[166] As might be expected, the molecular weight data show considerable scatter and, intriguingly, the standard deviation of the mean molecular weights also increased with age. Data were also placed into groups according to life style, with the abstinent group (non-smokers, etc.) scoring the least damage. This investigation indicates that muscle tissue is a particularly good model system for studying postmitotic changes in DNA, and more work should address age changes in mammalian muscle since their nuclei do not enter S-phase after birth. Furthermore, a number of studies indicate that as muscle cells differentiate they lose much of their ability to repair different forms of DNA damage.[175-178]

Bergtold and Lett[174] examined alterations in chromosomal DNA of retinal photoreceptor cells from New Zealand white rabbits, using reorienting gradient zonal ultracentrifugation. They selected the retina as a model system because these cells remain postmitotic throughout the life span and if lost are not replaced by stem cells. Furthermore, the samples represent a single type of differentiated cell (photoreceptor rod cells); retinas can easily be removed surgically; the total cell population of a retina can be measured in one gradient; and there are two retinas per animal, allowing one to serve as a control for experimental manipulation of the other.[174] The results were consistent with DNA strand scissions, and possibly alkaline-sensitive sites, accumulating with age.[174] The age-specific frequency of DNA single-strand breaks was nonlinear. The aging effects were noted only in the older photoreceptor cells, after the median life span of the animal. In addition, the effects could be accelerated by X-irradiation. Interestingly, the age-related alterations of chromosomal DNA were not accompanied by a decrease in the ability of older photoreceptor cells to rejoin strand breaks induced by γ-photons.

If DNA repair processes for strand break ligation are not impaired in senescent photoreceptor cells, why were the spontaneous DNA strand scissions not rejoined? The answer may lie in the type of lesion, e.g., gaps or alkali-sensitive sites vs. single-strand breaks, or in changes in chromatin that make the lesions inaccessible to repair.[174] Another explanation is that breaks are occurring with greater frequency in the old cells.[128] Architectural rearrangements changing the tertiary and quaternary structure of chromosomal DNA could be coupled to an age-related accumulation of a complex spectrum of DNA damages, perhaps resulting from normal cellular metabolism or chemical instability of DNA.[174,179] Alterations in chromatin, accruing with age, could lead to a negative feedback loop in limiting overall repair efficiency. Single-strand breaks might inhibit repair proteins that track DNA laterally, and reduced negative supercoiling in a chromatin domain would seemingly make helicase opening of duplex regions carrying a lesion more difficult.[128,180] Single-strand breaks could lead to a reduction in transcription (collaboration) which is associated with preferential repair,[19-21] thus as transcription decreases with age[181] repair might decrease in tandem.[128,180]

3. Sequence Changes Including Rearrangements, Deletions, and Amplifications

When considering inheritable changes in the primary sequence of somatic cell DNA, there is a logical division into point mutations and macromutations, involving larger alterations. It is also convenient to discuss repetitive sequences and single- or low-copy sequences separately. To begin, large scale changes of repetitive sequences in postmitotic cells will be reviewed. Repetitive sequence families in mammals can be grouped into (1) highly repetitive, tandemly repetitive simple sequences, such as those associated with chromosomal centromeres and telomeres, (2) short-interspersed and long-interspersed repetitive sequences that appear to be evolutionary products of retroposons,[182,183] and (3) repetitive genes.

a. Telomeres

Olovnikov[33] suggested that dividing cells lose their ability to divide, and thus age because of the gradual loss of sequences from the ends of chromosomes due to the inability of DNA polymerases to completely replicate the 3′ ends of linear duplex DNA. In mammals the short sequence $(TTAGGG)_n$ is repeated in tandem thousands of times at the ends of the chromosomes to form specialized structures known as telomeres.[184,185] It is thought that telomeres protect and anchor chromosomes.[186] The simple repetitive sequences are synthesized by telomerase, which is a ribozyme containing an internal guide template that codes for the repeat.[187,188] Cellular levels of telomerase activity generally correlate directly with cellular proliferation.[189] The average size of telomeric DNA decreases during serial passage *in vitro* and also as a function of donor age for human fibroblasts.[190] Other somatic cells *in vivo*, such as epidermal cells and peripheral blood cells, also exhibit loss of telomeric repeats with age.[191,192] It has been suggested that telomere length predicts the replicative capacity for dividing cells,[193] and in the absence of sufficient telomerase, telomere shortening is associated with chromosomal instability, as indicated by chromosomal aberrations.[194] Thus, there is a shortening of telomeres associated with *in vivo* and *in vitro* aging of dividing cells, and this loss may be both necessary and sufficient to cause cellular aging.[193,195]

The question to be addressed here is are telomeric sequences unstable in nondividing cells? To our knowledge, no studies examining the *in vivo* loss of telomeric repeats with age have been carried out with postmitotic cells. Kipling and Cooke[196] measured telomere length in various inbred mouse strains. Randomly chosen mice were selected, and telomere tract sizes were determined for liver DNA. The tract sizes of telomeres in mice are 10 to 15 times larger than those of human, and individual restriction enzyme banding patterns are characteristic of an inbred strain but highly polymorphic within populations of a strain, suggesting an usually high mutation rate.[196] Liver DNA from a 17-month-old mouse showed a normal size distribution of telomere fragments that was representative of younger mice of the same strain.[196] This result, and the much longer telomeres of mice, indicates that telomere shortening is unlikely to have any causal role in aging of postmitotic rodent cells *in vivo*. Given the total size and G+C content of telomeres, however, this terminal repeat array represents a significant target for DNA damage, and it would be of considerable importance to learn whether DNA repair takes place in telomeres or if telomeres accumulate damage with age. There is some reason to think repair might be troublesome since telomeric DNA has an unusual structure, and some specialized proteins, in addition to core histones, bind to these sequences.[184,188] If telomeres do indeed accumulate DNA damage during aging of noncycling cells *in vivo* and such cells were induced to divide, e.g., as hepatocytes during liver regeneration, then damaged telomeres might either block cell cycle completion or lead to a multitude of chromosomal aberrations.

b. Satellite DNAs

Numerous studies indicate that tandemly repetitive sequences other than telomeres are unstable. Tandemly repetitive mammalian centromeric DNAs, classically referred to as satellite DNAs, are unstable in cultured cells[197,198] and appear to be lost during the replicative life span of human diploid fibroblasts.[199] Prashad and Cutler[200] determined the fraction of satellite DNA in different tissue preparations as a function of age for C57BL/6J mice. They reported that the percentage of total DNA that was satellite remained essentially constant at $11 \pm 1\%$ for spleen, kidney, and brain tissues from 10 to 780 days of age. However, the data clearly show that the oldest age group contained the lowest levels of satellite DNA. From 590 days of age to 780 days of age, the following decreases were observed — 10.5 to 9.0%, 12.0 to 9.5%, and 12.0 to 10.3% for spleen, kidney, and brain tissue, respectively.[200] Inasmuch as the reproducibility of quantification of DNA bands from the CsCl buoyant density gradients following equilibrium sedimentation was estimated to be less than 1%, the age differences reported are compatible with a physical loss of the these sequences from senescent mouse postmitotic genomes. In the same study a different trend was noted for liver tissue.[200] Until approximately 300 days of age, satellite DNA was underrepresented in the liver genome, averaging about 8%. Thereafter, the percentage of satellite DNA increased in liver cells until a maximum of 13% was reached at 780 days of age. It was during this latter increase that the liver cells underwent more extensive polyploidization.[200] A similar age-related increase was noted for the rRNA gene copy number in liver tissue of this inbred mouse strain.[201,202] A possible mechanism to account for these repetitive sequence differences in liver cells is through differential DNA replication during endoduplication processes of polyploid hepatocytes, i.e., some sequences are not replicated with the rest of the genome, and are therefore underrepresented.[202] Whatever replicative block existed earlier in their history, it apparently was relieved later as these cells acquire close to their normal complement of satellite and rRNA gene sequences.[200-202]

c. Minisatellites

Variable number of tandem repeats (VNTR), or minisatellite loci, are unstable genetic elements.[203,204] Minisatellite polymorphisms arise from variation in the number of repeat units at a locus, and new-length alleles are associated with high rates of germ-line mutations that result in the gain or loss of repeat units.[205] Hybridization probes, recognizing a core sequence common to many minisatellite loci, generate DNA fingerprints that are specific for an individual, but exceedingly variable in the population.[204,206] Kelley et al.[207] have characterized a highly unstable minisatellite locus in mice and presented evidence for somatic mutations occurring early in development. The hypervariable minisatellite loci was detected by cross hybridization with a human minisatellite probe. Genetic analysis revealed that the Ms6-hm loci was amplified within a member of the MT (mouse transcript) family of interspersed repetitive elements, and that allelic variation arose from the number of tandem repeats at this locus.[207] A nonparental or mutant allele was detected in somatic cells of the offspring at a frequency of 0.028. Two mosaic mice contained the same dosage of mutant allele in different adult tissues (brain, kidney, liver, lower jaw, midvertebral region, sternal region, and tail). To contribute equally to these somatic tissues, the mutational events affecting the Ms6-hm must have occurred very early during development.[207] It would be of interest to determine if these repetitive elements show continued instability in different cellular compartments of senescent mice.

The possibility of using hypervariable minisatellite sequences to track genomic instability in senescent somatic cells has been comprehensively reviewed by Vijg and associates.[208-212] Uitterlinden et al.[209] have advocated using a two-dimensional DNA typing technique for such studies, and Slagboom et al.[212] have employed this approach to study VNTR sequences in rat fibroblasts cloned from primary cultures of young and old rodents. An examination of more than 3,000 DNA fragments indicated a high somatic mutation rate at several loci. Surprisingly, though, no correlation with age was found. In fact, clones from young donor rats (6 months) had somewhat higher sequence variation frequencies than fibroblasts from old donor rats (30 months).[212] This might mean that somatic mutations at such loci are occurring at very early stages of development, when enzymes that induce such variability are present or at least more abundant.

d.   Interspersed Repetitive Sequences

A large fraction of the mammalian genome is occupied by interspersed repetitive sequences. There are hundreds of thousands of copies of short-interspersed-nucleotide-sequences, such as the 300-base-pair Alu family in primates and the related B1 family in rodents, that are dispersed amongst nonrepetitive DNA.[182] Long-interspersed-nucleotide-sequences, represented by the L1 family of repeat elements, also exist at high copy numbers and have a sequence organization resembling mammalian retroviruses.[183] It has been demonstrated that these repetitive elements can move to new chromosomal locations, and thus increase their number, through RNA intermediates, a process known as retrotransposition.[182,183] These elements, termed retroposons, would seem to be a likely source of genetic instability during senescence.

Murray[31] has proposed that during aging the number of transposons increases exponentially, thereby eventually inactivating essential genes and killing cells. An important phase for transposition of interspersed repetitive sequences is their expression, since RNA molecules are the templates required by reverse transcriptase. In differentiated somatic cells, however, transcription of short- and long-interspersed sequences is normally repressed. Transcription of short-interspersed repetitive sequences and long-interspersed repetitive sequences is often derepressed in transformed cells and relatively undifferentiated tissues.[213] Transcriptional derepression of these sequences could, in turn, lead to higher rates of retrotransposition and greater chromosome instability.[214] If senescent cells become more "undifferentiated", a similar scenario might happen as part of the aging process. In support of this theory, Servomaa and Rytomaa[215] have shown that rat chloroleukemia cells die when kept at a high cell density, and cell death is accompanied by an increase in an L1 element (L1Rn) dispersed into various locations in the genome. Subsequent studies indicated that UV light and ionizing radiation induced transpositions of the L1Rn element and caused rat chloroleukemia cell death.[216] Short-interspersed elements can also become unstable following DNA damaging events. For example, it has been shown that DNA-advanced glycosylation end products induced transposition of an Alu-containing element in murine lymphoid cells.[217] The rat chloroleukemia and murine lymphoid cells appear to be very good systems for studying the mechanisms of retrotransposition, but the relevance of this phenomenon and others to aging of normal diploid cells remains to be established, and similar examples of genetic instability in postmitotic mammalian cells have not been described.

e.   Tandemly Repeated Genes

Evidence supporting an instability of tandemly duplicated genes in mammalian chromosomes is also known. Most of these studies have focused on ribosomal RNA genes which are repeated in tandem at several different loci in mammalian cells. Strehler and co-workers[32,218-222] have described an age-related loss of rRNA genes in heart, skeletal muscle, and brain tissues from beagle dogs, human cardiac tissue, and human cerebral cortex cells. The same laboratory found no significant differences in rRNA gene dosage as a function of age in liver, kidney, and spleen tissues of beagle dogs.[219] To buttress the argument that rRNA genes are lost during aging of nonreplenishing cells, Strehler has pointed out that there is a loss of nucleolar organizing regions (NORs, or sites of rRNA gene transcription) that paralleled the measured loss of genes.[32] In other studies, the rRNA gene dosage remained constant for brain, liver, spleen, and kidney tissues throughout most of the adult life span of C57BL/6J mice, but showed a rather remarkable decrease in rRNA gene hybridization after 26 months of age — roughly 60% of the life span potential of this mouse strain.[201,202] Liver tissue was the lone exception in these experiments; rRNA genes were initially underrepresented, then the dosage was compensated for following maturity (see above). Although various mechanisms could account for these observations, age-dependent gene excision from the chromosomal DNA, mediated through intrastrand recombination between tandemly repeated genes, has received the most attention.[218,219] In contrast to this mechanism, the possibility has been raised that rRNA genes were not physically lost from the genome but, instead, some genes became inaccessible to hybridization probes after they were masked by protein or other crosslinks.[202] There is some experimental support for this latter view,[34,202,223] and the issue has not yet been resolved. Furthermore, it is now known that epigenetic mechanisms, i.e., gene methylation, might cause an age-related loss of NORs in rodent postmitotic cells by inactivating transcription.[224]

f.   Extrachromosomal DNAs

Another means of obtaining information about sequence stability is to monitor sequences in extrachromosomal circular DNAs (eccDNAs). All somatic cells investigated to date contain populations of eccDNA molecules of varying sizes and having many different types of chromosomal sequences which tend to be characteristic of a differentiated cell type.[213] However, the population of molecules can change in response to varying environmental conditions or during cellular differentiation.[213] The rationale for looking at eccDNAs as a biomarker for unstable chromosomal sequences, e.g., DNA rearrangements, is based on documented cases where eccDNA molecules were created by intrachromosomal recombination of repetitive elements[225] or by site-specific recombination of genes generating somatic cell diversity.[226] However, it should be mentioned that the mechanisms for eccDNA formation are uncertain concerning the creation of most of these molecules.[213]

An age-related increase in the abundance of eccDNAs has been observed in mouse and rat lymphocytes during *in vitro* and *in vivo* aging.[227,228] Similar observations have been made for human fibroblasts during serial culture and for human lymphocytes during aging.[228,229] Macieira-Coelho[229] has fit the production of eccDNAs into an overall model of chromatin reorganization that takes place during senescence of proliferating cells. For nondividing cells, analysis of eccDNAs in heart tissue from aging mice revealed similar amounts and size distributions of circular molecules at all ages, except that more discrete size classes and slightly larger circles were measured in senescent heart preparations.[230] Cloned repeats of murine B1, B2, L1, Intracisternal A-type particles (IAP), and major satellite sequence elements were used to look for age-related changes in eccDNAs from heart, brain, and liver tissues.[231] Together, these five repetitive sequence families make up about 15% of the mouse genome, and therefore should comprise sensitive probes for sequence variations. Hybridization experiments demonstrated that there were tissue-specific and age-related variations in repetitive sequences of mouse eccDNAs.[231] In cardiac tissue, satellite sequences decreased from 1 to 8 months of age but did not change thereafter, whereas the abundance of B1, B2, L1, and IAP sequences was the lowest in the oldest heart samples.[230] Alternatively, these repetitive sequences all decreased in brain and liver tissues during maturation but appeared to remain stable during older ages.[231]

Extrachromosomal circular DNAs are important intermediates in chromosomal gene amplification processes.[232,233] Although gene amplification is a common event involving oncogenes following somatic cell transformation,[234] and may occur during developmental stages of higher cells,[235] there are no data to suggest sequence amplification in the aging processes of postmitotic mammalian cells. Even eccDNAs, such as IAP elements, which can be intermediates in stable gene amplification do not appear to increase with age in postmitotic mouse cells.[213,214,230,231]

g. Low-Copy Sequences

There is little information available on the possibility of age-associated deletions, amplifications, and rearrangements or single-copy of low-copy DNA sequences. Ono et al.[236] studied DNA regions at, or flanking, nine cloned sequences that previously had been shown to undergo rearrangements or amplifications *in vivo* (usually through applying selective pressure). These regions encompassed the actin gene, dihydrofolate reductase gene, immunoglobulin μ constant gene, c-abl oncogene, c-ras oncogene, MMTV provirus, AKv provirus, and the VL30 retroviral-like sequences. No detectable age-related sequence changes were observed in these DNA regions for mouse liver, brain, and spleen tissues.[236] Of course, negative data do not mean that such changes do not take place — only that they were not detected by the methods used in the investigation. It seems that, in the absence of cell division, it would be highly unlikely that changes in low-copy DNA sequences will be uncovered by Southern hybridization or similar experiments. As another way to approach this same problem, newly developed PCR strategies might make age-related analyses of low-copy sequences a worthwhile endeavor.[237]

h. Gene Mutations

There are virtually no data on spontaneous point mutation frequencies in nondividing mammalian cells. Although mutations are likely to accumulate in the diploid genome of somatic mammalian cells, it has remained difficult to measure these "background" levels given the cellular and genomic complexities of a nondividing cell base in postmitotic tissues. What data are available are derived from somatic cells that can be stimulated to divide in culture. Mutations are measured indirectly through phenotypic changes in clonogenic assays wherein mutant cells are selected.

The most widely used method is the HPRT (hypoxanthine-guanine phosphoribosyl transferase) assay.[238] HPRT is an X-linked gene; so only one allele will be expressed in a somatic cell. An inactive HPRT allele will confer resistance to cells when grown in a medium containing 6-thioguanine. Slagboom and Vijg[49] and Vijg and Gossen[50] have recently reviewed results of mutational studies using the HPRT assay and other assays. Mutation frequencies at the HPRT loci are in the range 10^{-6} to 10^{-5}, depending on the cell type, and apparently increase with age.

With the plethora of modern molecular and cellular techniques now available,[239] there has been a renaissance in thinking about somatic mutations. Gossen and Vijg[240,241] have promoted transgenic mice as a model to study spontaneous and induced mutagenicity and somatic mutation rates. Gossen et al.[242] have created transgenic mouse strains carrying multiple copies of tandemly integrated lambda shuttle vectors, each with a copy of the bacterial lacZ gene as a target for mutagenesis. The transgene is retrieved from chromosomal DNA of different tissues, either untreated, or at various intervals following chemical mutagen treatment. The gene is rescued either by *in vitro* packaging in lambda heads or circularization of restriction fragments with subsequent transformation of competent bacterial cells.[50] Mutations are scored as colorless plaques or white colonies (mutants) when grown on X-gal, a chromogenic indicator that turns blue when metabolized by β-galactosidase (wild-type). Mutation frequencies are then determined as the ratio of mutants per total plaques or colonies.[240-243] At least three results have emerged from this work so far: (1) spontaneous mutation rates vary 10- to 100-fold among different transgenic mouse strains (presumably, mutation rates depend upon the chromosomal integration site),[243,244] (2) tissues with higher mitotic activities tend to have relatively higher spontaneous mutation frequencies,[50,211] and (3) in general (excluding one exception), mutation frequencies are about 10^{-5},[50,211,241-244] a value consistent with frequencies measured by the HPRT assay using primary cultures of proliferating cells. DNA sequencing of mutant lacZ genes has revealed a mutation spectrum coming out of the rodent somatic cell genomes. Transitions of the GC to AT type were the predominant point mutation detected.[244] These mutations tended to cluster at CpG dinucleotides, suggesting that deaminations of 5-methylcytosines were promutagenic lesions in the mutagenic process. Deletion mutations were a minor fraction of the total scored.[244] However, the bacteriophage lambda-shuttle vector system used in the analysis effectively selected against larger deletions.

The transgenic mouse model systems offer a truly remarkable new way to analyze the impact of aging on genomic stability, as well as environmental and nutritional modulations of intrinsic mutagenesis and DNA repair pathways. With animals carrying various combinations of transgenes and lacZ "mutagenes", one could now test some aspects of mutational theories of aging. To consider the possibilities, for instance, Orr and Sohal[245] recently reported that transgenic *Drosophila* carrying additional copies of the Zn/Cu superoxide dismutase and catalase genes showed an impressive increase in life span over parental strains. If these transgenic organisms had also been bearing the lacZ shuttle vector, it might have been possible to correlate longevity with spontaneous mutation rates of somatic cells *in vivo*. Alternatively, reciprocal experiments could be performed with mutagenes, in conjunction with knockout genetics,[246] to inactivate a component of the oxidation defense system or a DNA repair pathway. Thus, it might be feasible to determine the force of mortality in relation to somatic mutation frequencies. At the present time, mutation frequencies as a function of age have not yet been reported, but such data should be emerging soon and is eagerly awaited.

There are certain caveats associated with the transgenic model system. The small target size of the lacZ gene seems to be greatly influenced by the integration site.[243,244] The background type of changes measured may not apply to specialized types of sequences, i.e., repetitive elements, or be representative of total mutational events in *in vivo* aging. It would seem wise to separate postmitotic cells from replicating cells prior to marker rescue, so as to clarify the origin of the somatic mutations. Considering that the bulk of the DNA derived from the mouse tissues studied thus far represents mostly nonproliferating cells, the mutational spectra observed with rescued lacZ shuttle vectors may reflect, in part, *E. coli's* handling of promutagenic lesions incurred in the mouse tissue. The question of whether these mutations were fixed *in vivo* before the DNA was introduced into the bacterial cells is valid, since steady-state levels of different indigenous damages are present, may increase with aging, and can persist for long times (see Section II.B). Such damages, when presented to *E. coli*, could be processed by the bacterial repair enzymes systems, or lead directly to misincorporations via replication, e.g., O^6-methylguanine-induced GC to AT transitions.[68-72] Thus, the resultant mutational spectra is ambiguous. It might be possible to treat the rescued DNA with repair enzymes *in vitro* prior to transformation or transduction to remove a class of damage and compare mutation frequencies between treated and untreated samples. For example, DNA from EMU-treated mice could be assayed following incubation with O^6-alkylguanine alkyl-DNA transferase to remove alkyl groups adduced to exocyclic oxygens;[70-72] DNA ligase could be used to seal single-strand breaks before rescue, etc.

A different type of approach to study the role of somatic mutations in the aging process is to use nucleoside or base analogs in developing rodents.[247,248] The thymidine analog, 5-bromo-2'-deoxyuridine (BrdUrd), can be incorporated into replicating DNA and base pair normally with adenosine. Less frequently, the tautomeric enol form of BrdUrd can base pair with guanosine, giving rise to a transition mutation.[249] BrdUrd is not a known substrate for DNA repair and persists for long periods *in vivo*.[250] Model shuttle vector systems have shown a high degree of sequence specificity for BrdUrd-induced GC to AT transitions.[251] Anisimov and Osipova[247] and Craddock[248] have observed a dose-dependent reduction in the mean life span of neonatal rats treated with BrdUrd. BrdUrd administration led to substantial increases in the frequency of chromosomal aberrations and sister chromatid exchanges in dividing cells. The data could be interpreted as support for the somatic mutation theory of aging. However, the available evidence can not rule out the possible role of toxic, epigenetic, or metabolic effects in shortening the life span, and somatic mutation frequencies in postmitotic cells have not been assessed.[247,248]

C. Epigenetic Instability

1. DNA Methylation

In all vertebrates, a fraction of cytosine residues in DNA is methylated at the fifth carbon.[23-28] Methylation involves the enzymatic conversion of cytosine in DNA to 5-methylcytosine. This modification is carried out by DNA methyltransferases, using *S*-adenosylmethionine as a methyl donor.[54] The preferred substrate for DNA methylation in mammals is the dinucleotide CpG.[24,25] DNA methylation provides one mechanism for stably altering the local structure of a gene. The methyl group that is added projects into the major groove of DNA, and this strategic positioning can affect DNA protein interactions.[252] In fact, DNA methylation can stably repress transcription, perhaps by interfering with DNA binding proteins.[27,252] Methylation at the 5' end of genes in regions rich in CpG clusters (CpG islands) has been correlated with inhibition of gene expression.[24-27,252] Although there are exceptions to this general rule, an important determinant of repression is the density of methyl-CpGs near a promoter sequence.[24] Thus, covalent modification of mammalian DNA may confer some level of gene control to a cell.

In addition to transcriptional regulation, other roles have been proposed for DNA methylation. Several articles have evaluated alternative roles of DNA methylation in genomic imprinting,[253] chromosome inactivation,[254] chromosome condensation during mitosis,[26] and chromosomal stability.[255] One of the best characterized aspects of DNA methylation is in mutagenesis. More than one-third of all point mutations that are associated with human genetic diseases are transitions of CpG to TpG,[256,257] despite the relative rarity of CpG dinucleotides and the presence of a dedicated repair system to protect methylation status.[258] Mechanistically, spontaneous deamination of 5-methylcytosine in DNA will create deoxythymidine, which will base pair with deoxyadenosine during DNA synthesis to yield the transition mutation described above.[23,28] Therefore, there is good reason to think that CpG sequences will be hot spots for mutagenesis; and the frequency of events, i.e., deaminations, is time-dependent and will increase with age.

In general, the inheritance of methylation patterns is stable and reproducibly transferred from generation to generation at each cell division. This may be achieved by a maintenance methylase which conserves the methylation pattern after replication following the action of a *de novo* methylase which initiates a new pattern of methylation.[253,259] Specific methyl-acceptor sites have been found to be modulated during differentiation of the organism in a programmed manner such that transcriptionally active genes are undermethylated in tissues in which they are expressed.[27, 260] These observations are consistent with a model in which discrete changes in methylation patterns dictate the characteristics of differentiated cells. In fact, recent work with transgenic mice have shown that DNA methylation is essential to normal murine development.[261] It has been suggested that if DNA methylation exemplifies a developmental program, then demethylation during senescence represents a loss of that program, and as such is a dedifferentiation process.[26,262] Cutler[262] has called this process dysdifferentiation. One of the signal ideas of dysdifferentiation is that genetic regulation will break down in old cells and, as an indicator of deregulation, cells start to express proteins and other markers that are not tissue specific. Evidence for the dysdifferentiation theory of aging has been brought together by Cutler.[262]

Studies on mammalian DNA methylation have revealed that total genomic 5-methylcytosine levels change with age. Most organisms exhibit a global loss of 5-methyldeoxycytidine as a function of age *in vivo* and *in vitro*. When normal diploid fibroblasts from mice, hamsters, and humans were grown in culture, the 5-methylcytosine content of their genomes markedly decreased.[263] The greatest rate of loss was observed with the mouse cells which survived the least number of divisions. On the other hand, immortal mouse cell lines had more stable levels of methylation.[263] Replicating human cells apparently lose methyl groups from DNA *in vivo*, too.[264-266]

Wilson et al.[266] have presented data that showed significant age-dependent losses of 5-methyldeoxycytidine residues from DNAs of C57BL/6J mouse brain, liver, and small intestine mucosa tissues and from DNAs of *Peromyscus leucopus* (white-footed mice) liver and small intestine tissues. Similar losses in genomic 5-methyldeoxycytidine were also shown to correlate with donor age of cultured normal human bronchial epithelial cells.[266] Methylation levels in these experiments were quantified by ^{32}P-postlabeling techniques. The most important finding to come out of this work is that the rate of 5-methyldeoxycytidine loss from nuclear DNA appeared to be inversely proportional to maximum life span for three different mammalian species.[266] The results suggested that the age-related reductions in 5-methyldeoxycytidine were not connected to mitotic activity *in vivo* since three different tissues, ranging from nondividing to actively dividing tissues, exhibited similar rates of loss.[266] Analytical HPLC methods used by Singhal et al.[267] also found a gradual decline in mouse liver DNA 5-methyldeoxycytidine content up to 24 months of age. No further decrease in methylated residues occurred after 24 months and the data, in fact, indicated an increase after that age. This latter result is puzzling because C57BL/6J male mice from the same colony were used in both Wilson et al.[266] and Singhal et al.[267] studies, which suggests that these discordant results might stem from different experimental methods. A possible late onset of increased deoxycytidine methylation is in agreement with an age-related increase in chromosome-specific methylation of rRNA gene clusters in mouse tissues.[224]

Negative data have also been reported. Excluding studies before 1980, when less sensitive methods of analysis were used to investigate DNA methylation, several groups have found either no change or rather insignificant differences in DNA methylation as a function of age. No significant differences in total 5-methyldeoxycytidine levels were detected during aging of human liver,[268] rat liver,[269] or mouse brain tissues.[270] There are many reasons why various studies do not reach the same conclusions. To point out just one complicating factor, 5-methyldeoxycytidine levels can be modulated by diet or compounds that affect methylation metabolism.[271-273] (Cooney[54] has recently reviewed the interplay of methylation metabolism and senescence on DNA methylation.) Even considering the negative results, there is still a clear consensus in favor of an age-related genomic decrease in 5-methyldeoxycytidine content.

Sequence-specific methylation sites have been examined by comparing DNA fragment sizes generated by isoschizomer restriction enzymes. The most commonly used pair of restriction enzymes have been HpaII (methylation-sensitive) and MspI (methylation-resistant) which both recognize the same sequence — CCGG. MspI cleaves whether or not CCGG is methylated at the internal C, whereas HpaII cleaves only unmethylated CCGG. Following enzyme digestion and Southern hybridization to the probe of interest, methylation sites can be deduced by comparing band patterns between the two DNA digests. Studies have shown decreased DNA methylation of L1Md and IAP repetitive sequence families with aging in one or more mouse organs.[274,275] Endogenous murine retroviral genomes also become hypomethylated during aging.[276] Satellite sequences that are normally highly methylated in postmitotic tissues become undermethylated in senescent organisms.[277]

Methyl groups can be lost from DNA by both active and passive systems, such as demethylases and spontaneous glycolytic release of 5-methyldeoxycytosine, respectively.[259] If repair of these lesions is incomplete, then genomic loss of methylated residues will ensue. Part of the genomic methylation losses might be explained by some type of selective deletion of highly repetitive DNA sequences which are hypermethylated. HPLC analysis of mouse satellite DNA, however, showed that the mole percent fraction of 5-methyldeoxycytidine decreased in satellite DNA to the same extent as main band (nonsatellite) DNA, which demonstrated that selective loss of this highly repetitive sequence could not be responsible for decreased DNA methylation in senescent tissues.[277] Therefore, DNA methylation levels associated with various repetitive sequence families seem to correlate well with total genomic levels and decline with age.

In contrast to genome-wide demethylation during aging, studies of individual genes have indicated no general pattern of methylation changes with age.[49] For the most part, methylation patterns are generally well maintained in stably differentiated cell *in vivo*.[49,278] *In vitro* methylation patterns on single-copy sequences of normal human diploid fibroblasts, however, do show variability between and within subclones of such fibroblasts as a function of population doublings.[279-281] Mice carrying an X-autosomal translocation have been used to study age-related reactivation of X-linked genes *in vivo*.[282] Histochemical analysis has demonstrated a progressive age-related reactivation of the ornithine carbamoyl transferase locus on the inactive normal X chromosome, presumably due to changes in DNA methylation.[282] Other data[283] indicate that an age-related reactivation of genes may not be a feature of all X-linked loci, continuing the trend of mixed results from individual gene methylation studies.

As part of the aging process, random loss of methyl groups in DNA may lead to aberrant epigenetic changes in gene expression and perhaps affect chromosomal stability. For genes that do exhibit age-related changes in methylation status, there have been no consistent correlations with changes in gene expression.[49,54] One caveat to correlations between site-specific methylation and gene expression is the uncertainty of whether some sites exert a stronger influence on transcriptional regulation than others.[24-27] Therefore, until good correlations are in hand, the argument that transcriptional control is diminished with aging due to aberrant DNA methylation is rather weak.

2. Chromatin

Mechanisms of genomic instability that may be involved in intrinsic aging processes of somatic cells extend into interphase chromatin — the nucleoprotein complex inside the cell nucleus. This complex contains RNAs, histone, and nonhistone proteins and DNA molecules in various ratios. The biochemical composition of chromatin varies from cell type to cell type, changes during development and aging, fluctuates with biorhythms, and is modulated by diet, temperature, etc.[284] It is not the intention here to comment on the multitude of chromatin changes that mammalian postmitotic tissues display during aging, but to discuss two topics that seem propitious regarding epigenetic aging processes, i.e., the nuclear matrix and poly(ADP)ribosylation of nuclear proteins.

a. Nuclear Matrix

The nuclear matrix is an insoluble skeletal framework of the nucleus which directs the functional organization of DNA into domains and furnishes sites for genetic regulation and nucleic acid metabolism.[285-287] It is composed of the nuclear lamina and interior nuclear proteins that resist digestion with nucleases, extraction with detergents, and extraction with high salts. Age-related alterations in the nuclear matrix could affect not only the structure of the nucleus, but also DNA replication/repair and RNA synthesis and processing.[285-287] Relatively few studies have examined the effects of aging on the nuclear matrix. For dividing cells, Macieira-Coelho[229] has made measurements of chromatin structures throughout the proliferative life span of human fibroblasts. A number of architectural and morphological changes occurred as a function of population doubling levels. One of the more prominent chromatin alterations was in the spacing and density of the 30-nm fiber. Results showed that the 30-nm fiber underwent a decondensation during *in vitro* aging. Macieira-Coelho[229] proposed that age-related reorganization of chromatin was accompanied by, and perhaps arose from, changes in the nuclear matrix. Pienta et al.[288] attempted to study nuclear matrix alterations in early-passage, primary cultures of human skin fibroblasts from donors of different ages. Their results showed that the nucleus increased in size and became more rounded with age, consistent with expectations of chromatin decondensation. Although there appeared to be some quantitative changes in nuclear matrix proteins of senescent fibroblasts, the qualitative pattern of these proteins did not change in a major way.[288]

One of the earliest studies to look at chromatin reorganization in postmitotic cells as a function of age is also one of the most informative. Murty et al.[289] examined the transcriptional activity and matrix association of $\alpha_{2\mu}$-globulin genes in the rat liver during maturation and aging. Synthesis of $\alpha_{2\mu}$-globulin in the male rat begins at puberty and ceases at about 800 days of age. Age-dependent changes in protein synthesis correlated directly with the rates of transcription of the $\alpha_{2\mu}$-globulin family and the levels of hepatic mRNA.[289] Transcriptional activation and deactivation were linked to an association and dissociation of this gene domain with the nuclear matrix, suggesting a regulatory role for the nuclear matrix in $\alpha_{2\mu}$-globulin gene expression. Therefore, transcriptional cessation during senescence was associated with the release of this gene from the nuclear matrix.[289] What determines gene-specific connections with the nuclear matrix is not clear, but it seems that this area is fertile ground for future inquiries. In contrast to gene-specific studies, no significant differences in the organization of bulk chromatin or its association with the nuclear matrix was ascertained in aging cerebellar neurons of Fischer 344 rats.[290] This latter result probably underscores the need to perform more sequence-specific experiments.

b. Poly(ADP-Ribosyl)ation

DNA damaging agents may participate in epigenetic mechanisms that alter chromatin structure, gene expression, and DNA metabolism, e.g., recombination. An example of epigenetic effects resulting from DNA damage is poly(ADP-ribosyl)ation of chromosomal proteins. Poly(ADP-ribose)polymerase is a nuclear enzyme that is activated by single- and double-strand breaks in DNA.[291] The activated polymerase synthesizes ADP-ribose homopolymers covalently anchored to nuclear proteins. The physiological role(s) of poly(ADP-ribose)polymerase are unknown, which has led to wide speculation about its possible function. However, it seems clear that extensive DNA damage can cause cell death via poly(ADP-ribose)polymerase- mediated activity.[291,292] The enzyme utilizes NAD$^+$ as a substrate, and excessive poly(ADP-ribosyl)ation can deplete the intracellular stores of NAD$^+$ (and ATP), thereby contributing to the suicide of damaged cells.[291,292] Since this phenomenon could be interpreted as programmed cell death, it is natural to think of poly(ADP)ribosylation of proteins as a factor in aging processes. Recent results[293] indicate that the unmodified polymerase binds tightly to DNA strand breaks, then covalently modifies itself; auto-poly(ADP-ribosyl)ation of the protein leads to its release, presumably to allow entry of DNA ligase or other DNA repair enzymes into the site. This proposed model of action could have the benefit of holding strand breaks in place for repair enzymes, and thus prevent double-strand breaks from moving apart. An alternative scenario related to this model is that during senescence, the polymerase loses its ability to auto-poly(ADP-ribosyl)ate itself, thereby blocking repair of the lesion. This latter scenario might explain, in part, why single-strand breaks accumulate with age.

To put this cellular activity into perspective with other aging phenomena, nucleotide modifications and DNA strand breaks increase with age for some cell types (see Section II.B); postmitotic cell death *in vivo* is a well-characterized occurrence for some senescent mammalian tissues (Sections I.A and I.B, above); functional decrements during aging could be tied to the loss of cells with time. Therefore, this posttranslational protein modification mechanistically potentially ties together various aging changes from the molecular level to the organismal level. Monti et al.[294] have summarized results in favor of the hypothesis that poly(ADP-ribose)polymerase is involved in senescence. These results include the finding that poly(ADP-ribose)polymerase activity in mononuclear leukocytes of 13 different mammalian species correlates strongly with a species-specific life span.[295] Furthermore, inhibitors of poly(ADP-ribose)polymerase exert a protective effect on cell death induced by oxidative stress.[296] The majority of studies done to date, however, have focused on replicating cells where alterations in enzyme activities appear to remain stable or decline modestly during aging *in vitro* and *in vivo*.[295] How, or even if, these activities change in fixed postmitotic cells as a function of age is not known.

III. MITOCHONDRIAL GENOMIC INSTABILITY

Mammalian mitochondrial DNA (mtDNA) is a closed circular molecule of less than 20 kb. Just about all the genome codes for functional products, in part because mitochondrial genes lack introns.[297] The human mitochondrial genome carries the information for 13 mRNAs encoding various subunits of respiratory enzymes, an incomplete set of 22 tRNAs, one copy each of 12S and 16S rRNAs, and an origin of replication.[298] Other respiratory enzyme subunits and enzymes involved in the flow and maintenance of mitochondrial genetic information are encoded in the nuclear compartment.[299] Its small size makes the mitochondrial genome more amenable than the nuclear genome to probe for mutations at the sequence level. Each mitochondrion contains several copies of mtDNA, and individual cells have a thousand or more apparently identical mtDNA molecules.[300] Since these molecules are replicating in dividing and nondividing cells, the possibility exists that mutant genomes might be lost in the process, but mitochondrial myopathies in humans show that some mtDNA mutations can be inherited in somatic cells.[301] Fleming et al.[42,43] proposed that damage accumulation in mtDNA might be a mechanism for aging of postmitotic cells. In lower eukaryotes there is some precedent for this hypothesis. Indeed, the paradigm for mtDNA-dependent senescence can be found in the fungus *Podospora*. DNA sequences called sen-DNAs are excised from the mitochondrial genome and become selectively amplified.[302] These sequences then become integrated into the nuclear genome and mtDNA, causing mutations and cell death. Aging of mammalian cells could conceivably occur by similar mechanisms if analogous processes emanate from their mitochondrial compartments.[303,304]

It would seem reasonable to think that mtDNA is particularly at risk to damage by oxygen free radicals, malonaldehyde, and liperoxides generated during respiration.[305] Data agree with reason in that mature rat liver mtDNA contained 16 times more 8-hydroxydeoxyguanosine (an oxidized nucleoside residue of DNA) than nuclear DNA.[134] Studies have also demonstrated that mtDNA is more vulnerable than nuclear DNA to exogenous mutagens and carcinogens,[305,306] perhaps because mtDNA is not protected by the binding of histone proteins. Less efficient or limited DNA repair capabilities,[307] in conjunction with an apparently high error rate of DNA polymerase γ,[308] help fuel the perception that mtDNA has a high mutation rate. Recent results[301] confirm that mtDNA damage and mutations accumulate with age, and thus have reinforced the notion that aging results from genetic instability.

Electron microscopy studies by Piko and colleagues[309-311] showed senescent nondividing rodent cells exhibited higher levels of complex structural forms of mtDNA. The frequency of double-length circles increased with aging, and evidence was presented for an increased frequency of deletions and insertions in senescent mtDNA from rats and mice. The alkyl adduct 7-methylguanine appeared to accumulate in rat liver mtDNA with age,[126]and I-compounds also increased in mtDNA during maturation.[312] It would be of interest to know if I-compounds continue to increase later in life.

Sequence-specific deletions of mtDNA are present at high levels in skeletal muscle and other tissues of patients with the neuromuscular diseases, Kearns-Sayre syndrome, and progressive external ophthalmoplegia.[301] Using PCR strategies, a specific mtDNA deletion was detected in heart muscle and brain tissue of older humans.[313] This deletion was not found in fetal brain or heart cells. Subsequently, it was demonstrated that myocardial mtDNA contained a population of molecules with a 7,436-base-pair deletion that was present in senescent human subjects.[314] The number of genomes with this deletion increased exponentially with age and was estimated to be 3 and 9% of total mtDNA in 80-year-old and 90-year-old subjects, respectively.[314] The deleted sequences encode 7 subunits of the ATP generation system and were bordered by 12 base pair direct repeats. An age-associated exponential accumulation of 8-hydroxydeoxyguanosine in mtDNA of human diaphragms has been observed to correlate with multiple mtDNA deletions in this muscle[315] and with a 7.4-kb mtDNA deletion in human hearts during aging.[316] Even larger deletions have been observed in a few late-onset human diseases of unknown etiology.[317]

In humans, the most commonly detected mtDNA deletion is a segment of 4,977 base pairs flanked by 13 base pair direct repeats, and considerable effort has been expended to show that these deletions were not artifacts related to PCR methodology.[318] This deletion is associated with a number of different age-related pathologies and becomes more abundant in senescent brain, liver, and muscle tissues.[301, 317-320] Some studies have indicated that fixed postmitotics, such as brain and muscles, have much higher deletion frequencies than renewing tissues (e.g., skin) or partially renewing tissues (e.g., spleen and liver),[318] and the age-related onset frequency for PCR detection appears to be about age 35 in humans.[318,320]

Aging cells can carry mixtures of mutants and wild-type mtDNAs (known as heteroplasmy), but homoplasmic mutations are also known for humans, as are point mutations.[301] Myoclonic epilepsy and ragged-red fiber disease result from a heteroplasmic mtDNA point mutation in a tRNA gene.[317] Respiratory deficiencies are associated with defects in mitochondrial protein synthesis. It has been recognized that deletion mutations, such as those described above, might have a replicative advantage due to their smaller size, and thus become selectively amplified over normal-length mtDNA as a function of age. A similar age-dependent selection process would not be anticipated for mtDNA point mutations. Nonetheless, various point mutation in tRNA genes of mtDNA appear to be more frequent with age in some human muscle tissues.[321] These tRNA sequence changes may represent hot spots for mutations in the mitochondrial genome.

The mechanisms by which these deletions arise remain obscure, but it seems that short direct DNA repeats are involved. Homologous intramolecular recombination or replication bypass of DNA single-strand loops, formed by slippage and intrastrand base pairing of the repeat sequences, are two mechanisms that could account for direct repeat-associated mtDNA deletions. However, there is no direct evidence that recombination enzymes are present in mammalian mitochondria, which leaves the slippage mechanism as a prime candidate. It has been argued by some that DNA damage plays a role in generating mtDNA deletions, perhaps by inducing alterations in DNA structure.[315,316] The age correlates between oxidative adducts and deletions in mtDNA are consistent with this idea. In addition, chronic cardiac ischemia has been associated with an immense increase in the 4,977-base-pair deletion.[322]

How are these mtDNA mutations linked to aging and what do they mean for the bioenergy of the cell? One of the potential outcomes associated with an age-related accumulation of mtDNA damage and mutations is a reduction in oxidative phosphorylation. Oxidative phosphorylation does indeed decrease during the aging of many mammalian postmitotic tissues, and the data have recently been summarized by Wallace.[301,317] Mitochondrial respiratory activities, protein synthesis, and RNA synthesis appear to decline substantially with age in nondividing tissues of rodents and humans.[323-326] Alterations in cristae structure are observed more frequently in older postmitotic cells.[326] DNA damage and mtDNA mutations might lead to a loss of normal oxidative metabolism on the one hand, and an increase of cytotoxic oxygen species on the other hand. There is indirect evidence to support this idea. Mitochondria from the hearts of old rats released 30% more H_2O_2 and O_2^- than those isolated from young rats.[327] This effect was also apparent in senescent rat brain tissue.

The threshold level to produce a physiological deficit is currently not known, but clearly mitochondrial mutations can exist at low levels in apparently normal human tissues. The fraction of mtDNA mutants in senescent tissues, described above, is quite a bit lower than the proportion of deleted mtDNA seen in skeletal muscle of patients with Kearns-Sayre syndrome or progressive external ophthalmoplegia, where ranges from 20 to 90% have been reported.[301,313,317,319] Only a single type of deletion was measured as a function of age in most studies, however. If all mutation and damages were tallied, then the total might be quite significant. Furthermore, it is not known if these mutations are randomly distributed among all the cells of a tissue or if some cells in a tissue have a much higher frequency of mutations.[325] Therefore, the data to date suggest that mitochondrial genomic instability is a major factor in aging, and this instability may cause functional deficits in nonrenewing tissues, e.g., brain and heart, that have high energy demands and oxygen consumption.

IV. CONCLUSIONS

This review has focused on **what** happens to the genetic information of mammalian cells during their life span, not on **why** various genetic entities change during aging. In the Introduction, various sources for genetic alterations were briefly mentioned. The sources of genetic damage have been reviewed many times[2,3,44,45,55-64] and have changed little over the years because there seems to be general agreement on what sorts of things affect DNA stability, although there is not necessarily agreement on the relative importance of individual sources. The types of instability that can be found in the genome have been fairly well documented, but again, the relative significance of different types of lesions or mutations is in dispute. It was also stated that the working premise behind genomic instability was that pernicious DNA damage and mutations are continuously introduced into the genomes of all cells and eventually, over time, there is a losing battle to maintain the original cellular information. This leads to an age-related increase in damage and mutations. Why the battle is lost is not known, but it is sure to be as complex in its roots as it is in its manifestations. Obviously, DNA repair and other cellular repair and defense mechanisms play a crucial role in fighting the battle,[67-72] but it is not at all clear how DNA repair functions during aging of postmitotic cells. To gain a better understanding of the influence of aging on the ability of a nondividing cell to maintain differentiated function for many years, it is important to consider gene-specific damage and expression. In mammalian cells, DNA repair exhibits intragenomic heterogeneity — with some DNA sequences being repaired more efficiently than others.[19-21] In some cases, preferential repair is strand specific.[331] Studies have shown that gene-specific repair provides the most useful information regarding the functional consequences of unrepaired DNA damage for a cell.[21,328-331] Sequence-specific repair studies on working genes in senescent postmitotic cells is one approach that may lead to a better understanding of the fundamental mechanisms of aging. Future studies should also try to correlate individual gene damage levels (and damage repair) with gene expression levels and gene regulation.

One of the original goals of this chapter was to ask whether the data show clear patterns. Therefore, the different sections of the review will be summarized to determine if they conform to a pattern or trend, and some experimental options that might shed additional light on a subject or consolidate the existing data will be proposed.

Chromosomal instability. Chromosomal instability is clearly an aging index for dividing and nondividing cells. Comparing young and old animals, frequencies of aberrations are higher in normally nonproliferating cells than in proliferating cells.[86-93] Liver cells appear to be a paradigm for nondividing cells. The spontaneous frequency of chromosomal aberration of a normally nonreplicating hepatocyte increases as a function of chronological age.[81-87] The results show that lesions accumulate at a fairly constant rate, which is characteristic for a species. The rate of development of chromosomal abnormalities is inversely proportional to an animal's life span for several mammalian species, suggesting a close relationship to basic aging processes. There are numerous studies that show induction of chromosome aberrations per se do not mimic natural senescence, which is difficult to reconcile with the spontaneous aberration results.[4,14,15] Whereas additional experiments comparing more species and more cell types would be interesting, it is doubtful that any additional mechanistic insight would be gained. Experiments using fluorescent-*in-situ*-hybridization with chromosome- or gene-specific probes to obtain sequence-related information on chromosome aberrations might help in revealing the relevance of these events. Furthermore, an attempt should be made to correlate chromosomal aberrations with histological evidence of cell death or mutations.

Genetic instability. When sensitive methods have been used, studies have demonstrated that a variety of modified bases and DNA adducts increase during aging on nondividing tissues *in vivo*. The observations are most apparent for liver, kidney, and muscle tissue in which alkyl adducts, oxygen additions, and strand breaks increased during aging[124,126-128,135] (see also Table 2). Base cross-linkages have also been reported for mammalian liver tissue.[150] Therefore, there is a pattern for liver, brain, and kidney tissues. This pattern suggests that other related lesions will also be found to accumulate in the genome of these tissues with age. The results have been less obvious in the brain. An analysis of the data indicates that brain DNA is more resistant to damage accumulation than these other three tissues. It should also be emphasized that the levels of measured damages are not trivial. For a more quantitative treatment of the subject, the reader can consult Mullaart et al.[44]

One question, that may be rhetorical, pertains to whether damages accumulate with age or whether their steady-state levels change with age. Mechanistically, there is a distinction between the two alternatives. If damages accumulate, it might signify that repair enzymes can not get in contact with the lesions for a variety of reasons, including biochemical and structural changes to chromatin. If steady-state levels increase as a function of age, the implications might differ. Either a decline in damage processing efficiency or an increase in damage induction would be sufficient to cause an increase in steady-state amounts of damage. For a lesion to accumulate with time, it must be stable. DNA strand breaks are stable, and therefore, may accrue with age. On the other hand, 7-methylguanine, and 8-hydroxydeoxyguanosine are relatively unstable. It seems logical to think that these base damages increased as a function of age because of steady-state changes, but there are no definitive experiments to show what changes with age other than the measured levels, and future experiments should seek to address this question. In discussing the repair of intrinsic DNA lesions, Lindahl[332] has argued that some chemically stable base modifications, such as xanthine, and 1-methyladenine, should indeed accumulate as a function of age. Powerful methods, such as ^{32}P-postlabeling, monoclonal antibodies, and chromatography coupled with electrochemical or mass spectrometry detection, could be employed to determine if these damages increase in senescent nondividing cells, as predicted.

A rationale was given in the Introduction that contended single-strand DNA breaks are among the most abundant and informative lesions in the genome, and that the biological effects of unrepaired breaks are probably more severe than most other, but not all, lesions. There have been more studies examining DNA strand breaks during aging of cells than any others. It is therefore rather astounding that no age-related studies have investigated DNA ligase activity in senescent, nondividing cells. Experiments have examined strand rejoining *in vivo* following DNA damage induction, but an actual examination of the complexities and activities of the ligases themselves has not been carried out. Furthermore, the effects of age on the interplay of DNA ligases and poly(ADP-ribose)polymerase,[293] which binds strand breaks, is an intriguing but unstudied problem.

The comprehensive data do not firmly support mutations, sequence rearrangements, deletions, or amplifications occurring in the nuclear genome to any appreciable extent in aging postmitotic cells. Sequence changes probably do take place in senescent cells, but in the absence of replication they are unique for the cells that harbor them and are therefore quantitatively insignificant in a tissue. However, there is hope on the horizon for measuring somatic mutations due to the advent of transgenic mice and other model systems. The use of the transgenic mouse strains, developed by Vijg and associates[240-244] to test some aspects of somatic mutation theories of aging, has already been discussed and will not be repeated here. This is also true for methods devised to analyze genomic instability of hypervariable minisatellite sequences.[204-212] Lastly, there are PCR-based strategies that might bring positive results to studies of sequence rearrangement, deletions, and point mutations in nondividing cells.[237]

Epigenetic instability. The consensus of the evidence points to an age-related decline in total genomic methylation in postmitotic mammalian cells. Whether or not a positive correlation exists between decreased methylation and aberrant gene regulation has not been established. Future experiments to accelerate or decelerate genomic demethylation may be fruitful. Cooney[54] has discussed various strategies for manipulating DNA methylation that may affect longevity. Methylase mutants, if they are viable, seem to be a valid approach to study cause and effect.[261] Other gaps in our knowledge are data on maintenance transmethylases and other methylation-related enzymes during aging. Do the activities or specificities of these enzymes change with age? The data on nuclear matrix and poly(ADP-ribosyl)ation are too meager to define any pattern or trend. More analyses of gene-specific nuclear matrix associations need to be carried out, and experiments that describe activities of poly(ADP-ribose)polymerase as a function of age have yet to be done in postmitotic cells.

Mitochondrial genomic instability. The data supporting the view that mitochondrial genomic instability is the primary reason postmitotic cells age seems to be strong,[301] and future experiments should be promising. Base damages, point mutations, and various deletions of mtDNA increased in senescent tissues.[311-321] The aging changes in mtDNA appear to be more conspicuous in fixed postmitotic cells, such as cardiac and neural tissues. The levels of measured *single* lesions might appear to be insufficient to account for major functional decrements, given the genomic and cellular redundancies of mammalian cells, but the totality of all lesions combined may be more than sufficient to cause cellular senescence. Thus, there needs to be an adding up of all the damages and mutations. Concerning informational gaps, we clearly need to know more about mtDNA repair enzymes and systems. The distribution of mtDNA deletions, etc., among different cell types in aging tissues is of importance. Clearer correlation between mitochondrial function and mitochondrial genomic instability are of more importance, but experimentally may be difficult to show due to heteroplasmy. Although not yet attempted, creation of recombinant mtDNA genomes, and mitochondrial genome replacement experiments seem to be exciting future possibilities.

Summary. The experimental results do not show that genomic instability causes senescence of somatic cells. What we have are numerous descriptions and correlations. Examples of instability at the chromosomal level, at the epigenetic level, and at the mitochondrial genome level correlate with life span and more generally with the decreasing functions of aging, nondividing cells. These genome-based changes might be the causes of various physiological decrements characteristic of aging mammals, but there is no proof of this at the present time. However, there is reason to be optimistic that more mechanistic experiments will be forthcoming soon. With the use of transgenic animals, and techniques to inactivate individual genes in the germ cells, the roles of various components of the aging process (or anti-aging mechanisms) can be dissected.

REFERENCES

1. Hayflick, L., Theories of biological aging, *Exp. Gerontol.*, 20, 145, 1985.
2. Burnet, F. M., *Intrinsic Mutagenesis: A Genetic Approach to Aging*, John Wiley & Sons, New York, 1974.
3. Burnet, F. M., *Immunology, Aging and Cancer*, W. H. Freeman, San Francisco, 1976, 94.
4. Casarett, G. W., Similarities and contrasts between radiation and time pathology, *Adv. Gerontol. Res.*, 1, 109, 1964.
5. Failla, G., The aging process and carcinogenesis, *Ann. N.Y. Acad. Sci.*, 71, 1124, 1958.
6. Szilard, L., On the nature of the aging process, *Proc. Natl. Acad. Sci. U.S.A.*, 45, 30, 1959.
7. Maynard Smith, J., Review lectures on senescence. I. The causes of ageing, *Proc. R. Soc. London Ser. B*, 157, 115, 1962.
8. Kirkwood, T. B. L., Evolution and ageing, *Nature*, 270, 301, 1977.
9. Kirkwood, T. B. L., Comparative and evolutionary aspects of longevity, in *Handbook of the Biology of Aging*, 2nd ed., Finch, C. E. and Schneider, E. L., Eds., Van Nostrand Reinhold, New York, 1985, 27.
10. Kirkwood, T. B. L., DNA, mutations and aging, *Mutat. Res.*, 219, 1, 1989.
11. Kirkwood, T. B. L. and Holliday, R., Ageing as a consequence of natural selection, in *The Biology of Human Ageing*, Collins, K. J. and Bittles, A. H., Eds., Cambridge University Press, Cambridge, 1986, 1.
12. Curtis, H. J., Biological mechanisms underlying the aging process, *Science*, 141, 686, 1963.
13. Curtis, H. J., Genetic factors in aging, *Adv. Genet.*, 16, 305, 1971.
14. Walburg, H. E., Jr., Radiation-induced life shortening and premature aging, *Adv. Radiat. Biol.*, 5, 145, 1975.
15. Alexander, P., The role of DNA lesions in processes leading to aging in mice, *Symp. Soc. Exp. Biol.*, 21, 29, 1967.
16. Gensler, H. L. and Bernstein, H., DNA damage as the primary cause of aging, *Q. Rev. Biol.*, 56, 279, 1981.
17. Bernstein, H. and Gensler, H. L., DNA damage and aging, in *Free Radicals in Aging*, Yu, B. P., Ed., CRC Press, Boca Raton, FL, 1993, 89.
18. Yielding, E. L., A model for aging based on differential repair of somatic mutational damage, *Perspect. Biol. Med.*, 17, 201, 1974.
19. Bohr, V. A., Okumoto, D. S., and Hanawalt, P. C., Survival of UV-irradiated mammalian cells correlates with efficient DNA repair in an essential gene, *Proc. Natl. Acad. Sci. U.S.A.*, 83, 3830, 1986.

20. Smith, C. A. and Mellon, I., Clues to the organization of DNA repair systems gained from studies of intragenomic repair heterogeneity, *Adv. Mutagen Res.*, 1, 153, 1990.

21. Bohr, V. A., Gene specific DNA repair, *Carcinogenesis*, 12, 1983, 1991.

22. Orgel, L., The maintenance of accuracy of protein synthesis and its relevance to aging, *Proc. Natl. Acad. Sci. U.S.A.*, 49, 517, 1963.

23. Holliday, R., The significance of DNA methylation in cellular aging, in *The Molecular Biology of Aging: Basic Life Sciences*, Vol. 35, Woodhead, A. D., Blackett, A. D., and Hollaender, A., Eds., Plenum Press, New York, 1984, 269.

24. Antequera, F. and Bird, A., CpG islands in *DNA Methylation: Molecular Biology and Biological Significance*, Jost, J. P. and Saluz, H. P., Eds., Birkhauser Verlag, Basel, 1993, 169.

25. Bird, A., The essentials of DNA methylation, *Cell*, 70, 5, 1992.

26. Mays-Hoopes, L. L., Age-related changes in DNA methylation. Do they represent continued developmental changes?, *Intl. Rev. Cytol.*, 114, 181, 1989.

27. Cedar, H., DNA methylation and gene activity, *Cell*, 53, 3, 1988.

28. Holliday, R., The inheritance of epigenetic defects, *Science*, 238, 163, 1987.

29. Harman, D., Role of free radicals in mutation, cancer, aging, and the maintenance of life, *Radiat. Res.*, 16, 753, 1962.

30. Harman, D., The aging process, *Proc. Natl. Acad. Sci. U.S.A.*, 78, 7124, 1981.

31. Murray, V., Are transposons a cause of ageing?, *Mutat. Res.*, 237, 59, 1990.

32. Strehler, B. L., Genetic instability as the primary cause of human aging, *Exp. Gerontol.*, 21, 283, 1986.

33. Olovnikov, A. M., A theory of marginotomy, *J. Theor. Biol.*, 41, 181, 1973.

34. Cutler, R. G., Cross-linking hypothesis of aging: DNA adducts in chromatin as a primary aging process, in *Aging, Carcinogenesis and Radiation Biology, The Role of Nucleic Acid Addition Reactions*, Smith, K. C., Ed., Plenum Press, New York, 1976, 443.

35. Cutler, R. G., Nature of aging and life maintenance processes, *Interdiscipl. Topics Gerontol.*, 9, 83, 1976.

36. Cutler, R. G., Redundancy of information content in the genome of mammalian species as a protective mechanism determining aging rate, *Mech. Ageing Dev.*, 2, 381, 1973.

37. Linn, S., Kairis, M., and Holliday, R., Decreased fidelity of DNA polymerase activity isolated from aging human fibroblasts, *Proc. Natl. Acad. Sci. U.S.A.*, 73, 2818, 1976.

38. Srivastava, V. K. and Bushee, D. L., Decreased fidelity of DNA polymerases and decreased excision repair in aging mice: effects of caloric restriction, *Biochem. Biophys. Res. Commun.*, 182, 712, 1992.

39. Hart, R. W. and Setlow, R. B., Correlation between deoxyribonucleic acid excision-repair and life-span in a number of mammalian species, *Proc. Natl. Acad. Sci. U.S.A.*, 71, 2169, 1974.

40. Hart, R. W., D'Ambrosio, S. M, Ng, N. K., and Modak, S. P., Longevity, stability and DNA repair, *Mech. Ageing Dev.*, 9, 203, 1979.

41. Cutler, R. G., Antioxidants, aging, and longevity, in *Free Radicals in Biology*, Vol. VI, Pryor, W. A., Ed., Academic Press, New York, 1984, 371.

42. Fleming, J. E., Miquel, J., Cottrell, S. F., Yengoyan, L. S., and Economos, A. C., Is cell aging caused by respiration-dependent injury to the mitochondrial genome?, *Gerontology*, 28, 44, 1982.

43. Miquel, J. and Fleming, J. E., A two-step hypothesis on the mechanisms of in vitro aging: cell differentiation followed by intrinsic mitochondrial mutagenesis, *Exp. Gerontol.*, 19, 31, 1984.

44. Mullaart, E., Lohman, P. H. M., Berends, F., and Vijg, J., DNA damage metabolism and aging, *Mutat. Res.*, 237, 189, 1990.

45. Ames, B. N. and Gold, L. S., Endogenous mutagens and the causes of aging and cancer, *Mutat. Res.*, 250, 3, 1991.

46. Vijg, J., DNA sequence changes in aging: how frequent, how important?, *Aging*, 2, 105, 1990.

47. Rao, K. S. and Loeb, L. A., DNA damage and repair in brain: relationship to aging, *Mutat. Res.*, 275, 317, 1992.

48. Martin, G. M., Genetic and environmental modulations of chromosomal stability: their roles in aging and oncogenesis, *Ann. N.Y. Acad. Sci.*, 621, 401, 1991.

49. Slagboom, P. E. and Vijg, J., Genetic instability and aging: theories, facts, and future perspectives, *Genome*, 31, 373, 1989.

50. Vijg, J. and Gossen, J. A., Somatic mutations and cellular aging, *Comp. Biochem. Physiol.*, 104B, 429, 1993.

51. Holmes, G. E., Bernstein, C., and Bernstein, H., Oxidative and other DNA damages as the basis of aging: a review, *Mutat. Res.*, 275, 305, 1992.

52. Slagboom, P. E., The aging genome: determinant or target?, *Mutat. Res.*, 237, 183, 1990.

53. Rao, K. S., Genomic damage and its repair in young and aging brain, *Mol. Neurobiol.*, 7, 23, 1993.

54. Cooney, C. A., Are somatic cells inherently deficient in methylation metabolism? A proposed mechanism for DNA methylation loss, senescence and aging, *Growth, Dev. Aging*, 57, 261, 1993.

55. Tice, R. R. and Setlow, R. B., DNA repair and replication in aging organisms and cells, in *Handbook of the Biology of Aging*, Finch, C. E. and Schneider, E.L., Eds., Van Nostrand Reinhold, New York, 1985, 173.

56. Saul, R. L., Gee, P., and Ames, B. N., Free radicals, DNA damage and aging, in *Modern Biological Theories of Aging*, Warner, R. H., Butler, R. N., Sprott, R. S., and Schneider, E. L., Eds., Raven Press, New York, 1987, 113.

57. Gensler, H. L., Hall, J. D., and Bernstein, H., The DNA damage hypothesis of aging: importance of oxidative damage, in *Review of Biological Research in Aging*, Vol. 3, Rothstein, M., Ed., Alan R. Liss, New York, 1987, 451.

58. Singer, S. and Kusmierek, J. T., Chemical mutagenesis, *Ann. Rev. Biochem.*, 51, 655, 1982.

59. Ryberg, B. and Lindahl, T., Nonenzymatic methylation of DNA by the intracellular methyl group donor S-adenosyl-L-methionine is a potentially mutagenic reaction, *EMBO J.*, 1, 211, 1982.

60. Ames, B. N., Endogenous DNA damage as related to cancer and aging, *Mutat. Res.*, 214, 41, 1989.

61. Aucher, M. C., Hazards of nitrate, nitrite, and N-nitroso compounds in human nutrition, in *Nutritional Toxicology*, Hathcock, J. N., Ed., Academic Press, New York, 1982, 328.

62. Ames, B. N., Dietary carcinogens and anticarcinogens: oxygen radicals and degenerative diseases, *Science*, 221, 1256, 1983.

63. Saul, R. L. and Ames, B. N., Background levels of DNA damage in the population, in *Mechanisms of DNA Damage and Repair*, Simic, M. G., Grossman, L., and Upton, A. C., Eds., Plenum Press, New York, 1986, 529.

64. Overvik, E. and Gustafsson, J., Cooked-food mutagens: current knowledge of formation and biological significance, *Mutagenesis*, 5, 437, 1990.

65. Brash, D. E. and Hart, R. W., DNA damage and repair *in vivo*, *J. Environ. Pathol. Toxicol.*, 2, 79, 1978.

66. Friedberg, C. E., *DNA-Repair*, W.H. Freeman, New York, 1985.

67. Sancar, A. and Sancar, G. B., DNA-repair enzymes, *Ann. Rev. Biochem.*, 57, 29, 1988.

68. Hanawalt, P. C., Concepts and models for DNA repair: from *Escherichia coli* to mammalian cells, *Environ. Mol. Mutagen.*, 14, 90, 1989.
69. Warner, H. R. and Price, A. R., Involvement of DNA-repair in cancer and aging, *J. Gerontol.*, 44, 45, 1989.
70. Friedberg, E. C., The enzymology of DNA-repair, *Mutat. Res.*, 236, 145, 1990.
71. Friedberg, E. C., Eukaryotic DNA-repair: glimpses through the yeast *Saccharomyces cerevisiae*, *Bioessays*, 13, 295, 1991.
72. Safhill, R., Margison, P. G., and O'Connor, P. J., Mechanisms of carcinogenesis induced by alkylating agents, *Biochim. Biophys. Acta*, 823, 111, 1985.
73. Cameron, I. L. and Thrasher, J. D., Cell renewal and cell loss in the tissues of aging mammalians, *Interdiscip. Top. Gerontol.*, 10, 108, 1976.
74. Crine, P. and Verly, W. G., A study of DNA spontaneous degradation, *Biochim. Biophys. Acta*, 442, 50, 1976.
75. Lindahl, T. and Nyberg, B., Rate of depurination of native deoxyribonucleic acid, *Biochemistry*, 11, 3610, 1972.
76. Lindahl, T. and Karlstrom, O., Heat-induced depyrimidination of deoxyribonucleic acid in neutral solutions, *Biochemistry*, 12, 5151, 1973.
77. Caldecott, R. S., Seedling height, oxygen availability, storage and temperature; their relationship to radiation induced genetic injury in barley, in *Effects of Ionizing Radiations on Seeds*, International Atomic Energy Agency, Vienna, 1961, 3.
78. Berenblum, I. and Trainin, N., New evidence on the mechanism of radiation leukemogenesis, in *Cellular Basis and Aetiology of Late Somatic Effects of Ionizing Radiation*, Harris, R. J. C., Ed., Academic Press, New York, 1963, 41.
79. Maini, M. M. and Stich, H. F., Chromosomes of tumor cells. II. Effect of various liver carcinogens on mitosis of hepatic cells, *J. Natl. Cancer Inst.*, 26, 1413, 1961.
80. Conklin, J. W., Upton, A. C., Christenberry, K. W., and McDonald, T. P., Comparative late somatic effects of some radiomimetic agents and X-rays, *Radiat. Res.*, 19, 156, 1963.
81. Stevenson, K. G. and Curtis, H. J., Chromosome aberrations in irradiated and nitrogen mustard treated mice, *Radiat. Res.*, 15, 774, 1961.
82. Crowley, C. and Curtis, H. J., The development of somatic mutations in mice with age, *Proc. Natl. Acad. Sci. U.S.A.*, 49, 626, 1963.
83. Curtis, H. and Crowley, C., Chromosome aberrations in the liver cells in relation to the somatic mutation theory of aging, *Radiation Res.*, 19, 337, 1963.
84. Curtis, H. J., Leith, J., and Tilley, J., Chromosome aberrations in liver cells of dogs of different ages, *J. Gerontol.*, 21, 268, 1966.
85. Curtis, H. J. and Miller, K., Chromosome aberrations in liver cells of guinea pigs, *J. Gerontol.*, 26, 292, 1971.
86. Brooks, A. L., Mead, D. K., and Peters, R. F., Effect of aging on frequency of metaphase chromosome aberrations in the liver of the Chinese hamster, *J. Gerontol.*, 28, 452, 1973.
87. Martin, G. M., Smith, A. C., Ketterer, D. J., Ogburn, C. E., and Disteche, C. M., Increased chromosomal aberrations in the first metaphase of cells isolated from the kidneys of aged mice, *Isr. J. Med. Sci.*, 21, 296, 1985.
88. Richard, F., Muleris, M., and Dureillaux, B., The frequency of micronuclei with X chromosome increases with age in human females, *Mutat. Res.*, 316, 1, 1994.
89. Grist, S. A., McCarron, M., Kutlaca, A., Turner, D. R., and Morley, A. A., In vivo human somatic mutation: frequency and spectrum with age, *Mutat. Res.*, 266, 189, 1992.
90. Gauguly, B. B., Cell division, chromosomal damage and micronucleus formation in peripheral lymphocytes of healthy donors: related to donor's age, *Mutat. Res.*, 295, 135, 1993.

91. Schneider, E. L., Buckings, C. K., and Sternberg, H., Aging and sister chromatid exchanges. VII. Effects of aging on background SEC *in vivo, Cytogenet. Cell Genet.,* 33, 249, 1982.
92. Martin, G. M., Fry, M., and Loeb, L. A., Somatic mutation and aging in mammalian cells, in *Molecular Biology of Aging: Gene Stability and Gene Expression,* Sohal, R. S., Bernbaum, L. S., and Cutler, R. G., Eds., Raven Press, New York, 1985, 7.
93. Ellsworth, J. F. and Schimke, R. T., On the frequency of metaphase chromosome aberrations in the small intestine of aged rats, *J. Gerontol.,* 45, B94, 1990.
94. Curtis, H. J., Tilley, J., Crowley, C., and Fuller M., The role of genetic factors in the aging process, *J. Gerontol.,* 21, 365, 1966.
95. Takeda, T., Hosokawa, M., Takeshita, S., Irino, M., Higuchi, K., Matsushita, T., Tomita, Y., Yasuhira, K., Hamamoto, H., Shimizu, K., Ishii, M., and Yamamuro, T., A new murine model of accelerated senescence, *Mech. Ageing Dev.,* 17, 183, 1981.
96. Nisitani, S., Hosokawa, M., Sasaki, M. S., Yasuoka, K., Naiki, H., Matsushita, T., and Takeda, T., Acceleration of chromosomes aberrations in senescence-accelerated strains of mice, *Mutat. Res.,* 237, 221, 1990.
97. Salk, D., Werner's syndrome: a review of recent research with an analysis of connective tissue metabolism, growth control of cultured cells, and chromosomal aberrations, *Hum. Genet.,* 62, 1, 1982.
98. Webb, T., Harden, D. G., and Harding, M., The chromosome analysis and susceptibility to transformation by simian virus of fibroblasts from ataxia telangiectasis, *Cancer Res.,* 37, 997, 1977.
99. Thweatt, R. and Goldstein, S., Werner syndrome and biological ageing: a molecular genetic hypothesis, *BioEssays,* 15, 421, 1993.
100. Martin, G. M., Genetic syndromes in man with potential relevance to the pathobiology of aging, *Birth Defects: Orig. Article Ser.,* 14, 5, 1978.
101. Martin, G. M., Sprague, C.A., and Epstein, C. J., Replicative life-span of cultivated human cells. Effects of donor's age tissue and genotype, *Lab. Invest.,* 23, 86, 1970.
102. Hoehn, H., Bryant, E. M., Au, K., Norwood, T. H., Boman, H., and Mortin, G. M., Variegated translocation mosaicism in human skin fibroblasts, *Cytogenet. Cell Genet.,* 15, 282, 1975.
103. Salk, D., Au, K., Hoehn, H., and Martin, G. M., Cytogenetics of Werner's syndrome cultured skin fibroblasts: variegated translocation mosaicism, *Cytogenet. Cell Genet.,* 30, 92, 1981.
104. Fuchuchi, K., Martin, G. M., and Monnat, R. J., Mutator phenotype of Werner's syndrome is characterized by extensive deletions, *Proc. Natl. Acad. Sci. U.S.A.,* 86, 5893, 1989.
105. Salk, D., Au, K., Hoehn, H., and Martin, G. M., Cytogenetic aspects of Werner's syndrome, *Adv. Exp. Med. Biol.,* 190, 541, 1985.
106. Fuchuchi, K., Tanaka, K., Kumahara, Y., Marumo, K., Pride, M. B., and Martin, G. M., Increased frequency of 6-thioguanine-resistant peripheral blood lymphocytes in Werner's syndrome patients, *Hum. Genet.,* 84, 249, 1990.
107. Cohen, M. M. and Leby, H. P., Chromosome instability syndromes, *Adv. Hum. Genet.,* 18, 43, 1989.
108. Alexander, P. and Connell, D. I., Shortening of the life-span of mice by irradiation with X-rays and treatment with radiometric compounds, *Radiat. Res.,* 12, 38, 1960.
109. Dunjic, A., Shortening of the span of life of rats by 'Myleran', *Nature,* 203, 887, 1964.
110. Kodell, R. L., Farmer, J. H., and Littlefield, N. A., Analysis of life-shortening effects in female BALB/C mice fed 2-Acetylaminofluorene, *J. Environ. Pathol. Toxicol.,* 3, 69, 1980.

111. Richards, R. I. and Sutherland, G. R., Fragile X syndrome: the molecular picture comes into focus, *Trends Genet.*, 8, 249, 1992.
112. Caskey, C. T., Pizzuti, A., Fu, Y. H., Fenwick, R. G., Jr., and Nelson, D. L., Triplet repeat mutations in human diseases, *Science*, 256, 784, 1992.
113. Natarajan, A. T., Darroudi, F., Mullenders, L. H. F., and Meijers, M., The nature and repair of DNA lesions that lead to chromosomal aberrations induced by ionizing radiations, *Mutat. Res.*, 160, 231, 1986.
114. Bryant, P. E., 9-Beta-D-arabinofuranosyladenine increases the frequency of X-ray induced chromosome abnormalities in mammalian cells, *Int. J. Radiat. Biol.*, 3, 459, 1983.
115. Mirzayans, R. and Paterson, M. C., Differential repair of 1-β-D-arabinofuranosylcytosine-detectable sites in DNA of fibroblasts exposed to ultraviolet light and 4-nitroquinoline 1-oxide, *Mutat. Res.*, 255, 57. 1991.
116. Natarajan, A. T., Mutagenesis and chromosome changes, in *Radiation Research. Proc. 7th Int. Congr. Rad. Res.*, Broerse, J. J., Barendsen, G. W., Kal, H. B., and van der Kogel, A. J., Eds., Plenum Press, New York, 1983, 239.
117. Natarajan, A. T. and Obe, G., Molecular mechanisms involved in the production of chromosomal aberrations. III. Restriction endonucleases, *Chromosoma*, 90, 120, 1984.
118. Bryant, P. E., Enzymatic restriction of mammalian cell DNA using PvuII and BamHI evidence for the double strand break origin of chromosomal aberrations, *Int. J. Radiat. Biol.*, 46, 57, 1984.
119. Gille, J. J. P., Mullaart, E., Vijg, J., Leyva, A. L., Arwert, F., and Joenje, H., Chromosomal instability in an oxygen-tolerant variant of Chinese hamster ovary cells, *Mutat. Res.*, 219, 17, 1989.
120. Manca, A., Korn, B., Poustka, A., Yu, S., Sutherland, G. R., and Mulley, J. C., Fragile X syndrome without CCG amplification has an FMR1 deletion, *Nature Genet.*, 1, 341, 1992.
121. Richards, R. I. and Sutherland, G. R., Dynamic mutations: a new class of mutations causing human disease, *Cell*, 70, 709, 1992.
122. Rubinstein, D. C., Barton, D. E., Davidson, B. C., and Ferguson-Smith, M. A., Analysis of the Huntington gene reveals a trinucleotide-length polymorphism in the region of the gene that contains two CCG-rich stretches and a correlation between decreased age of onset of Huntington's disease and CAG repeat number, *Hum. Mol. Genet.*, 2, 1713, 1993.
123. Kohwi, Y., Wang, H., and Kohwi-Shigematsu, T., A single trinucleotide, 5'AGC3'/5'GCT3', of the triplet-repeat disease genes confers metal ion-induced non-B DNA structure, *Nucleic Acids Res.*, 21, 5651, 1993.
124. Gaubatz, J. W., DNA damage during aging of mouse myocardium, *J. Mol. Cell Cardiol.*, 18, 1317, 1986.
125. Pegg, A. E., Alkylation and subsequent repair of DNA after exposure to dimethylnitrosamine and related carcinogens, *Rev. Biochem. Toxicol.*, 5, 83, 1983.
126. Park, J. W. and Ames, B. N., 7-Methylguanine adducts in DNA are normally present at high levels and increase on aging: analysis by HPLC with electrochemical detection, *Proc. Natl. Acad. Sci. U.S.A.*, 85, 7467, 1988.
127. Park, J. W. and Ames, B. N., Correction, *Proc. Natl. Acad. Sci. U.S.A.*, 85, 9508, 1988.
128. Tan, B. H., Bancsath, A., and Gaubatz, J. W., Steady-state levels of 7-methylguanine increase in nuclear DNA of postmitotic mouse tissues during aging, *Mutat. Res.*, 237, 229, 1990.
129. Mustonen, R., Forsti, A., Hietanen, P., and Hemminki, K., Measurement by ^{32}P-postlabeling of 7-methylguanine levels in white blood cell DNA of healthy individuals and cancer patients treated with dacarbazine and procarbazine. Human data and method development for 7-alkylguanines, *Carcinogenesis*, 12, 1423, 1991.

130. Barrows, L. R. and Magee, P. N., Nonenzymatic methylation of DNA by S-adenosyl methionine in vitro, *Carcinogenesis*, 3, 349, 1982.

131. Xiao, W. and Samson, L., In vivo evidence for endogenous DNA alkylation damage as a source of spontaneous mutations in eukaryotic cells, *Proc. Natl. Acad. Sci. U.S.A.*, 90, 2117, 1993.

132. Adelman, R., Saul, R. L., and Ames, B. N., Oxidative damage to DNA: relation to species metabolic rate and life span, *Proc. Natl. Acad. Sci. U.S.A.*, 85, 2706, 1988.

133. Park, J., Cundy, K. C., and Ames, B. N., Detection of DNA adducts by high-performance chromatography with electrochemical detection, *Carcinogenesis*, 10, 827, 1989.

134. Richter, C., Park, J. W., and Ames, B. N., Normal oxidative damage to mitochondrial and nuclear DNA is extensive, *Proc. Natl. Acad. Sci. U.S.A.*, 85, 6465, 1988.

135. Fraga, C. G., Shigenaga, M. K., Park, J. W., Degan, P., and Ames, B. N., Oxidative damage to DNA during aging: 8-hydroxy-2′-deoxyguanosine in rat organ DNA and urine, *Proc. Natl. Acad. Sci. U.S.A.*, 87, 4533, 1990.

136. Iverson, L. L., The chemistry of the brain, *Sci. Am.*, 241, 118, 1979.

137. Randerath, K., Reddy, M. V., and Disher, R. M., Age- and tissue-related DNA modifications in untreated rats. Detection by ^{32}P-postlabeling assay and possible significance for spontaneous tumor induction and aging, *Carcinogenesis*, 7, 1615, 1986.

138. Randerath, K., Liehr, J. G., Gladek, A., and Randerath, E., Age-dependent covalent DNA alterations (I-compounds) in rodent tissues: species, tissue, and sex specificities, *Mutat. Res.*, 219, 121, 1989.

139. Li, D. and Randerath, K., Modulation of DNA modification (I-compound) levels in rat liver and kidney by dietary carbohydrate, protein, fat, vitamin, and mineral content, *Mutat. Res.*, 275, 47, 1992.

140. Randerath, K., Li, D., and Randerath, E., Age-related DNA modifications (I-compounds). Modulation by physiological and pathological processes, *Mutat. Res.*, 238, 245, 1990.

141. Li, D., Xu, D., Chandar, N., Lombardi, B., and Randerath, K., Persistent reduction of indigenous DNA modification (I-compound) levels in liver DNA from male Fischer rats fed choline-devoid diet and in DNA of resulting neoplasms, *Cancer Res.*, 50, 7577, 1990.

142. Li, D. and Randerath, K., Association between diet and age-related DNA modifications (I-compounds) in rat liver and kidney, *Cancer Res.*, 50, 3991, 1990.

143. Randerath, K., Putman, K. L., Osterburg, H. H., Johnson, S. A., Morgan, D. G., and Finch, C. E., Age-dependent increases of DNA adducts (I-compounds) in human and rat brain DNA, *Mutat. Res.*, 295, 11, 1993.

144. Randerath, K., Hart, R. W., Zhou, G. D., Reddy, R., Danna, T. F., and Randerath, E., Enhancement of age-related increases in DNA I-compound levels by calorie restriction: comparison of male B-N and F-344 rats, *Mutat. Res.*, 295, 31, 1993.

145. Randerath, E., Randerath, K., Reddy, R., Rao, M.S., and Reddy, J. K., Rat liver DNA alterations induced by the peroxisome proliferator ciprofibrate, *Proc. Am. Assoc. Cancer Res.*, 30, 146, 1989.

146. Randerath, K., Putman, K. L., Randerath, E., Mason, G., Kelley, M., and Safe, S., Organ-specific effects of long term feeding of 2,3,7,8-tetrachlorodibenzo-p-dioxin and 1,2,3,7,8-pentachlorodibenzo-p-dioxin on I-compounds in hepatic and renal DNA of female Sprague-Dawley rats, *Carcinogenesis*, 9, 2285, 1988.

147. Gaubatz, J. W., Postlabeling analysis of indigenous aromatic DNA adducts in mouse myocardium during aging, *Arch. Gerontol. Geriatr.*, 8, 47, 1989.

148. Sharma, R. C. and Yamamoto, O., Base modification in adult animal liver DNA and similarity to radiation-induced base modification, *Biochem. Biophys. Res. Commun.*, 96, 662, 1980.

149. Mandal, P. C. and Yamamoto, O., Changes of fluorescence spectra of 2'-deoxyguanosine in aqueous solution by radiation, *Biochem. Int.*, 12, 255, 1986.
150. Yamamoto, 0., Fuji, I., Yoshida, T., Cox, A. B., and Lett, J. T., Age dependency of base modification in rabbit liver DNA, *J. Gerontol.*, 43, B132, 1988.
151. Kirsh, M. E., Cutler, R. G., and Hartman, P. E., Absence of deoxyuridine and 5-hyroxymethyldeoxyuridine in the DNA from three tissues of mice of various ages, *Mech. Ageing Dev.*, 35, 71, 1986.
152. Setlow, R. B., Regan, J. D., German, J., and Carrier, W. L., Evidence that xeroderma pigmentosum cells do not perform the first step in the repair of ultraviolet damage to their DNA, *Proc. Natl. Acad. Sci. U.S.A.*, 64, 1035, 1969.
153. Kohn, K.W., Erickson, L. C., Ewig, R. A. G., and Friedman, C. A., Fractionation of DNA from mammalian cells by alkaline elution, *Biochemistry*, 15, 4629, 1976.
154. Birnboim, H. C. and Jevcak, J. J., Fluorometric method for rapid detection of DNA strand breaks in human white blood cells produced by low doses of radiation, *Cancer Res.*, 41, 1889, 1981.
155. Mullaart, E., Boerrigter, M. E. T. I., Boer, G. J., and Vijg, J., Spontaneous DNA breaks in the rat brain during development and aging, *Mutat. Res.*, 237, 9, 1990.
156. Hartnell, J. M., Storrie, M. C., and Mooradian, The tissue specificity of the age-related changes in alkali-induced DNA unwinding, *Mutat. Res.*, 219, 187, 1989.
157. Fu, C. S., Harris, S. B., Wilhelmi, P., and Walford, R.L., Lack of effect of age and dietary restriction on DNA single-strand breaks in brain, liver, and kidney of (C3HX C57BL/10) F1 mice, *J. Gerontol.*, 46, B78, 1991.
158. Price, G. B., Modak, S. P., and Makinodan, T., Age-associated changes in the DNA of mouse tissue, *Science*, 171, 917, 1971.
159. Modak, S. P. and Price, G. B., Exogenous DNA polymerase-catalyzed incorporation of deoxyribonucleotide monophosphates in nuclei of fixed mouse-brain cells, *Exp. Cell Res.*, 65, 289, 1971.
160. Chetsanga, C. J., Boyd, V., Peterson, L., and Rushlow, K., Single-stranded regions in DNA of old mice, *Nature*, 253, 130, 1975.
161. Dean, R. G. and Cutler, R. G., Absence of significant age-dependant increase of single stranded DNA extracted from mouse liver nuclei, *Exp. Gerontol.*, 13, 287, 1978.
162. Finch, C. E., Susceptibility of mouse liver DNA to digestion by S1 nuclease: absence of age-related change, *Age*, 2, 45, 1979.
163. Mori, N. and Goto, S., Estimation of the single stranded region in the nuclear DNA of mouse tissues during aging with special reference to the brain, *Arch. Gerontol. Geriatr.*, 1, 143, 1982.
164. Chetsanga, C. J., Tuttle, M., and Jacobini, A., Changes in structural integrity of heart DNA from aging mice, *Life Sci.*, 18, 1405, 1976.
165. Chetsanga, C. J., Tuttle, M., Jacobini, A., and Johnson, C., Age-associated structural alterations in senescent mouse brain DNA, *Biochim. Biophys. Acta*, 474, 180, 1977.
166. Zahn, R. K., Reinmuller, J., Beyer, R., and Pondeljak, V., Age-correlated DNA damage in human muscle tissue, *Mech. Ageing Dev.*, 41, 73, 1987.
167. Nakanishi, K., Shima, A., Fukuda, M., and Fujita, S., Age associated increase of single-stranded regions in the DNA of mouse brain and liver cells, *Mech. Ageing Dev.*, 10, 273, 1979.
168. Massie, H. R., Baird, M. B., Nicolosi, R. J., and Samis, H. V., Changes in the structure of rat liver DNA in relation to age, *Arch. Biochem. Biophys.*, 153, 736, 1972.
169. Ono, T., Okada, S., and Sugahara, T., Comparative studies of DNA size in various tissues of mice during the aging process, *Exp. Gerontol.*, 11, 127, 1976.
170. Su, C. M., Brash, D. E., Turturro, A., and Hart, R. W., Longevity-dependant organ-specific accumulation of DNA damage in two closely related murine species, *Mech. Ageing Dev.*, 27, 239, 1984.

171. Wheeler, K. T. and Lett, J. T., On the possibility that DNA repair is related to age in non-dividing cells, *Proc. Natl. Acad. Sci. U.S.A.*, 71, 1862, 1974.

172. Lawson, T. and Stohs, S., Changes in endogenous DNA damage in aging mice in response to butylated hydroxyanisole and oltipraz, *Mech. Ageing Dev.*, 30, 179, 1985.

173. Mullaart, E., Boerrigter, M. E. T. I., Brouwer, A., Berends, F., and Vijg, J., Age-dependant accumulation of alkali-labile sites in DNA of postmitotic but not in that of mitotic rat liver cells, *Mech. Ageing Dev.*, 45, 41, 1988.

174. Bergtold, D. S. and Lett, J. T., Alterations in chromosomal DNA and aging: an overview, in *Molecular Biology of Aging: Gene Stability and Gene Expression*, Sohal, R. S., Bernbaum, L. S., and Cutler, R. G., Eds., Raven Press, New York, 1985, 23.

175. Hahn, G. M., King, D., and Yang, S. J., Quantitative changes in unscheduled DNA synthesis in rat muscle after differentiation, *Nature New Biol.*, 230, 242, 1971.

176. Stockdale, F. F. and O'Neill, M. C., Repair synthesis in differentiated embryonic muscle cells, *J. Cell Biol.*, 52, 589, 1972.

177. Karran, P. and Ormerod, M. G., Is the ability to repair damage to DNA related to the proliferative capacity of a cell? The rejoining of X-ray-produced strand breaks, *Biochim. Biophys. Acta*, 299, 54, 1973.

178. Ho, L. and Hanawalt, P. H., Gene-specific repair in terminally differentiating rat myoblasts, *Mutat. Res.*, 255, 123, 1991.

179. Gaubatz, J. W. and Tan, B. H., Aging affects the levels of DNA damage in postmitotic cells, *Ann. N.Y. Acad. Sci.*, 719, 97, 1994.

180. Lipetz, P. D., DNA superstructure, differentiation, and aging, in *Biological Mechanisms of Aging*, Schimke, R. T., Ed., NIH Publ. No. 81–2194, Department of Health and Rehabilitative Services, Washington, D.C., 1981, chap. 3.

181. Richardson, A., Roberts, M. S., and Rutherford, M. S., Aging and gene expression, in *Review of Biological Research in Aging*, Vol. 2, Rothstein, M., Ed., Alan R. Liss, New York, 1985, 395.

182. Rogers, J., The origin and evolution of retroposons, *Int. Rev. Cytol.*, 93, 231, 1985.

183. Weiner, A. M., Deininger, P. L., and Efstratiadis, A., Non-viral retroposons: genes, pseudogenes, and transposable elements generated by reverse flow of genetic information, *Ann. Rev. Biochem.*, 55, 631, 1986.

184. Blackburn, E. H., Structure and function of telomeres, *Nature*, 350, 569, 1991.

185. Moyzis, R. K., Buckingham, J. M., Cram, L. S., Dani, M., Deaven, L. L., Jones, M. D., Meyne, J., Ratcliff, and Wu, J. R., A highly conserved repetitive DNA sequence, (TTAGGG)n is present at the telomeres of human chromosomes, *Proc. Natl. Acad. Sci. U.S.A.*, 85, 6622, 1988.

186. Agard, D. A. and Sedat, J. W., The three-dimensional architecture of a polytene nucleus, *Nature*, 302, 676, 1983.

187. Morin, G. B., The human telomere terminal transferase is a ribonucleoprotein that synthesizes TTAGGG repeats, *Cell*, 59, 521, 1989.

188. Greider, C. W., Telomeres, telomerase, and senescence, *BioEssays*, 12, 363, 1990.

189. Counter, C. M., Avillion, A. A., LeFeuvre, C. E., Stewart, N. G., Greider, C. W., Harley, C. B., and Bacchetti, S., Telomere shortening associated with chromosome instability is arrested in immortal cells which express telomerase activity, *EMBO J.*, 11, 1921, 1992.

190. Harley, C. B., Futcher, A. B., and Greider, C. W., Telomeres shorten during aging of human fibroblasts, *Nature*, 345, 458, 1990.

191. Lindsey, J., McGill, N. I., Lindsey, L. A., Green, D. K., and Cooke, H. J., In vivo loss of telomeric repeats with age in humans, *Mutat. Res.*, 256, 45, 1991.

192. Hastie, N. D., Dempster, M., Dunlop, M. G., Thompson, A. M., Green, D. K., and Allshire, R. C., Telomere reduction in human colorectal carcinoma and with aging, *Nature*, 346, 866, 1990.
193. Allsopp, R. C., Vaziri, H., Patterson, C., Goldstein, S., Younglai, E. V., Futcher, A. B., Greider, C. W., and Harley, C. B., Telomere length predicts replicative capacity of human fibroblasts, *Proc. Natl. Acad. Sci. U.S.A.*, 89, 10114, 1992.
194. Sherwood, S. W., Rush, D., Ellsworth, J. L., and Schimke, R. T., Defining cellular senescence in IMR-90 cells: a flow cytometric analysis, *Proc. Natl. Acad. Sci. U.S.A.*, 85, 9086, 1989.
195. Levy, M. Z., Allsopp, R. C., Futcher, A. B., Greider, C. W., and Harley, C. B., Telomere end-replication problem and cell aging, *J. Mol. Biol.*, 225, 951, 1992.
196. Kipling, D. and Cooke, H. J., Hypervariable ultra-long telomeres in mice, *Nature*, 347, 400, 1990.
197. Butner, K. A. and Lo, C. W., High frequency DNA rearrangements associated with mouse centromeric satellite DNA, *J. Mol. Biol.*, 187, 547, 1986.
198. Chatterjee, B. and Lo, C. W., Chromosomal recombination and breakage associated with instability in mouse centromeric satellite DNA, *J. Mol. Biol.*, 210, 303, 1989.
199. Shmookler Reis, R. J. and Goldstein, S., Loss of reiterated DNA sequences during serial passage of human diploid fibroblasts, *Cell*, 21, 739, 1980.
200. Prashad, N. and Cutler, R. G., Percent satellite DNA as a function of tissue and age of mice, *Biochim. Biophys. Acta*, 418, 1, 1976.
201. Gaubatz, J., Prashad, N., and Cutler, R. G., Ribosomal RNA gene dosage as a function of tissue and age for mouse and human, *Biochim. Biophys. Acta*, 418, 358, 1976.
202. Gaubatz, J. M. and Cutler, R. G., Age-related differences in the number of ribosomal RNA genes of mouse tissues, *Gerontology*, 24, 179, 1978.
203. Jeffreys, A. J., Wilson, V., and Thein, S. L., Hypervariable 'minisatellite' regions in human DNA, *Nature*, 318, 67, 1985.
204. Jeffreys, A. J., Wilson, V., Wong, Z., Royle, N., Patel, I., Kelly, R., and Clarkson, R., Highly variable minisatellites and DNA fingerprints, *Biochem. Soc. Symp.*, 53, 165, 1987.
205. Jeffreys, A. J., Royle, N. J., Wilson, V., and Wong, Z., Spontaneous mutation rates to new length alleles at tandem-repetitive hypervariable loci in human DNA, *Nature*, 322, 278, 1988.
206. Jeffreys, A. J., Wilson, V., Thein, S. L., Weatherall, D. J., and Ponder, B. A. J., DNA 'fingerprints' and segregation analysis of multiple markers in human pedigrees, *Am. J. Hum. Genet.*, 39, 11, 1986.
207. Kelly, R., Bulfield, G., Collick, A., Gibbs, M., and Jeffreys, A. J., Characterization of a highly unstable mouse mini-satellite locus: evidence for somatic mutation during early development, *Genomics*, 5, 844, 1989.
208. Vijg, J. and Uitterlinden, A. G., A search for DNA alterations in the aging mammalian genome. An experimental strategy, *Mech. Ageing Dev.*, 41, 47, 1987.
209. Uitterlinden, A. G., Slagboom, P. E., Knook, D. L., and Vijg, J., Two-dimensional DNA fingerprinting of human individuals, *Proc. Natl. Acad. Sci. U.S.A.*, 86, 2742, 1989.
210. Vijg, J., Gossen, J. A., Slagboom, P. E., and Uitterlinden, A. G., New methods for the detection of DNA sequence variation. Applications on molecular genetic studies on aging in *Molecular Biology of Aging*, Vol. 123, Finch, C. E. and Johnson, T. E., Eds., Wiley-Liss, New York, 1990, 103.
211. Vijg, J., Gossen, J. A., De Leeuw, W. J. F., Mullaart, E., Slagboom, P. E., and Uitterlinden, A. G., DNA processing, aging, and cancer, *Ann. N.Y. Acad. Sci.*, 621, 53, 1991.

212. Slagboom, P. E. and Vijg, J., The dynamics of genome organization and expression during the aging process, *Ann. N.Y. Acad. Sci.*, 673, 58, 1992.

213. Gaubatz, J. W., Extrachromosomal circular DNAs and genomic sequence plasticity in eukaryotic cells, *Mutat. Res.*, 237, 271, 1991.

214. Gaubatz, J. W., Arcement, B., and Cutler, R. G., Gene expression of an endogenous retrovirus-like element during murine development and aging, *Mech. Ageing Dev.*, 57, 71, 1991.

215. Servomaa, K. and Rytomaa, T., Suicidal death of rat chloroleukemia cells by activation of the long interspersed repetitive DNA (L1Rn), *Cell Tissue Kinet.*, 21, 33, 1988.

216. Servomaa, K. and Rytomaa, T., UV light and ionizing radiations cause programmed death of rat chloroleukaemia cells by inducing retropositions of a mobile DNA element (L1Rn), *Int. J. Radiat. Biol.*, 57, 331, 1990.

217. Bucala, R., Lee, A. T., Rourke, L., and Cerami, A., Transposition of an Alu-containing element induced by DNA-advanced glycosylation endproducts, *Proc. Natl. Acad. Sci. U.S.A.*, 90, 2666, 1993.

218. Johnson, R. and Strehler, B. L., Loss of genes coding for ribosomal RNA in aging brain cells, *Nature*, 240, 412, 1972.

219. Johnson, R., Chrisp, C., and Strehler, B. L., Selective loss of ribosomal RNA genes during the aging of post-mitotic tissues, *Mech. Ageing Dev.*, 1, 183, 1972.

220. Johnson, L. K., Johnson, R. W., and Strehler B. L., Cardiac hypertrophy, aging and changes in ribosomal RNA gene dosage in man, *J. Mol. Cell Cardiol.*, 7, 125, 1975.

221. Strehler, B. L., Chang, M., and Johnson, L. K., Loss of hybridizable ribosomal RNA from human post-mitotic tissues during aging. I. Age-dependent loss in human myocardium, *Mech. Ageing Dev.*, 11, 371, 1979.

222. Strehler, B. L. and Chang, M., Loss of hybridizable ribosomal DNA from human post-mitotic tissues during aging. II. Age dependent loss in human sensory cortex comparison, *Mech. Ageing Dev.*, 11, 379, 1979.

223. Peterson, C. R. D., Cryar, J. R., and Gaubatz, J. W., Constancy of ribosomal RNA genes during aging of mouse heart cells and during serial passage of WI-38 cells, *Arch. Gerontol. Geriatr.*, 3, 115, 1984.

224. Swisshelm, K., Disteche, C. M., Thorvaldsen, J., Nelson, A., and Salk, D., Age-related increase in methylation of ribosomal genes and inactivation of chromosome-specific rRNA gene clusters in mouse, *Mutat. Res.*, 237, 131, 1990.

225. Flavell, A. J. and Ish-Horowicz, D., The origin of extrachromosomal circular copia elements, *Cell*, 34, 415, 1983.

226. Lieber, M. R., Site-specific recombination in the immune system, *FASEB J.*, 5, 2934, 1991.

227. Yamagishi, H., Kunisada, T., and Takeda, T., Amplification of extrachromosomal small circular DNAs in a murine model of accelerated senescence. A brief note, *Mech. Ageing Dev.*, 29, 101, 1985.

228. Kunisada, T., Yamagishi, H., Ogita, Z., Kirakawa, T., and Mitsui, Y., Appearance of extrachromosomal circular DNAs during in vivo and in vitro ageing of mammalian cells, *Mech. Ageing Dev.*, 29, 89, 1985.

229. Macieira-Coelho, A., Chromatin reorganization during senescence of proliferating cells, *Mutat. Res.*, 256, 81, 1991.

230. Flores, S. C., Sunnerhagen, P., Moore, T. K., and Gaubatz, J. W., Characterization of repetitive sequence families in mouse heart small polydispersed circular DNAs: age-related studies, *Nucleic Acids Res.*, 16, 3889, 1988.

231. Gaubatz, J. W. and Flores, S. C., Tissue-specific and age-related variations in repetitive sequences of mouse extrachromosomal circular DNAs, *Mutat. Res.*, 237, 29, 1990.

232. Wahl, G. M., The importance of circular DNA in mammalian gene amplification, *Cancer Res.*, 49, 1333, 1989.
233. Windle, B. E. and Wahl, G. M., Molecular dissection of mammalian gene amplification: new mechanistic insights revealed by analyses of very early events, *Mutat. Res.*, 276, 199, 1992.
234. Alitalo, D. and Schwab, M., Oncogene amplification in tumor cells, *Adv. Cancer Res.*, 47, 235, 1986.
235. Stark, G. R. and Wahl, G. M., Gene amplification, *Ann. Rev. Biochem.*, 53, 447, 1984.
236. Ono, T., Okada, S., Kawakami, T., Honjo, T., and Getz, M. J., Absence of gross change in primary DNA sequence during aging process of mice, *Mech. Ageing Dev.*, 32, 227, 1985.
237. Cortopassi, G. A. and Arnheim, N., Using the polymerase chain reaction to estimate mutation frequencies and rates in human cells, *Mutat. Res.*, 277, 239, 1992.
238. Horn, P. L., Turker, M. S., Ogburn, C. E., Disteche, C. M., and Martin, G. M., A cloning assay for 6-thioguanine resistance provides evidence against certain somatic mutational theories of aging, *J. Cell. Physiol.*, 121, 309, 1984.
239. Marx, J. L., Detecting mutations in human genes, *Science*, 243, 737, 1989.
240. Gossen, J. A. and Vijg, J., Transgenic mice as a model to study gene mutations: applications as a short-term mutagenicity assay, in *Mutation and the Environment*, Part A: Basic Mechanisms, Mendelsohn, M. L. and Albertini, R. J., Eds., Wiley-Liss, New York, 1990, 347.
241. Gossen, J. A. and Vijg, J., Transgenic mice as model systems for studying gene mutations in vivo, *Trends Genet.*, January, 34, 1993.
242. Gossen, J. A., De Leeuw, W. J. F., Tan, C. H. T., Zwarthoff, E. C., Berends, F., Lohman, P. H. M., Knook, D. L., and Vijg, J., Efficient rescue of integrated shuttle vectors from transgenic mice. A model for studying mutations in vivo, *Proc. Natl. Acad. Sci. U.S.A.*, 86, 7971, 1989.
243. Vijg, J., De Leeuw, W. J. F., Douglas, G. R., and Gossen, J. A., Transgenic mice and age-related mutations, *Ann. N.Y. Acad. Sci.*, 663, 26, 1992.
244. Gossen, J. A., de Leeuw, W. J. F., Verwest, A., Lohman, P. H. M., and Vijg, J., High somatic mutation frequencies in a LacZ transgene integrated on the mouse X-chromosome, *Mutat. Res.*, 250, 423, 1991.
245. Orr, W. C. and Sohal, R. S., Extension of life-span by overexpression of superoxide dismutase and catalase in *Drosophila melanogaster*, *Science*, 263, 1128, 1994.
246. Steinmetz, M. and Haas, W., Recent experiments with knock-out mice: more questions than answers, *Bioessays*, 15, 613, 1993.
247. Anisimov, V. N. and Osipova, G. Y., Effect of neonatal exposure to 5-bromo-2'-deoxyuridine on life span, estrus function and tumor development in rats — an argument in favor of the mutation theory of aging?, *Mutat. Res.*, 275, 97, 1992.
248. Craddock, V. M., Shortening of the life span caused by administration of 5-bromodeoxyuridine to neonatal rats, *Chem. Biol. Interact.*, 35, 139, 1981.
249. Maier, P., Weibel, B., and Zbinden, G., The mutagenic activity of 5-bromo-2'-deoxyuridine (BrdUrd) in vivo in rats, *Environ. Mutagen.*, 5, 695, 1983.
250. Likhachev, A. J., Tomatis, L., and Margison, G. P., Incorporation and persistence of 5-bromodeoxyuridine in new-born rat tissue DNA, *Chem. Biol. Interact.*, 46, 31, 1983.
251. Davidson, R. L., Broeker, P., and Ashman, C. R., DNA base sequence changes and sequence specificity of bromodeoxyuridine-induced mutations in mammalian cells, *Proc. Natl. Acad. Sci. U.S.A.*, 85, 4406, 1988.
252. Tate, P. H. and Bird, A. P., Effects of DNA methylation on DNA-binding proteins and gene expression, *Curr. Opinion Genet. Dev.*, 3, 226, 1993.

253. Peterson, K. and Sapienza, C., Imprinting the genome: imprinted genes, imprinting genes, and a hypothesis for their interaction, *Ann. Rev. Genet.*, 27, 7, 1993.

254. Cooney, C. A. and Bradury, E. M., DNA methylation and chromosome organization in eukaryotes, in *The Eukaryotic Nucleus: Molecular Biochemistry and Macromolecular Assemblies*, Vol. 2, Strauss, P. and Wilson, S., Eds., Telford Press, Caldwell, NJ, 1990, 813.

255. Engler, P., Weng, A., and Storb, U., Influence of CpG methylation and target spacing on V(D)J recombination in a transgenic substrate, *Mol. Cell. Biol.*, 13, 571, 1993.

256. Cooper, D. N. and Krawczak, M., Cytosine methylation and the fate of CpG dinucleotides in vertebrate genomes, *Hum. Genet.*, 83, 181, 1989.

257. Rideout, W. M., III, Coetzee, G. A., Olumi, A. F., and Jones, P. A., 5-Methylcytosine as an endogenous mutagen in the human LDL receptor and p53 genes, *Science*, 249, 1288, 1990.

258. Jones, P. A., Wolkowicz, M. J., Rideout, W. M., III, Gonzales, F. A., Marziasz, C. M., Coetzee, G. A., and Tapscott, S. J., De novo methylation of the MyoD1 CpG island during the establishment of immortal cell lines, *Proc. Natl. Acad. Sci. U.S.A.*, 87, 6117, 1990.

259. Razin, A. and Cedar, H., DNA methylation and embryogenesis in *DNA Methylation: Molecular Biology and Biological Significance*, Jost, J. P. and Saluz, H. P., Eds., Birkhauser Verlag, Basel, 1993, 343.

260. Bird, A.P., CpG-rich islands and the function of DNA methylation, *Nature*, 321, 209, 1986.

261. Li, E., Bestor, T. H., and Jaenisch, R., Targeted mutation of the DNA methyltransferase gene results in embryonic lethality, *Cell*, 69, 915, 1992.

262. Cutler, R. G., Dysdifferentation hypothesis of aging: a review, in *Molecular Biology of Aging: Gene Stability and Gene Expression*, Sohal, R. S., Bernbaum, L. S., and Cutler, R. G., Eds., Raven Press, New York, 1985, 307.

263. Wilson, V. L. and Jones, P. A., DNA methylation decreases in aging but not immortal cells, *Science*, 220, 1055, 1983.

264. Drinkwater, R. D., Blake, T. J., Morley A. A., and Turner, D. R., Human lymphocytes aged in vivo have reduced levels of methylation in transcriptionally active and inactive DNA, *Mutat. Res.*, 219, 29, 1989.

265. Golbus, J., Palella, T. D., and Richardson, B. C., Quantitative changes in T cell DNA methylation occur during differentiation and ageing, *Eur. J. Immunol.*, 20, 1869, 1990.

266. Wilson, V. L., Smith, R. A., Ma, S., and Cutler, R. G., Genomic 5-methyldeoxycytidine decreases with age, *J. Biol. Chem.*, 262, 9948, 1987.

267. Singhal, R. P., Mays-Hoopes, L. L., and Eichhorn, G. L., DNA methylation in aging of mice, *Mech. Ageing Dev.*, 41, 199, 1987.

268. Tawa, R., Ueno, S., Yamamoto, K., Yamamoto, Y., Sagisaka, K., Katakura, R., Kayama, T., Yoshimoto, T., Sakuri, H., and Ono, T., Methylated cytosine level in human liver DNA does not decline in aging process, *Mech. Ageing Dev.*, 62, 255, 1992.

269. Zhavoronkova, E. N. and Vanyushin, B. F., Methylation of DNA and its interaction with rat liver glucocorticoid-receptor complexes, *Biochemistry*, 52, 748, 1987.

270. Tawa, R., Ono, T., Kurishita, A., Okada, S., and Hirose, S., Changes on DNA methylation level during pre- and postnatal periods in mice, *Differentiation*, 45, 44, 1990.

271. Rogers, A. E., Zeisel, S. H., and Akhtar, R., Choline, methionine, folate and chemical carcinogenesis in *Vitamins and Minerals in the Prevention and Treatment of Cancer*, Jacobs, M. M., Ed., CRC Press, Boca Raton, FL, 1991, 123.

272. Shivapurkar, N., Wilson, M. J., and Poirier, L. A., Hypomethylation of DNA in ethionine-fed rats, *Carcinogenesis*, 5, 989, 1984.
273. Miyamura, Y., Tawa, R., Koizumi, A., Uehara, Y., Kurishita, A., Sakurai, H., Kamiyama, S., and Ono, T., Effects of energy restriction on age-associated changes of DNA methylation in mouse liver, *Mutat. Res.*, 295, 63, 1993.
274. Mays-Hoopes, L. L., Brown, A., and Huang, R. C. C., Methylation and rearrangement of mouse intracisternal A particle genes in development, aging and myeloma, *Mol. Cell. Biol.*, 3, 1371, 1983.
275. Mays-Hoopes, L. L., Chao, W., Butcher, H. C., and Huang, C. C., Decreased methylation of the major long interspersed repeated DNA during aging and in myeloma cells, *Dev. Genet.*, 7, 65, 1986.
276. Ono, T., Shinya, K., Uehara, Y., and Okada, S., Endogenous virus genomes become hypomethylated tissue specifically during aging process in C57BL mice, *Mech. Ageing Dev.*, 50, 27, 1989.
277. Howlett, D., Dalrymple, S., and Mays-Hoopes, L. L., Age-related demethylation of mouse satellite DNA is easily detectable by HPLC but not by restriction endonucleases, *Mutat. Res.*, 219, 101, 1989.
278. Slagboom, P. E., de Leeuw, W. J. F., and Vijg, J., Messenger RNA levels and methylation patterns of GAPDH and β-actin genes in rat liver, spleen and brain in relation to aging, *Mech. Ageing Dev.*, 53, 243, 1990.
279. Shmookler Reis, R. J. and Goldstein, S., Interclonal variation in methylation patterns for expressed and non-expressed genes, *Nucleic Acids Res.*, 10, 4293, 1982.
280. Shmookler Reis, R. J. and Goldstein, S., Variability of DNA methylation patterns during serial passage of human diploid fibroblasts, *Proc. Natl. Acad. Sci. U.S.A.*, 79, 3949, 1982.
281. Shmookler Reis, R. J., Finn, G. K., Smith, K., and Goldstein, S., Clonal variation in gene methylation: c-H-ras and α-hCG regions vary independently in human fibroblast linkages, *Mutat. Res.*, 237, 45, 1990.
282. Wareham, K. A., Lyon, M. F., Glenister, P. H., and Williams, E. D., Age related reactivation of an X-linked gene, *Nature*, 327, 725, 1987.
283. Pagani, F., Toniolo, D., and Vergani, C., Stability of DNA methylation of X-chromosome genes during aging, *Somatic Cell Mol. Genet.*, 16, 79, 1990.
284. Thakur, M. K., Age-related changes in the structure and function of chromatin: a review, *Mech. Ageing Dev.*, 27, 263, 1984.
285. Nelson, W. G., Pienta, K. J., Barrack, E. R., and Coffey, D. S., The role of the nuclear matrix in the organization and function of DNA, *Ann. Rev. Biophys. Chem.*, 15, 457, 1986.
286. Getzenberg, R. H., Pienta, K. J., and Coffey, D. S., The tissue matrix: cell dynamics and hormone action, *End. Rev.*, 11, 399, 1990.
287. Pienta, K. J., Partin, A. W., and Coffey, D. S., Cancer as a disease of DNA organization and dynamic cell structure, *Cell. Res.*, 49, 2525, 1989.
288. Pienta, K. J., Getzenberg, R. H., and Coffey, D. S., Characterization of nuclear morphology and nuclear matrices in ageing human fibroblasts, *Mech. Ageing Dev.*, 62, 13, 1992.
289. Murty, C. V. R., Mancini, M. A., Chatterjee, B., and Roy, A. K., Changes in transcriptional activity and matrix association of α_{2u}-globulin gene family in the rat liver during maturation and aging, *Biochim. Biophys. Acta*, 949, 27, 1988.
290. Jaberaboansari, A., Fletcher, C., Wallen, C. A., and Wheeler, K. T., Organization of DNA in cerebellar neurons of ageing unirradiated and irradiated rats, *Mech. Ageing Dev.*, 50, 257, 1989.
291. Boulikas, T., Relationship between carcinogenesis, chromatin structure, and poly(ADP-ribosyl)ation, *Anticancer Res.*, 11, 489, 1991.

292. Althaus, F. R. and Richter, C., *ADP-ribosylation of proteins: enzymology and biological significance, Molecular Biology, Biochemistry, and Biophysics*, Vol. 27, Springer, Berlin, 1987.

293. Satoh, M. S. and Lindahl, T., Role of poly(ADP-ribose) formation in DNA repair, *Nature*, 356, 356, 1992.

294. Monti, D., Grassilli, E., Troiano, L., Cossarizza, A., Salvioli, S., Barbieri, D., Agnesini, C., Bettuzzi, S., Ingletti, M. C., Corti, A., and Franceschi, C., Senescence, immortalization, and apoptosis, *Ann. N.Y. Acad. Sci.*, 673, 70, 1992.

295. Grube, K. and Burkle, A., Poly(ADP-ribose) polymerase activity in mononuclear leukocytes of 13 mammalian species correlates with species-specific life span, *Proc. Natl. Acad. Sci. U.S.A.*, 89, 11759, 1992.

296. Marini, M., Zunica, S., Tamba, M., Cossarizza, A., Monti, D., and Franceschi, C., Recovery of human lymphocytes damaged with gamma radiation or enzymatically-produced oxygen radicals: different effects of poly(ADP-ribosyl)polymerase inhibitors, *Int. J. Radiat. Biol.*, 58, 279, 1990.

297. Attardi, G., Organization and expression of the mammalian mitochondrial genome: a lesson in economy, *TIBS*, 6, 100, 1981.

298. Rosamond, J., The molecular biology of the mitochondrion, *Biochem. J.*, 202, 1, 1982.

299. Tzagoloff, A. and Myers, A. M., Genetics of mitochondrial biogenesis, *Ann. Rev. Biochem.*, 55, 249, 1986.

300. Bogenhagen, D. and Clayton, D. A., The number of mitochondrial deoxyribonucleic acid genomes in mouse L and human HeLa cells, *J. Biol. Chem.*, 249, 7991, 1974.

301. Wallace, D. C., Mitochondrial genetics: a paradigm for aging and degenerative diseases, *Science*, 256, 628, 1992.

302. Osiewacz, H. D., Molecular analysis of aging processes in fungi, *Mutat. Res.*, 237, 1, 1990.

303. Picard-Bennoun, M., Introns, protein synthesis and aging, *FEBS Lett.*, 184, 1, 1985.

304. Osiewacz, H. D. and Hermanns, J., The role of mitochondrial DNA in aging and human diseases, *Aging*, 4, 273, 1992.

305. Bandy, B. and Davidson, A. J., Mitochondrial mutations may increase oxidative stress: implications for carcinogenesis and aging?, *Free Radical Biol. Med.*, 8, 523, 1990.

306. Myers, K. A., Saffhill, R., and O'Connor, P. J., Repair of alkylated purines in the hepatic DNA of mitochondria and nuclei of the rat, *Carcinogenesis*, 9, 285, 1988.

307. Miyaki, M., Yatagai, K., and Ono, T., Strand breaks of mammalian mitochondrial DNA induced by carcinogens, *Chem. Biol. Interact.*, 17, 321, 1977.

308. Kunkel, T. A. and Loeb, L. A., Fidelity of mammalian DNA polymerases, *Science*, 213, 765, 1981.

309. Bullpitt, K. J. and Piko, L., Variation in the frequency of complex forms of mitochondrial DNA in different brain regions of senescent mice, *Brain Res.*, 300, 41, 1984.

310. Piko, L., Bullpitt, K. J., and Meyer, R., Structural and replicative forms of mitochondrial DNA in tissues from adult and senescent BALB/c mice and Fisher 344 rats, *Mech. Ageing Dev.*, 26, 113, 1984.

311. Piko, L., Hougham, A. J., and Bullpitt, K. J., Studies of sequence heterogeneity frequency of deletions/additions with aging, *Mech. Ageing Dev.*, 43, 279, 1988.

312. Gupta, K. P., Van Golen, K. L., Randerath, E., and Randerath, K., Age-dependent covalent DNA alterations (I-compounds) in rat liver mitochondrial DNA, *Mutat. Res.*, 237, 17, 1990.

313. Cortopassi, G. A. and Arnheim, N., Detection of a specific mitochondrial DNA deletion in tissues of older humans, *Nucleic Acids Res.*, 18, 6927, 1990.

314. Sugiyama, S., Hattori, K., Hayakawa, M., and Ozawa, T., Quantitative analysis of age-associated accumulation of mitochondrial DNA with deletion in human hearts, *Biochem. Biophys. Res. Commun.*, 180, 894, 1991.

315. Hayakawa, M., Torii, K., Sugiyama, S., Tanaka, M., and Ozawa, T., Age-associated accumulation of 8-hydroxydeoxyguanosine in mitochondrial DNA of human diaphragm, *Biochem. Biophys. Res. Commun.*, 179, 1023, 1991.

316. Hayakawa, M., Hattori, K., Sugiyama, S., and Ozawa, T., Age-associated oxygen damage and mutations in mitochondrial DNA in human hearts, *Biochem. Biophys. Res. Commun.*, 189, 979, 1992.

317. Wallace, D. C., Diseases of the mitochondrial DNA, *Ann. Rev. Biochem.*, 61, 1175, 1992.

318. Cortopassi, G. A., Shibata, D., Soong, N. W., and Arnheim, N., A pattern of accumulation of a somatic deletion of mitochondrial DNA in aging human tissues, *Proc. Natl. Acad. Sci. U.S.A.*, 89, 7370, 1992.

319. Mita, S., Schmidt, B., Schon, E. A., DiMauro, S., and Bonilla, E., Detection of "deleted" mitochondrial genomes in cytochrome-c oxidase-deficient muscle fibers of a patient with Kearns-Sayre syndrome, *Proc. Natl. Acad. Sci. U.S.A.*, 86, 9509, 1989.

320. Yen, T. C., Su, J. H., King, K. L., and Wei, Y. H., Ageing-associated 5 kb deletion in human liver mitochondrial DNA, *Biochem. Biophys. Res. Commun.*, 178, 124, 1991.

321. Munscher, C., Muller-Hocker, J., and Kadenbach, B., Human aging is associated with various point mutations in tRNA genes of mitochondrial DNA, *Biol. Chem.*, 374, 1099, 1993.

322. Corral-Debrinski, M., Stepien, G., Shoffner, J. M., Lott, M. T., Kanter, K., and Wallace, D. C., Hypoxemia is associated with mitochondrial DNA damage and gene induction: implications for cardiac disease, *J. Am. Med. Assoc.*, 266, 1812, 1991.

323. Trounce, I., Byrne, E., and Marzuki, S., Decline in skeletal muscle mitochondrial respiratory chain function: possible factor in ageing, *Lancet*, 1, 637, 1989.

324. Fernandez-Silva, P., Petruzzella, V., Fracasso, F., Badaleta, M. N., and Cantatore, P., Reduced synthesis of mtRNA in isolated mitochondria of senescent rat brain, *Biochem. Biophys. Res. Commun.*, 176, 645, 1991.

325. Nagley, P., Makay, I. R., Baumer, A., Maxwell, R. J., Vaillant, F., Wang, Z. X., Zhang, C., and Linnane, A. W., Mitochondrial DNA mutation associated with aging and degenerative disease, *Ann. N.Y. Acad. Sci.*, 673, 92, 1992.

326. Miquel, J., Economos, A. C., Fleming, J., and Johnson, J. E., Jr., Mitochondria role in cell aging, *Exp. Gerontol.*, 15, 575, 1980.

327. Sawada, M. and Carlson, J. C., Changes in superoxide radical and lipid peroxide formation in the brain, heart, and liver during the lifetime of the rat, *Mech. Ageing Dev.*, 41, 125, 1987.

328. Bohr, V. A., DNA repair at the level of the gene: molecular and clinical considerations, *J. Cancer Res. Clin. Oncol.*, 116, 384, 1990.

329. Link, C. J., Burt, B. K., and Bohr, V. A., Gene-specific repair of DNA damage induced by UV irradiation and cancer chemotherapeutics, *Cancer Cells*, 3, 427, 1991.

330. Madhani, H. D., Bohr, V. A., and Hanawalt, P. C., Differential repair in transcriptionally active and inactive proto-oncogenes: c-abl and c-mos, *Cell*, 45, 417, 1986.

331. Mellon, I.M., Spivak, G., and Hanawalt, P. C., Selective removal of transcription blocking DNA damage from the transcribed strand of the mammalian DHFR gene, *Cell*, 51, 241, 1987.

332. Lindahl, T., Repair of intrinsic DNA lesions, *Mutat. Res.*, 238, 305, 1990.

Chapter **3**

DNA REPAIR DURING AGING

H. Niedermüller

CONTENTS

0-8493-4786-6/95/$0.00+$.50
© 1995 by CRC Press, Inc.

I. AIM AND PURPOSE OF DNA REPAIR

"Nobody is perfect" — this saying can also apply to the processes of intermediary metabolism and, in a more remote sense, to every organism existing in this world. Especially, the genetic material of the cell of an organism should be perfect in order to guarantee the optimum function of the cell. On the other hand, if there had not been some errors during or even before the replication of the DNA, no evolution of the organism would have taken place.[1] These organisms have always been exposed to influences that have the power to damage structures necessary for optimum function and survival. We will not be so presumptuous as to maintain that structural damages might be the only cause of aging, but they are a powerful instrument that contributes to the aging process. As is more extensively explained later (Section III) we are convinced that aging, in its true essence, is substantially "stochastic", in all matter of the universe. In living multicellular job-sharing organisms these "stochastic" damages are interacting with a high number of functional elements at different levels of organization and are counteracted by programmed longevity determinant strategies.[2-5]

The first comprehensive reviews on the matter of DNA repair and aging were published by Hart and Trosko,[6] Tice,[7] Strehler and Freeman,[8] and Tice and Setlow.[9] The first intensive investigation on DNA repair and aging *in vivo* (rats) was carried out by Niedermüller.[10]

A. Damages

In this chapter we shall refer exclusively to damages and repairs concerning DNA, unless noted otherwise; these damages can have either an *endogenous* or an *exogenous* origin.

Damages are physically distinct alterations and therefore different from mutations. Damage causes an abnormal structure of the DNA while a mutation normally refers to a DNA sequence change. Of course, damages that are not repaired can eventually become mutations. In opposition to mutations, damages cannot be replicated nor inherited. Mutations cannot be repaired, damages can. A damage changes DNA structure to an abnormal one that can be recognized by enzymes, removed, and replaced, and therefore repaired.

One of the most prominent endogenous causes is error-prone replication,[11,12] estimated by interactions in base pairing to cause about 10^{-3} damages per replicated base pair, but many of these errors are corrected in bacteria by proofreading.[13-15] Proofreading reduced the probability of damages to 10^{-10} per base pair. To date, proofreading has not been found in eukaryotes, which surely must possess another mechanism of control or we would not exist.

Other endogenous sources can be temperature, which causes single-strand breaks (SSB) and the loss of bases or of functional groups of bases.[16-18] Kinetic theory of heat defines temperature as the mean kinetic energy per degree of freedom of the single smallest component of a system. The kinetic energies of these components obey Maxwell's "Law of the Distribution of Molecular Velocities". Therefore, at any given temperature there exists a spectrum of molecules ranging from low to high velocities. Molecules possessing high velocities may destroy DNA.

Further damage comes from the action of free radicals being generated in the normal oxygen metabolism.[19,20] They cause total base damages, SSBs, double-strand breaks (DSBs), and probably cross links.[21-24] Finally, glycation[25,26] and alkylation of bases may occur by normal metabolic processes.[27,28]

Exogenous sources can be of natural and/or artificial origin and consist mainly of irradiation (UV, ionizing) and chemicals. With the exception of the formation of pyrimidine dimers, damages are of the same nature as caused by endogenous sources.[29] One difference consists in the amount of damages: while endogenous events cause only up to $4 \cdot 10^4$ damages per cell per day, up to 10^6 damages per cell per day can be induced by natural influences and of course an unlimited amount can be traced to artificial action (atomic bomb explosion!).[30]

We want to refer to the comprehensive and detailed reviews on DNA damages by Friedberg[31] and Mullaart et al.[32] From these expositions it becomes evident that it is extremely necessary to remove this high number of damages. Organisms developed mechanisms in the early beginning of their existence through evolution, that are able to repair DNA damages (we also know of such mechanisms to repair RNA damages, because the first organisms probably had a single-stranded RNA genome).[33]

B. Historical Background

In 1935 Hollaender and Curtis[34] published a paper on the effect of sublethal doses of UV irradiation on *E. coli* suspensions. They discovered that:

1. The retarded growth (lag) phase of the irradiated bacteria was extended considerably over the control. This extension apparently depends on the energy applied to the suspension. When the bacteria had completed their growth, the suspension with the control and that with the irradiated bacteria contained the same number of organisms, and

2. A careful determination of the lag phase revealed that where the control culture changed little in number of bacteria during this phase, the culture which had survived irradiation increased in number quite rapidly in the earlier part of the lag phase and then slowed down more or less for a certain time before it came into the log phase, thus producing a modified extension of the lag phase. The growth curve of the control rising in the beginning of the lag phase actually crossed the curve of the exposed culture and in the end an extension of the lag phase was induced by the radiation. The total number of viable bacteria of the exposed culture had increased during the lag phase. These increases were so pronounced that in the time during which the control culture showed a change in number of not more than 10 to 15%, the exposed culture had increased up to, or more than, 100%.

The authors ascribed this phenomenon to a stimulation of mitosis by certain substances, but did not exclude completely the possibility of recovery of the cells. This was essentially the first report on DNA repair, and preceded by nearly two decades the discovery of the DNA structure by Watson and Crick.[35] Therefore, it was impossible for Hollaender and Curtis to draw the right inferences from their findings. In 1962 Howard-Flanders et al.[36] reported on the control of reactivation of UV-photoproducts in *E. coli*. They concluded that a repair mechanism must exist and founded the research on DNA repair.

II. MECHANISMS OF REPAIR AND METHODS OF ITS DETERMINATION

A. Mechanisms

Mechanisms of repair are extensively and broadly discussed and described by Friedberg.[31] There are only a few recent new thoughts and investigations beyond that today. We shall give a short overview on the most important mechanisms, concentrating on repair processes in cells of organisms that age.

There are six repair systems that have been characterized reasonably well.[37-40] Until now, not all of the enzymological details of these repair systems were known and these systems are not completely independent of each other. First of all we can discriminate between repair of single- and double-strand DNA damages.

The systems to be considered for single-strand damages are

- Base excision repair
- Nucleotide excision repair
- Repair of single-strand breaks (SSB)
- Direct reversal processes (photoreactivation and repair of O^6-alkyl-guanine)
- Postreplication and error-prone repair

Those concerning double strand damages:

- Repair of double-strand breaks (DSB)

These systems repair different types of damages produced by a variety of exogenous or endogenous sources.

Genomes containing dsDNA have built-in informational redundancy because of complementarity. Damage within a single strand can be repaired by excising the damage and replacing the lost information by copying. One of the best-investigated processes that can serve as an example for all excision repair mechanisms is the repair of a thymine dimer in phage T4.[41,42]

1. Base Excision Repair

This is a repair pathway based on the action of glycosylases. A DNA glycosylase catalyzes the hydrolysis of the N-glycosylic bonds linking bases to the deoxyribose-phosphate backbone, leaving a base-free site (AP site). The removal of such a site requires the action of an AP endonuclease that incises the DNA. Many such enzymes have been characterized in mammals.[43] They remove uracil, hypoxanthine, 3-methyladenine, 7-methylguanine, urea, hydroxymethyluracil, and thymine-glycol in different organs of the mouse, rat, calf, and humans. An AP site formed by these enzymes can be removed by the sequential action of a 5'-acting and a 3'-acting AP endonuclease. The resulting gap is enlarged by the action of an exonuclease in both directions that is not specifically repair directed. The gap is filled in by a polymerase and the last nick ligated. Some of these enzymes exhibit both a glycosylase and an AP endonuclease activity, especially those that remove bases damaged by oxidation.

Nucleotide excision involves an initial attack on the polynucleotide backbone; base excision repair does not. There exist three major subdivisions of this repair scheme. Alkylation damage and, in particular, O^6-alkylguanine products (see Section II.A.4) may be repaired by direct dealkylation through transfer of the alkyl group to an acceptor protein, which converts the DNA to its original unaffected form. This repair cannot be measured by unscheduled DNA synthesis (UDS, see Section II.B.1) or by repair replication. A second base excision repair pathway involves the removal of the affected base itself without touching the polynucleotide strand. By one pathway a new base is inserted in place of the old one, while by another there is an endonuclease attack on the AP site, as already described.

Either the patch size is one, i.e., only a single nucleotide has been removed, (since the inserted base is usually a purine, UDS using ^{3}H-dThd would measure a patch of zero), or the patch size will be short. Hence, UDS is not a good measure of base excision repair, especially since O^6-alkylguanine, the major mutational product, is repaired with zero patch size.

Another interesting way is the removal of pyrimidine dimers in mammals, analogous to that described in phage T4. Mellon et al.[44] demonstrated a strong preferential rate of removal of dimers from transcriptionally active genes as compared to that in total DNA. Their results indicate the great importance of the removal of dimers from active genes in mammals. Possibly the chromatin structure of active sequences is more accessible to repair enzymes because of its open conformation, or transcription might be directly coupled with repair.

2. Nucleotide Excision Repair

One class of endonucleases recognizes conformational distortions of the DNA by many other damages. This type of repair might be the most universal, has been extensively studied in *E.coli,* and should be widely applied in mammals. Recently, genes have been identified in mammals which are partially homologous to the uvrA and uvrC genes of *E. coli* that code for an endonuclease.[45] These genes seem to be highly conserved during evolution. Louda and Niedermüller isolated this gene from rats.[46] Hybridization studies comparing the genes of young with those of old rats, besides other explanations, indicated the possibility of sequence changes during aging.

The prototype damage is represented by pyrimidine dimers resulting from UV irradiation. Irradiation produces dimers between adjacent pyrimidines in the same strand, and such lesions are recognized by specific endonucleases or glycosylases that initiate a rather complicated series of reactions which result in the removal of the damaged section of DNA and its replacement by normal nucleotides. In mammalian cells, the average size of the repaired section is large — 25 to 100 nucleotides, depending on the method used — and seems independent of species.

During the process of nucleotide excision repair, there is an increase followed by a subsequent decrease in the number of single-strand nicks in cellular DNA. This fact is used to measure the repair extent.

3. Repair of Single-Strand Breaks

As already mentioned, large numbers of single-strand breaks are induced in cells, in part from unknown metabolic reactions (e.g., oxidative processes) and in part probably as a result of enzymological actions near depurinated regions of the DNA regions that accumulate as a result of temperature (see Section I.A). When such breaks are introduced into cells by ionizing radiation or radiomimetic chemicals (endogenous breaks do not arise in significant numbers from background ionizing radiation), they are quickly repaired. Thus, mammalian cells are capable of repairing about $2 \cdot 10^5$ single-strand breaks per hour.

4. Direct Reversal Processes (Photoreactivation, O^6-Alkylguanine)

Direct repair is an infrequent event. The simple removal or canceling of the damage belongs to these mechanisms. Photoreactivation repair is specific for pyrimidine dimers.[47] It involves binding of enzyme to the damaged DNA, absorption of visible light by the enzyme-DNA complex, monomerization of the dimer, and dissociation of the enzyme from what is now unaltered DNA. The repair system is useful analytically because it gives one an indication of the fraction of UV damage that may be ascribed to dimers.

One type of dimer results from covalent linkage between two neighboring pyrimidine bases and forms a cyclobutane ring. The DNA photolyase directly opens the ring in a light-dependent process.[48] This photolyase was found in bacteria, plants and animals — with the highest significance probably in plants. Interestingly, this enzyme was found in internal organs which never get in contact with exogenous UV. Possibly it is used to remove damages caused by endogenous UV that is produced together with visible light inside the cells.[49]

O[6]-alkylguanine repair, again, is best investigated in *E. coli*. If the methyl and ethyl derivatives are not repaired they are highly mutagenic. An enzyme was found in mammals that transfers these groups to cysteine of a protein.[50-52] The properties of the bacterial and mammalian enzymes are similar; transferase and acceptor activities uniting in one protein.

Because of the mutagenic force of remaining residues the repair activity may be important to avoid neoplasms, but in nonreplicating cells these damages have less significance, therefore being less important for aging.

5. Postreplication and Error-Prone Repair

What happens when the DNA polymerase, during the course of replication, meets a bulky DNA damage? If one of the repair systems just discussed has not completed the repair before DNA synthesis, replication may be attempted on a damaged template. If the changes in DNA are small (e.g., the presence of an O[6]-alkylguanine or an apurinic site), miscoding may take place. If the changes are bulky ones (e.g., a pyrimidine dimer), then the replication fork may stop, at least temporarily, near the site of damage. If the fork passes the damage, a gap is left in the Okazaki fragment that is blocked, which leaves a gap in the newly synthesized strand. The gaps are eventually filled in by a mechanism called postreplication repair which is not clearly understood for eukaryotic systems. One model was presented by Villani et al.[53] DNA polymerase idles at a damaged site, inserting nucleotides opposite the damage in the new strand, but then removing them by its proofreading exonuclease. The enzyme works according to two mechanisms and continues replication after an arrest. Firstly, DNA synthesis is reinitiated downstream of the block. This results in gaps within the daughter strands which are filled in afterwards. Secondly, after an initial arrest, replication runs past the damage continuously, causing error-prone DNA synthesis. Both mechanisms improve cell survival.[53]

Gaps can be filled in by repair with relaxed proofreading, resulting in an error-prone synthesis or, as proposed by Rupp et al.,[54] by recombinational repair, a mechanism that is less conclusive for mammals. However, Kaufmann found evidence for recombinational repair in mitotic cells.[55]

Error-prone repair uses tolerance systems. They could represent a possibility to read a damaged template, in certain cases at the price of a relatively high error frequency. Probably, they are especially important in cells of higher eukaryotes where a complete repair of the big genome is very unlikely. Kaufmann reviewed extensively the possibility of error-prone repair in mammals.[55] It might play a role in producing focal lesions that arise by mutation and therefore contribute to aging.

6. Repair of Double-Strand Breaks

Double-strand breaks are rare events compared to single-strand ones. These damages are characterized in that both strands are altered at the same position so that neither strand can be used as an accurate template. They may arise from ionizing radiation, from the action of certain chemicals, or from a combination of single-strand nicks plus endonucleolytic attack on the strand opposite the nick. Such breaks are readily repaired in mammalian cells, but perhaps less readily than single-strand breaks. Besides these breaks, we find DNA-DNA interstrand and DNA-protein cross-links as the results of double-strand damages.

Ward et al.[56] concluded that in order to produce lethal events for cells DSBs are required and these lethal effects reflect double-strand damages. One single DSB remaining unrepaired after 2 hours of incubation is lethal for a cell.[57]

The source of information redundancy for this repair must be a second DNA-intact and information-identical molecule, and information is exchanged by recombination. This must occur within a short time after the damage, especially in postmitotic cells, otherwise the cell dies. DSB repair seems to have greater relevance to aging as compared to SSB repair, although the normal endogenous frequency of breaks is fairly low (8.8/cell/day).

B. Measurement

The methods of the measurement of the different repair mechanisms and the extent of DNA damages are listed along with accurate procedure descriptions in the comprehensive two-volume laboratory manual edited by Friedberg and Hanawalt.[58]

We shall limit ourselves here to a short description of methods especially used for eukaryotic cells of higher multicellular organisms. This enables us to discover repair changes during aging in whole organs, cells *in vivo* and *in vitro*, and in isolated nuclei.

1. Excision Repair

This type of repair may be measured in a number of ways, each of which has its virtues and experimental difficulties. If particular products such as pyrimidine dimers are known, it is possible to measure their loss from DNA by chromatographic procedures.[59-61]

The measurement of smaller numbers of lesions per unit length can be done by the determination of the loss of sites sensitive to damage-specific endonucleases. The endonuclease introduces single-strand nicks into the DNA, and the nicks are quantified by sedimentation in alkali. These methods were developed by Ganesan et al.[62] and Paterson et al.[63]

A variation of the latter procedure is to render cells permeable so that an exogenous endonuclease can be introduced to probe for the regions sensitive to enzymic action. This technique, in conjunction with experiments on purified DNA, would measure the accessibility of the lesions in chromatin to nucleases. Such nicks can also be measured by sedimentation in alkali. These methods will be discussed in the next section, concerning SSBs.

A commonly used way of measuring repair is to determine the incorporation of an isotope such as ^{3}H-dThd into parental DNA. The repaired DNA represents so-called unscheduled DNA synthesis (UDS; i.e., synthesis during the non-S phase of the cell cycle). Such measurements are usually made in one of two ways: either by the measurement of the radioactivity incorporated,[64,65] or by autoradiography, as the number of grains per nucleus.[66]

Complications in the quantitative interpretation of such measurements might arise but can be met by the determination of the specific activity of the radioisotope, since there may well be unlabeled thymidine in the growth medium, or because the cells may have an endogenous pool of thymidine metabolites that compete with the exogenous label. The latter can be minimized by shutting off the endogenous pathway for DNA synthesis by use of the inhibitor fluorodeoxyuridine (FdUrd). Another complication of the interpretation of UDS can be met by suppression of the "normal" DNA synthesis. The scheduled incorporation of radioactive label may far outweigh the unscheduled. Hence, it is customary to inhibit scheduled synthesis by antimetabolic agents such as hydroxyurea, with the hope that this inhibitor will not affect unscheduled DNA synthesis. In actual practice, too low a concentration of inhibitor permits too much scheduled DNA synthesis, and too high a concentration of inhibitor tends to inhibit unscheduled DNA synthesis. The optimum concentration between these two extremes is difficult to determine. In studies of excision repair in postmitotic or long G_1-phase cells the use of inhibitors is not necessary, in other studies they should not be used. Measurement of UDS by autoradiography permits the unique identification of cells doing scheduled synthesis.

Measurements of UDS do not provide direct evidence that the incorporated label is going into parental DNA. The measurements of repair replication in which cells are permitted to repair in the presence of a radioactive dense isotope such as tritium-labeled bromodeoxyuridine (BrdUrd), avoids this difficulty. By isopycnic sedimentation, replicated DNA can be separated from unreplicated, and the amount of incorporation into parental DNA measured uniquely.[67]

A variation on this latter technique uses the photochemical sensitivity of BrdUrd incorporated into DNA (light of wavelength 313 nm specifically makes single-strand nicks in DNA containing BrdUrd) to measure both the number and, in many cases, the patch size of the repaired regions.[68]

A completely different way of measuring DNA repair, and one that is essentially applicable to all repair pathways, is host cell reactivation of DNA-containing viruses.[69] If viruses are inactivated by a DNA-damaging agent, the level of inactivation depends upon the ability of the host cells on which they will be grown to repair damage to the viral DNA. Cells proficient in repair show much higher viral survival than cells deficient in repair. The technique is important not only because of its sensitivity but because its use eliminates the possibility that differences in chemical metabolism and/or transport may be responsible for an apparent change in cellular sensitivity to specific chemical agents.

2. Single-Strand Break Repair

Such repair measurements are made by several techniques. Most of them use the fragmentation of DNA by alkali.[65,70-72]

Other techniques use labeling with radioactivity so as to detect the DNA in subsequent analytical steps,[73] also using nitrocellulose membrane filtration,[74] or the DNA can be detected by fluorescence after absorption of a fluorescent dye.[75]

The cells are lysed in alkali, which causes the DNA to unwind. The rate of unwinding depends upon the number of single-strand nicks in the DNA, since the unwinding of the DNA duplex starts at such breaks. In one technique — sedimentation in alkali — the unwinding reaction is allowed to go to completion, and the molecular weight distribution of the resulting DNA is determined by sedimentation in alkali. From the average molecular weight, one can calculate the number of single-strand nicks in the DNA as the reciprocal of the average molecular weight. In a second technique, the reaction is stopped part way through the unwinding by neutralizing the solution, and the fraction of DNA that has reformed the double helix is determined either by chromatographic techniques or by resistance to digestion by a single-strand nuclease. In a third technique, alkaline elution, cells are lysed on filters and the DNA is eluted with mild alkali to give an estimate of the rate of DNA unwinding. The alkaline sucrose technique, although very easy to do, can only measure breaks at the levels of several $\times 10^8$ Da, whereas the other techniques have sensitivities in the neighborhood of several $\times 10^{10}$ Da. Measurements made at different times after the introduction of single-strand breaks indicate that the breaks disappear rapidly. As a practical matter, sedimentation in alkali is only a useful technique for cells that have accumulated single-strand breaks resulting from the equivalent of 50 Gy or more, whereas the techniques that depend upon the rate of unwinding may be used in the biological range of several Gy.

Nucleoid sedimentation also is a very useful test system for repair of SSBs and other types of damage. It was first developed by Cook and Brazell,[76] and used by Niedermüller for the discrimination between several repair mechanisms in relation to aging.[65] Mattern used this system to determine the damage-changed DNA structure.[77]

3. Postreplication Repair

This type of repair is usually measured by pulse labeling the newly synthesized DNA and determining the distribution of its molecular weight in alkaline sucrose gradients.[78,79] Such distributions permit one to determine whether the newly synthesized DNA is chased into parental size material as rapidly as that made on a normal template. They also allow one to determine if replicon initiation is inhibited, because if it is a pulse label will only add on to large replicating DNA and have a high sedimentation rate.

4. Double-Strand Break Repair

They can be measured because of the already existing fragmentation of DNA by sedimentation in neutral gradients or by elution from filters after cell lysis at about pH 9. The DSB repair rate is proportional to the rejoining rate of fragments.[65,80]

III. AGING AND LONGEVITY DETERMINANT STRATEGIES

A. Aging

In a proper and essential sense concerning living organisms aging is a normal, physiological event that appears without exception in all surviving individuals of a species, progressively reduces all functional capacities, and must inevitably lead to death. The concept of biological age (BA) is based on the assumption that in the course of normal aging each chronological age is characterized by a certain functional and morphological state of the organism as a whole.[2] Multicellular aging follows a fixed pattern that seems to be the result of fundamental aging processes at the molecular level and the effect these have on the homeostatic system.[81] These effects include biosenescent and antibiosenescent processes at all levels of organization.[82] Aging in an *extensive* sense is a universal phenomenon observed in inorganic and in animated and dead organic matter. In a more restricted sense we characterize with **"aging"** the changes, observable in the course of senescence, in a multicellular organism that divides its labor, and in a very narrow sense changes in mammals, because these processes take a very uniform and homogeneous course.

In a discussion about aging, couples of opposites always emerge: *stochastic-programmed, adaptive-nonadaptive, regular-accidental,* and also overlapping themselves to some extent. Which of these attributes can we ascribe to aging, or are all of them divided in a proportional, different extent?

One cause of "aging" which manifests itself in dead matter (breaking of glassware in the laboratory) and also in wildlife populations is seen mathematically as a result of accidents. It results in a decreasing exponential function, containing one or more exponential terms. This function represents the respective fraction of surviving structures, systems, organisms or individuals. However, this is a statistical concept of aging and can only be applied to populations and not to the individual — the latter may die without aging, that is, while still **young**! Hence such courses don't tell us what concerns the virtual aging that is an utmost complex process as a change of structure and function. This aging we naturally can investigate only *where it occurs* — in those individuals who still are alive after the stochastic-statistical individuals already have died — if therefore the population does *not* decrease according to the above-mentioned accidental-regular exponential function!

This is the case in all individuals and populations that can withdraw from those stochastic exogenous influences which had led to death before senescence.

Starting from these considerations, predictions about the nature of the aging process can be made:

Result of an accumulation of somatic damage

Species with different maximum life span potentials (MLP, the maximum life span attainable by an individual of a species) should show similar differences in repair

In germ cells special maintenance processes should occur (also fast elimination of damaged cells — transfer of repair capacity of the ovum to the sperm cell[83]).

One process of repair, that of DNA, shows this correlation with MLP, and furthermore it also shows a decrease with aging within the species (see Sections IV, V, and VI)

B. Stochastic Aging Processes

1. Definition of "Stochastic"

Stochastic dependence is said to derive from several chance values which are not independent of one another. Stochastic events are statistical and are chance dependent events of statistical trials, values of chance quantities, and so on. It is possible to adjoin certain probabilities to stochastic events, determined by a distribution function, if a sufficiently large number of trials exist. A stochastic process is a chance process — an arbitrary, not completely determined event — for instance, the course of a physical quantity underlying statistical variations. A stationary stochastic process exists if its distribution function is time-independent (MARKOW-process). In stochastic systems the relation between an influencing input and the system's answer (output) possesses chance character, and the transition to a new state only happens with a certain probability.

2. Stochastic and Chance

From these definitions we see that stochastic does not mean totally accidental, and as we shall see later, aging is stochastic, but not accidental.

In any case, in a very severe and strict sense, we have to characterize the aging process as causal and regular, because nothing happens without cause and what we characterize as an accident is simply an expression of our temporary helplessness to explain the phenomenon.

However, this preliminary helplessness must remain preliminary forever, because every new cognition or knowledge raises infinite new problems and we shall remain at these traditionally consensual styles of the above-mentioned couples of opposites.

C. Adaptive — Nonadaptive

To explain the development towards greater longevity on this basis it might be necessary to consider the following, because we cannot simply say that aging does not need an evolutionary explanation since it is an intrinsic inevitable quality of multicellular organisms. One group of hypotheses states that aging would be favored by selection and would therefore be a positive adaptation for itself — competition for food, living space, and so on. These are summarized as "adaptive hypotheses". A second group postulates that aging would be harmful to the fitness of an organism or, at best, selectively neutral. These "nonadaptive" hypotheses must explain the evolution of aging indirectly: either the power of selection decreases with aging and finally is too weak to inhibit senescence, or senescence is a "trade-off" of other adaptive characteristics.[84,85]

1. Adaptive

The adaptive hypotheses have the advantage over the nonadaptive ones to see aging as a *programmed-regular* process under its own strict genetic control. Apart from the fact that no experimental hints exist for these hypotheses, logical arguments also contradict them: in wildlife populations there are nearly no senile animals (being exposed to natural selection) and therefore no competition and, furthermore, the selection in favor of the species or group must have been much more effective than the selection among the individuals within one group — which is not true! There are many more arguments against adaptive hypotheses.

2. Nonadaptive

Numerous nonadaptive explanations have been presented. Genes with a later onset of age-specific effects are selected for much less than those with an earlier onset, because of the smaller fraction of older individuals. Thus, senescence would be the result of an accidental accumulation of harmful mutations with late age-specific effects, because they were not subject to negative selection. Extended, this hypothesis means that aging can be ascribed to pleiotropic genes, positively selected very early in life; aging therefore being a trade-off of the selection for other characteristics. Although this hypothesis was elaborated only recently in a subtle and comprehensive way, in its present form it already explains something:

- Pleiotropy, genes control the maintenance of the soma
- Stochastic events, as there are free radicals, somatic mutations, errors of protein synthesis, cross-linking
- Biosenescent and antibiosenescent processes, and it enables further systematic research starting points.

A more extensive hypothesis with a more comprehensive mode of explanation is the disposable soma theory.[86] Shortly summarized, it states that the individual only possesses a limited amount of energy that it must invest optimally into the maintenance of the soma and into the increase of the number of offspring, respectively. If too little energy is invested into the prevention or repair of damages, the individual dies before reproduction, but more investment as necessary for the wild-type lifetime also is wasteful, because fitness rather is achieved by energy for a higher number of offspring. Fitness therefore is maximized at a repair extent that is lower than necessary for an infinite survival. Once a soma had evolved, there are two alternative strategies for survival:

1. To develop to adulthood, start to reproduce, maintain the soma in a steady state (by **repair**, replacement of cells, tissue regeneration) with continuing propagation of the germ line. This holds for simple organisms, such as *coelenterates and flatworms*. In these individuals early and late acting genes have no reality because the soma is not aging.
2. To evolve a soma that cannot survive indefinitely, so inevitably it will age. For instance, *Drosophila melanogaster* has very limited or no powers

of cell replacement and tissue repair. It is unreasonable to expect postmitotic cells to survive indefinitely. Sooner or later they will die from terminal events (lethal mutations, loss of mitochondrial function, failure to replace defective proteins). Thus, the already evolved physiological and anatomical design of the organism is the origin of aging, not antagonistic pleiotropy, or any related genetic mechanism. The design has evolved because it increases the reproductive advantage of the species, in comparison to those that invest resources in a fruitless attempt to maintain the soma indefinitely.

Early- and late-acting genes are only relevant to the modulation of aging, or the evolution of longevity, not the evolution of aging per se.

D. Longevity Determinant Genes

The more important question is whether the identification of genes that modulate aging will provide the greatest insight into the physiological or biochemical basis of aging. The organism invests energy in "maintenance systems" that are controlled by longevity genes, until reproduction is guaranteed, but not longer.[87] A change of these genes can only be achieved by genetic engineering.

E. Consequences

Following the last field of explanation (Sections III.C.2 and III.D) we now are able to postulate that aging is not subject to selection, being an error-accumulating process, and that it is stochastic, nevertheless antibiosenescent processes counteract this aging and are subject to selection.

Our hypothesis is that a class of processes then can be estimated as a cause of aging, if it is expressed in the dynamics of aging of an organism as a whole, therefore in the dynamics of its biological age (BA).

F. Intervention into the Aging Process

Under these conditions, intervention into or modulation of the aging process only seems possible in systems of antibiosenescent strategies; no intervention might be possible into stochastic processes. Perhaps this postulate explains the failures of attempts to prolong life with antioxidants or radical scavengers. DNA repair certainly is a longevity determinant strategy, therefore it would be a very promising project to search for intervention strategies in this field.

IV. REPAIR MECHANISMS AND AGING

A. *In Vitro* Repair Studies

Aging *in vitro* is expressed by the growth potential of cultivated cells and the bulk of metabolic changes occurring in these cells during this process. The limitations and problems inherent in *in vivo* experimentation have prompted the development of *in vitro* mammalian models of aging. One *in vitro* system frequently utilized for aging studies employs the characteristic pattern of growth of fibroblast cells derived from human embryonic lung as a correlate for aging *in vivo*.[88] After a period of rapid, sustained growth (known as Phase I), these cells with successive passages enter a period of gradually decreasing proliferation (Phase II), followed by complete cessation of growth (Phase III).[89] This cessation of growth is followed by a short terminal phase, corresponding to the last three or four doublings, that was called Phase IV by Macieira-Coelho and Taboury.[90]

Whether or not this *in vitro* model of aging is a valid one (for instance, see Reference 91) a number of studies have assessed different types of DNA repair competency and/or the accumulation of unrepaired damage in these cells as a function of passage number.

1. *DNA Damages Resulting in Chromosomal Aberrations*

Chromosomal aberrations can be formed "spontaneously" by the action of endogenous causes and they can be induced by DNA damaging agents. As an indicator of age-related DNA repair capacity, several investigators have examined the "spontaneous" level of chromosomal aberrations in metaphase cells of mammalian cultures as a function of *in vitro* passage level. Chromosomal aberrations can result from the presence of unrepaired DNA lesions.[92,93] Many types of DNA lesions can induce the same general classes of aberrations.[94-96] Consequently, a decline in the efficiency of any DNA repair process may give rise to an increase in the level of spontaneous aberrations. A decrease in DNA repair capability is not, however, the only possible mechanism by which increased levels of spontaneous aberrations could arise. Chromosomal aberrations could also occur as a result of interference with normal DNA synthesis and, by extrapolation, as a result of a decline in the competency of DNA synthesis.[97]

Several investigators have detected an increase in the frequency of spontaneous chromosomal aberrations in human fibroblasts aging *in vitro*.[98-102] Others have not observed such increases.[103-105] Where an increase in the frequency of chromosomal aberrations was observed, the aberration type largely involved an increased incidence of dicentric chromosomes. An increase in dicentric chromosomes could result from a delay in single-strand break rejoining, which offers a greater opportunity for open breaks to interact, or from an increase in the number of breaks formed due to more damage and/or to better repair recognition of existing damage. The increased occurrence of chromosomal aberrations in senescent cells has also been suggested to be a consequence of defective proteins and not a major cause of senescence.[105]

The spontaneous frequency of sister chromatid exchanges (SCE) as an indicator of mutagenicity and carcinogenicity is another cytogenetic phenomenon with possible relevance to the existence of DNA lesions and/or to DNA repair competency.[106] Schneider et al.[107] present a comprehensive survey on SCEs in mice and man, presenting data on spontaneous as well as on induced SCEs with aging. A significant reduction of induced SCEs was observed in late passage fibroblasts, while baseline SCE frequencies remain relatively stable. *In vivo*, the same results are found in bone marrow and spleen cells. In lymphocytes of humans, on the contrary, Schmidt and Sanger demonstrated a significant increase of SCE frequency with age.[108] More recent studies performed with trimethyltin and zirconium oxychloride could not establish such a correlation.[109,110]

Only a few studies in the induction of chromosomal aberrations in mammalian cell strains as a function of *in vitro* life span have been reported.[111] They could not find a correlation in human lymphocyte cultures of different population doublings (PD), whereas Kishi et al.[112] discovered an increase of dicentric and ring chromosomes in these cells during aging, as did Hartwig.[113] There is also reported a distinct increase of aberration frequencies induced by caffeine in human lymphocytes, paralleled by a longer G_2 duration.[114]

2. Excision Repair (ER)

The complex multienzyme system for excision repair can only be induced by genotoxic agents causing DNA damage. The principal agent for assessing nucleotide excision repair competency has been UV, but later on UV-like chemicals causing damages that are repaired by a similar long-patch repair were used. In proliferating human fibroblast cultures, excision repair capacity as measured by UDS declined at late passages.[115-117] Oxygen-induced damages in late passage human fibroblasts were not repaired at all.[118] However, in confluent cultures, UDS was observed to be independent of age.[119,120]

A problem with the interpretation of the experiments involving proliferating cells lies in the heterogeneity of the repair response among cells at late passages.[121] At later passages, not all cells are equally competent in UDS. This was also confirmed in mice by Kempf et al.,[122] who also found a significant decrease of UDS with the donor's age.

The correlation of ER with aging is to date a controversial issue, because there are numerous studies supporting it and as many refuting it. It seems that in the last decade the supporters prevailed. Vijg et al.[123] established a significant age-related decrease in the initial rate of rat fibroblast UDS — but not in the end level — a phenomenon that we also know from other enzymes. The ability to incise UV lesions in human peripheral lymphocytes was determined to be impaired in older age.[124] Neurons from human donors of different ages were used *in vitro* and the response of aging neurons to UV light was found limited.[125] A decrease of ER with aging in a subpopulation of human lymphocytes, but not in all cells, was established, an indication not to rely only on overall repair measurements.[126] If mice lymphocytes were treated with nicotinamide after UV irradiation, besides a decrease of UDS in untreated cells, an increase in the cells derived of both young and old mice was found.[127] The authors suggested that one of the limiting factors affecting the DNA repair activity is the level of intracellular NAD^+. The same authors investigated the age dependency of UDS in the lymphocytes of two strains of mice with different longevity.[128] Not only was an age-associated decline in both strains found, but also an earlier impairment of ER in the short-lived strain was determined.

One really big exception to the above-demonstrated body of "pros" is the work of Hasegawa et al.,[129] who maintained that human fibroblasts at a high population doubling level (PDL) incorporated the double label as compared to low PDL — but they arrested cells in the G_1 phase by lowering serum concentration.

There might be a connection between replication and excision repair, because in many investigations it was found that as the amount of scheduled synthesis of the culture decreased, so did the amount of UDS following UV irradiation. To determine if this correlation at the culture level also held at the cell level, the amount of both scheduled and unscheduled synthesis was measured by double-label radioautography in the same cell. These results indicate that there are two broad classes of cells at later passages: those that undergo a considerable degree of both syntheses, and those that undergo very little scheduled or unscheduled synthesis. Such data make it difficult to conclude that the failure of DNA repair is a cause of aging; rather they suggest that DNA synthesis and nucleotide excision repair decline coordinately. The respective reason might be the removal of preexisting DNA lesions, which would otherwise interfere with replication.[130]

Another type of lesion, however, does not appear to be removed at all in late passage cells. Mattern and Cerutti examined aging WI-38 cell nuclei and nuclear sonicates for their ability to specifically excise osmium tetroxide- or γ-ray-induced 5,6-dihydroxydihydrothymine residues.[131] Late passage cells exhibited a complete loss in their ability to excise these lesions.

In mouse embryo fibroblast cultures, UV-induced UDS and pyrimidine dimer release declined only in terminally senescent cultures.[132-134] These changes were reversed by spontaneous transformation of the cultures. However, primary rat fibroblasts underwent a loss in 4-nitroquinoline-1-oxide-induced repair synthesis and in the formation and repair of excision repair-related single-strand breaks by the third subculture.[132] UV- and γ-induced UDS in primary hamster embryo cultures were investigated. In agreement with the results observed in mouse embryo cells, active UV- and γ-induced UDS was present throughout their *in vitro* life span, ceasing only in terminally senescent cultures.[135] Also, transformed cells retained both the UDS activity and the single-strand break rejoining rates of early passage cells. Using host cell reactivation, an increase in reactivation, of UV-treated herpes simplex virus in UV-pretreated African green monkey kidney cells until passage 60 was detected, followed by a decline in reactivation.[136] Finally, in a chick fibroblast system a decline in UV-induced UDS in middle and late passage cells, in comparison with early passage populations, was observed.[137]

Possibly, DNA repair can be stimulated or repressed by the cell, depending on the situation. This would imply that a cell can tolerate a certain level of damage and will remove it only when it is necessary. This was the case in the above-mentioned correlation of replication and repair and might also be the case in the preferential repair of transcribed strands.[138] Mainly, the parts essential for survival are repaired. There also seems to exist a coupling between repair and transcription.[139]

3. Single- and Double-Strand Break Repair

Aging hypotheses assume that the accumulation of DNA damage result in strand breaks. Damage, as measured by single-strand breaks and estimated by alkaline elution techniques, accumulated in human fibroblasts cells aging *in vitro*, but the accumulation was only appreciable at passages close to senescence.[140] In agreement with this observation in human cells, an increase in single-strand breaks (measured by alkaline sucrose gradient centrifugation) but not of double-strand breaks (measured by neutral gradient centrifugation) in late passage fibroblasts was detected.[141] Qualitatively similar results — an accumulation of single-strand breaks at late passage levels — have also been obtained in mouse cell strains *in vitro*.[142]

Repair after γ-induced damage only occurred in stimulated lymphocytes and showed an age-associated decline.[128] The rate of rejoining of induced breakage has been extensively examined in human fibroblast cells at different *in vitro* passage levels. Clarkson and Painter examined X-ray-induced single-strand break rejoining in aging human embryonic lung fibroblast cells (WI-38) using alkaline sucrose gradient centrifugation.[143]

The rate of repair remained constant throughout the *in vitro* life span of the cell strain. The same results were obtained by Mayer et al.[144] They investigated human fibroblasts. Normal rates of single-strand break rejoining for WI-38 cells were also reported by Bradley et al.[145] using alkaline elution and alkaline sedimentation techniques. Suzuki et al.[140] found normal rates of break rejoining until the fibroblast cultures had reached very near the end of their *in vitro* life span, where a slight decrease was observed. Furthermore, cell survival, a measure of strand break rejoining capacity in combination with other repair systems, remained unaltered during the *in vitro* life span of these cells after exposure to X-rays and neutrons.[146,147] Using mild hypo- and hyperthermia, Mayer et al.[148] were not able to find an age-related change of repair as well as of strand breaks.

The following studies in human skin fibroblasts, lymphocytes, and leukocytes attained similar results. A decline in the rate of strand rejoining measured by alkaline sucrose gradient centrifugation as the cells approached senescence was observed.[149-151] While this decline in DNA repair capacity was more marked in cells at the end of their *in vitro* life span, it appeared to commence prior to any indication of terminal senescence.[135] This decline in single-strand break rejoining in midpassage (Phase II) cells was also observed in primary hamster embryo cultures.[135] Lymphocyte studies yielded not only a decrease in the repair of alkylating agent-induced damage that was neither cell cycle dependent nor correlated with the CD4+/CD8+ ratio, but also a decrease of DSB rejoining that was more pronounced in older women than men.[152,153] Leukocytes from older human donors following X-irradiation showed greater residual damage and less repair as compared to those of younger donors.[154] The authors used the technique of premature chromosome condensation for the measurement of chromatid repair in interphase nuclei.

A very important aspect of repair, only recently developed, should be mentioned here. The accumulation of DNA lesions and their repair is not a homogeneous process throughout the whole genome, but heterogeneous with respect to different genomic domains. That means, repair occurs selectively in expressed genes. While Kunisada et al.[155] reported no change in repair with age in transcribed sequences, using transfection of both fetal lung and of primary culture lung and skin human fibroblasts, Hanawalt et al.[156] pointed out that determination of overall genomic repair capacities does not give any information about preferential repair in selected genes. They put forward some experimental evidence: in differentiated rat myoblasts and PC12 neuron-like cells several expressed genes are repaired relatively efficiently but without strand specificity; and in human HT1080 fibroblasts differentiating in the presence of dexamethasone, they demonstrated enhanced repair in the induced gene for plasminogen activator inhibitor I, but a reduced repair rate in the suppressed urokinase plasminogen activator gene. The authors concluded that any attempted correlation of repair with aging should focus on the relevant genes in the tissue of interest. Therefore, Louda and Niedermüller attempted to isolate specific genes thought of as coding for longevity determinant strategies for the determination of their instability and of remaining damage with aging.[46]

V. SPECIES, MAXIMUM LIFE SPAN POTENTIAL (MLP), AND DNA REPAIR

The first investigation into a correlation of repair capacity with MLP was done by Hart and Setlow, who determined the initial rate and the maximum level of UDS in fetal mammalian fibroblasts.[157] If aging is a consequence of the accumulation of damage to DNA, animals with long life spans should have more efficient DNA repair systems. Hence, a number of experiments have been carried out in attempts to correlate life span with DNA repair proficiency. As a matter of fact, wide differences have been reported in the ability of cells from animals with different life spans to repair UV damage to their DNA. The usual measure of such repair has been UDS. UV has been used as the damaging agent in most studies for historical reasons: it was the first repair system to be carefully analyzed, the level of damage does not depend on metabolic activation, and the repair of this damage by nucleotide excision results in long patches of repair synthesis, thus making the amount of repair easy to estimate by UDS. However, repair measured by scintillation counting of incorporated ^{3}H-dThd depends on the endogenous nucleotide pool sizes, the average patch size, and the number of repaired regions per cell. Despite the fact that there have been many experiments attempting to correlate UDS after UV irradiation with life span, UV is probably a poor model for such studies since it is not a stress on existing species. Even in humans, skin cancer is a disease of old age, and it is hard to see how proficiency in UV repair would have any selective reproductive advantage. However, one could argue that the nucleotide excision repair elicited by UV damage is typical of that detected after many of the damages induced by chemicals such as polycyclic aromatic hydrocarbons.[158] A high level of UV repair would also imply a high level of repair of the DNA adducts induced by chemical compounds. These UV-mimetic adducts could affect cells in tissues other than skin; therefore, an efficient repair system of this type could have a selective advantage. On the other hand, the available epidemiological data on humans deficient in UV repair — xeroderma pigmentosum individuals — do *not* indicate that they have large numbers of internal cancers.[159] There is an inverse correlation between life span and the ability of fibroblasts from animals with different life spans to metabolize polycyclic aromatic hydrocarbons.[160,161] Short-lived animals would probably suffer from more DNA damage as a result of exposure to exogenous UV-mimetic chemicals requiring metabolic activation.

The following studies not only dealt with the comparison of different species, but also compared different strains of the same species and the comparison of diseased with normal individuals. The low excision repair of mouse compared to human not only is a property of fibroblasts *in vitro* but is also observed in skin.[162,163] It was shown that fibroblasts from three inbred mouse strains, ranging in life span from 300 to 900 days, showed UDS increasing with life span.[164] On the other hand, there was no observed difference in the amount of UV excision repair between embryonic cells from congeneic mouse strains differing by 30 to 40% in life span.[165] However, as judged from UDS measurements on lymphocytes, there may well be an interrelationship among three quantities — the histocompatibility complex, repair of UV damage, and life span — which could obscure a simple relationship between two of them.[166] Hart et al. showed that there was a large difference in UDS after UV irradiation in fibroblasts from *Mus* (3.4 years) and *Peromyscus* (8.2 years), the latter having about 2.5-fold more UDS than the former.[167] Moreover, the patch size for repair in the two sets of cells was the same, which indicated that there was probably a real difference in the numbers of UV photoproducts excised per cell. No difference was found between the two species in their ability to repair single-strand breaks introduced by γ-rays. Considering differences between diseased individuals with a shorter MLP and normal ones, Rebhorn and Pfeiffenberger found a marked reduction in repair capacities, as well as reduced *in vitro* life spans of trisomic fibroblast cultures, following damage by UV light.[168]

Three other extensive experiments have been completed which support the association between excision repair of UV damage and life span. One study was by Hart and Daniel, who measured repair among a number of primate species.[169] The data showed an excellent correlation with life span. The other was by Francis et al.,[170] who carefully examined the amount of excision repair from cells, usually fibroblasts, of 21 different species. They used the BrdUrd photolysis technique to measure both the number of repaired regions per 108 Da of DNA and the patch size. Again, there was a correlation between the number of repaired regions and the life span. These data give a good correlation on linear scales, whereas the data of Hart and Daniel for primates give a good relation between the logarithm of the life span and repair.[169] Moreover, it should be clear that a second difference between these experiments is the numbers chosen for life span: Hart and Daniel used 100 years as the life span of humans; Francis et al. used 80 years. Note also that the two studies give significantly different values for the repair by gorilla compared to human. Other authors established an earlier impairment of both proliferative and repair (UV- and γ-induced damage) in short-lived as compared to long-lived mouse strains.[128] A third series of measurements measured UDS in epithelial cells of the lenses of five species:[171] the correlation was excellent. The same was observed in isolated hepatocytes from species of different longevities for the lowest fluences, whereas this finding could not be confirmed for higher fluence levels.[172]

There are two large experimental exceptions to these correlations. The first exception involves the extensive data of Kato et al.[173] in which UV-induced UDS was investigated in fibroblast cells from 34 species representing 11 orders. Most of the cells investigated were derived from lung tissue explants obtained from animals of unknown ages. That represents a problem for the interpretation of the results, because other authors compared fetal fibroblasts. Obviously, there is no correlation between UDS and life span. Two orders of species destroy any correlation that might exist. If we omit Chiroptera and Primates from the data of Kato et al.,[173] there is a reasonable correlation between UDS and life span. We should not compare very different species, for instance, mammals and reptiles: excision repair in cells of the box turtle was measured.[174] Despite the 100-year life span of the box turtle, its excision repair is less than that of the mouse.

There were no publications on this matter found in the literature after 1985. It is unfortunate that there are no systematic data on the repair of the kinds of damages that arise from endogenous reactions. In one example, the level of repair activity of O^6-methylguanine activity in human liver is about tenfold greater than that in rat liver.[175] Thus, this repair system also conforms to the correlation between life span and repair. However, before generalizing these data to a correlation between life span and repair, the levels of endogenous reactions involved in alkylating DNA in humans and rats should also be known. Consequently, provided one does not go over too broad a range of mammalian species, there can be a close correlation between the excision repair of UV damage and life span. Although it is attractive to think that this correlation may have some causal relationship to aging, no good theoretical or experimental reasons have been advanced to support this point of view. It could be that many different types of repair activities are coordinately expressed, and that the findings for UV repair are only an indication that other, presumably more important, repair systems for living are correlated with life span.

VI. ORGANS AND SYSTEMS, AGING RATES, AND DNA REPAIR

A. In Vivo Repair Studies

The most prominent studied systems and organs are the skin, the liver and the brain. Several authors also examined repair in the heart, the kidney, the lung, the spleen, the skeletal muscle and the duodenum, and some groups investigated cells derived from individuals of different ages.

1. Damages Resulting in Chromosomal Aberrations

In vivo, three cellular systems have been examined for spontaneous chromosomal aberrations as a function of age. Two of the systems involve tissues which are normally quiescent — liver and peripheral lymphocytes — but which can be forced into active mitosis under the appropriate stimulus. The liver system was initially chosen because it offered an opportunity to examine a tissue that would have the potential of accumulating DNA lesions without their loss due to normal cellular turnover.[176] This system involves the partial destruction of the liver, either by subcutaneous injections of carbon tetrachloride or by partial hepatectomy.[177,178] While the liver is subsequently undergoing regeneration, metaphase or anaphase cells can be examined for chromosomal aberrations. Several investigators have observed an age-dependent increase in chromosomal aberrations in the liver of mice,[177] dogs,[179] guinea pigs,[180] and Chinese hamsters.[178] This age-dependent increase was inversely proportional to life span, increasing at a faster rate in inbred mouse strains with shorter life spans than in inbred mouse strains with longer life spans.[181] While this proportionality also held true for mice, guinea pigs, and dogs, Chinese hamsters appeared to be an exception. This discrepancy, however, could have been due to differences in the method of ascertainment.

In another *in vivo* cellular system, peripheral lymphocytes, no significant changes in the frequency of aberrations were found in the first years of investigations.[9] The peripheral blood lymphocyte system is extremely complex, however, and there are significant differences between the replicative rates of stimulated cells obtained from young and aged donors.[182] Consequently, differences in spontaneous aberration frequencies might be attributable to proliferative differences and not to the presence of unrepaired lesions in DNA. Other repair and aberration studies on lymphocytes were reported in Section IV.A.1, related to *in vitro* studies of lymphocyte cultures.

These studies were mostly related to the determination of chromosomal aberrations in humans as a function of age. In humans they have been limited to two cellular systems: skin fibroblasts and peripheral lymphocytes. In studies also involving ionizing radiation, an increase in aberration yields in peripheral blood lymphocytes from aged humans was observed.[183] Also, in a comparative approach, adult lung fibroblast contained more chromosomal aberrations after X-ray and neutron exposure *in vitro* than did comparably exposed embryonic lung fibroblasts.[184]

Chemical agents also can provoke the induction of chromosomal aberrations in lymphocyte cultures. Because peripheral blood lymphocytes from young and aged donor are stimulated and subsequently cycle at different rates, apparent differences in chromosomal aberration yields could be explained trivially by the differences in growth characteristics.[182] In experiments primarily directed at assessing the frequency of mitomycin

C-induced sister chromatid exchanges (SCE) in fibroblasts as a function of donor age, a greater incidence of chromosomal aberrations was observed in first-generation metaphase cells in cultures obtained from aged individuals (>75 years) than in cultures obtained from young ones (<25 years).[185] Similar results in human lymphocytes from donors of different ages are reported by Musilova et al.,[186] who found no age-dependent spontaneous SCE frequency, but a significantly induced SCE rate in old donors. Whether the result is due to greater chemical damage or to decreased repair capability is not known.[187] The findings of Lil'p on SCE induction in mouse bone marrow cells were not so clear, probably because she used two mouse strains that differed in repair capacity.[188]

2. Excision Repair

Excision repair is the best-studied repair system *in vivo*. Especially interesting is the comparison of different repair systems between mitotic and postmitotic cells. DNA damage would be particularly serious for postmitotic cells, as these include heart and brain cells. Therefore, myocardial cells isolated from newborn and adult rats were among the first cell types to be compared for UV-induced UDS. The adult cell exhibited a complete loss of repair capability.[189] However, because the newborn rat myocardial cells still evidenced some normal DNA synthesis, this observation could be attributed to the normal process of differentiation and not to aging. UV can only be used as a DNA damaging agent if cells are isolated from the organs and cultivated. To measure repair in the whole organ, other agents (alkylating) must be used. A more recent study that determined the number of alkylated nucleotides in mouse heart tissue found a 9-fold increase between 2 and 39 months.[190] This is in agreement with the findings of Niedermüller, who determined a significant reduction of ER capacity of about 50% from 9 to 28 months of age after damage by N-nitroso-methylurea (MNU).[65] MNU also was used as a damaging agent by other investigators to measure ER by UDS determination in mice bone marrow cells: a marked decrease of UDS from 10 to 74 weeks of age was noticed.[191] The completion of repair after stressors was measured in the hearts of rats of different age by Vasiliev and Meerson, who found the repair completed in young hearts 2 days and in adult hearts 3 days after exposure to stress — unfortunately, the authors did not dispose of aged rats.[192]

Retinal cells constitute another postmitotic cell system. Unfortunately, only the cells of chicken embryos were used for repair determination, and the results only reflect development and not aging. As a general rule, embryonic chicken cells are not very proficient in nucleotide excision repair.[137] A different result was obtained with rat retinal ganglion cells treated in organ culture with a number of chemical carcinogens and then assayed for UDS. There was no significant age-associated change in repair measured radioautographically.[193] Lens epithelial cells in rats also retained their UDS capacity throughout the life span of the animal.[194]

The third group of postmitotic cells investigated are those of the brain. Only recently the first reliable studies were published. De Sousa et al.[195] found decreases of UDS of up to 73% in mice neurons with aging. On the contrary, another group, determining DNA β-polymerase activity, found the highest polymerase activity in rat neurons as compared with other cells that did not change remarkably during aging.[196] The same was reported following studies of several repair enzymes in rat cerebral cortex neurons.[197] In two recently published reviews the same author conceded conflicting results regarding the age-dependent decline in repair capacity, but reported a high accumulation of damages in cerebral neurons.[198,199]

ER, measured by the incorporation of labeled precursors into DNA and UDS, measured by autoradiography, has been followed in the cells of several organs of species of different ages. UDS changes in several organs of hamsters between 8 and 520 days of age were reported; even at the older ages, only about 30% of the cells were labeled, indicating that the population was either heterogeneous in its repair capability or heterogeneous in its exposure to UV radiation.[200] This heterogeneity might present a problem if we investigate overall organ repair, because a change in a small number could be veiled by the unchanged main part of cells or genes. Nevertheless, Niedermüller could establish a significant decrease of ER capacity in some organs of the rat with aging.[65] DNA was damaged by MNU and 24 h later ER was measured. A significant decrease during aging from 9 to 28 months was found in the spleen, the lung, and the heart, but from 18 to 28 months only in the liver, the kidney, the testes, and the brain. No change was observed in the duodenum and skeletal muscle. On the other side, in one of the largest studies so far published on human DNA damage and aging, Zahn et al.[201] found an increase of damages with age in the DNA of human muscle tissue. These results show that it is not so easy to associate repair capacity with either mitotic or postmitotic cells, especially since in the same study SSB repair was reduced just in the testes and the brain only! When investigating spontaneous DNA breaks in rat brain and liver, an almost 2-fold increase in liver DNA from 6 to 36 months of age, but no change in brain DNA, was found.[202]

Primary hepatocyte cultures of rats of different age showed a markedly decreased incorporation of ^{3}H-thymidine with aging after damage by UV or bleomycin.[203] In contrast, following treatment with carcinogens and UV light, Sawada and Ishikawa could not find a decrease of UDS with aging in rat hepatocytes, but the cells revealed a significantly lower scheduled synthesis.[204]

Surprisingly, in human lymphocytes exposed to chemical agents such as AAAF and dimethylbenzanthracene, UDS tended to increase with donor age.[205] The investigators interpreted their results as indicating greater damage, but not greater repair, in the lymphocytes from older individuals. On the other hand, there seems to be an age-related decrease in UDS in human leukocytes (at least in subjects over 60 years) exposed to UV.[205] The correlation appeared to be a clear one, but the most impressive observation about these experiments on almost 60 individuals was the wide variation in UDS levels among individuals, independent of age. Such experiments were carried out in the presence of hydroxyurea and were done on a heterogeneous population of cells in which the estimate of UDS was made by scintillation counting. This experimental design would not permit the detection of wide variations among cell types. Similar results consistent with a decline in UDS capacity in humans with increasing subject age have also been reported.[206] The relationship between age and UDS in human peripheral blood lymphocytes after UV or after a UV-mimetic chemical is complicated in that there seem to be two kinetic components of UDS. One of the components correlates positively with age, the other negatively.[207] The wide variation in DNA repair capacity among lymphocytes indicates that there are parameters other than age or sex that are the major determinants of repair measured by UDS. Also, the levels of UV-induced excision repair in this system depend on the degree and extent of lymphocyte stimulation.[208] Consequently, these results might be artifactual and not reflect the true state of DNA repair capacity. Furthermore, cell survival of UV-exposed lymphocytes from aged individuals (60 to 90 years) appeared to equal the survival of comparably exposed lymphocytes from young individuals (17 to 40 years).[209] See also Section IV.A.2 for a comparison with *in vitro* aging of lymphocytes.

Studying parts of the intestinum as an example for mitotically active cells, several investigations are of interest. Decreases in repair after alkylation treatment have been observed in colonic mucosal cells of aging rats and in the liver cells from newborn and adult rats.[210,211] However, since the measures of repair were alkaline sucrose gradients in the former study and UDS in the latter, and since one of the most important alkylation products — O^6-methylguanine — gives no strand breakage or unscheduled synthesis upon repair, the significance of these observations is not apparent. Perhaps, the assays measure steps subsequent to the depurination of the alkylated DNA as a result of other methylation products. Removal of carcinogens was significantly reduced in liver and kidney of mice aged 14 months as compared to those aged 2 months.[212] Niedermüller could not find any change of ER capacity (or of SSB or DSB repair) up to this age in liver and kidney during the aging of the rat.[65] Using an assay system to measure the activity of the methyl acceptor protein specific for the repair of O^6-methylguanine damage, a process not capable of eliciting UDS, Waldstein et al.[213] detected comparable levels of activity in extracts of lymphocytes from individuals 60 years or younger. Older individuals have not yet been included in the study.

Removal of alkylated bases also was investigated in several organs of mice and rats. Following the determination of the activities of a glycosylase and a methyltransferase, a decrease of the glycosylase activity in liver, lungs, brain, and ovaries of mice during aging was found, but O^6-methylguanine-DNA methyltransferase did not change.[214] Likhachev et al.[215] could establish a decrease of alkyltransferase activity in liver, but not in kidney and leukocytes of rats with aging, kidney displayed the highest activity. The same O^6-methylguanine-DNA methyltransferase activity showed a significant decrease in rat liver with age.[216] And, finally, the removal of 7-methylguanine from DNA of mouse kidney decreased substantially with aging.[217] For the interpretation of these results we must establish that, with the exception of the last study, the authors determined baseline enzyme activities; in most of the cases comparing baseline with induced activities we find differences in favor of age changes of the latter ones. Most of the results raise the possibility that the older animals are at a higher risk than young adults following exposure to alkylating mutagens.

There exists a body of studies concerning repair in skin, either using whole skin or explanting fibroblasts in culture. Goldstein has published data in which DNA repair levels were compared in skin fibroblast cultures derived from young and aged donors.[115] He examined cell survival after UV exposure to early passage cultures of fetal, newborn, young, and aged origins and observed no significant differences in UV sensitivity. In agreement, Hall et al.[218] observed similar levels of colony forming ability in skin fibroblast cultures from young (3 days to 3 years) and old (84 to 94 years) donors exposed *in vitro* in UV.[218] These investigators also observed an equal ability to reactivate UV, MMS, or 4,5,8-trimethylpsoralen plus light-treated herpes simplex virus among these young and aged fibroblast cultures. Finally, in limited studies involving epidermal keratinocyte cultures established from a newborn and from aged adults (72 and 90 years of age), no significant differences in UV-induced rates of repair replication were detected,[219] and no significant differences were found in UV-induced UDS in cultures of chondrocytes derived from 23-, 43-, or 63-year-old adults or between chondrocytes from 3-month-old and 2-year-old rabbits,[220] although the rabbit chondrocytes were less proficient in UV repair than were human ones.[221] More recent studies yielded a diminished repair rate of *in vivo* irradiated (electrons) skin with aging.[222] The same authors examined the relationship between this finding and sensitivity of epidermal cells to the cytotoxic effect of the radiation. The greatest sensitivity was found in rats aged 2 and 728 days.[223] These results are in accordance with those of Niedermüller, who found the time course of ER capacity following damage by UV to be a Bateman function.[65] Using high UV doses the UDS level decreased markedly in mouse skin with age, whereas low UV doses or treatment with 4-hydroxyaminoquinoline-1-oxide brought about no age-dependent repair.[224] Finally, Mullaart et al.[225] reported that when using low UV doses skin cells (fibroblasts and keratinocytes) from young and old rats equally well removed pyrimidine dimers — this again could be a baseline effect.

3. Single- and Double-Strand Break Repair

While many types of unrepaired damages may be present in DNA, most *in vivo* investigations have been largely concerned with assessing the presence of single- or double-strand breaks. The first strong evidence that there might be an accumulation of DNA damage in the cells of older animals came from the work of Price et al.[226] and Modak and Price[227] on liver, heart, and brain cells from old and young mice. Single-strand DNA breaks could act as initiation points for DNA synthesis detected radioautographically by the incorporation of tritium-labeled triphosphate into acid insoluble material. Acid denaturation was used to possibly enhance the expression of such breaks. Denaturation increased the template activity in cells from both young and old animals, but appreciably more so in cells from old ones. Without denaturation, only brain cells exhibited an age-related increase in polymerase activity. The molecular weight of both single- and double-stranded DNA isolated from rat liver cells as a function of animal age was measured hydrodynamically.[228] Average molecular weight decreased approximately tenfold with increasing age, demonstrating an increase in single- and double-strand breaks. This result might appear to be indicative of a decline in strand break repair with age.

The alkaline sucrose sedimentation technique was used to detect the accumulation of single-strand breaks in aging animals.[229] Strand breaks accumulated in the muscle cells of older (i.e., 28 days vs. 1 day) rats and in the red blood cells of older chickens. As the authors suggested, this apparent increase in single-strand breaks might have reflected developmental changes or have been the result of the preparative procedure, and may not reflect *in vivo* aging. Wheeler and Lett used zonal centrifugation in alkali to investigate DNA from young and old dog neurons.[230] With age, the DNA was found to have a decreased molecular weight, indicative of a possible accumulation of unrepaired single-strand breaks. Alkaline sucrose gradient centrifugation to examine DNA isolated from aging mouse liver, spleen, thymus, and cerebellum for strand breakage was used.[231] Only hepatic DNA was observed to decrease in molecular weight with age. This decrease in molecular weight occurred, however, in mice between 1 to 2 and 14 months old. There was no further significant decrease in molecular weight after 14 months of age. All these results must be interpreted very cautiously because we know that the difference between the results obtained by using two different methods can be very high: Mullaart et al.[202] determined DNA breaks by the methods of alkaline sucrose gradient centrifugation and alkaline elution assay. The first method rendered up to 50,000 and the second only 800 breaks per liver cell of mice aged 6 months.

Other experiments showed that the DNA isolated from the liver of older mice acted as if it had many more single-stranded regions than the DNA from the liver of younger animals.[232] The amount of single-stranded DNA increased in the liver of older animals (i.e., after one-half of their life span) to as much as 25% of the total, making it improbable that this finding could result from only a small fraction of dead cells. Chetsanga and colleagues subsequently also examined the S_1 nuclease sensitivity of DNA from heart and brain of aging mice.[233,234] DNA from both organs exhibited an age-related increased sensitivity to S_1 digestion, but to a lesser extent than that observed for liver.[232] The increased S_1 sensitivity in aged mouse brain DNA correlated with a decrease in molecular weight detected by alkaline sucrose gradient centrifugation.[234] These results were not confirmed by Dean and Cutler.[235] These investigators observed a constant level of S_1 nuclease sensitivity and the same molecular weight in DNA obtained from liver, brain, spleen, and kidney of aging mice: discrepant data which remain unresolved.

Several investigations using other species (rabbits, dog neurons, mice brain, spleen, and liver cells) could not find a change of the number of SSBs.[230,236,237] In agreement with these results, the repair of strand breaks in hepatic DNA from young and aged rats treated with bleomycin is the same.[238] The survival of X-ray-exposed colonic cells in young (6 months) and old (24 months) mice also is identical.[239] On the other hand, in a study involving the survival of X-irradiated human lymphocytes obtained from donors of different ages, lymphocytes from aged individuals (60 to 90 years) were approximately twice as sensitive as lymphocytes from young individuals (17 to 40 years).[209] Singh et al.[240] examined basal DNA damage in human lymphocytes from aged donors and found a small overall increase but a high heterogeneity: in a subpopulation of highly damaged lymphocytes the increase was fivefold!

VII. SPECIAL PROBLEMS OF REPAIR

Within the limited space of such a review it is impossible to enter into, albeit important, other aspects of DNA repair. There is modulation of repair capacity (by chemicals, environmental influences, caloric restrictions or special diet, and so on), repair and diseases, repair and apoptosis, and repair in lower organisms or in mitochondria. A very interesting subject also would be the role of repair and aging in development of the organisms, recombination and gender differences during phylogeny and evolution. We take the liberty to politely refer to the literature on the subject.

VIII. DISCUSSION

If we carefully study the literature on repair and aging the evidence for and against a correlation of these events is nearly balanced until the middle of the 1980s. A slight predominance for such a correlation is obtained by additional studies relating repair capacity to the MLP and to certain genetic diseases. From 1985 through the present time many more experimental findings indicate a decrease of the capacity of several DNA repair mechanisms with aging than do not.

Surely we must discriminate between different repair processes. Thus, excision repair seems to have a good age dependency, SSB repair is probably maintained at a high level over a long period of the lifetime and reduced only in very old animals, whereas DSB repair is maintained during all of life; if one DSB is not repaired in a cell within 2 hours this cell would die.[57] Those cells would not contribute to the measured repair anymore — therefore the repair capacity related to the amount of DNA would always be the same. Postreplication repair has not yet been proved in mammalian DNA, but was suggested by Park and Cleaver.[241] Surely this repair has no significance in postmitotic cells or cells with a long G_1-phase (most of the cells in mammals).[241]

Next, we must direct our attention to the difference between baseline repair and induced repair. As we have seen, baseline repair in most cases does not show any age dependency, whereas induced repair capacity often is reduced during aging. Lindahl investigated repair systems for DNA damage by endogenous causes and found nearly no repair capacity for alkylated DNA, so that these damages therefore possibly accumulate with age.[242] On the other side, Mullaart et al.[243] reported that lesions produced by endogenous sources, as are base damages, apurinic sites, or single-strand breaks, are repaired rapidly and those of exogenous sources remain for a longer time in DNA, especially in older individuals. It is a common fact of most aging hypotheses that basic functions are maintained up to old age, while during any kind of stress that can lead to the death of senescent cells or organisms because the energy of vitality decreased below the energy value of the stressor the adaptation is reduced. Therefore, most of the induced reactions show a decreased performance with aging — the adaptive age parameters (for instance kidney, lung, heart, and immune function, the induction of heat shock proteins, and also repair).

The statistical variation of the repair activity — especially among old organisms and cells — is another problem that must be considered as to the interpretation of the results. Variation between species is not only correlated with MLP, but that it can also occur between species of the same MLP is very difficult to explain.

Agreement exists with regard to the sometimes large differences of the repair capacities between organs that change with aging. Possibly, organs with less repair capacity possess some spare systems to prevent DNA from damages (antioxidants, radical scavengers, enzymatic defense systems), or there also exists a high redundancy of functional elements within the DNA. Another possibility to substitute for highly efficient repair systems is a high replication rate of the DNA.

Finally we must consider the difference between *in vitro* and *in vivo* repair and the sometimes different results obtained. We are not convinced that *in vitro* studies are good models for *in vivo* investigations — too many control and regulation systems are missing, therefore conflicting results following use of even the same cells in these different systems might be true and must be interpreted specifically. Still, todays methodology raises some problems, because some methods are only suitable for *in vitro* determinations and many methods possibly cause artifacts, especially those that require previous isolation of DNA. Alkaline sucrose centrifugation for the determination of SSBs causes many more artificial breaks than do alkaline elution or nucleoid sedimentation that is done with homogenates of cells.

Because we know that DNA lesions accumulate with aging, we may interpret this fact either by an increased rate of damage induction caused by an overall impairment of metabolic events like protein synthesis and others, accompanied by constant levels of repair or/and by reduced repair capacity. Reduced protein synthesis might expose the proteins to post-translational damages, for instance glycation, on account of their longer half-life. We have reported evidence for both mechanisms. Final consequences might not only be changes in gene expression and impairment of important cell functions leading to aging phenomena, but also DNA sequence changes resulting from unrepaired lesions by following replication. Only recently, subtle methods for the determination of such mutations were developed.[244,245] The development of more sensitive assays will give us better information in the future.

Molecular defense systems, including DNA repair, must also have a certain degree of imperfection on account of system theoretical considerations.[246] From this view, and from the huge body of experimental results, we conclude that there exists a correlation between repair and aging. It might be impossible to decide if repair processes are dependent on aging or repair deficiency is the cause of aging (of course not the only cause) and responsible for aging and disease phenomena. But surely we can establish that repair events are — besides others — life maintenance systems and therefore belong to longevity determinant strategies.[87] A modulation and a desired retardation of the aging rate can only be achieved by specifically aimed interventions into these systems. One first goal could be equipping the genome of low-repair and short-lived organisms like the rat with a correct pattern of the repair genes of a long-lived species like humans by newly developed recombinant DNA techniques. Other more obvious procedures are to enhance the repair capacity by exogenous influences (caloric reduction already has proved to enhance repair and to prolong the life span). If it will be possible to improve DNA repair capacity in humans, who are possibly optimized to a perfect degree by evolution, we do not know — but we shall try!

REFERENCES

1. Kirkwood, T. B. L., Repair and its evolution. Survival versus reproduction, in *Physiological Ecology: An Evolutionary Approach to Resource Use*, Townsend, C.R. and Calow, P., Eds., Blackwell, London, 1981, 165.
2. Hofecker, G., Skalicky, M., Kment, A., and Niedermüller, H., Models of the biological age of the rat. A factor model of age parameters, *Mech. Ageing Dev.*, 14, 345, 1980.
3. Niedermüller, H., Skalicky, M., and Hofecker, G., Biological parameters of normal ageing using animal experiments, *Z. Gerontopsychol-psychiatr.*, 2, 201, 1989.
4. Hofecker, G., Niedermüller, H., and Skalicky, M., Assessment of modifications of the rate of aging in the rat, Arch. Gerontol. Geriatr., 12, 273, 1991.
5. Hofecker, G., Skalicky, M., and Niedermüller, H., What animal experiments can tell us about human biological age, in *Practical Handbook of Human Biological Age Determination*, Balin, A.K., Ed., CRC Press, Boca Raton, FL, 1994, 419.
6. Hart, R. W. and Trosko, J. E., DNA repair processes in mammals, in *Cellular Ageing: Concepts and Mechanisms*, Part I, Cutler, R.G., Ed., Karger, Basel, 1976, 134.
7. Tice, R. R., Aging and DNA-repair capability, in *The Genetics of Aging*, Schneider, E.L., Ed., Plenum Press, New York, 1978, 53.
8. Strehler, B. L. and Freeman, M. R., Randomness, redundancy and repair: roles and relevance to biological aging, *Mech. Ageing Dev.*, 14, 15, 1980.
9. Tice, R. R. and Setlow, R. B., DNA repair and replication in aging organisms and cells, in *Handbook of the Biology of Aging*, Finch, C.E. and Schneider, E.L., Eds, Van Nostrand Reinhold, New York, 1985, 173.
10. Niedermüller, H., Experimentell-gerontologische Untersuchungen zur DNA-Reparaturkapazität von Ratten, Habil.Schr., (thesis), Vet. Med. Univ. Vienna, 1977.
11. Kornberg, A., *DNA Replication*, W.H. Freeman, San Francisco, 1980.
12. Campbell, J. L., Eukaryotic DNA replication, *Ann. Rev. Biochem.*, 55, 733, 1986.
13. Kunkel, T. A., Schaaper, R. M., Beckman, R. A., and Loeb, L. A., On the fidelity of DNA replication. Effect of the next nucleotide on proofreading, *J. Biol. Chem.*, 256, 9883, 1981.

14. Loeb, L. A. and Kunkel, T. A., Fidelity of DNA synthesis, *Ann. Rev. Biochem.*, 52, 429, 1981.
15. Kunkel, T. A., Exonucleolytic proofreading, *Cell*, 53, 837, 1988.
16. Crine, P. and Verly, W. G., A study of DNA spontaneous degradation, *Biochim. Biophys. Acta*, 442, 50, 1976.
17. Saul, R. L. and Ames, B. N., Background levels of DNA damage in the population, in *Mechanisms of DNA Damage and Repair*, Simic, M., Grossman, L., and Upton, A., Eds., Plenum Press, New York, 1985, 529.
18. Lindahl, T., DNA repair enzymes acting on spontaneous lesions in DNA, in *DNA Repair Processes*, Nichols, W.W. and Murphy, D.G., Eds., Symposia Specialists, Miami, 1977, 225.
19. Harman, D., Aging: a theory based on free radical and radiation chemistry, *J. Gerontol.*, 11, 298, 1956.
20. Harman, D., The aging process, *Proc. Natl. Acad. Sci. U.S.A.*, 78, 7124, 1981.
21. Loeb, L. A., Endogenous carcinogenesis: molecular oncology into the twenty-first century. Presidential address, *Cancer Res.*, 49, 5489, 1989.
22. Saul, R. L., Gee, P., and Ames, B. N., Free Radicals, DNA damage and aging, in *Modern Biological Theories of Aging*, Warren, H.R., Butler, R.N., Sprott, R.L., and Schneider, E.L., Eds., Raven Press, New York, 1987, 113.
23. Cathcart, R., Schwiers, E., Saul, R. L., and Ames, B.N., Thymine glycol and thymidine glycol in human and rat urine: a possible assay for oxidative DNA damage, *Proc. Natl. Acad. Sci. U.S.A.*, 81, 5633, 1984.
24. Shigenaga, M. K., Gimeno, C. J., and Ames, B. N., Urinary 8-hydroxy-2'-deoxyguanosine as a biomarker of *in vivo* oxidative DNA damage, *Proc. Natl. Acad. Sci. U.S.A.*, 86, 9697, 1989.
25. Cerami, A., Aging of proteins and nucleic acids: what is the role of glucose?, *Trends Biochem. Sci.*, 11, 311, 1986.
26. Lee, T. A. and Cerami, A., Modification of proteins and nucleic acids by reducing sugars: possible role in aging, in *Handbook of the Biology of Aging*, Schneider, E.L. and Rowe, J.W., Academic Press, San Diego, 1990, 116.
27. Rydberg, B. and Lindahl, T., Nonenzymatic methylation of DNA by intracellular methyl group donor S-adenosyl-L-methionine is a potentially mutagenic reaction, *EMBO J.*, 1, 211, 1982.
28. Park, J.-W. and Ames, B. N., 7-Methylguanine adducts in DNA are normally present at high levels and increase on aging. Analysis by HPLC with electro-chemical detection, *Proc. Natl. Acad. Sci. U.S.A.*, 85, 7467, 1988.
29. Setlow, R. B., DNA repair, aging and cancer, *Natl. Cancer Inst. Monogr.*, 60, 259, 1982.
30. Fry, R. J. M., Grahn, D., Griem, M.L., and Rust, J. H., *Late Effects of Radiation*, Taylor & Francis, London, 1970.
31. Friedberg, E. C., *DNA Repair*, W.H. Freeman, New York, 1985, 1.
32. Mullaart, E., Lohman, P. H. M., Berends, F., and Vijg, J., DNA damage metabolism and aging, *Mutat. Res.*, 237, 189, 1990.
33. Woese, C. R., The primary lines of descent and the universal ancestor, in *Evolution from Molecules to Man*, Bendall, D.S., Ed., Cambridge University Press, London, 1983.
34. Hollaender, A. and Curtis, J. T., Effect of sublethal doses of monochromatic ultraviolet radiation on bacteria in liquid suspensions, *Proc. Soc. Exp. Biol. Med.*, 33, 61, 1935.
35. Watson, J. D. and Crick, F. H. C., Molecular structure of nucleic acids: a structure for deoxynucleic acids, *Nature*, 171, 737, 1953.
36. Howard-Flanders, P., Boyce, R. P., Simson, E., and Theriot, L., A genetic locus in E. coli K12 that controls the reactivation of UV-photoproducts associated with thymine in DNA, *Proc. Natl. Acad. Sci. U.S.A.*, 48, 2109, 1962.

37. Setlow, R. B. and Setlow, J. K., Effects of radiation on polynucleotides, *Ann. Rev. Biophys. Bioeng.*, 1, 293, 1972.
38. Hanawalt, P. C., Cooper, P. K., Ganesan, A. K., and Smith, C. A., DNA repair in bacteria and mammalian cells, *Ann. Rev. Biochem.*, 48, 783, 1979.
39. Friedberg, E. C., Ehmann, U. K., and Williams, J. , Human diseases associated with defective DNA repair, *Adv. Radiat. Biol.*, 8, 85, 1979.
40. Seeberg, E. and Kleppe, K., Eds., *Chromosome Damage and Repair*, Plenum Press, New York, 1981.
41. Bernstein, C. and Wallace, S. S., DNA repair, in *Bacteriophage T4*, Mathews, C.K., Kutter, E.M., Mosig, G., and Berget, P.B. Eds., American Society for Microbiology, Washington, D.C., 1983, 138.
42. Grossman, L., Caron, P. R., Mazur, S. J., and Oh, E. Y., Repair of DNA-containing pyrimidine dimers, *FASEB J.*, 2, 2696, 1988.
43. Wallace, S. S., AP endonucleases and DNA glycosylases that recognize oxidative DNA damage, *Environ. Molec. Mutagenesis*, 12, 431, 1988.
44. Mellon, , Bohr, V. A., Smith, C. A., and Hanawalt, P. C., Preferential DNA repair of an active gene in human cells, *Proc. Natl. Acad. Sci. U.S.A.*, 83, 8878, 1986.
45. VanDuin, M., van den Tol, J., Warmerdam, P., Odijk, H., Meijer, D., Westerveld, A., Bootsma, D., and Hoeijmakers, J. H. J., Evolution and mutagenesis of the mammalian excision repair gene ERCC-1, *Nucl. Acids Res.*, 16, 5305, 1988.
46. Louda, N. and Niedermüller, H., Age changes within the genome, in *Aspects of Aging and Disease*, Vienna Aging Series 4, Knook, D.L. and Hofecker, G., Eds., Facultas, Vienna, 1994, 61.
47. Sutherland, B. M., Photoreactivating enzymes, *The Enzymes*, 14, 481, 1981.
48. Rupert, C. S., Enzymatic photoreactivation. Overview, in *Molecular Mechanisms for Repair of DNA*, Part A, Hanawalt, P.C. and Setlow, R.B., Eds., Plenum Press, New York, 1975, 73.
49. Popp, F. A., Photon storage in biological systems, in *Electromagnetic Bio-Information*, Popp, F.A., Becker, G., König, H.L., and Peschka, W., Eds., Urban & Schwarzenberg, Baltimore, 1979, 123.
50. Yarosh, D. B., Rice, M., Ziolkowski, C. H., Day, R. S., III, and Scudiero, D. A., O⁶-methylguanine-DNA methyltransferase in human tumor cells, in *Cellular Responses to DNA Damage*, Friedberg, E.C. and Bridges, B.A., Eds., Alan R. Liss, New York, 1983, 261.
51. Renard, A., Lemaitre, M., and Verly, W. G., The O⁶-alkylguanine transferase activity in rat liver chromatin, in *Cellular Responses to DNA Damage*, Friedberg, E.C. and Bridges, B.A., Eds., Alan R. Liss, New York, 1983, 255.
52. Harris, A., Karran, P., and Lindahl, T., O⁶-methylguanine-DNA methyltransferase of human lymphoid cells, *Cancer Res.*, 43, 3247, 1983.
53. Villani, G., Boiteux, S., and Radman, M., Mechanism of ultraviolet-induced mutagenesis: extent and fidelity of in vitro DNA synthesis on irradiated templates, *Proc. Natl. Acad. Sci. U.S.A.*, 75, 3037, 1978.
54. Rupp, W. D., Wilde, C. E., III, Reno, D. L., and Howard-Flanders, P., Exchanges between DNA strands in ultraviolet-irradiated *Escherichia coli*, *J. Mol. Biol.*, 61, 25, 1971.
55. Kaufmann, W. K., Pathways of human cell post-replication repair, *Carcinogenesis*, 10, 1, 1989.
56. Ward, J. E., Blakely, W. F., and Jones, E. , Mammalian cells are not killed by DNA single-strand breaks caused by hydroxyl radicals from hydrogen peroxide, *Radiat. Res.*, 103, 383, 1985.
57. Van der Schans, G. P., Centen, H. P., and Lohman, P. H. M., DNA lesions induced by ionizing radiation, *Progr. Mut. Res.*, 4, 285, 1982.

58. Friedberg, E. C. and Hanawalt, P. C., *DNA Repair. A Laboratory Manual for Research Procedures*, Marcel Dekker, New York, 1981.

59. Carrier, W. L., Measurement of pyrimidine dimers by paper chromatography, in *DNA Repair. A Laboratory Manual for Research Procedures I*, Friedberg, E.C. and Hanawalt, P.C., Eds., Marcel Dekker, New York, 1981, 3.

60. Reynolds, R. J., Cook, K. H., and Friedberg, E. C., Measurement of thymine containing pyrimidine dimers by one-dimensional thin-layer chromatography, in *DNA Repair. A Laboratory Manual for Research Procedures I*, Friedberg, E.C. and Hanawalt, P.C., Eds., Marcel Dekker, New York, 1981, 11.

61. Sekiguchi, M. and Shimizu, K., Measurement of pyrimidine dimers by ion-exchange chromatography, in *DNA Repair. A Laboratory Manual for Research Procedures I*, Friedberg, E.C. and Hanawalt, P.C., Eds., Marcel Dekker, New York, 1981, 23.

62. Ganesan, A., Smith, C. A., and van Zeeland, A. A., Measurement of the pyrimidine dimer content of DNA in permeabilized bacterial or mammalian cells with endonuclease V of bacteriophage T4, in *DNA Repair. A Laboratory Manual for Research Procedures I*, Friedberg, E.C. and Hanawalt, P.C., Eds., Marcel Dekker, New York, 1981, 89.

63. Paterson, M. C., Smith, B. P., and Smith, P. J., Measurement of enzyme-sensitive sites in UV- or γ-irradiated human cells using *Micrococcus luteus* extracts, in *DNA Repair. A Laboratory Manual for Research Procedures I*, Friedberg, E.C. and Hanawalt, P.C., Eds., Marcel Dekker, New York, 1981, 99.

64. Niedermüller, H., Age dependency of DNA repair in rats after DNA damage by carcinogens, *Mech. Ageing Dev.*, 19, 259, 1982.

65. Niedermüller, H., DNA repair during aging, in *Molecular Biology of Aging. Gene Stability and Gene Expression*, Sohal, R.S., Birnbaum, L.S., and Cutler, R.G., Eds., Raven Press, New York, 1985, 173.

66. Cleaver, J. E. and Thomas, G. H., Measurement of unscheduled synthesis by autoradiography, in *DNA Repair. A Laboratory Manual for Research Procedures I*, Friedberg, E.C. and Hanawalt, P.C., Eds., Marcel Dekker, New York, 1981, 277.

67. Smith, C. A., Cooper, P. K., and Hanawalt, P. C., Measurement of repair replication by equilibrium sedimentation, in *DNA Repair. A Laboratory Manual for Research Procedures I*, Friedberg, E.C. and Hanawalt, P.C., Eds., Marcel Dekker, New York, 1981, 289.

68. Setlow, R. B. and Regan, J. D., Measurement of repair synthesis by photolysis of bromouracil, in *DNA Repair. A Laboratory Manual for Research Procedures I*, Friedberg, E.C. and Hanawalt, P.C., Eds., Marcel Dekker, New York, 1981, 307.

69. Day, R. F., III, Use of human adenoviruses 2 and 5. Purification, plaque assay and inactivation, in *DNA Repair. A Laboratory Manual for Research Procedures I*, Friedberg, E.C. and Hanawalt, P.C., Eds., Marcel Dekker, New York, 1981, 587.

70. Lett, J. T., Measurement of single-strand breaks by sedimentation in alkaline sucrose gradients, in *DNA Repair. A Laboratory Manual for Research Procedures I*, Friedberg, E.C. and Hanawalt, P.C., Eds., Marcel Dekker, New York, 1981, 363.

71. Kohn, K. W., Ewig, R. A. G., Erickson, L. C., and Zwelling, L. A., Measurements of strand breaks and cross-links by alkaline elution, in *DNA Repair. A Laboratory Manual for Research Procedures I*, Friedberg, E.C. and Hanawalt, P.C., Eds., Marcel Dekker, New York, 1981, 379.

72. Ahnström, G. and Erixon, K., Measurement of strand breaks by alkaline denaturation and hydroxyapatite chromatography, in *DNA Repair. A Laboratory Manual for Research Procedures I*, Friedberg, E.C. and Hanawalt, P.C., Eds., Marcel Dekker, New York, 1981, 403.

73. Hagen, U. F. W., Measurement of strand breaks by end labeling, in *DNA Repair. A Laboratory Manual for Research Procedures I*, Friedberg, E.C. and Hanawalt, P.C., Eds., Marcel Dekker, New York, 1981, 431.

74. Braun, A., Measurement of strand breaks by nitrocellulose membrane filtration, in *DNA Repair. A Laboratory Manual for Research Procedures I*, Friedberg, E.C. and Hanawalt, P.C., Eds., Marcel Dekker, New York, 1981, 447.

75. Wolff, S., Measurement of sister chromatid exchange in mammalian cells, in *DNA Repair. A Laboratory Manual for Research Procedures I*, Friedberg, E.C. and Hanawalt, P.C., Eds., Marcel Dekker, New York, 1981, 575.

76. Cook, P. R. and Brazell, A., Detection and repair of single-strand breaks in nuclear DNA, *Nature*, 263, 679, 1976.

77. Mattern, M. R., The relation of three-dimensional DNA structure to DNA repair as studied by nucleoid sedimentation, in *DNA Repair and its Inhibition*, Collins, A., Downes, C.S., and Johnson, R.T., Eds., IRL Press, Oxford, 1984, 35.

78. Lehmann, A. R., Measurement of postreplication repair in mammalian cells, in *DNA Repair. A Laboratory Manual for Research Procedures I*, Friedberg, E.C. and Hanawalt, P.C., Eds., Dekker, New York, 1981, 471.

79. Meyn, R. E. and Fletcher, S. E., Measurement of postreplication repair by alkaline elution, in *DNA Repair. A Laboratory Manual for Research Procedures I*, Friedberg, E.C. and Hanawalt, P.C., Eds., Marcel Dekker, New York, 1981, 487.

80. Lehmann, A. R. and Stevens, S., The production and repair of double strand breaks in cells from normal humans and from patients with ataxia telangiectasia, *Biochim. Biophys. Acta*, 474, 49, 1977.

81. Strehler, B. L., *Time, Cells and Aging*, Academic Press, New York, 1977, 10.

82. Cutler, R. G., Evolutionary biology of senescence, in *The Biology of Senescence*, Behnke, J.A., Finch, C.E., and Moment, G.B., Eds., Plenum Press, New York, 1978, 311.

83. Generoso, W. M., Cain, K. T., Krishna, M., and Huff, S. W., Genetic lesions induced by chemicals in spermatozoa and spermatids of mice are repaired in the egg, *Proc. Natl. Acad. Sci. U.S.A.*, 76, 435, 1979.

84. Kirkwood, T. B. L., The nature and causes of ageing, in *Research and the Ageing Population*, Evered, D. and Whelan, J., Eds., Wiley, Chichester, 1988, 193.

85. Kirkwood, T. B. L., DNA, mutations, and aging. Review, *Mutat. Res.*, 219, 1, 1988.

86. Kirkwood, T. B. L., Comparative and evolutionary aspects of longevity, in *Handbook of the Biology of Aging*, Finch, C.E. and Schneider, E.L., Eds., Van Nostrand Reinhold, New York, 1985, 27.

87. Cutler, R. G., Longevity is determined by specific genes: testing the hypothesis, in *Testing the Theories of Aging*, Adelman, R. and Roth, G., Eds., CRC Press, Boca Raton, FL, 1982, 25.

88. Hayflick, L., Current theories of biological ageing, *Fed. Proc., Fed. Am. Soc. Exp. Biol.*, 34, 9, 1975.

89. Hayflick, L., The limited in vitro lifespan of human diploid cell strains, *Exp. Cell. Res.*, 37, 614, 1965.

90. Macieira-Coelho, A. and Taboury, F., A reevaluation of the changes in proliferation in human fibroblasts during aging in vitro, *Cell. Tiss. Kinet.*, 15, 213, 1982.

91. Mitsui, Y. and Schneider, E. L., Characterization of fractionated human diploid fibroblast populations, *Exp. Cell Res.*, 103, 23, 1976.

92. Parrington, J. M., Delhanty, J. D. A., and Baden, H. P.,Unscheduled DNA synthesis, UV-induced chromosome aberrations and SV40 transformation in cultured cells from xeroderma pigmentosum, *Ann. Human Gen.*, 35, 149, 1971.

93. Sasaki, M. S., DNA repair capacity and susceptibility to chromosome breakage in xeroderma pigmentosum cells, *Mutat. Res.*, 20, 291, 1973.

94. Bender, M. A., Griggs, H. G., and Walker, P. L. Mechanism of chromosomal aberration production. Aberration induction by ultra-violet light, *Mutat. Res.*, 20, 387, 1973.

95. Bender, M. A., Bedford, J. S., and Mitchell, J. B., Mechanism of chromosomal aberration production. II. Aberrations induced by S-bromodeoxyuridine and visible light, *Mutat. Res.*, 20, 403, 1973.

96. Bender, M. A., Griggs, H. G., and Bedford, J. S., Mechanism of chromosomal aberration. III. Chemicals and ionizing radiation, *Mutat. Res.*, 23, 197, 1974.

97. Kihlman, B. A., *Actions of Chemicals on Dividing Cells*, Prentice-Hall, Englewood Cliffs, NJ, 1966.

98. Sax, H. J. and Passano, K. N., Spontaneous chromosome aberrations in human tissue cells, *Am. Nat.*, 95, 97, 1961.

99. Saksela, E. and Moorhead, P. S., Aneuploidy in the degenerative phase of serial cultivation of human cell strains, *Proc. Natl. Acad. Sci. U.S.A.*, 50, 390, 1963.

100. Thompson, K. V. A. and Holliday, R., Chromosome changes during the in vitro ageing of MRC-5 human fibroblasts, *Exp. Cell Res.*, 96, 1, 1975.

101. Benn, P. A., Specific chromosome aberrations in senescent fibroblast cell lines derived from human embryos, *Am. J. Hum. Genet.*, 28, 465, 1976.

102. Miller, R. C., Nichols, W. W., Pottash, J., and Aronson, M. M., In vitro aging. Cytogenetic comparison of diploid human fibroblasts and epithelial cell lines, *Exp. Cell Res.*, 110, 63, 1977.

103. Kadanka, Z. K., Sparkes, J. D., and Macmorine, H. G., A study of the cytogenetics of the human cell strain WI-38, *In Vitro*, 8, 353, 1973.

104. Chen, T. R. and Ruddle, F. H., Chromosome changes revealed by the Q-band staining method during cell senescence of WI-38, *Proc. Soc. Exp. Biol. Med.*, 147, 533, 1974.

105. Reis, R. J. S. and Goldstein, S., Loss of reiterated DNA sequences during serial passage of human diploid fibroblasts, *Cell*, 21, 739, 1980.

106. Wolff, S., Sister chromatid exchange, *Ann. Rev. Genet.*, 11, 183, 1977.

107. Schneider, E. L., Kram, D., Tice, R. R., Nakanishi, Y., Monticone, R. E., Bickings, C. K., and Gilman, B. A., Sister chromatid exchange in mice and man, in *Conference on Structural Pathology in DNA and the Biology of Ageing*, Verlag Chemie, Weinheim, 1980, 96.

108. Schmidt, M. A. and Sanger, W. G., Sister chromatid exchange in aged human lymphocytes. A brief note, *Mech. Ageing Dev.*, 16, 67, 1981.

109. Ghosh, B. B., Talukder, G., and Sharma, A., Frequency of sister chromatid exchanges induced by trimethyltin chloride in human peripheral blood lymphocytes as related to age of donors. A brief report, *Mech. Ageing Dev.*, 50, 95, 1989.

110. Ghosh, S., Talukder, G., and Sharma, A., Chromosomal alterations and sister chromatid exchanges induced by zirconium oxychloride in human lymphocytes in vitro with relation to age of donors, *Mech. Ageing Dev.*, 62, 245, 1992.

111. Fenech, M. and Morley, A. A., Ageing in vivo does not influence micronucleus induction in human lymphocytes by X-irradiation, *Mech. Ageing Dev.*, 39, 113, 1987.

112. Kishi, K., Homma, A., Kawa, A., and Kadowaki, K., Age related change in the frequency of ara C-induced chromosome aberrations in human peripheral blood lymphocytes, *Mech. Ageing Dev.*, 37, 211, 1987.

113. Hartwig, M., Altersabhängige strukturelle und funktionelle Änderungen in der DNA von menschlichen Lymphozyten, *Z. Alternsforsch.*, 41, 251, 1986.

114. Pincheira, J., Gallo, C., Bravo, M., Navarrete, M. H., and Lopez-Saez, J. F., G_2 repair and aging: influence of donor age on chromosomal aberrations in human lymphocytes, *Mutat. Res.*, 295, 55, 1993.

115. Goldstein, S., The role of DNA repair in aging of cultured fibroblasts from xeroderma pigmentosum and normals, *Proc. Soc. Exp. Biol. Med.*, 137, 730, 1971.

116. Painter, R. B., Clarkson, J. M., and Young, B. R., Ultraviolet-induced repair replication in aging diploid human cells, *Radiat. Res.*, 56, 560, 1973.

117. Bowman, P. D., Meek, R. L., and Daniel, C. W., Decreased unscheduled DNA synthesis in nondividing aged WI38 cells, *Mech. Ageing Dev.*, 5, 251, 1976.

118. Honda, S. and Matsuo, M., Lack of recovery from oxygen-induced damage to colony formation and DNA synthesis in senescent human diploid fibroblasts, *Mech. Ageing Dev.*, 40, 81, 1987.

119. Dell'Orco, R. T. and Whittle, W. L., Unscheduled DNA synthesis in confluent and mitotically arrested populations of aging human diploid fibroblasts, *Mech. Ageing Dev.*, 8, 269, 1978.

120. Dell'Orco, R. T. and Anderson, L. E., Unscheduled DNA synthesis in human diploid cells of different donor ages, *Cell Biol.-Intern. Rep.*, 5, 359, 1981.

121. Hart, R. W. and Setlow, R. B., DNA repair in late-passage human cells, *Mech. Ageing Dev.*, 5, 67, 1976.

122. Kempf, C., Schmitt, M., Danse, J. M., and Kempf, J., Correlation of DNA repair synthesis with aging in mice, evidenced by quantitative autoradiography, *Mech. Ageing Dev.*, 26, 183, 1984.

123. Vijg, J., Mullaart, E., Lohman, P. H., and Knook, D. L., UV-induced unscheduled DNA synthesis in fibroblasts of aging inbred rats, *Mutat. Res.*, 146, 197, 1985.

124. Hartwig, M. and Körner, J., Age-related changes of DNA winding and repair in human peripheral lymphocytes, *Mech. Ageing Dev.*, 38, 73, 1987.

125. Subrahmanyam, K. and Rao, K. S., UV light-induced unscheduled DNA synthesis in isolated neurons of rat brain of different ages, *Mech. Ageing Dev.*, 57, 283, 1991.

126. Singh, N. P., Danner, D. B., Tice, R. R., Brant, L., and Schneider, E. L., DNA damage and repair with age in individual human lymphocytes, *Mutat., Res.*, 237, 123, 1990.

127. Licastro, F. and Walford, R. L., Modulatory effect of nicotinamide on unscheduled DNA synthesis in lymphocytes from young and old mice, *Mech. Ageing Dev.*, 35, 123, 1986.

128. Licastro, F., and Walford, R. L., Proliferative potential and DNA repair in lymphocytes from short-lived and long-lived strains of mice, relation to aging, *Mech. Ageing Dev.*, 31, 171, 1985.

129. Hasegawa, N., Hanaoka, F., and Yamada, M.-A., Increased unscheduled DNA synthesis in aged human diploid fibroblasts, *Mech. Ageing Dev.*, 25, 297, 1984.

130. Gupta, P. K. and Sirover, M. A., Sequential stimulation of DNA repair and DNA replication in normal human cells, *Mutat. Res.*, 72, 273, 1980.

131. Mattern, M. R. and Cerutti, P. A., Age-dependent excision repair of damaged thymine from gamma-irradiated DNA by isolated nuclei from human fibroblasts, *Nature*, 254, 450, 1975.

132. Ben-Ishai, R. and Peleg, L., Excision-repair in primary cultures of mouse embryo cells and its decline in progressive passages and established cell lines, in *Molecular Mechanisms for Repair of DNA*, Hanawalt, P. and Setlow, R., Eds., Plenum Press, New York, 1975, 607.

133. Meek, R. L., Rebeiro, T., and Daniel, C. W., Patterns of unscheduled DNA synthesis in mouse embryo cells associated with in vitro aging and with spontaneous transformation to a continuous cell line, *Exp. Cell. Res.*, 129, 265, 1980.

134. Chan, A. C. and Walker, G., Loss of DNA repair capacity during successive subcultures of primary rat fibroblasts, *J. Cell. Biol.*, 74, 365, 1977.

135. Little, J. B., Relationship between DNA repair capacity and cellular aging, *Gerontology*, 22, 28, 1976.

136. Moore, S. P. and Coohill, T. P., An effect of cell culture passage on ultraviolet-enhanced viral reactivation by mammalian cells, *Mutat. Res.*, 62, 417, 1979.

137. Paterson, M. C., Lohman, P. H. M., and deWeerd-Kastelein, E. A., Photoreactivation and excision repair of ultraviolet radiation-injured DNA in primary embryonic chick cells, *Biophys. J.*, 14, 454, 1974.

138. Mellon, Spivak, G., and Hanawalt, P. C., Selective removal of transcription blocking DNA damage from the transcribed strand of the mammalian DHFR gene, *Cell*, 51, 241, 1987.

139. Mellon, and Hanawalt, P. C., Induction of the *Escherichia coli* lactose operon selectively increases repair of its transcribed DNA strand, *Nature*, 342, 95, 1989.

140. Suzuki, F., Watanabe, E., and Horikawa, M., Repair of X-ray-induced DNA damage in aging human diploid cells, *Exp. Cell. Res.*, 127, 299, 1980.

141. Icard, C., Beaupain, R., Diatloff, C., and Macieira-Coelho, A., Effects of low dose rate irradiation on the division potential of cells in vitro. VI. Changes in DNA and in radiosensitivity during aging of human fibroblasts, *Mech. Ageing Dev.*, 11, 269, 1979.

142. Beaupain, B., Icard, C., and Macieira-Coelho, A., Changes in DNA alkali-sensitive sites during senescence and establishment of fibroblasts in vitro, *Biochim. Biophys. Acta*, 606, 251, 1980.

143. Clarkson, J. M. and Painter, R. B., Repair of X-ray damage in ageing WI-38 cells, *Mutat. Res.*, 23, 107, 1974.

144. Mayer, P. J., Bradley, M. O., and Nichols, W. W., No change in DNA damage or repair of single- and double-strand breaks as human diploid fibroblasts age in vitro, *Exp. Cell Res.*, 166, 497, 1986.

145. Bradley, M. O., Erickson, L. C., and Kohn, K. W., Normal DNA strand rejoining and absence of DNA crosslinking in progeroid and aging human cells, *Mutat. Res.*, 37, 279, 1976.

146. Ban, S., Nikaido, O., and Sugahara, T., Acute and late effects of a single exposure of ionizing radiation on cultured human diploid cell populations, *Radiat. Res.*, 81, 120, 1980.

147. Ban, S., Ikushima, T., and Sugahara, T., Reduction in proliferative life span of human diploid cells after exposure to a reactor radiation beam, *Radiat. Res.*, 87, 1, 1981.

148. Mayer, P. J., Bradley, M. O., and Nichols, W. W., The effect of mild hypothermia (34°C) and mild hyperthermia (39°C) on DNA damage, repair and aging of human diploid fibroblasts, *Mech. Ageing Dev.*, 39, 203, 1987.

149. Epstein, J., Williams, J. R., and Little, J. B., Deficient DNA repair in human progeriod cells, *Proc. Natl. Acad. Sci. U.S.A.*, 70, 977, 1973.

150. Epstein, J., Williams, J. R., and Little, J. B., Role of DNA repair in progeric and normal human fibroblasts, *Biochem. Biophys. Res. Commun.*, 59, 850, 1974.

151. Little, J. B., Epstein, J., and Williams, J. R., Repair of DNA strand breaks in progeric fibroblasts and aging human diploid cells, in *Molecular Mechanisms for Repair of DNA*, Hanawalt, P.C. and Setlow, R.R., Eds., Plenum Press, New York, 1975, 793.

152. Hartshorn, J. N. and Robison, S. H., The relationship between DNA repair after alkylation damage and in vitro aging in human T-lymphocytes, *Mutat. Res.*, 237, 153, 1990.

153. Mayer, P. J., Lange, C. S., Bradley, M. O., and Nichols W. W., Gender differences in age-related decline in DNA double-strand break damage and repair in lymphocytes, *Ann. Hum. Biol.*, 18, 405, 1991.

154. Maillie, H. D., Baker, J. V., Simon, W., Watts, R. J., and Quinn, B. R., Age related rejoining of broken chromosomes in human leukocytes following X-irradiation, *Mech. Ageing Dev.*, 65, 229, 1992.

155. Kunisada, T., Miller, C. D., and Schneider, E. L., Ultraviolet light-induced DNA damage in transcribed sequences: no change in repair with age, *Mutat. Res.*, 237, 75, 1990.

156. Hanawalt, P. C., Gee, P., Ho, L., Hsu, R. K., and Kane, C. J., Genomic heterogeneity of DNA repair. Role in aging?, *Ann. N.Y. Acad. Sci.*, 663, 17, 1992.

157. Hart, R. W. and Setlow, R. B., Correlation between deoxynucleic acid excision repair and lifespan in a number of mammalian species, *Proc. Natl. Acad. Sci. U.S.A.*, 71, 2169, 1974.

158. Setlow, R. B., Repair-deficient human disorders and cancer, *Nature*, 271, 713, 1978.

159. Cairns, J., The origin of human cancers, *Nature*, 289, 353, 1981.

160. Moore, C. J. and Schwartz, A. G., Inverse correlation between species life span and capacity of cultured fibroblasts to convert benzo[a]pyrene to water-soluble metabolites, *Exp. Cell Res.*, 116, 359, 1978.

161. Schwartz, A. G. and Moore, C. J., Inverse correlation between species life span and capacity of cultured fibroblasts to bind 7,12-dimethylbenz[a]anthracence to DNA, *Exp. Cell Res.*, 109, 448, 1977.

162. Ley, R. D., Sedita, B. A., Grube, D. D., and Fry, R. J. M., Induction and persistence of pyrimidine dimers in the epidermal DNA of two strains uf hairless mice, *Cancer Res.*, 37, 3243, 1977.

163. Sutherland, B. M., Harber, L. C., and Kochevar, E., Pyrimidine dimer formation and repair in human skin, *Cancer Res.*, 40, 3181, 1980.

164. Paffenholz, V., Correlation between DNA repair of embryonic fibroblasts and different life span of 3 inbred mouse strains, *Mech. Ageing Dev.*, 7, 131, 1978.

165. Collier, E., Popp, D. M., Lee, W. H., and Regan, J. D., DNA repair in a congeneic repair of mice with different longevities, *Mech. Ageing Dev.*, 19, 141, 1982.

166. Hall, K. Y., Bergman, K., and Walford, R. L., DNA repair, H-2, and aging in NZB and CBA mice, *Tissue Antigens*, 16, 104, 1981.

167. Hart, R. W., Sacher, G. A., and Hoskins, T. L., DNA repair in a short- and a long-lived rodent species, *J. Gerontol.*, 34, 808, 1979.

168. Rebhorn, H. and Pfeiffenberger, H., In vitro life span and "unscheduled DNA synthesis" in subconfluent cultures and clones of trisomic and normal diploid fibroblasts, *Mech. Ageing Dev.*, 18, 201, 1981.

169. Hart, R. W. and Daniel, F. B., Genetic stability in vitro and in vivo, *Adv. Pathobiol.*, 7, 123, 1980.

170. Francis, A. A., Lee, W. H., and Regan, J. D., The relationship of DNA excision repair of ultraviolet induced lesions to the maximum life span of mammals, *Mech. Ageing Dev.*, 16, 181, 1981.

171. Treton, J. A. and Courtois, Y., Correlation between DNA excision repair and mammalian lifespan in lens epithelial cells, *Cell Biol. Int. Rep.*, 6, 253, 1982.

172. Maslansky, C. J. and Williams, G. M., Ultraviolet light-induced DNA repair synthesis in hepatocytes from species of different longevities, *Mech. Ageing Dev.*, 29, 191, 1985.

173. Kato, H., Harada, M., Tsuchija, K., and Moriwaki, K., Absence of correlation between DNA repair in ultraviolet irradiated mammalian cells and life span of the donor species, *Jpn. J. Genet.*, 55, 99, 1980.

174. Woodhead, A. D., Setlow, R. B., and Grist, E., DNA repair and longevity in three species of cold-blooded vertebrates, *Exp. Gerontol.*, 15, 301, 1980.

175. Montesano, R., Bresil, H., Likhachev, A., vonBahr, C., Roberfroid, M., and Pegg, A. E., Removal from DNA of O^6-methylguanine (O^6-MeG) by human liver fractions, *Proc. Am. Assoc. Cancer Res.*, 23, 11, 1982.

176. Curtis, H. J., Biological mechanisms underlying the aging process, *Science*, 141, 686, 1963.

177. Stevenson, K. G. and Curtis, H. J., Chromosome aberrations in irradiated and nitrogen mustard treated mice, *Radiat. Res.*, 15, 774, 1961.
178. Brooks, A. L., Mead, D. K., and Peters, R. F., Effect of ageing on the frequency of metaphase chromosome aberrations in the liver of the Chinese hamster, *J. Gerontol.*, 28, 452, 1973.
179. Curtis, H . J., Leith, J., and Tilley, J., Chromosome aberrations in liver cells of dogs of different ages, *J. Gerontol.*, 21, 268, 1966.
180. Curtis, H. J. and Miller, K., Chromosome aberrations in liver cells of guinea pigs, *J. Gerontol.*, 26, 292, 1971.
181. Crowley, C. and Curtis, H. J., The development of somatic mutations in mice with age, *Proc. Natl. Acad. Sci. U.S.A.*, 49, 626, 1963.
182. Tice, R. R., Schneider, E. L., Kram, D., and Thorne, P., Cytokinetic analysis of the impaired proliferative response of peripheral lymphocytes from aged humans to phytohemagglutinin, *J. Exp. Med.*, 140, 1029, 1979.
183. Deknudt, G. and Leonard, A., Aging and radiosensitivity of human somatic chromosomes, *Exp. Geront.*, 12, 237, 1977.
184. Bourgeois, C. A., Raynaud, N., Diatloff-Zito, C., and Macieira-Coelho, A., Effect of low dose ionizing radiation on the division potential of cells in vitro. VIII. Cytogenetic analysis of human fibroblasts, *Mech. Ageing Dev.*, 17, 225, 1981.
185. Schneider, E. L. and Gilman, B., Sister chromatid exchanges and aging. III. The effect of donor age on mutagen induced sister chromatid exchanges in human diploid fibroblasts, *Hum. Genet.*, 46, 57, 1979.
186. Musilova, J., Michalova, K., and Pacovsky, V., Induction of sister chromatid exchanges by mitomycin C in lymphocytes of young and old human donors, *Gerontology*, 30, 365, 1984.
187. Pero, R. W., Bryngelsson, C., Mitelman, F., Kornfalt, R., Thulin, J., and Norden, A., Interindividual variation in the responses of cultured human lymphocytes to exposure from DNA damaging chemical agents, *Mutat. Res.*, 53, 327, 1978.
188. Lil'p, I. G., The influence of age and genotype on the levels of sister chromatid exchanges in mouse bone marrow cells, *Genetika*, 20, 260, 1984.
189. Lampidis, T. J. and Shaiberger, G. E., Age-related loss of DNA repair synthesis in isolated rat myocardial cells, *Exp. Cell. Res.*, 96, 412, 1975.
190. Gaubatz, J. W., DNA damage during aging of mouse myocardium, *J. Mol. Cell Cardiol.*, 18, 1317, 1986.
191. Bond, S. L. and Singh, S. M., Methyl nitrosourea induced unscheduled DNA synthesis in vivo in mice. Effects of background genotype on excision repair during aging, *Mech. Ageing Dev.*, 41, 177, 1987.
192. Vasiliev, V. K. and Meerson, F. Z., Age-associated features of poststressor repair of myocardial DNA, *Byull. Eksp. Biol. Med.*, 98, 649, 1984.
193. Ishikawa, T., Takayama, S., and Kitagawa, T., DNA repair synthesis in rat retinal ganglion cells treated with chemical carcinogens or ultraviolet light in vitro with special reference to aging and repair level, *J. Natl. Cancer Inst.*, 61, 1101, 1978.
194. Treton, J. A. and Courtois, Y., Evolution of the distribution, proliferation and ultraviolet repair capacity of rat lens epithelial cells as a function of maturation and aging, *Mech. Ageing Dev.*, 15, 251, 1981.
195. De Sousa, J., de Boni, U., and Cinader, B., Age-related decrease in ultraviolet induced DNA repair in neurons but not in lymph node cells of inbred mice, *Mech. Ageing Dev.*, 36, 1, 1986.
196. Subrahmanyam, K. and Rao, K. S., On the type of DNA polymerase activity in neuronal, astroglial, and oligodendroglial cell fractions from young, adult and old rat brains, *Biochem. Int.*, 16, 1111, 1988.
197. Rao, K. S., DNA repair in developing and aging brain, *Proc. Indian Natl. Sci. Acad., Part B*, 56, 141, 1990.

198. Rao, K. S. and Loeb, L. A., DNA damage and repair in brain: relationship to aging, *Mutat. Res.*, 275, 317, 1992.

199. Rao, K. S., Genomic damage and its repair in young and aging brain, *Mol. Neurobiol.*, 7, 23, 1993.

200. Gensler, H. L., The effect of hamster age on U.V.-induced unscheduled DNA synthesis in freshly isolated lung and kidney cells, *Exp. Gerontol.*, 16, 59, 1981.

201. Zahn, R. K., Reinmüller, J., Beyer, R., and Pondeljak, V., Age-correlated DNA damage in human muscle tissue, *Mech. Ageing Dev.*, 41, 73, 1987.

202. Mullaart, E., Boerrigter, M. E. T. , Boer, G. J., and Vijg, J., Spontaneous DNA breaks in the rat brain during development and aging, *Mutat. Res.*, 237, 9, 1990.

203. Kennah, H. E., II, Coetzee, M. L., and Ove, P., A comparison of DNA repair synthesis in primary hepatocytes from young and old rats, *Mech. Ageing Dev.*, 29, 283, 1985.

204. Sawada, N. and Ishikawa, T., Reduction of potential for replicative but not unscheduled DNA synthesis in hepatocytes isolated from aged as compared to young rats, *Cancer Res.*, 48, 1618, 1988.

205. Lambert, B., Ringborg, U., and Skoog, L., Age-related decrease of ultraviolet light-induced DNA repair synthesis in human peripheral leukocytes, *Cancer Res.*, 39, 2792, 1979.

206. Lezhava, T. A., Prokofjeva, V. V., and Mikhelson, V. M., Reduction in UV-induced unscheduled DNA synthesis in human lymphocytes at an extreme age, *Tsitologica*, 11, 1360, 1979.

207. Pero, R. W. and Ostlund, C., Direct comparison in human resting lymphocytes of the inter-individual variations in unscheduled DNA synthesis induced by N-acetoxy-2-acetylaminofluorene and ultraviolet radiation, *Mutat. Res.*, 73, 349, 1980.

208. Darzynkiewicz, Z., Radiation induced DNA synthesis in normal and stimulated human lymphocytes, *Exp. Cell. Res.*, 69, 356, 1971.

209. Kutlaca, R., Seshadri, R., and Mosley, A. A., Effect of age on sensitivity of human lymphocytes to radiation. A brief note, *Mech. Ageing Dev.*, 19, 97, 1982.

210. Kanagalingam, K. and Balis, M. E., In vivo repair of rat intestinal DNA damage by alkylating agents, *Cancer*, 36, 2364, 1975.

211. Prodi, G., Arfellini, G., and Grilli, S., DNA repair in newborns, *Proc. Perugia Quadren. Int. Conf. Cancer*, 803, 1977.

212. Ball, S. S., Neshat, M. S., Mickey, M. R., and Walford, R. L., DNA damage and repair in female C57BL/10 mice of different ages injected with the carcinogen benzo[a]pyrene-trans-7,8-diol, *Mutat. Res.*, 219, 241, 1989.

213. Waldstein, E. A., Cao, E.-H., Bender, M. A., and Setlow, R. B., Abilities of extracts of human lymphocytes to remove O^6-methylguanine from DNA, *Mutat. Res.*, 95, 405, 1982.

214. Washington, W. J., Foote, R. S., Dunn, W. C., Generoso, W. M., and Mitra, S., Age-dependent modulation of tissue-specific repair activity for 3-methyladenine and O^6-methylguanine in DNA in inbred mice, *Mech. Ageing Dev.*, 48, 43, 1989.

215. Likhachev, A., Zhukovskaia, N. V., Anisimov, V. N., and Hall, J., The age-related dynamics of the activity of the DNA repair enzyme O^6-alkylguanine-DNA alkyltransferase in different organs of rats, *Vopr. Onkol.*, 37, 197, 1991.

216. Pardini, C., Mariani, L., Voliani, M., Rainaldi, G., and Citti, L., The ability of liver extracts from different-aged rats to repair 'mis-instructive' and 'non-instructive' lesions of DNA, *Mutat. Res.*, 275, 1, 1992.

217. Gaubatz, J. W. and Tan, B. H., Age-related studies on the removal of 7-methylguanine from DNA of mouse kidney tissue following N-methyl-N-nitrosourea treatment, *Mutat. Res.*, 295, 81, 1993.

218. Hall, J. D., Almy, R. E., and Scherer, K. L., DNA repair in cultured human fibroblasts does not decline with donor age, *Exp. Cell Res.*, 139, 351, 1982.
219. Liu, S. C. C., Parsons, C. S., and Hanawalt, P. C., DNA repair response in human epidermal keratinocytes from donors of different ages, *J. Invest. Dermatol.*, 79, 330, 1982.
220. Krystal, G., Morris, G. M., Lipman, J. M., and Sokoloff, L., DNA repair in articular chondrocytes. Unscheduled DNA synthesis following ultraviolet irradiation in monolayer culture, *Mech. Ageing Dev.*, 21, 83, 1983.
221. Setlow, R. B., Lipman, J. M., and Sokoloff, L., DNA repair by articular chondrocytes. II. Direct measurements of repair of ultraviolet and X-ray damage in monolayer cultures, *Mech. Ageing Dev.*, 21, 97, 1983.
222. Sargent, E. V. and Burns, F. J., Repair of radiation-induced DNA damage in rat epidermis as a function of age, *Radiat. Res.*, 102, 176, 1985.
223. Sargent, E. V. and Burns, F. J., Radioautographic measurement of radiation-induced epidermal kinetic effects in different aged rats, *J. Invest. Dermatol.*, 88, 320, 1987.
224. Ishikawa, T. and Sakurai, J., In vivo studies on age-dependency of DNA repair with age in mouse skin, *Cancer Res.*, 46, 1344, 1986.
225. Mullaart, E., Roza, L., Lohman, P. H. M., and Vijg, J., The removal of UV-induced pyrimidine dimers from DNA of rat skin cells in vitro and in vivo in relation to aging, *Mech. Ageing Dev.*, 47, 253, 1989.
226. Price, G. B., Modak, S. P., and Makinodan, T., Age-associated changes in the DNA of mouse tissue, *Science*, 171, 917, 1971.
227. Modak, S. P. and Price, G. B., Exogenous DNA polymerase-catalyzed incorporation of deoxyribo-nucleotide monophosphates in nuclei of fixed mouse-brain cells, *Exp. Cell Res.*, 65, 289, 1971.
228. Massie, H. R., Baird, M. B., Nicolosi, R. J., and Samis, H. V., Changes in the structure of rat liver DNA in relation to age, *Arch. Biochem. Biophys.*, 153, 736, 1972.
229. Karran, P. and Ormerod, M. G., Is the ability to repair damages to DNA related to the proliferative capacity of a cell? The rejoining of X-ray-produced strand breaks, *Biochim. Biophys. Acta*, 229, 54, 1973.
230. Wheeler, K. T. and Lett, J. T., On the possibility that DNA repair is related to age in nondividing cells, *Proc. Natl. Acad. Sci. U.S.A.*, 71, 1862, 1974.
231. Ono, T., Okada, S., and Sugahara, T., Comparative studies of DNA size in various tissues of mice during the aging process, *Exp. Gerontol.*, 11, 127, 1976.
232. Chetsanga, C. J., Boyd, V., Peterson, L., and Rushlow, K., Single-stranded regions in DNA of old mice, *Nature*, 253, 130, 1975.
233. Chetsanga, C. J., Tuttle, M., and Jacoboni, A., Changes in structural integrity of heart DNA from aging mice, *Life Sci.*, 18, 1405, 1976.
234. Chetsanga, C. J., Tuttle, M., Jacoboni, A., and Johnson, C., Age-associated structural alterations in senescent mouse brain DNA, *Biochim. Biophys. Acta*, 474, 180, 1977.
235. Dean, R. G. and Cutler, R. G., Absence of significant age-dependent increase of single-stranded DNA extracted from mouse liver nuclei, *Exp. Geront.*, 13, 287, 1978.
236. Lett, J. T., Keng, P. C., and Sun, C., Rejoining of DNA strand breaks in nondividing cells irradiated in situ, in *DNA Repair Mechanisms*, Hanawalt, P.C., Friedberg, E.C., and Fox, C.F., Eds., Academic Press, New York, 1978, 481.
237. Ono, T. and Okada, S., Does the capacity to rejoin radiation-induced DNA breaks decline in senescent mice?, *Int. J. Radiat. Biol.*, 33, 403, 1978.

238. Ove, P. and Coetzee, M. L., A difference in bleomycin-induced DNA synthesis between liver nuclei from mature and old rats, *Mech. Ageing Dev.*, 8, 363, 1978.

239. Hamilton, E. and Franks, L. M., Cell proliferation and ageing in mouse colon. II. Late effects of repeated X-irradiation in young and old mice, *Eur. J. Cancer*, 16, 663, 1980.

240. Singh, N. P., Danner, D. B., Tice, R. R., Pearson, J. D., Brant, L. J., Morrell, C. H., and Schneider, E. L., Basal DNA damage in individual human lymphocytes with age, *Mutat. Res.*, 256, 1, 1991.

241. Park, S. D. and Cleaver, J. E., Postreplication repair: questions of its definition and possible alteration in xeroderma pigmentosum cell strains, *Proc. Natl. Acad. Sci. U.S.A.*, 76, 3927, 1979.

242. Lindahl, T., Repair of intrinsic lesions, *Mutat. Res.*, 238, 305, 1990.

243. Mullaart, E., Boerrigter, M. E. T., Lohman, P. H. M., and Vijg, J., Age-related induction and disappearance of carcinogen-DNA-adducts in livers of rats exposed to low levels of 2-acetylaminofluorene, *Chem.-Biol. Interact.*, 69, 373, 1989.

244. Uitterlinden, A. G., Slagboom, P. E., Knook, D. L., and Vijg, J., Two-dimensional DNA fingerprinting of human individuals, *Proc. Natl. Acad. Sci. U.S.A.*, 86, 2742, 1989.

245. Kovar, H., Jug, G., Auer, H., Skern, T., and Blaas, D., Two-dimensional single-strand conformation polymorphism analysis: a useful tool for the detection of mutations in long DNA fragments, *Nucl. Acids Res.*, 19, 3507, 1991.

246. Rosen, R., Feedforwards and global system failure. A general mechanism for senescence, *J. Theor. Biol.*, 74, 579, 1978.

Chapter **4**

CHANGES IN GENE EXPRESSION DURING AGING OF MAMMALS

M. S. Kanungo

CONTENTS

0-8493-4786-6/95/$0.00+$.50
© 1995 by CRC Press, Inc.

I. INTRODUCTION

Several phenotypic changes occur in a mammal after it attains adulthood. These are the results of the changes in the levels and activities of proteins/enzymes that are coded by specific genes. For example, a decrease in the level of the enzyme tyrosinase leads to graying of hair in old age. The level of collagenase declines, leading to a decreasing turnover of collagen. This increases cross-linking between collagen fibrils and, in turn, an increase in the tensile strength of collagen. Wrinkling of the skin in the elderly is the result of these changes. The changes in the cell membrane that alter its permeability may be due to changes in its lipid components which are synthesized by specific enzymes. The levels of several enzymes are known to decrease with age, leading to a decline in metabolism and organ function, and deterioration of functions of the organism. Thus, the functional changes that occur after adulthood at the molecular, cellular, and organic levels are due to changes in the activities of specific enzymes/ proteins that are coded by specific genes. Nutrition, environmental and intrinsic factors, and stresses of various kinds such as temperature, radiation, pollution, and psychological stress, however, influence the rate and degree of such changes in different individuals of the same species. Hence, one finds variability in the rates of aging of different organs, and in different individuals of a species. The fact that all individuals of a species have the same pattern of life span indicates that the primary reason for a functional change is due to one or more genes that code for enzymes/ proteins responsible for the change. Hence, an understanding of the changes in gene expression during aging may give insight into the basic cause of aging. This may help in postponing the onset of old age or prolonging the period of adulthood.

Beginning from the early 1980s, researchers have been engaged in studying the changes in the expression of various genes of rats and mice as they age. However, whether the genes being studied are crucial for aging is not known. The basic question is: are there one or several genes that cause aging? If so, where are they located, and how and when are they expressed? It is unlikely that one gene alone is responsible for aging because if a single gene that caused aging appeared during evolution, it might have been selected out or eliminated as it would be detrimental for the perpetuation of the species. It is more likely that expression of several genes may be involved, i.e., different genes in different organs of a mammal are implicated in the aging process. Neither the number nor the identity of these gene is known at present. These are the questions which the biochemists and molecular biologists seek to answer. The use of genetic engineering techniques to quantitate specific messenger RNAs (mRNAs), understanding the role of promoter regions, especially of the *cis*-acting elements, in the regulation of gene expression, the role of modification of bases, etc., are beginning to throw much light on the types of changes that occur in the expression of genes as an animal ages. The alterations that occur in the expression of genes during aging in various animals and the factors that influence them have been described recently by Kanungo.[1]

II. GENE EXPRESSION *IN VIVO*

It is comparatively easy to study the changes in the expression of genes during early development as the changes are rapid, generally localized, and specifically timed in each organ of an embryo. On the other hand, the changes that occur after adulthood are slower, and vary among individuals both in location and timing. Moreover, the total number of genes being expressed in the embryo is relatively small. In adulthood the number of genes being expressed in all the organs of an organism is enormous, and to single out from this large number the genes whose expressions are changing is extremely difficult. Cells of different organs, especially those having postmitotic and differentiated cells, differ in the types of genes that are expressed in them, though certain housekeeping genes may be common. Is the functional decline or aging in these organs due to the genes that are being expressed in all of them, or due to the unique genes that confer differentiated status to each of them? If it is the former, a common gene may be found that is switched on or off at a specific time in each organ. If it is the latter, the reason for aging of different organs, especially those having postmitotic differentiated cells, at different times in the life span of the animal, and the reason for different rates of their aging, may be found by studying the expression of these unique genes. Thus, the search for a common gene or a common set of genes that causes aging may be futile. A more desirable approach may be to compare the changes in the organ-specific genes as a function of age. So far, it has not been possible to carry out such extensive studies because of the enormous number of genes that are expressed in each organ, and the lack of sufficiently sensitive techniques. Hence, certain genes which have been cloned and are inducible have been studied.

Three types of changes may occur in the expression of genes as an organism ages: those whose expression decreases, those whose expression increases, and those whose expression does not change. Moreover, certain genes that are not expressed up to adulthood may become activated after this stage and begin to be expressed. Examples of the above category of genes are described below.

A. Genes for Enzymes

Cytochrome P-450s are microsomal enzymes that range in molecular weight from 50 to 60 kilodaltons (kDa). They are multisubstrate monooxygenases that are involved in the biosynthesis and degradation of steroids, fatty acids, prostaglandins, biogenic amines, pheromones, phytolexins, etc. They also metabolize most drugs, chemical carcinogens, mutagens, and several environmental pollutants.[2] Mammalian liver contains high levels of these enzymes. They are also present in extrahepatic tissues. At least 5 cytochrome P-450 gene families, each consisting of 2 or more than 20 genes and pseudogenes, have been reported.[3] They have a protective role for the organism as they metabolize and detoxify various pollutants. Cytochrome P-450s also have several biosynthetic functions. Other interesting features of these enzymes are their inducibility by several xenobiotics, such as phenobarbital (PB) and β-naphthoflavone (β-NF) and their sex differences.

Horbach and van Bezooijen[4] measured the mRNA levels of cytochrome P-450IIB1 and B2 in the liver of 3-, 12-, 24-, and 36-month-old male rats by solution hybridization. No significant differences were seen in the mRNA levels. However, the inducibility of its gene by PB in the 36-month-old rats was only one-third of that of 12-month-old rats. Also, in the old rats there was a longer lag period for the induction of the enzymes and for them to reach the maximum level. A similar decrease in induction was seen for cytochrome P-450 IIA1 and A2 mRNAs.

Since feeding a restricted diet has been shown to prolong life span of rats,[5] its effect on induction of cytochrome P-450 mRNA was studied.[4] Those given food *ad libitum* lived up to 22 to 30 months, and those given restricted (60%) diet lived to 36 to 45 months. The level of the enzyme was also higher in the rats given a restricted diet, which indicated that the drug metabolizing capacity may be higher in these rats. This is consistent with the finding that the level of mRNA for cytochrome P-450 BII1 and BII2 was nearly twofold higher in the rats given the restricted diet.

Rath and Kanungo[6] studied the induction of cytochrome P-450(b+e) gene in 21- and 120-week-old female rats. The gene is induced in the liver, but not in the brain and kidney. Its induction by PB is far greater in the young female than in the older rats. On the other hand, the level of cytochrome P-450(b+e) mRNA decreases with increasing age in male rats.[7] Also, its inducibility by PB is lower in the old. Young and old male rats

Figure 1
Southern hybridization of DNA fragments with the 5' cytochrome P-450 gene. Nuclei of the liver of young and old rats that had been administered phenobarbital were digested with different concentrations of MNase (2, 5, 10, and 20 units/mg DNA). The DNA fragments were resolved in 1.7% agarose gel, transferred to a nytran filter, and hybridized to a ^{32}P-labeled 1.1 kbp fragment of the promoter region of the gene.[1] (From Kanùngo, M. S., *Genes and Aging,* Cambridge University Press, New York, 1994. With permission.)

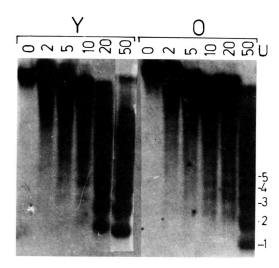

were administered PB, then nuclei were purified from the liver and digested by micrococcal nuclease (MNase). The DNA fragments were resolved by gel electrophoresis. Southern hybridization with a 1.0-kilobase pair (kbp) labeled probe containing 800 bp of the promoter region and the first exon of cytochrome P-450(b+e) gene showed that, after PB administration, nucleosomes in the promoter region relax more in the young than in the old[7] (Figure 1). Hence, the nucleosomal organization of the promoter region of the gene may be more compact in the old, which may be the reason for the lower induction by PB. Furthermore, it was also shown that there are three DNase I hypersensitive (DH) sites in the promoter region of the gene in young rats, but only two in the old. The presence of DH-sites have been correlated with expression of genes. Thus, the lower expression and induction of the cytochrome P-450(b+e) gene in old rats is due to conformational changes in the chromatin containing the promoter region of the gene.

The expression of the genes for acetyl CoA carboxylase and fatty acid synthetase has been studied in the liver of rats as a function of age.[8] The time course of transcription of the two genes was measured after refeeding a fat-free diet to fasted rats. The levels of the two mRNAs in the liver of old rats (18 months) were 40 to 70% of those of young (1.5 months) rats. Transcriptional rates increased within 1 h in young rats after refeeding, but after a lag of 6 h in old rats. The mRNA concentrations reached the highest level after 16 h in the young, but after 24 h in the old. There was no difference, however, in the rate of translation of the mRNA in young and old rats. Hence the decrease in the induction of the two enzymes is due to the decrease in the transcription of their genes.

Since free radicals have been implicated in the aging process due to their deleterious effects on macromolecules,[9] the enzymes that scavenge and detoxify free radicals have received considerable attention in aging studies. These enzymes are superoxide dismutase (SOD), catalase, and glutathione reductase. Mammalian SOD is a 32-kDa dimer with two copper and two zinc atoms (Cu-Zn SOD). Superoxide radical ($\cdot O_2^-$) is produced by the reaction

$$O_2 + e^\cdot \rightarrow \cdot O_2^-$$

$\cdot O_2^-$ is very toxic and harmful to tissues as it inactivates proteins and nucleic acids. It is neutralized by SOD as follows:

$$\cdot O_2^- + \cdot O_2^- + 2H^+ \rightarrow 2H_2O_2 + O_2$$

H_2O_2 is less toxic and is neutralized by catalase as follows:

$$2H_2O_2 \rightarrow 2H_2O + O_2$$

Thus, SOD is essential for neutralization of the superoxide radical which is constantly produced in mitochondria.

Tolmasoff et al.[10] have shown that there is a positive correlation between the specific activity of SOD, the metabolic rate, and the maximum life span potential of different mammalian species. That is, mammals with a long life span have higher SOD activity per metabolic rate. Semsei et al.[11] found that not only the activities of SOD and catalase decrease in the liver of the rat with increasing age, but also the levels of their mRNAs, and run-on transcription of the genes are lower in the old. However, if the rats are kept under dietary restriction (60% normal diet), then both nuclear run-on transcription and the levels of mRNAs increase. Also, the average life span of the rats increases by 30% when they are kept under restricted diet.

B. Genes for Other Proteins

Fibronectins (FNT) are high molecular weight glycoproteins having two nonidentical subunits, each of 220 to 240 kDa. They are linked by –S–S– bonds. FNTs are involved in differentiation, migration, adhesion of cells, and also wound healing, hemostasis, and tumor metastasis.[12] They are synthesized in the liver and secreted to the plasma. A single FNT gene is present per haploid genome in rodents and mammals. It is located in chromosome 2 in the rat, spans ~70 kbp, and has 50 exons. Subunit variants of FNTs are generated by alternative splicing of primary transcripts.[13] The promoter region of the gene contains several *cis*-acting

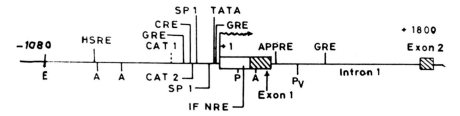

Figure 2

Map of the rat fibronectin gene showing *cis*-acting elements and restriction sites in the 5' region. Restriction sites: A, Ava I; E, EcoRI; P, PstI; Pv, PvuI. Hatched box exon: CRE, cAMP response element; CAT, CCAAT; GRE, glucocorticoid response element; IFNRE, interferon response element; Sp1, Sp1 protein binding site.[1] (From Kanungo, M. S., *Genes and Aging*, Cambridge University Press, New York, 1994. With permission.)

elements including TATAA, CCAAT, GGGCGG, and responsive element for cAMP (CRE), glucocorticoid (GRE), and heat shock (HSRE) that take part in transcriptional regulation[14] (Figure 2).

Expression of the FNT gene in the rat liver as a function of age of the rat has been studied by Singh and Kanungo.[15,16] The level of FNT protein in the plasma of a 125-week-old rat is significantly lower than that of a 20-week-old rat. This may be due to a lower rate of transcription as seen by run-on nuclear transcription, and a lower steady-state level of mRNA as measured by slot-blot hybridization with a labeled complementary DNA (cDNA) probe. Digestion of nuclei of liver by DNAase I, followed by restriction of the DNA and Southern hybridization with a 1.2-kbp probe encompassing the promoter region of the gene, revealed three DH-sites, one overlapping the CRE, the second in the TATA region, and the third in the first intron. The DH-sites in the promoter are more susceptible to DNAase I in the young than in the old. There is no difference in the methylation status of 5'-CCGG-3' sequences of the promoter of young and old rats, as seen by MspI/HpaII digestion of nuclei followed by Southern hybridization with the probe.

The FNT mRNA is about 8.0 kb long. Nuclear run-on transcription assay shows that its transcription in the liver is less than 10% of that of albumin.[16] Cyclic AMP is known to stimulate the expression of the gene. This is brought about by cAMP binding to *trans*-acting factors which then bind to the CRE in the promoter. Whether or not the levels of *trans*-acting factors change with age was studied by using a labeled 25-bp-long (25-mer) synthetic double-stranded DNA (dsDNA) containing the CRE sequence (TGACGTCA). It was incubated with nuclear extract of the liver from 2-, 25-, and 110-week-old male rats, and the number of *trans*-acting factors that bind to it, and their levels, were assayed by gel mobility shift. Three specific proteins were found to bind to the 25-mer DNA, and their levels were significantly lower in the older rat (Figure 3). The expression

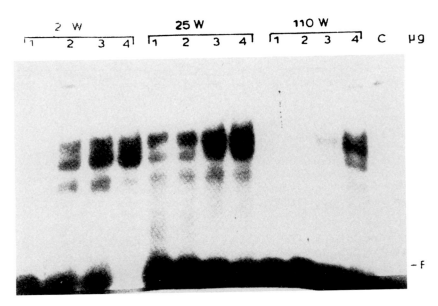

Figure 3
Mobility shift assay of 25-base-pair-long (25-mer) double-stranded DNA (dsDNA) containing the cAMP response element (–TGACGTCA–) present in the promoter region of the fibronectin gene. Nuclear extract (1 to 4 µg) of the liver of 2-, 25-, and 110-week-old male rats was titrated with the 25-mer dsDNA, electrophoresed, blotted, and autoradiographed.[1] (From Kanugo, M.S., *Genes and Aging*, Cambridge University Press, New York, 1994. With permission.)

of the FNT gene was significantly higher in the young. This is the first report on the role of a promoter in the age-related expression of an important gene that codes for a multifunctional protein. It shows that the lower expression of the FNT gene in the older rat may be due to the decrease in the *trans*-acting factors that bind to a *cis*-acting element (CRE) in the promoter, and are required for stimulation of its transcription. Also, conformational changes in the chromatin regions in the promoter, as revealed by DNAase I digestion, may alter the expression of the gene.

Roy et al.[17] have studied the expression of α2µ-globulin genes which are not only age specific but also are hormone responsive. These plasma proteins of ~18.5 kDa are coded by a cluster of genes present in chromosome 5 of the rat. They are synthesized in the liver and secreted to the blood. Northern blot hybridization using poly-A[+] mRNAs and cDNA probe for the gene showed that the gene is expressed from about day 40 in the liver of male rats, and its expression totally ceases after about day 900 (Figure 4). There is a corresponding decrease in α2µ-globulin synthesis in the liver. The protein has five variants. Variant 2 is the dominant

75   750   900

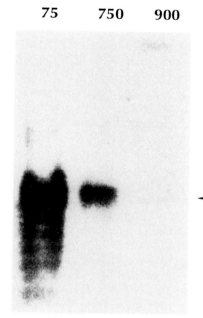

Figure 4
Decline in hepatic α2μ-globulin mRNA during aging. Autoradiograph shows the extent of hybridization of a ^{32}P-labeled cloned α2μ-globulin cDNA probe with electrophoretically separated hepatic mRNA obtained from 75-, 750-, and 900-day-old male rats. (From Roy, A. K., Nath, T. S., Motwani, N. M., and Chatterjee, B., *J. Biol. Chem.*, 258, 10123, 1983. With permission.)

form which appears first at puberty. Variant 4 is the last to disappear at senescence. Thus, the genes in the cluster may be differentially regulated. Richardson et al.[18] showed that if rats are kept on a 40% restricted diet, both the transcription and the level of α2μ-globulin mRNA increase. Thus, the decrease in the protein that occurs with increasing age is due to lower transcription of the gene.

The age-dependent expression of the α2μ-globulin gene correlates well with the appearance and disappearance of cytoplasmic androgen-binding protein (AR) in the liver. AR is absent before day 40, and disappears after about day 800. It was shown that its gene becomes sensitive to DNAase I after about day 20 and retains the sensitivity for the rest of the life span.[19] The gene is not expressed after about day 900. Hence DNAase I sensitivity is not the only requirement for its expression.

Song et al.[20] found that AR is expressed in the hepatocytes. The steady-state level of AR mRNA correlates with the three phases of hepatic androgen sensitivity, that is, insensitivity to androgen during prepuberty, responsiveness during adulthood, and gradual loss of responsiveness during aging. Both prepubertal and senescent rats are relatively insensitive to the induction of α2μ-globulin. The age-dependent decline in AR mRNA can be delayed by reducing caloric intake by 40%. Thus, it appears that changes in androgen sensitivity of the liver during aging is due to the age-dependent expression of AR-mRNA and the level of AR. The expression of the AR gene appears to be due to a *cis*-acting element present in its promoter.[21] It has two contiguous sites, one of 19 bp that binds to a nuclear androgen-dependent factor (ADF), and another of 25 bp that binds to an associated factor (AF). ADF appears to be ubiquitous and is evolutionarily conserved, whereas AF is tissue specific. Thus the age-dependent androgen responsiveness of the gene appears to be modulated through this sequence.

The expression of two other genes of the liver of the rat that code for age-related proteins, senescence marker proteins SMP-1 and SMP-2, have also been studied by Roy and co-workers.[22] SMP-1 is 34 kDa and SMP-2 is 31 kDa. SMP-1, an androgen-responsive gene, begins to be expressed from day 40 and its expression stops after 750 days. However, SMP-2 is expressed until 40 days after birth and is then repressed. Its expression is restored after 750 days. Thus it is androgen repressible. Its expression, however, is high in young and adult females. Thus, whereas the expression of SMP-1 decreases during senescence due to the decrease in androgen level, that of SMP-2 increases. Fujita et al.[23] have detected a 30-kDa protein in the soluble fraction of the liver of the rat which decreases with age, independent of androgen. It has been designated senescence marker protein-30 (SMP-30). Its expression is not altered by castration or treatment with testosterone after castration. It is also present in female rats. This protein is distinct from SMP-1 and SMP-2 mentioned above.

Kanungo and co-workers[24] have shown by dot-blot hybridization of a 1.0-kbp cDNA probe for albumin with the RNA purified from the liver of male rats, and by nuclear run-on transcription, that the level of albumin mRNA and the expression of its gene decrease up to 85 weeks. This is consistent with their finding that the DNAase I sensitivity of its promoter decreases with age. There is also an increase in cytosine methylation in the –CCGG– sequences of the promoter region of the gene as revealed by digestion of the chromatin by restriction enzymes, MspI and HpaII, followed by Southern hybridization with the probe. The level of α-fetoprotein mRNA of the liver of young (6 months) rat, however, is not different from that of old (29 months) rat.[25]

The expression of calbindins (calcium-binding proteins) is regulated by 1,25-dihydroxyvitamin D_3. They are present in large amounts in the proximal intestine (calbindin D-9K) and kidney (calbindin D-28K), and are involved in calcium transport. Absorption of Ca^{2+} declines in the intestine and kidney with increasing age. Armbrecht et al.[26] found that the level of D-9K mRNA declines from ages 2 to 6 months in the intestine, as does the level of the proteins. Surprisingly, the level of its mRNA increases between 13 to 24 months, but the level of the protein continues to decline. Apparently, translation of the mRNA is deficient. In the kidney, the level of the mRNA for calbindin D-28K declines between 2 to 13 months, then plateaus, as does the level of the protein. No changes, however, are seen in the expression of the gene for calmodulin, which is also involved in calcium transport.

The expression of the calbindin-28K gene not only changes during aging, but also in neurodegenerative diseases.[27] The levels of its mRNA and protein decrease by 60 to 80% in different ages of the brain. It also decreases in the areas that are implicated in specific diseases such as substantia nigra in Parkinson's disease, nucleus basalis in Alzheimer's disease, and both the hippocampus and nucleus raphe dorsalis in Parkinson's, Huntington's, and Alzheimer's diseases. The decrease in the expression of the calbindin gene and lower levels of calbindin may impair calcium buffering or intraneuronal calcium homeostasis, which may contribute to calcium-mediated cytotoxic effects during aging, and pathogenesis of neurodegenerative diseases.

Friedman et al.[28] have reported significant changes in the expression of five genes in old age. They prepared cDNA libraries from 3- and 27-month-old whole mice using poly-A[+] mRNAs. The mRNAs were screened by hybridization with cDNAs of various tissues from these mice. Though the functions of these genes are not known, such approaches are useful in identifying changes in the tissue-specific expression of genes.

The level of epidermal growth factor mRNA has been shown to decrease by 75% between 12 to 27 months of age in male mice.[29] Whittenmore et al.[30] found that β-nerve growth factor (β-NGF) mRNA level increases up to 47 weeks in the brain and then decreases. Goss et al.[31] have reported a significant increase in the level of mRNA for glial fibrillary acidic protein which is astrocyte specific. There is, however, no change in the level of mRNA of glutamine synthetase which is also astrocyte specific. Astrocytes are involved in several brain functions such as neurotransmitter uptake, synthesis of trophic factors and hormones, regulation of synaptic density, regulation of cerebral blood flow, etc. Since glial cells outnumber neurons in the brain, research on age-related changes in these cells may throw much light on the aging of the brain, and of the organism.

The role of gonadotropin-releasing hormone (GnRH), and β-endorphin (βE), an opioid peptide derived from proopiomelanocortin (POMC), in reproductive functions of male rats has been studied.[32] βE has a toxic effect on GnRH. The POMC mRNA level decreases significantly in old age. Also, the number of neurons expressing the POMC gene decreases with age. Hence βE synthesis also decreases with age.

Wismer et al.[33] studied the expression of β-actin and β-tubulin genes in the rat brain using cDNA probes for these genes. Northern and dot-blot hybridization of their mRNAs with the labeled probes do not show any significant change in their levels as a function of age. The levels of these mRNAs are different in different regions of the brain, but no age-related differences are seen in their levels in any region.

C. Stress-Induced Genes

1. Acute Phase Reactants

Infection, wounding, or chronic diseases cause inflammation in an animal resulting in significant changes in the levels of plasma proteins. This response takes place primarily in the liver and is called "acute phase reaction", in which hepatic genes are stimulated leading to production of proteins that enter the blood. Several plasma proteins, such as T-kininogen, fibrinogen, α-1-acid glycoprotein, C-reactive protein, hemopexin, ceruloplasmin, and haptoglobin increase in level. These are called "positive acute phase reactants". Certain proteins such as albumin, transthyretin, 2-HS-glycoprotein, transferrin, and apolipoprotein A-1 decrease in level. They are "negative acute phase reactants".

Sierra et al.[34] have identified genes that specifically change in expression during aging. They constructed a cDNA library from the mRNA of the liver of an old rat (24 months), and by differential screening with those of young rats (10 months) found that the expression of the T-kininogen gene is higher in the old rats. Its product, T-kininogen, is a positive acute phase protein which is also called cysteine proteinase inhibitor or thiostatin. Nuclear elongation experiments showed that the increase in its expression in the old liver is transcriptionally regulated. They have also studied the expression of the T-kininogen gene in young and old rats after administration of turpentine, which causes acute phase reaction. No significant change in the expression of the gene or the level of the protein in the plasma was noticed as a function of age after 24 h. On the other hand, the level of another acute phase protein, γ_2-macroglobulin, significantly decreased both during aging and after acute phase reaction.

The expression of the T-kininogen gene appears to be age related since it is silent up to 18 months in the rat[34,35] and abruptly increases thereafter. The level of T-kininogen in the serum is also higher in the old rat. There is no change in the methylation status of the gene, such as hypomethylation of –CCGG– sequences, which may account for its higher expression. It is likely that its age dependent increase may be due to humoral factors because no differences are seen in its expression when hepatocytes of young and old rats are cultured *in vitro*. A subunit of cytochrome oxidase also increases with age, but it does not show the abrupt increase in expression that is seen for T-kininogen. Though the role of the T-kininogen protein in acute phase reaction is not known, it is evident from these studies that the response of some genes to stress in old animals is different from that of young animals. This may destabilize the physiology of the animal in old age and lead to functional decline.

Haptoglobin, another positive acute phase protein present in plasma, binds to free hemoglobin released from ruptured red cells. It is synthesized in the liver. Its mRNA level increases by twofold in 16-month-old mice and by fourfold in 28-month-old mice after inflammation, though their albumin mRNA level does not change appreciably.[36] The ceruloplasmin mRNA level also increases like that of haptoglobin. Ceruloplasmin binds to free copper, and protects the brain from copper toxicity. The elevation of ceruloplasmin and haptoglobin mRNA levels indicate that these are related to age and to inflammatory responses.

2. Heat Stress

Genes that respond to heat stress have been studied in relation to age. They are expressed under heat stress and code for heat shock proteins (HSPs). Other stresses such as heavy metals, free radicals, and amino acid analogs also cause expression of these genes. They are highly conserved. Their major role is to maintain the tertiary structures of proteins, prevent denaturation of sensitive proteins, and thus protect cells from death. Several *hsp* genes are known that code for 60-, 70-, and 90-kDa proteins. Hence these proteins are called HSP-60, HSP-70, and HSP-90, respectively. Of these, the *hsp*-70 gene has been extensively studied.

Blake et al.[37] found that when young and old rats are exposed to 40°C for various durations, the rise in colonic temperature in old rats is slower than in young rats. The expression of the *hsp*-70 gene is lower in the brain, lung, and skin of old rats after a specific time period. However, when the colonic temperature of the old rat reaches 42°C, it produces the same amount of *hsp*-70 mRNA as that of young rat at 40°C.

Since the *hsp*-70 gene is expressed after exposure to stresses other than temperature, its expression after subjecting rats to mobility restraint stress has also been studied.[38] Rats were restricted from mobility for 30 min to 6 h, RNA was purified from various tissues, and expression of *hsp*-70 mRNA was assayed by northern blot hybridization. Its expression was greatly enhanced in the adrenal and pituitary, but no significant differences were seen in the brain, muscle, liver, heart, kidney, spleen, and thymus. Hypophysectomy suppressed its expression after stress. Administration of ACTH induced its expression in the adrenal. So ACTH is a physiologic regulator of the expression of *hsp*-70 in the adrenal. Restraint-induced expression of *hsp*-70 declines with age. It has also been shown that a cellular protein, heat shock factor (HSF), which binds to the heat shock element (HSE) in the promoter region of the *hsp*-70 gene, is induced in the adrenal after restraint stress. Whether the induction of HSF alters with age needs to be studied.

The expression of the *hsp*-70 gene in the hepatocytes of rats kept on a restricted diet that extended their life span by 30%, was studied by Wu et al.[39] Hepatocytes from 6- and 28-month-old rats were incubated for 30 min at 42.5°C to induce a heat-shock response, and were then returned to 37°C. The induction of *hsp* mRNA in old hepatocytes was 40 to 50% of that of young rats (Figure 5). This was found to be due to a decline in transcription. The age-related decline is reversed if the rats are kept under a calorie-

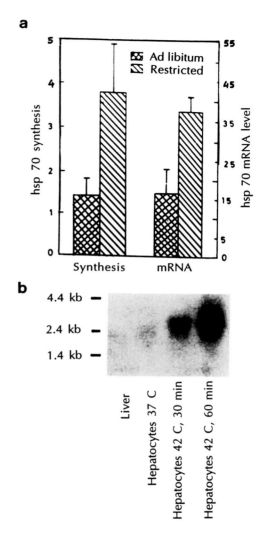

Figure 5
(a) Induction of HSP70 synthesis and mRNA levels by heat shock in hepatocytes isolated from 28-month-old rats fed an *ad libitum* or calorie restricted diet. (b) Comparison of hsp mRNA levels in liver and hepatocytes before and after heat shock. Northern blot of RNA isolated from liver and hepatocytes incubated at 37°C and 42°C. (From Wu, B., Heydari, A. R., Conrad, C. C., and Richardson, A., *Liver and Aging*, Kitani, K., Ed., Excerpta Medica, Amsterdam, 1991. With permission.)

restricted diet. Gel-shift assay shows that the binding of the transcription factor to the HSE decreases with age and is significantly higher in the heat-shocked hepatocytes of rats fed a restricted diet.[40] Hepatocytes of old (28-months) rats kept on *ad libitum* diet or restricted diet (60% of the *ad lib* diet) were then used for induction of HSP-70 protein by examining the incorporation of ^{35}S-methionine. It was found to be twofold higher in the hepatocytes of 28-month-old rats fed calorie-restricted diets in comparison to those of 28-month-old rats given *ad lib* diets.[40] Thus, dietary restriction enhances induction of *hsp*-70 genes and enables hepatocytes to respond to heat stress better. How a restricted diet induces this better response is not known.

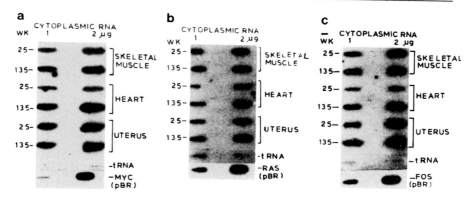

Figure 6

Determination of the levels of mRNA of (a) c-*myc*, (b) c-Ha-*ras*, and (c) c-*fos* in the skeletal muscle, heart, and uterus of young (25-week) and old (135-week) female rats by slot-blot hybridization. Cytoplasmic RNA, 1 and 2 μg, was used. tRNA was used as negative control. pBR containing c-*myc*, c-*fos*, and c-Has-*ras* was used with respective blots as positive control. (Jaiswal, Y. K. and Kanungo, M. S., unpublished data).

D. Oncogenes

Several oncogenes have been implicated in tumor growth. Since the frequency of occurrence of tumors is reported to be higher in old age, Kanungo and co-workers studied the expression of several oncogenes in various tissues of young and old rats by dot-blot hybridization (Y. K. Jaiswal and M. S. Kanungo, unpublished, Figure 6). They found that the mRNA levels of the oncogenes, c-*fos*, c-*myc*, and c-Ha-*ras*, are higher in the old heart. Such overexpression of oncogenes may make the heart more prone to hypertrophy. The expression of c-*fos* and c-*myc* oncogenes also was found to be higher in the brain and liver of old rats.

Fujita and Maruyama[41] measured the mRNA levels of c-*jun* and c-*fos* oncogenes in the liver of 6- to 7- and 24- to 25-month-old male and female rats by northern hybridization. The levels of both the mRNAs were significantly higher in old rats. The protein coded by the c-*fos* oncogene has been implicated in cell proliferation. It is likely that its expression gets stimulated in old rats due to certain unknown factors. Likewise, the *myc* family of oncogenes has been shown to be expressed in several tissues of old mice.[42]

E. Expression of *trans*-genes

Transgenic mice have been used as models to study the types of changes that occur in genes during aging, and the way the responses of genes alter under various types of stress. The responses of human genes to stress after insertion in the mouse genome have been studied.[43,44] Human plasma protein gene promoters have been fused with the bacterial chloramphenicol acetyltransferase (CAT) reporter gene, and the chimeric gene then transfected into a mouse egg to study the regulatory role of promoters of human genes as the mouse developed and aged. Also, the responses of the human genes to hormones, heavy metals, and inflammation have been examined. The expression of several human plasma proteins such as α1-antitrypsin, transthyretin, transferrin. C-reactive protein, and apolipoprotein A-1 have been studied.

Transferrin gene codes for the plasma protein, transferrin, that binds to ferric ion and transports it to target organs. Different segments of the promoter of the human transferrin gene were fused to the bacterial CAT gene, and introduced into the mouse genome.[43] Since the assay of CAT gene activity is easy, it was used as the reporter gene to study the regulatory role of the promoter of the transferrin gene in the expression of the CAT gene. The transgenic mice carrying the transferrin promoter –CAT construct were given lipopolysaccharide (LPS) intraperitoneally, which produces inflammatory response. In humans, transferrin is a negative acute phase reactant and decreases during inflammation, but in rodents it is a positive acute phase reactant. In the transgenic mice, administration of LPS lowered the CAT activity, but the transferrin level increased. This opposite effect may be due to differences in the regulatory *cis*-acting sequences of the mouse and human transferrin genes, and also to *trans*-acting factors that interact with these sequences. Furthermore, it was seen that the CAT activity in the liver of 24-month-old transgenic mice was only 65% of that of 6-month-old transgenic mice. However, the CAT activity was higher in the old brain. Such studies are useful in examining the expression of human genes during aging.

Reveillaud et al.[45] produced transgenic strains of the fruitfly, *Drosophila*, that overproduce the mammalian Cu-Zn superoxide dismutase (SOD) enzyme. This was achieved by microinjecting *Drosophila* embryo with P-elements containing bovine Cu-Zn SOD cDNA. Adult flies produced both *Drosophila* and bovine SOD. There was a slight but significant increase in the mean life span of the transgenic flies. The level of SOD in the adult flies was 1.6-fold higher than that of normal flies. The extension of the life span may be due to more efficient removal of free radicals by a higher level of SOD.

III. GENE EXPRESSION *IN VITRO*

Human diploid fibroblasts (HDF) have been used since 1961 for the study of senescence of cells after Hayflick and Moorhead[46] discovered that these cells have limited replicative activity *in vitro*. HDFs *in vitro* are not subjected to the same environmental influence as HDFs *in vivo*, and hence these data cannot explain fully the mechanism of *in vivo* aging. Nevertheless, these studies have provided useful insights into the expression of genes and mechanism of aging *in vitro*.[47,48]

Animal cells have a finite life span phenotype; that is, they have an intrinsic limit to their proliferative capacity. Aging at the organismal level may be a manifestation of cellular aging, because for a given population of cells, the maximum number of times the cells can divide (population doubling) is generally directly proportional to the maximum life span of the species.[49] Also, cells derived from donors with heritable premature aging syndromes, such as Werner's syndrome and progeria, divide for a lesser number of times and senesce sooner than age-matched cells of normal donors. So cellular senescence appears to be a mechanism for restricting the growth of the organism and production of tumors, because it is found that genetic events that confer an infinite life span (immortal) phenotype to cells also increase their susceptibility to tumorigenic transformation. The malignant tumor cells generally have an immortal phenotype. Thus, it appears that the finite life span phenotype is under genetic control.

A. Nature of Cellular Senescence

Several workers have fused normal and immortal human cells and have found that the hybrid cells have a limited life span.[50,51] This showed that the senescence phenotype of cells is dominant over its immortal phenotype, and that immortality results from recessive changes in growth-regulatory genes of normal cells. This observation is strengthened by the finding that when a heterokaryon cell hybrid is formed by having one old and one young HDF nuclei in a single cytoplasm, initiation of DNA synthesis in the young nucleus, which was actively proliferating, gets inhibited, though its ongoing DNA synthesis is not inhibited.[52] If the senescent cells are treated with inhibitors of protein synthesis before fusion, inhibition of DNA synthesis in young nuclei is prevented. It appears that this inhibitory effect is due to protein(s). This is supported by the finding that when poly-A[+] mRNA from senescent HDF is microinjected into proliferating HDF, DNA synthesis is inhibited.[53] So cellular senescence is dominant, and that immortality results from recessive changes in growth inhibitory genes. It is likely that immortalization requires the loss of both alleles of a dominant gene. Since the frequency of immortalization is very low and it is recessive, it is unlikely that the senescent phenotype is under the control of a single locus.

Sugawara et al.[54] have found that the human chromosome 1 induces senescence in an immortal hamster cell line. On the other hand, chromosome 4 limits the proliferative life span of three immortal human tumor cell lines.[55] In cell hybrids formed between HDF and an immortal Syrian hamster cell line, most cells exhibit a limited life span comparable to that of HDF. This indicates that cellular senescence is dominant in these hybrids. The hybrid clones that do not senesce do not have both copies of human chromosome 1, whereas all other chromosomes are present in at least some of the immortal hybrids. Furthermore, the introduction of a single copy of human chromosome 1 to the immortal hamster cell by microcell fusion causes typical signs of cellular senescence, whereas transfer of chromosome 2 has no effect on the growth of cells. These data, therefore, suggest that a gene(s) in chromosome 1 in humans has a role in cellular senescence, and that aging has a genetic basis.

B. Protooncogenes and Cellular Senescence

Protooncogenes encode positive growth regulators, whereas tumor suppressor genes encode growth inhibitors. When quiescent fibroblasts are stimulated to proliferate by mitogens, three protooncogenes: c-fos, c-myc, and c-ras are induced before DNA synthesis begins.[56,57] If antisense RNAs of the protooncogenes are transfected, or antibodies against their protein products are microinjected, proliferation of the cells is inhibited. Especially, their DNA synthesis is inhibited. Seshadri and Campisi[58] found that the expression of c-fos is repressed at the transcriptional step in senescent fibroblasts, though the expression of several other genes is the same as those of early passage cells. However, for c-myc and c-ras protooncogenes, the basal and growth-factor-inducible expression do not change as the fibroblasts senesce in culture. It appears, therefore, that senescence is due to selective repression of a few genes, and is not due to the general breakdown of the entire transcription machinery.

The protooncogene, c-fos, encodes a nuclear protein which is an essential component of the activator protein (AP-1) family of transcriptional regulatory complexes. When fibroblasts are stimulated by a mitogen, the expression of c-fos increases within minutes, but quickly returns to the low basal level that is characteristic of quiescent and proliferating cells. It is likely, therefore, that it may control the expression of other genes that are required for proliferation of cells following induction of c-fos. However, when c-fos expression vector is microinjected into senescent fibroblasts, a high level of Fos protein is attained in the nuclei, but DNA synthesis is not stimulated.[48] On the other hand, microinjection of SV40 T-antigen vector stimulates DNA synthesis in all fibroblasts and immortalizes the cells.[59,60] Therefore, repression of c-fos expression in senescent cells may be one of the many regulatory changes that are responsible for irreversibly blocking proliferation. Besides the repression of c-fos protooncogene, the thymidine kinase gene is also reported to be repressed.[61] Whether it is the cause or consequence of growth arrest is not known.

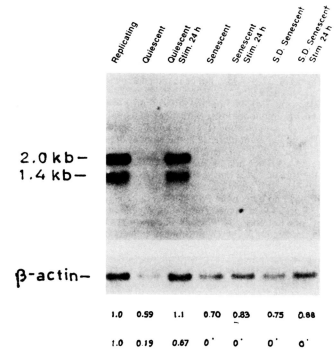

Figure 7
Steady-state levels of *cdc*-2 transcripts in senescent, quiescent, and replicating IMR-90 cells. Poly-A⁺ mRNA was prepared from IMR-90 cells in different growth states and analyzed for the presence of cdc 2 transcripts by northern blot analysis. Amount of cdc 2 mRNA in each sample was normalized to the amount of cytoplasmic β-actin in that sample. Relative amounts of β-actin and of cdc 2 β-actin are given at the bottom of the figure. (From Stein, G. H., Drullinger, L. F., Robetorye, R. S., Pereira-Smith, O. M., and Smith, J. R., *Proc. Natl. Acad. Sci. U.S.A.*, 88, 11012, 1991. With permission.)

The protein, cdc2 (p34) kinase, which is involved in regulation of the cell cycle, has also been implicated in fibroblast proliferation and senescence. It is a highly conserved protein, both structurally and functionally. Its expression increases several hours after mitogenic stimulation of early passage HDF and several hours after the decline of c-*fos* expression.[62] Its expression is not seen after the fibroblasts senesce[63] (Figure 7). Young quiescent HDF have low levels of cdc2 mRNA and protein, but if serum-stimulated, they begin to produce cdc2 mRNA and proteins, synthesize DNA, and undergo mitosis. On the other hand, if senescent cells are serum stimulated, no cdc2 mRNA accumulates, and they do not undergo mitosis. If cdc2 DNA is microinjected into senescent HDF, the cells still do not synthesize DNA. These cells are deficient in cyclins A and B, which are cofactors of the protein kinase activity of p34 protein. These deficiencies may be responsible for the lack of DNA synthesis in senescent HDF. Whether or not the repression of c-*fos* and cdc2 proteins occurs by the same or different mechanisms is not known. It is clear, however, that failure of senescent fibroblasts to respond to growth stimulatory signals occurs due to a selective block of gene expression and it is not due to a global block of expression of genes.

Pignolo et al.[64] have isolated a gene, EPC-1, from lung-derived WI-38 cells which is expressed 100-fold higher in serum-starved confluent cells in comparison to senescent cells. Sequencing of its cDNA indicates that it codes for a mammalian serine protease inhibitor. They have shown that the expression of the EPC-1 gene is associated with Go growth arrest in W1–38 cells. Its mRNA accumulates in density-arrested and/or unstarved young cells but not in log phase, low density young cells. Its expression is negligible in senescent cells.

Metallothioneins (MT) are low molecular weight, cysteine-rich proteins that are induced by heavy metals like cadmium. They are also induced by dexamethasone. HDF were exposed to $CdCl_2$ for 18 h to study the induction of MT gene. Even though the old cells have a higher level of MTs, the inducibility of MT in old cells by $CdCl_2$ was significantly lower. However, the induction of MT by dexamethasone was the same in both young and old cells.[65] Likewise, the induction of the heat shock protein was also reduced in old cells.

The expression of proliferation-associated genes cdc2 and E2F-1, and squamous specific genes, transglutaminase type 1 and cornfin, was studied in senescing human epidermal keratinocytes. Keratinocytes in *in vitro* culture undergo 34 population doublings before senescing when the expression of cdc2 and E2F-1 genes declines. As senescence proceeds, the expression of the cornfin gene which is specific for squamous differentiation begins. Thus, events regulating senescence are linked to squamous differentiation.[66]

Seshadri et al.[67] have reported that the mRNA for the L7 protein, which is a component of the large subunit of eukaryotic ribosomes, is abundant in presenescent human fetal or foreskin fibroblasts, but its level is five- to tenfold lower in senescent cells. Both quiescent and senescent cells synthesize protein at similar rates, but only the latter show a decline in L7 mRNA. The mRNAs encoding other ribosomal proteins, L5, S3, S6, and S10, show a similar pattern. Thus, senescence-associated decline in L7 and other ribosomal protein mRNAs is unrelated to the growth state or the rate of protein synthesis. It appears, therefore, that senescence and quiescence of cells *in vitro* are dissimilar.

Though, in general, the expression of most of the genes becomes increasingly downregulated with increasing age of HDF, there are a few genes which get overexpressed. One such gene that codes for a cytoplasmic smooth muscle protein of 22.5 kDa has been detected by Thweatt et al.[68] by differential screening of a cDNA library constructed from mRNA of subjects suffering from Werner's syndrome (WS). The steady-state level of this mRNA is higher not only in late passage cells of HDF, but also in WS. They have detected nine genes which are overexpressed both in WS and in old HDF.

Activation of the AP-1 complex is one of the earliest nuclear responses to mitogenic stimuli. Riabowol et al.[69] have shown that the activity of AP-1 complex is lower in HDF prior to their entering the senescent phase. Also, the level of Fos protein which binds to Jun to form a heterodimer before binding to AP-1 sites in the promoter of genes is also reduced. The composition of AP-1 complex also changes, in that the old cells produce predominantly Jun-Jun homodimers instead of Fos-Jun heterodimers. This may be due to changes in posttranslational modifications of the Fos protein that impair its binding to Jun.

Another gene which gets overexpressed in old HDF is metalloproteinase.[70] Interestingly, concomitant with the increase in the level of its mRNA, the level of mRNA of the gene that codes for the protein that represses this gene decreases. A similar type of change is seen for the two genes in WS cells. However, cells obtained from patients suffering from progeria do not show such changes. Though WS and progeria are genetic diseases and are due to defects in autosomal genes, obviously the pathways for their manifestation are different.

C. Response of Fibroblasts to Heat Shock

Response of IMR-90 fibroblast cells to heat shock was studied by giving heat shock at 42°C for different periods.[71] The presence of protein factors in the supernatant obtained from the cells at 100,000 g was analyzed by gel retardation studies using a 24-mer dsDNA containing a heat shock element (HSE). A distinct decrease in the level of a protein of 83 kDa that binds to the HSE was found in old fibroblasts. It was also seen that the heat shock protein (HSP) is involved in transcriptional activation of *hsp* genes in IMR-90 cells. A lower level of HSP protein in old fibroblasts may be responsible for the decrease in its cellular functions.[72]

The induction of *hsp*-70 mRNA and protein in lung and skin fibroblasts of 24-month-old rats is also reported to be lower than that of 5-month-old rats after the cells are exposed to heat stress at 42.5°C for 90 min.[73] Freshly excised lung tissue from old rats also shows a lower response to heat stress. Thus the decrease in the response to heat stress in old age is controlled at the level of the gene and is not a random process.

D. Inhibitors of Cellular Proliferation

The retinoblastoma (Rb) gene codes for a 110-kDa tumor suppressor and cell cycle regulator protein which is absent or mutated in many human tumors.[74] Expression of wild-type Rb protein through retrovirus-mediated gene transfer suppresses the tumorigenicity of many neoplastic cell lines that contain Rb mutations. Microinjection of Rb protein into synchronized cells inhibits S-phase progression. Rb protein is nuclear and is phosphorylated. It is relatively hypophosphorylated during G1, and gets increasingly phosphorylated until the end of G2, and is then dephosphorylated at mitosis. It is associated with nuclear matrix proteins such as lamin A and C.[75] When cell proliferation is stimulated by a mitogen the Rb protein gets phosphorylated, so underphosphorylation of Rb protein presumably inhibits cell proliferation. Stein et al.[76] found that the Rb protein fails to get phosphorylated in senescent fibroblast cells. Thus, it appears that these cells contain a constitutively active growth-inhibitory Rb protein that inhibits DNA synthesis. This is supported by the finding that oncogenes that immortalize cells encode proteins that bind, and possibly inactivate, at least two cellular proteins that are tumor-suppressor gene products, the p53 protein and Rb susceptibility gene product. The cdc2 kinase phosphorylates Rb protein as well as other proteins.[77] This enzyme is induced when phosphorylation of Rb protein occurs just prior to DNA synthesis. The discovery that the 5′ promoter region of the c-*fos* gene has a negative-acting Rb response element[78] suggests that the repression of c-*fos*, expression of cdc2, and underphosphorylation of Rb protein in senescent cells may be interrelated.

IV. REACTIVATION OF GENES IN OLD AGE

Cattanach[79] reported that a gene that is dormant in the adult may become activated later in life. During the developmental period of female mammals, one of the two X-chromosomes is randomly inactivated in each cell. This inactivation is stably inherited by cells that arise by mitotic division, so that all descendants have the same active X-chromosome, either paternal or maternal, and the same inactive one. So each adult female is a mosaic with regard to the X-chromosome. An autosomal gene translocated into an X-chromosome is also subject to inactivation if that X-chromosome becomes inactive.

The tyrosinase gene is responsible for pigmentation of hair in mammals. It is autosomal and is located in chromosome 7. In the mutant mouse, in which the gene is translocated to the inactive X-chromosome and is inactivated, the mouse becomes an albino. Cattanach[79] found that as the mouse grows older the tyrosinase gene is reactivated and its hair becomes pigmented. This is the reverse of what is found in normal aging when dark hair becomes white. How this gene gets reactivated in an inactive chromosome while other genes of the inactive X-chromosome remain inactive is not known.

Wareham et al.[80] studied the X-linked *spf* (sparse fur) mutation in the gene coding for ornithine carbamoyl transferase (OCT). A mutation in the OCT gene located in the inactive X-chromosome produces an abnormal OCT. The normal enzyme is positive in the histochemical test at pH 7, but the enzyme of mutant mice tests negative at pH 7. They found that the gene is reactivated with increasing age in mice. Reactivation is not linear with age, but is an all-or-none process, because no cells with intermediate stain are found. Thus, the OCT gene becomes fully active or remains inactive.

Whether or not the reactivation is due to demethylation of –C^mCGG– sequences is not known. It is possible that the methylation status of –CCGG– sequences at critical sites of the gene may turn the gene 'on' or 'off'. The demethylating agent, 5-azacytidine (AZT), a potent inhibitor of methylation, can reactivate genes in the inactive chromosome in somatic cell hybrids,[81] and there is convincing evidence that X-chromosome inactivation is related to differential methylation of cytosine in the DNA of the two X-chromosomes.[82] It would be interesting to find out which –CCGG– sequence(s) in the inactive OCT gene undergoes demethylation and whether this is due to an increase in the level of demethylase. Whatever the mechanism, it is clear that the reactivation of the gene is due to its destabilization by a random event. If such reactivation is random, it is difficult to comprehend how such events would cause 'normal' aging, because aging is more or less a gradual process. The normal mouse that does not have this mutation also ages. Hence, random destabilization or dysdifferentiation is unlikely to lead to 'normal' aging.

V. INCREASED ACTIVATION OF OTHER GENES

Certain genes that have low activity in an adult tissue become increasingly active in older tissue, and certain genes get expressed in nontarget tissues in old age. Jaiswal and Kanungo[83] measured the level of α-skeletal actin (α-SKA) mRNA in the heart of young and old rats by RNA-DNA slot-blot hybridization using a cDNA probe for α-SKA. The level was found to be higher in the heart of old rats (Figure 8). However, nuclear run-on transcription was not found to be different. α-SKA is the major isoform of skeletal actin of the fetal cardiac ventricle, whereas a different isoform is predominant in the adult heart.[84] Under experimental aortic coarctation in the adult, α-SKA gene is rapidly reexpressed followed by hypertrophy of the heart. Hypertrophy occurs due to an increase in cell size without cell division. The continuous pressure overload of the heart throughout the life span may stimulate increased expression of the α-SKA gene which, in turn, may lead to hypertrophy of the heart. This may lead to lower contractibility of the heart and affect its function. This is consistent

Figure 8
Levels of α-skeletal actin mRNA in the skeletal muscle, heart, and uterus of young (25-week) and old (135-week) female rats as determined by slot-blot hybridization. Level is higher in the heart but lower in skeletal muscle and uterus of old rats. (From Jaiswal, Y. K. and Kanungo, M. S., *Biochem. Biophys. Res. Commun.*, 168, 71, 1990. With permission.)

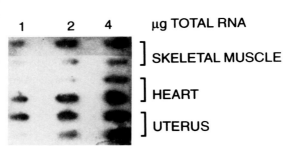

with the finding that c-*myc*, c-*fos*, and *hsp*-70 genes are activated first as an early response to pressure overload, and this is followed by overexpression of the α-SKA gene.[84]

The c-*myc* family of oncogenes is reported to be expressed in several tissues of old mice.[42] Also, studies on the expression of satellite DNA, which is highly methylated and is believed not to be transcribed, show that these sequences begin to be transcribed after adulthood only in the heart and not in other tissues of mice.[85] This may be due to the demethylation of these sequences that is reported to occur in old age.[86] Whether there is tissue- and age-specific demethylation of satellite DNA during aging is not known.

VI.   METHYLATION

Methylation of cytosine is the only modification that is so far known to occur in the DNA. Thus, changes in cytosine methylation during aging have been studied by several workers. There is a direct correlation between cytosine methylation and inactivation of genes, though there are examples of genes which may get inactivated even though no change in their methylation status has occurred. There are also cases in which a gene may be hypomethylated and inactivated; so it is not fully known whether changes in cytosine methylation are the cause or effect of aging.

Cytosine residues of mammalian genomes, especially in the CpG doublets, are known to be methylated. Two models have been proposed to explain the mechanism of action of methylated and demethylated doublets. In one, it is postulated that transcription factors are unable to bind if the site is methylated, and hence the gene is repressed. Certain transcription factors are sensitive to methylation, for example, the cAMP-responsive element (CRE) binding protein (CREB).[87] However, not all transcription factors are methyl sensitive. Sp1 binds to its site and activates the gene regardless of methylation of the site.[88] In the second model it is postulated that methylated DNA is bound to a nuclear protein(s) which prevents transcription factors from interacting with the gene. This is supported by the finding that transcriptional inhibition that is seen at low template concentrations can be overcome by addition of methylated competitor DNA, which perhaps mops up the mediator of inhibition leaving the template free to interact with the transcriptional machinery. Such a protein factor (CpG binding protein, MeCP-1) has been identified.[89]

Methylation of the –CCGG– sequences and CpG doublets in the genome and in specific genes has been implicated in overall transcription of specific genes. Studies on the effect of methylation of the tyrosine amino transferase (TAT) gene on its transcription show that the TAT mRNA level of the liver of 24- and 36-month-old female rats is nearly 65% lower than that of 6-month-old rats.[90] It was also seen by MspI/HpaII digestion followed by Southern hybridization that six CpG sites in the TAT gene are hypomethylated. Thus hypomethylation of the TAT gene lowers its transcription. The TAT gene may be rather an exception in that it becomes hypomethylated in old age, because it is seen that both mCpG and mCpC doublets are found in greater amounts in old brain, and an age-related increase in DNA methylation occurs both at –CCGG– sites of repetitive DNA sequences and in the entire genome.[91]

VII. ALTERATIONS IN MITOCHONDRIAL DNA

Mitochondrial DNA (mtDNA) is small in comparison to nuclear DNA, is naked, has no introns, and replicates autonomously. A mitochondrion may have two or three copies of mtDNA, and each cell may have hundreds of mitochondria. Mammalian mtDNA is a circular 16.5-kbp dsDNA. Except for a short noncoding region, the remaining mtDNA codes for two rRNAs (12S and 16S), 22 tRNAs, and 13 mRNAs for 13 enzymes of the electron transport system. The other proteins required for oxidative phosphorylation are coded by nuclear DNA. The mutation ratio of mtDNA is higher than that of nuclear DNA as it is unprotected by histones.[92] It has no proofreading or DNA repair system. Any damage to it is expected to impair energy production in the cell. Hence, damage, modifications, mutations, and deletions in mtDNA during the life span may affect energy production and contribute to aging.

Oxidative phosphorylation in human mitochondria is reported to decrease with age.[93] Hayakawa et al.[94] found that the occurrence of 8-OH-dG in mtDNA of human diaphragm muscle increases with age. In subjects below 55 years, the 8-OH-dG level is below 0.02% of the total dG, but it continues to increase after 65 years of age at a rate of 0.25%/10 years, reaching 0.51% at 85. It is also seen that multiple deletions occur in the mtDNA of human heart which can be detected by electrophoresis after amplification by polymerase chain reaction (PCR).[95] It is possible that the lower level of 8-OH-dG in the young is due to the high replication rate of mtDNA which dilutes out its number. In the old, its replication rate is slower, which may lead to accumulation of 8-OH-dG. The presence of modified guanine may be one of the causes of deletions in mtDNA.

The mitochondrial DNA of all subjects over 70 years has been found to have a 7,436-bp deletion.[95] The percentage of mtDNA with this deletion increases in old age. It is 3% at age 80 and 9% at age 90. This segment of mtDNA codes for five subunits of complex I and one subunit each of complexes III, IV, and V. Likewise, mtDNA of the striatum of the brain of patients suffering from Parkinson's disease and of elderly control subjects have a 4,977-bp deletion.[96] Mitochondrial DNA of the liver of old men also has a deletion of 4,977 bp, either between 8,469 and 13,447 bp, or between 8,482 and 13,460 bp.[97] The frequency of this deletion increases with age, being 5 out of 8 between 31 and 40 years, 9 out of 11 between 41 and 50 years, and in all men above 50 years. The loss of such a large fragment may decrease mitochondrial function as it is likely that it codes for some essential proteins.

Corral-Debrinski et al.[98] and Arnheim and Cortopassi[99] have quantitated the accumulation of a 4,977-bp deletion in mtDNA in different parts of old human brain. There is a significant increase in the deletion in elderly persons. In the cortex, the deleted to total mtDNA ratio ranges from 0.00023 to 0.012 in the 69- to 77-year-old brains, but in those over 80 years it is 0.034. Cortopassi et al.[100] have reported that the deletion of the 4,977-bp fragment occurs between two 13-bp direct repeats. This deletion increases at least 100-fold with age in human heart and brain of individuals without ailments. In the brain, the highest level of deletion is found in the caudate, putamen, and substantia nigra, which are characterized by high dopamine metabolism. Breakdown of dopamine by mitochondrial monoaminoxidase produces H_2O_2, which can lead to formation of the oxygen radical. This, in turn, may contribute to the deletion.[101] Another deletion, 7,436 bp, also occurs in the brain mtDNA and also shows a similar type of increase. Loss of such large segments of mtDNA may contribute to the neurological impairment often associated with aging.[102,103]

It has been reported that the steady-state levels of 12S mRNA, and mRNA for subunit 1 of cytochrome oxidase in the brain and heart of senescent rats are significantly lower than those of adult rats.[104] No such change is seen in the liver. Mitochondria from the cerebral hemisphere of old rats have 50% lower level of mitochondrial RNA than those of young rats. This is due to a lower rate of transcription. Biggs et al.[105] found that the level of cytochrome c mRNA in the heart of old rats is nearly 22% lower than that of young rats.

Despite the findings that significant deletions and decreases in transcription occur in mtDNA, it is unlikely that alterations in mtDNA are the principal cause of aging since the nuclear DNA is far in excess of the mtDNA, and codes for most of the vital enzymes and proteins.

VIII. ALTERNATIVE SPLICING OF PRE-mRNA

Alternative splicing of pre-mRNA is known to produce different mRNAs that are translated into different isoforms of a protein. Most pre-mRNAs transcribed from split genes are spliced in such a way that the original order of arrangement of the exons are maintained in the mature mRNAs. This is constitutive splicing. Some pre-mRNAs, however, are spliced in more than one way, thereby yielding a family of structurally related mRNAs that are translated into a family of protein isoforms. This is alternative splicing. Such splicing is seen in all organisms including humans, and occurs in several types of transcripts that encode varieties of proteins. This is a means of diversifying the output from a single gene without altering its genomic organization. In some cases, alternatively spliced mRNAs are produced concurrently in the same tissue, and several protein isoforms may perform the same or different functions. For example, four myelin basic protein isoforms derived from a single gene are all components of the myelin sheath. Some gene transcripts are spliced differently in different tissues. For example, the single mammalian calcitonin gene expresses calcitonin in the thyroid, but in the brain a different isoform is produced by a separate splicing pattern.

Alternative splicing of the rat and human FNT transcript is responsible for the production of 12 and 16 isoforms of FNTs in the rat and human, respectively.[13] Alternative splicing occurs at each of the three exons — extra domains A(ED-A), ED-B, and type III connecting sequence (IIICs). The FNT isoforms produced differ in properties. The ratios of FNT mRNAs with or without a given exon were determined in several rat tissues and IMR-9 human fibroblasts during aging *in vivo* and cellular senescence *in vitro*.[106] Statistically significant changes were found in both *in vivo* and *in vitro* aging. All three alternatively spliced exons were spliced out at a higher frequency as the animals and cells aged. However, major alterations leading to the absolute predominance of one form over another were not seen during aging. Whereas ED-A and ED-B mRNAs in adult tissues ranged from 0 to 25% and 0 to 10%, respectively, those of fibroblast cells in culture ranged from 50 to 60% and 15 to 25%, respectively. Factors such as serum deprivation, growth factors, and retinoic acid affect alternative splicing. Thus *in vivo* alternative splicing is not the same as that of *in vitro* splicing.

FNT synthesis increases in human skin fibroblasts after extensive passage in culture.[107] The FNT of late-passage fibroblasts is slightly longer, and its ability to bind to collagen is lower. In late passage cells of human foreskin fibroblasts an eightfold increase in the expression of the ED-A splicing variant relative to the sum of all other variants has been reported.[108]

It is likely that alternatively spliced transcripts of other genes, as well, undergo changes with age, and result in the production of different isoforms of proteins that have different properties. The transcript of the amyloid precursor protein (APP) gene is reported to be alternatively spliced to give three mRNAs.[109] More genes need to be studied to ascertain whether quantitative changes occur in mRNAs derived from a single transcript as an animal ages, because the effects of such changes would be enormous for the organism.

IX. CONCLUSIONS

The number of genes in an adult mammal is enormous, and to identify the few crucial genes that change in expression and contribute to aging, and the reason why they change, is indeed difficult. The postmitotic cells such as neurons, skeletal, and cardiac muscle cells have a long life span, and the timing of their senescence and death does not appear to be fixed, unlike those of embryonic cells and premitotic cells such as epithelial and bone marrow cells. Certain postmitotic cells live till the end of the life span of the organism, and certain cells die earlier. Is the trigger for their senescence the same as that of premitotic cells? Moreover, each type of postmitotic cell differs from another because it expresses certain unique genes that give the cell its own differentiated status. Do these unique genes have any role in its longevity, or do all cells, both premitotic and postmitotic, have a common set of genes whose expression/repression leads to aging?

Messenger RNAs of young and old rats have been used to construct cDNA libraries, and by subtractive hybridization certain genes, including T-kininogen, have been shown to increase in expression in old age. The significance of these genes in aging is not obvious, but such studies are useful in identifying genes that are either downregulated or upregulated as an animal ages. Studies on genes that encode enzymes/proteins, and genes that get expressed when the organism is under stress of different kinds such as inflammation and high temperature, are beginning to show how the expression of certain genes may be altered as a function of age. Attainment of adulthood and reproductive activity likewise may bring about changes in hormonal levels that may influence expression of specific genes. Such changes may destabilize the homeostatic balance of various functions, contribute to the decline of activity of the organism, and decrease its ability to adapt to changes in intrinsic and extrinsic factors.[1]

Cell fusion studies have provided evidence that senescence is a dominant phenotypic character, and chromosome 1 in humans may have a locus that controls cell proliferation. However, senescence is a gradual and

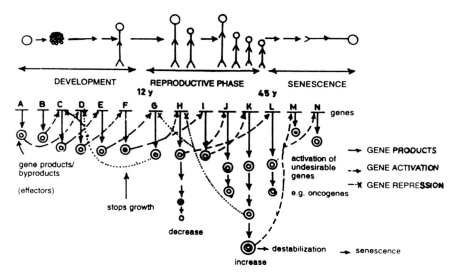

Figure 9

Model for Aging. (Top) Representation of various phases of the life span — development, reproduction, and senescence. (Bottom) The number of active genes have been kept to a minimum, and genes that are permanently repressed are not shown for sake of clarity. Developmental and reproductive phases are dependent on unique genes, A–F and G–L, respectively. They are activated in a sequential manner by the switching on of a gene by the product of a gene activated earlier. Growth ceases after a certain period by feedback repression of a growth-promoting gene. No gene for aging is depicted in the model. Continued reproduction and other stresses encountered during adulthood causes depletion of certain factors that are needed for maintenance of adulthood. Certain factors may also accumulate. Thus, there is a gradual destabilization of the homeostatic functioning of genes, resulting in deterioration of various functions and aging. (From Kanungo, M. S., *Biochemistry of Ageing*, Academic Press, London, 1990. With permission.)

progressive process, and it is likely that subtle changes in the expression of genes brought about through their promoters may be involved. The promoter has several *cis*-acting elements, some of which have stimulatory and others inhibitory roles in the expression of respective genes. These elements act in different combination and in a modular fashion. Despite the fact that all animals within a mammalian species have a more or less similar maximum life span, large variations in longevity among individual members within a species are seen. While the overall maximum life span of individual members may be determined by sequential activation and repression of genes as proposed in the gene regulation theory[110] (Figure 9), variations in the rate of aging and longevity among members of the species may occur due to changes in expression of vital genes brought about by effectors acting on various *cis*-acting elements in the promoter[1] (Figure 10).

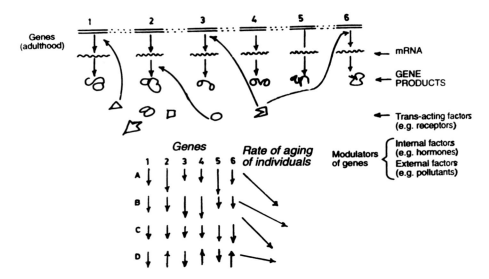

Figure 10
Model depicting how variations may occur in the rate of aging and longevity of different individuals of a species. Individuals differ in their genotype. Also, their nutrition may be different, and the stresses to which they are exposed during adulthood may be different. These affect the levels of *trans*-acting factors that modulate the expression of various genes. The sum total of the expression of an array of genes, say 1 to 6, in an organ affects its functioning. Another set of genes may affect another organ. This accounts for the variations in the pattern and rate of aging of different individuals (A–D) of a species. These are represented here as slopes (rate) of aging that account for the variations in longevity of different individuals. (From Kanugo, M.S., *Genes and Aging*, Cambridge University Press, New York, 1994. With permission.)

Studies on the promoter region of genes are beginning to yield data that show that gradual changes occur in the levels of *trans*-acting factors that bind to specific *cis*-acting elements. The levels of *trans*-acting factors, like those of other proteins, are likely to be influenced by changes in hormones, nutrients, and other effectors. This research should, in the next decade, bring deeper insight into the role of genes in the aging process and the cause of aging at the molecular level.

REFERENCES

1. Kanungo, M. S., *Genes and Aging*, Cambridge University Press, New York, 1994, 274.
2. Boobis, A., Caldwell, J., Dematteis, F., and Davis, D., *Microsomes and Drug Degradation*, Taylor and Francis Ltd., London, 1985, 85.

3. Nebert, D. W. and Gonzalez, F. J., Cytochrome P-450 gene expression and regulation, *Trends Pharmacol. Sci.*, 4, 1985, 160.
4. Horbach, G. J. M. J. and van Bezooijen, C. F. A., The effect of age on the synthesis of rat liver proteins, in *Liver and Aging*, Kitani, K., Ed., Elsevier, Amsterdam, 1991, 183.
5. McCay, C. M., Sperling, G., and Barnes, L. L., Growth, aging, chronic diseases and life span in rats, *Arch. Biochem.*, 2, 469, 1943.
6. Rath, P. C. and Kanungo, M. S., Age-related changes in the expression of cytochrome P-450 (b+e) gene in the rat after phenobarbitone administration, *Biochem. Biophys. Res. Commun.*, 157, 1403, 1988.
7. Kanungo, M. S., Singh, A., Singh, S., and Jaiswal, Y. K., Gene expression and aging, in *New Horizons in Aging Science*, Orimo, H., Fukuchi, Y., Kuramoto, K., and Iriki, M., Eds., University of Tokyo Press, Tokyo, 1992, 51.
8. Fukuda, H. and Iritani, N., Effect of aging on gene expression of acetyl-CoA carboxylase and fatty acid synthetase in rat liver, *J. Biochem.*, 112, 277, 1992.
9. Harman, D., Aging, a theory based on free radical and radiation, *J. Gerontol.*, 11, 298, 1956.
10. Tolmasoff, J. M., Ono, T., and Cutler, R. G., Superoxide dismutase: correlation with life span and specific metabolic rate in primate species, *Proc. Natl. Acad. Sci. U.S.A.*, 77, 2777, 1980.
11. Semsei, I., Rao, G., and Richardson, A., Changes in the expression of superoxide dismutase and catalase as a function of age and dietary restriction, *Biochem. Biophys. Res. Commun.*, 164, 620, 1989.
12. Hynes, R. O., *Fibronectins*, Springer-Verlag, New York, 1990, 12.
13. Schwarzbauer, J. E., Alternative splicing of fibronectin: three variants, three functions, *BioEssays*, 13, 527, 1991.
14. Patel, R. S., Odermatt, E., Schwarzbauer, J. E., and Hynes, R. O., Organisation of the fibronectin gene provides evidence for exon shuffling during evolution, *EMBO J.*, 6, 2565, 1987.
15. Singh, S. and Kanungo, M. S., DNase I hypersensitive sites of the 5′ region of the fibronectin gene of the liver of the rat, *Biochem. Biophys. Res. Commun.*, 181, 131, 1991.
16. Singh, S. and Kanungo, M. S., Changes in expression and CRE binding proteins of the fibronectin gene during aging of the rat, *Biochem. Biophys. Res. Commun.*, 193, 440, 1993.
17. Roy, A. K., Nath, T. S., Motwani, N. M., and Chatterjee, B., Age-dependent regulation of the polymorphic forms of α2μ-globulin, *J. Biol. Chem.*, 258, 10123, 1983.
18. Richardson, A., Butler, J. A., Rutherford, M. S., Semsei, I., Gu, M.-Z., Fernandes, G., and Chiang, W.-H., Effect of age and dietary restriction on the expression of α2μ-globulin, *J. Biol. Chem.*, 262, 12821, 1987.
19. Roy, A. K. and Chatterjee, B., Molecular aspects of aging, in *Molecular Aspects of Medicine*, Baum, H., Gergely, J., and Fanburg, B. L., Eds., Pergamon Press, Oxford, 1985, 1.
20. Song, C. S., Rao, T. R., Demyan, W. F., Mancini, M. A., Chatterjee, B., and Roy, A. K., Androgen receptor messenger ribonucleic acid (mRNA) in the rat liver: changes in mRNA levels during aging and caloric restriction, *Endocrinology*, 128, 349, 1991.
21. Supakar, P. C., Song, C. S., Jung, M. H., Slomczynska, M. A., Kim, J. M., Vellanoweth, R. L., Chatterjee, B., and Roy, A. K., A novel regulatory element associated with age-dependent expression of the rat androgen receptor gene, *J. Biol. Chem.*, 268, 26400, 1993.

22. Chatterjee, B., Majumdar, D., Ozbillan, O., Murty, C. V. R., and Roy, A. K., Molecular cloning and characterisation of the cDNA for androgen repressible rat liver protein SMP-2, *J. Biol. Chem.*, 262, 822, 1987.

23. Fujita, T., Uchida, K., and Maruyama, N., Purification of senescence-marker protein 30 (SMP-30) and its androgen-dependent decrease with age in the rat liver, *Biochem. Biophys. Acta,* 1116, 122, 1992.

24. Singh, A., Singh, S., and Kanungo, M. S., Conformation and expression of the albumin gene of young and old rats, *Mol. Biol. Rep.,* 14, 251, 1990.

25. Richardson, A., Rutherford, M. S., Birchenell-Sparks, M. C., Roberts, M. S., Wu, W. T., and Cheung, H. T., Levels of specific messenger RNA species as a function of age, in *Molecular Biology of Aging*, Sohal, R. S., Birnbaum, L. S., and Cutler, R. G., Eds., Raven Press, New York, 1985, 229.

26. Armbrecht, H. J., Boltz, M., Strong, R., Richardson, A., Bruns, M. E. H., and Christakos, S., Expression of calbindin-D decreases with age in intestine and kidney, *Endocrinology,* 125, 2950, 1989.

27. Iacopino, A. M. and Christakos, S., Specific reduction of calcium-binding protein (28-kilodalton calbindin D) gene expression in neurodegenerative diseases, *Proc. Natl. Acad. Sci. U.S.A.,* 87, 4078, 1990.

28. Friedman, V., Wagner, J., and Danner, D. O., Isolation and identification of aging related cDNAs in the mouse, *Mech. Ageing Dev.,* 52, 27, 1990.

29. Gresik, E. W., Wenk-Salamore, K., Onetti-Muda, A., Gubitts, R. M., and Shaw, R. A., Effect of advanced age on the induction by androgen or thyroid hormone of epidermal growth factor and epidermal growth factor mRNA in submandibular glands of C57 BL16 male mice, *Mech. Ageing Dev.,* 34, 175, 1986.

30. Whittenmore, S. R., Ebendal, T., Larkfors, L., Olson, L., Seiger, A., Stromberg, F., and Persson, H., *Proc. Natl. Acad. Sci. U.S.A.,* 83, 817, 1986.

31. Goss, J. R., Finch, C. E., and Morgan, D. G., Age-related changes in glial fibrillary acidic protein mRNA in the mouse brain, *Neurobiol. Aging,* 12, 165, 1991.

32. Gruenwald, D. A. and Matsumoto, A. M., Age-related decrease in proopiomelanocortin gene expression in the arcuate nucleus of the male rat brain, *Neurobiol. Aging,* 12, 113, 1991.

33. Wismer, C. T., Sherman, K. A., Zibart, M., and Richardson, A., *Central Nervous System Disorders of Aging,* Strong, R., Wood, W. B., and Burke, W. J., Eds., Raven Press, New York, 1988, 189.

34. Sierra, F., Fey, G. H., and Guigoz, Y., T-kininogen expression is induced during aging, *Mol. Cell. Biol.,* 9, 5610, 1989.

35. Sierra, F., Juillerat, Coeylaux, S., Ruffieux, C., and Guigoz, Y., T-kininogen gene expression: induction during aging and age-related changes during acute phase response, in *Liver and Aging,* Kitani, K., Ed., Excerpta Medica, Amsterdam, 1991, 123.

36. Milman, N., Graudel, N., and Andersen, H. C., Acute phase reactants in the elderly, *Clin. Chem. Acta,* 176, 59, 1988.

37. Blake, M., Elad, S., Epharti, E., Fargnoli, J., Rott, R., Holbrook, N., and Gershon, D., Studies on the expression of heat-shock proteins as a function of age, in *Liver and Aging,* Kitani, K., Ed., Excerpta Medica, Amsterdam, 1991, 213.

38. Blake, M. J., Udelsman, R., Feulner, G. J., Norton, D. D., and Holbrook, N. J., Stress induced heat shock protein 70 expression in adrenal cortex, an adrenocorticotropic hormone-sensitive age-dependent response, *Proc. Natl. Acad. Sci. U.S.A.,* 88, 9873, 1991.

39. Wu, B., Heydari, A. R., Conrad, C. C., and Richardson, A., The age-related decline in the induction of heat-shock protein is reversed by life-long dietary restriction, in *Liver and Aging,* Kitani, K., Ed., Excerpta Medica, Amsterdam, 1991, 197.

40. Heydari, A. R., Wu, B., Takahashi, R., Strong, R., and Richardson, A., Expression of heat-shock protein 70 is altered by age and diet at the level of transcription, *Mol. Cell. Biol.,* 13, 2909, 1993.
41. Fujita, T. and Maruyama, N., Elevated levels of c-*jun* and c-*fos* transcripts in the rat liver, *Biochem. Biophys. Res. Commun.,* 178, 1485, 1991.
42. Semsei, I., Ma, S., and Cutler, R. G., Tissue- and age-specific expression of the *myc* proto-oncogene family throughout the life span of C57BL/6J mouse strain, *Oncogene,* 4, 465, 1989.
43. Zakin, M. M., Regulation of transferrin gene expression, *FASEB J.,* 6, 3253, 1992.
44. Bowman, B. H., Yang, F., and Adrian, G. H., Expression of human plasma protein genes in ageing transgenic mice, *BioEssays,* 12, 317, 1990.
45. Reveillaud, I., Niedzniecki, A., Bensch, K. G., and Fleming, J. E., Expression of bovine superoxide dismutase in *Drosophila melanogaster* augments resistance to oxidation stress, *Mol. Cell. Biol.,* 11, 632, 1991.
46. Hayflick, L. and Moorhead, P., The serial cultivation of human diploid cell strains, *Exp. Cell Res.,* 25, 585, 1961.
47. Goldstein, S., Replicative senescence: the human fibroblast comes of age, *Science,* 249, 1129, 1990.
48. McCormick, A. and Campisi, J., Cellular ageing and senescence, *Curr. Op. Cell Biol.,* 3, 230, 1991.
49. Rohme, D., Evidence for relationship between longevity of mammalian species and life spans of normal fibroblasts in vitro and erythrocytes *in vivo, Proc. Natl. Acad. Sci. U.S.A.,* 78, 5009, 1981.
50. Pereira-Smith, O. M. and Smith, J. R., Evidence for the repressive nature of cellular immortality, *Science,* 221, 964, 1983.
51. Sager, R., Tumor suppressor genes: the puzzle and the promise, *Science,* 246, 1406, 1989.
52. Burmer, G. C., Ziegler, C. J., and Norwood, T. H., Evidence for endogenous polypeptide mediated inhibition of cell cycle transit in human diploid cells, *J. Cell Biol.,* 94, 187, 1982.
53. Lumpkin, C. K., Jr., McClung, J. K., Pereira-Smith, O. M., and Smith, J. R., Existence of high abundance antiproliferative messenger RNA in senescent human diploid fibroblasts, *Science,* 232, 393, 1986.
54. Sugawara, O., Oshimura, M., Koi, M., Annab, L. A., and Barrett, J. C., Induction of cellular senescence in immortalized cells by human chromosome 1, *Science,* 247, 707, 1990.
55. Ning, Y., Weber, J. L., Killary, A. M., Ledbetter, D. H., Smith, J. R., and Pereira-Smith, O. M., Genetic analysis of indefinite division in human cells: evidence for a cell senescence related gene(s) on human chromosome 4, *Proc. Natl. Acad. Sci. U.S.A.,* 88, 5635, 1991.
56. Riabowol, K., Vosatka, R. J., Ziff, E. B., Lamb, N. J., and Framisco, J. F., Micro-injection of *fos*-specific antibodies block DNA synthesis in fibroblast cells, *Mol. Cell Biol.,* 8, 1670, 1988.
57. Lu, K., Levine, R. A., and Campisi, J., C-ras-Ha gene expression is regulated by insulin-like growth factor and by epidermal growth factor in murine fibroblast, *Mol. Cell Biol.,* 9, 3411, 1989.
58. Seshadri, T. and Campisi, J., Repression of c-*fos* transcription and an altered genetic program in senescent human fibroblasts, *Science,* 247, 205, 1990.
59. Wright, W. E., Pereira-Smith, O. M., and Shay, J. W., Reversible cellular senescence: implications for immortalization of normal human diploid fibroblasts, *Mol. Cell Biol.,* 9, 3088, 1989.

60. Radna, R. L., Caton, Y., Jha, K. K., Kaplan, P., Li, G., Traganos, F., and Ozer, H. L., Growth of immortal simian virus 40ts A-transformed human fibroblasts is temperature dependent, *Mol. Cell Biol.*, 9, 3093, 1989.

61. Chang, Z. F. and Chen, K. Y., Regulation of ornithine decarboxylase and other cell cycle dependent genes during senescence of IMR 90 human diploid fibroblasts, *J. Biol. Chem.*, 263, 11431, 1988.

62. Lee, M. G., Norbury, C. J., Spurr, N. K., and Nurse, C., Regulated expression and phosphorylation of a possible mammalian cell cycle control protein, *Nature*, 333, 676, 1988.

63. Stein, G. H., Drullinger, L. F., Robetorye, R. S., Pereira-Smith, O. M., and Smith, J. R., Senescent cells fail to express cdc2, cyc A and cyc B in response to mitogen stimulation, *Proc. Natl. Acad. Sci. U.S.A.*, 88, 11012, 1991.

64. Pignolo, R. J., Cristofalo, V. J., and Rotenberg, M. O., Senescent W1–38 cells fail to express EPC-1, a gene induced in young cells upon entry into Go state, *J. Biol. Chem.*, 268, 8944, 1993.

65. Luce, M. C., Schyberg, J. P., and Bunn, C. L., Metallothionein expression and stress responses in aging human diploid fibroblasts, *Exp. Gerontol.*, 28, 17, 1993.

66. Saunders, N. A., Smith, R. J., and Jetten, A. M., Regulation of proliferation-specific and differentiation specific genes during senescence of human epidermal keratinocyte and mammary epithelial cells, *Biochem. Biophys. Res. Commun.*, 197, 46, 1993.

67. Seshadri, T., Uzman, J. A., Oshima, J., and Campisi, J., Identification of a transcript that is down-regulated in senescent human fibroblasts, *J. Biol. Chem.*, 268, 18474, 1993.

68. Thweatt, R., Lumpkin, C. K., and Goldstein, S., A novel gene encoding a smooth muscle protein is over-expressed in senescent human fibroblast, *Biochem. Biophys. Res. Commun.*, 187, 1, 1992.

69. Riabowol, K., Schiff, J., and Gilman, M. Z., Transcription factor AP-1 activity is required for initiation of DNA synthesis and is lost during cellular aging, *Proc. Natl. Acad. Sci. U.S.A.*, 89, 157, 1992.

70. Millis, A. J. T., Hoyle, M., McCue, H. M., and Martini, H., Differential expression of metalloproteinase and tissue inhibitor of metalloproteinase genes in aged human fibroblasts, *Exp. Cell Res.*, 201, 373, 1992.

71. Liu, A. Y.-C., Lin, Z., Chois, H. S., Sorhege, F., and Li, B., Attenuated induction of heat shock gene expression in aging diploid fibroblasts, *J. Biol. Chem.*, 264, 12037, 1989.

72. Choi, H. S., Lin, Z., Li, B., and Liu, A. Y.-C., Age-dependent decrease in heat inducible DNA sequence specific binding activity in human diploid fibroblasts, *J. Biol. Chem.*, 265, 18005, 1990.

73. Fragnoli, J., Kumisada, T., Fornace, A. J., Schneider, E. L., and Holbrook, N. J., Decreased expression of heat shock protein 70 mRNA and protein after heat treatment in cells of aged rats, *Proc. Natl. Acad. Sci. U.S.A.*, 87, 846, 1990.

74. Goodrich, D. W. and Lee, W.-H., Molecular characterisation of the retinoblastoma susceptibility gene (review), *Biochim. Biophys. Acta, Rev. Cancer*, 1155, 43, 1993.

75. Mancini, M. A., Shan, B., Nickerson, J. A., Penman, S., and Lee, W.-H., The retinoblastoma gene product is a cell cycle-dependent, nuclear matrix-associated protein, *Proc. Natl. Acad. Sci. U.S.A.*, 91, 418, 1994.

76. Stein, G. H., Beeson, M., and Gordon, L., Failure to phosphorylate the retinoblastoma gene product in senescent human fibroblasts, *Science*, 249, 666, 1989.

77. Pines, J. and Hunter, T., The S and M kinase?, *New Biologist*, 2, 399, 1990.

78. Robbins, P. D., Horowitz, J. M., and Mulligan, R. C., Negative regulation of human c-fos regulation by retinoblastoma gene product, *Nature*, 346, 668, 1990.

79. Cattanach, B. M., Position effect variation in the mouse, *Genet. Res.*, 23, 291, 1974.
80. Wareham, K. A., Lyon, M. F., Glenister, P. H., and Williams, E. D., Age-related reactivation of an X-linked gene, *Nature*, 327, 725, 1987.
81. Jones, P. A., Altering gene expression with 5-azacytidine, *Cell*, 40, 485, 1986.
82. Monk, M., Changes in DNA methylation during mouse embryonic development in relation to X-chromosome activity and imprinting, *Phil. Trans. R. Soc., London B*, 326, 299, 1990.
83. Jaiswal, Y. K. and Kanungo, M. S., Expression of actin and myosin heavy chain genes in skeletal, cardiac and uterine muscles of young and old rats, *Biochem. Biophys. Res. Commun.*, 168, 71, 1990.
84. Izumo, S., Nadal-Ginard, B., and Mahdavi, V., Proto-oncogene induction and reprogramming of cardiac gene expression by pressure overload, *Proc. Natl. Acad. Sci. U.S.A.*, 85, 339, 1988.
85. Gaubatz, J. W. and Cutler, R. G., Mouse satellite DNA is transcribed in senescent cardiac muscle, *J. Biol. Chem.*, 265, 17753, 1990.
86. Howlett, D., Dalrymple, S., and Mays-Hoopes, L. L., Age-related demethylation of mouse satellite DNA is easily detectable by HPLC but not by restriction endonucleases, *Mutat. Res.*, 219, 101, 1989.
87. Iguchi-Ariga, S. M. M. and Schaffner, W., CpG methylation of the cAMP responsive enhancer/promoter sequence TGACGTCA abolishes specific factor binding as well as transcriptional activation, *Genes Dev.*, 3, 612, 1989.
88. Holler, M., Westin, G., Jiricny, J., and Schaffner, W., Sp 1 transcription factor binds DNA and activates transcription even when binding site is CpG methylated, *Genes Dev.*, 2, 1127, 1988.
89. Meehan, R. R., Levis, J. D., Mckay, S., Kleiver, E. L., and Bird, A. P., Identification of a mammalian protein that binds specifically to DNA containing methylated CpGs, *Cell*, 58, 499, 1989.
90. Slagboom, P. E., deLeeuw, W. J. F., and Vijg, J., mRNA levels and methylation patterns of tyrosine aminotransferase gene in aging inbred rats, *FEBS Lett.*, 269, 128, 1990.
91. Rath, P. C. and Kanungo, M. S., Methylation of repetitive DNA sequences in the brain of the rat, *FEBS Lett.*, 244, 193, 1989.
92. Linnane, A. W., Maruzuki, S., Ozawa, T., and Tanaka, M., Mitochondrial DNA mutations as an important contribution to aging and degenerative diseases, *Lancet*, 1 (No. 8639), 642, 1989.
93. Trounce, I., Byrne, E., and Maruzuki, S., Decline in skeletal muscle mitochondrial respiratory chain function: possible factor in aging, *Lancet*, 1 (No. 8639), 637, 1989.
94. Hayakawa, M., Torii, K., Sugiyama, S., Tanaka, M., and Ozawa, T., Age-associated oxygen damage and mutations in mitochondrial DNA in human hearts, *Biochem. Biophys. Res. Commun.*, 179, 1023, 1991.
95. Sugiyama, S., Hattori, K., Hayakawa, M., and Ozawa, T., Quantitative analysis of age-associated accumulation of mitochondrial DNA with deletion in human hearts, *Biochem. Biophys. Res. Commun.*, 180, 894, 1991.
96. Ikebe, S., Tanaka, M., Ohno, K., Sato, W., Hattori, K., Kondo, T., Mizuno, Y., and Ozawa, T., Increase of deleted mitochondrial DNA in the striatum in Parkinson's disease and senescence, *Biochem. Biophys. Res. Commun.*, 179, 1044, 1990.
97. Yen, T. C., Su, J.-H., King, K.-L., and Wei, Y.-H., Liver mitochondrial respiratory functions decline with age, *Biochem. Biophys. Res. Commun.*, 165, 994, 1989.
98. Corral-Debrinski, M., Horton, T., Lotl, M. T., Shoffner, J. M., Beal, M. F., and Wallace, D. C., Mitochondrial DNA deletions in human brain: regional variability and increase with advanced age, *Nature Genetics*, 2, 324, 1992.

99. Arnheim, N. and Cortopassi, G., Deleterious mitochondrial DNA mutations accumulate in aging human tissues, *Mutat. Res.*, 275, 156, 1992.

100. Cortopassi, G. A., Shibata, D., Soong, N.-W., and Arnheim, N., A pattern of accumulation of somatic deletion of mitochondrial DNA in aging human tissues, *Proc. Natl. Acad. Sci. U.S.A.*, 89, 7370, 1992.

101. Soong, N.-W., Hinton, D. R., Cortopassi, G., and Arnheim, N., Mosaicism for specific somatic mitochondrial DNA mutation in adult human brain, *Nature Genetics*, 2, 318, 1992.

102. Muller-Hocker, J., Mitochondria and aging, *Brain Pathol.*, 2, 149, 1992.

103. Wei, Y.-H., Mitochondrial alterations as ageing associated molecular events, *Mutat. Res.*, 275, 145, 1992.

104. Fernandez-Silva, P., Petruzella, V., Fracasso, F., Gadaleta, M. N., and Contatore, P., Reduced synthesis of mtRNA in isolated mitochondria of senescent rat brain, *Biochem. Biophys. Res. Commun.*, 176, 645, 1991.

105. Biggs, R. B., Hanley, R. M., Morrison, P. R., and Booth, F. W., Cytochrome c mRNA levels decrease in senescent rat heart, *Mech. Ageing Dev.*, 60, 285, 1991.

106. Magnuson, V. L., Young, M., Schalterberg, D. G., Mancini, M. A., Chen, D., Steffensen, B., and Kleba, R. J., Is alternative splicing of fibronectin pre-mRNA altered during aging and in response to growth factors?, *J. Biol. Chem.*, 266, 14654, 1991.

107. Chandrasekhar, S., Sorrentino, J. A., and Mills, A. J. T., Interaction of fibronectin with collagen: age specific defect in the biological activity, *Proc. Natl. Acad. Sci. U.S.A.*, 80, 4747, 1983.

108. Burke, E. M. and Danner, D. B., Changes in fibronectin mRNA splicing with *in vitro* passage, *Biochem. Biophys. Res. Commun.*, 178, 620, 1991.

109. Goldgaber, D., Lerman, M. I., McBride, O. W., Saffoti, U., and Gajdusek, D. C., Characterisation and chromosomal localization of a cDNA encoding brain amyloid of Alzheimer's disease, *Science*, 235, 877, 1987.

110. Kanungo, M. S., *Biochemistry of Ageing*, Academic Press, London, 1980, 267.

Chapter 5

ROLE OF MITOCHONDRIA IN CELL AGING

Jaime Miquel

CONTENTS

0-8493-4786-6/95/$0.00+$.50
© 1995 by CRC Press, Inc.

I. INTRODUCTION

The aged population of the developed countries is fast increasing, but maximum life expectancy has barely changed in the last decades and many of the aged suffer from degenerative diseases of the cardiovascular and central nervous systems, which is very costly in terms of human suffering and requires huge economical and sanitary resources. Progress in life span extension and in the treatment and prevention of those age-related degenerative processes is hindered by a lack of agreement on the cellular and molecular mechanisms of senescence. According to Medvedev,[1] about 300 theories of aging have been proposed, but many gerontologists feel that a process as complex as senescence can not be explained by a single theory. We agree with this view and, on the basis of our finding of an age dependent loss of mitochondria,[2,3] with the resulting accumulation of age pigment from mitochondrial debris,[2-4] we have proposed an integrated *oxygen radical-mitochondrial injury* hypothesis of aging[2,4-8] that links this process to the attack by free radicals and other injurious oxygen species from the respiratory chain to mitochondrial membranes and mitochondrial DNA (mtDNA). Although mtDNA had been singled out before as one of the possible targets of free radical attack,[9] this early view mistakenly implied that mitochondrial genetic injury occurs in all cell types, which is in disagreement with our finding of normal mitochondria in fast-replicating cells.[2-4] Similar views on the key role of mitochondria in aging have been offered by other authors in order to explain the pathogenesis of normal senescence and of a number of degenerative diseases of the nervous and muscular systems[10-15] (Table 1).

In addition to a review of the fine structural and genetic aspects of the mitochondrial hypothesis of aging, we offer here related biochemical data and briefly discuss the bioenergetic and physiopathological implications of age-related mitochondrial dysfunction. We believe that the concept that senescence may derive, at least in part, from a mitochondrial bioenergetic dysfunction not only provides a reasonable explanation of age-related changes from the molecular to the physiological levels, but may also help to develop a preventive and therapeutic approach to many degenerative syndromes by pharmacological and nutritional modulation of energy-related metabolic pathways.

II. THE "MITOCHONDRIAL DAMAGE-ENERGY LOSS" HYPOTHESIS OF AGING

Our concept maintains that one of the primary causes of age-related injury in animals and humans is oxy-radical attack to mitochondrial membranes and genome rather than to nuclear DNA, as proposed by earlier somatic mutation theories of aging.[1] Mitochondrial injury occurs mainly

TABLE 1.

Hypotheses on the Role of Mitochondria in Aging[a]

Proposed Cause of Aging	Author	Year	Ref.
Free radical injury to mitochondria, including their DNA	Harman	1972	9
Oxy-radical or lipid peroxide-induced inactivation of the mitochondrial DNA of fixed postmitotic cells	Miquel et al.	1980	2
Irreversible injury to mtDNA	Fleming et al.	1982	5
Intrinsic mitochondrial mutagenesis in terminally differentiated cells	Miquel and Fleming	1986	12
Intranuclear accumulation of mitochondrial DNA fragments	Richter	1988	10
Accumulation of mitochondrial mutations and cytoplasmic segregation of these mutations	Linnane et al.	1989	11
Mitochondrial genetic and membrane damage as the result of a loss of regenerative mechanisms in irreversibly differentiated cells	Miquel	1991	6

[a]   Modified from Reference 6.

in differentiated cells, and especially in neurons and other fixed postmitotic cells because they can not regenerate their mitochondria as effectively as proliferating cells which renew their organelles each time they engage in mitosis. In addition, differentiated cells may be exposed to injurious oxy-radical stress because of the high levels of mitochondrial oxygen utilization needed to support their specialized physiological work.

If, as we propose, oxidative injury is not limited to mitochondrial membranes, but also occurs in mtDNA, the organelles which have sustained genome mutation, inactivation, or loss will be unable to turn over the macromolecules coded by this genome, namely the hydrophobic polypeptides of the electron transport chain and of ATP synthase as well as the mitochondrial rRNAs and tRNAs. This will lead to a progressive loss of the ability to rejuvenate the mitochondrial population, replacing with fully functional organelles the mitochondria damaged or lost because of lipid peroxidation and cross-linking reactions triggered by respiration-linked oxygen species. Because of the associated genome and membrane disorganization, the mitochondria will suffer autophagic breakdown with resulting formation of age pigment (Figure 1).

It is very important from a physiopathological and clinical viewpoint to recognize that, since most cellular energy is produced in mitochondria through the process of oxidative phosphorylation, the age-related dys-

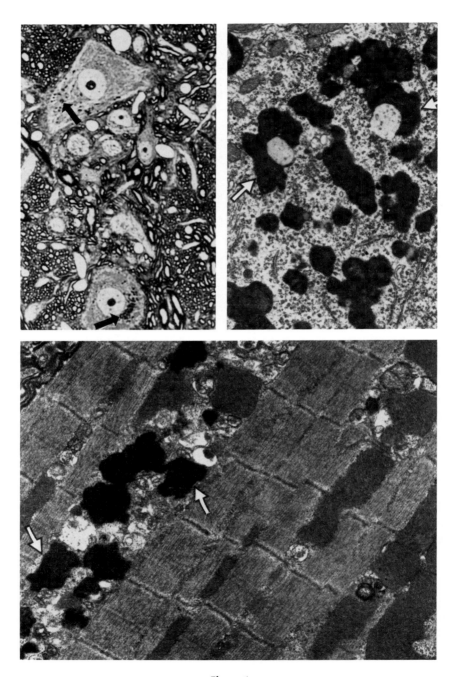

Figure 1

function and loss of these organelles must result in a bioenergetic decline. This may be compatible with the maintenance of health under nonstressful conditions, but impairs physiological performance and survival when high levels of ATP production are required to preserve homeostasis in the face of disease or environmental stress. Moreover, senescent mitochondrial breakdown and energy loss may play a role in the genesis of age-related degenerative diseases of the somatic tissues mainly composed of fixed postmitotic cells, such as the cardiac and skeletal muscle and the CNS. The liver, and other organs containing cells which occasionally engage in mitosis, will show a moderate loss of functional competence because of mitochondrial aging, while proliferating cells in the stem cell compartments and elsewhere will suffer little senescent change.

An important prediction of our hypothesis is that aging should be accompanied by progressive bioenergetic and functional decline, which may be slowed down and counteracted by compounds which protect mitochondria against oxy-radical attack, preserve the respiratory chain of the inner mitochondrial membrane, and "reenergize" aged mitochondria, thereby raising ATP synthesis in senescing differentiated cells.

III. THEORETICAL CONCEPTS AND EXPERIMENTAL DATA

A. Cell Differentiation as the Fundamental Cause of Mitochondrial and Cellular Aging

As first pointed out by Weissman,[18] multicellular organisms age because of the differentiation process, which resulted in the appearance of two different kinds of cells: the reproductive and the somatic. In his words: "Very soon the somatic cells surpassed the reproductive in num-

Figure 1
Lipofuscin age pigment accumulation is one of the most consistent age-related findings, not only in vertebrates but in invertebrates as well. Our data from *Drosophila* and mammalian research suggest that, in large proportion, this pigment derives from degenerating mitochondria. Therefore, its presence in high amounts may be associated with mitochondrial loss and bioenergetic decline. Upper left: lipofuscin granules (arrows) in the lateral vestibular nucleus of the brain of an 8-month-old rat. Magnification ×500. Upper right: structure of lipofuscin in a pyramidal neuron of the hypocampus of a 30-month-old mouse. The arrow points to a granule containing a lipid droplet. Magnification ×14,000. Bottom: myocardial cell of a 30-month-old mouse, showing abundant lipofuscin (arrows) in areas where, in young animals, rows of mitochondria are found. Magnification ×21,500. (The upper two electron micrographs are from Miquel, J., Johnson, J. E., and Cervos-Navarro, J., *Brain Aging: Neuropathology and Neuropharmacology*, Cervos-Navarro, J. and Sarkander, H.-I., Eds., Raven Press, New York, 1983; the lower micrograph is from Miquel, J., Economos, A. C., Bensch, K. G., Atlan, H., and Johnson, J. E., Jr., *Age*, 2, 78, 1979. With permission.)

ber, and during this increase they became more and more broken up by the principle of the division of labor into sharply separated systems of tissues. As these changes took place the power of reproducing large parts of the organism was lost, while the power of reproducing the whole individual became concentrated in the reproductive cells alone." These views are in agreement with the concept of another pioneer gerontologist, Charles Minot,[19] who stated that aging is the "price paid for cell differentiation."

Our mitochondrial hypothesis of aging is in agreement with the above, since it is well known that cell differentiation is accompanied by mitochondrial changes which include striking increases in cellular oxygen utilization,[20] and therefore in an increased formation of oxygen radicals which are side effects of the univalent reduction of oxygen in the mitochondrial respiratory chain,[21,22] thereby paving the way to mitochondrial peroxidative injury and concomitant cell aging.

At a higher level of biological organization, i.e., with focus on physiological, rather than cellular or molecular senescence, Pearl[23] proposed that the rate of aging is directly correlated with the *rate of living*, i.e., with organismic activity and metabolic rate. Likewise, the rate of aging of a particular cell may be explained in the framework of our oxy-radical-mitochondrial damage hypothesis of aging, since a higher rate of mitochondrial oxygen utilization (and resulting release of injurious free radicals) must lead to faster mitochondrial aging as the result of oxygen stress.

B. Physiological and Bioenergetic Decline

Since Shock's[24] pioneering work on human subjects ranging in age from 30 to 90 years who were studied for a period of up to 20 years, it is well known that aging is accompanied by functional and bioenergetic loss in every organ and physiological system. The senescent changes include the following:

1. Decreased exercise and work capacity measured as the maximal work load that a subject can perform with return to a normal heartbeat at 2 min after stopping the work.
2. Loss of hand grip strength from about 28 kg at 20 years to 20 kg at 75 years of age.
3. Impaired coordination of the organ systems which must work simultaneously to support complex physiological tasks such as physical exercise and sexual activity.
4. Decreased blood perfusion of the kidneys and decline of their detoxification capacity.

5. Neuroendocrine changes which have a detrimental effect on a wide range of physiological processes, from cellular metabolism to the regulation of the diameter of small blood vessels and, therefore, on the amount of blood which reaches the tissues.

These changes are accompanied by a decreased efficiency of the mechanisms that prevent the loss of homeostasis. Thus, as reported by Shock,[24] factors like the total blood volume, osmotic pressure, and protein and glucose levels in blood remain constant in both young and aged subjects under resting conditions. However, when they deviate from normal levels because of experimental manipulation, aged subjects need more time to return to the baseline values.

Of course, some of the above changes may be increased by unhealthy aspects of life style such as physical inactivity, drinking, drug abuse, poor nutrition, and smoking. Nevertheless, even in subjects adhering to the healthiest life style, aging is accompanied by a progressive loss of vigor and physiological competence, especially evident under conditions of disease, stress, and exhaustive work or sport activity, when there is a need to tap the reserve capacity of the organism.

The age-related decline in physiological performance and energy production that is probably linked to mitochondrial dysfunction is not only seen in human subjects, but is an universal characteristic of the metazoan phenotype as shown by data from our laboratory on the age-related loss of control of body weight,[25] neuromuscular coordination,[26] and immunological competence[27] in mice, as well as of negative geotaxis[28] and mating competence[29] in *Drosophila* fruit flies.

C. Oxidative Damage to the Nuclear and Mitochondrial Genomes

As pointed out elsewhere,[30] the first proponent of the DNA damage hypothesis of aging was careful to note the difference between DNA damage and mutation and emphasized that he considered nonmutagenic DNA damage, rather than mutation, as the primary cause of aging.[31] This concept was supported by the finding that administration of mutagenic substances to mice did not cause senescence-like physiological and pathological changes. According to Holmes et al.[30] the age-related changes caused by oxidative reactions on the DNA molecules of nonreplicating cells may block transcription of essential genes, resulting in decreased RNA and protein synthesis. Thus, mitochondrial biogenesis (which requires both mitochondrial and nuclear DNA) could be impaired and a decline in ATP synthesis would occur in the tissues of aged individuals as the result of oxidative damage to the nuclear genome.

In contrast to the above concept, we propose that mtDNA is a more probable target of age-related mutation or damage than nuclear DNA. As discussed elsewhere,[6,7] the reasons for assigning to the mitochondrial genome the role of the Achiles' heel responsible for metazoan aging are its rapid turnover rate and mutability, its relative lack of repair mechanisms, and its location in a highly mutagenic environment near the sites of formation of highly reactive oxy-radicals.

Recent studies support our hypothesis of senescent mtDNA injury, since deletions and other types of genetic damage have been shown in the organs of aged humans and animals. Thus, rat liver senescence is accompanied by strong binding of proteins or peptides to mtDNA, while no change was seen in the nuclear DNA.[32] Further, aging results in mtDNA deletions in human tissues and organs such as muscle and brain,[33] diaphragm muscle,[34] liver,[35] and heart,[36] while a study of respiratory chain proteins from human skeletal muscle suggests that the decrease in the respiratory efficiency of this tissue is due to mutations in structural mitochondrial DNA genes.[37]

On the basis of their own data, Yen et al.[35] and Linnane et al.[38] concur with our view[2,4] that mitochondrial genetic injury plays an important role in aging, contributing to the senescent decline in bioenergetic capacity. The mtDNA damage leads to organellar death as the result of homeostasis derangement, activation of endonucleases, proteases, and phospholipases, and concomitant autophagic breakdown. In essence, in normally aging fixed postmitotic cells the senescent energy decline may be linked to mitochondrial peroxidative DNA and membrane changes as well as to a decrease in the number of surviving organelles.

D. Age-Related Effects on Mitochondrial Biogenesis and Biochemistry

As previously reviewed,[7] our concept that aging results in a decreased rate of mitochondrial biogenesis is supported by the observation that physical training has a different effect on the mitochondria of leg skeletal muscle of young as compared to those of aged men.[39] In young subjects, it results in a 100% increase of the total mitochondrial volume, while the increase is only 20% for men over 50 years of age. This suggests that senescence is associated with a block in mitochondrial division in fixed postmitotic cells, such as those of muscle, since the larger mitochondrial volume found in the physically active young group was the result of an increase in the number of mitochondria without a change in their dimension, while in the older men the larger volume was associated with an increase in the size of the organelles without an increase in their amount.

An age-related impairment in mitochondria biosynthesis is also suggested by a computer-assisted morphometric study of the synaptic mitochondria of the cerebellar glomeruli of rats.[40] These data show that the synapses contain a higher number of mitochondria per tissue volume in adult as compared to young animals, and that this maturation-related increase is followed by a decrease in the number of organelles in aged rats. On the other hand, the mitochondria of old rats are larger in size and more elongated than those of young and adult rats. Previous work from the same laboratory had already shown that aging results in a decrease in the number of cerebellar and hippocampal synapses which, despite an age-related increase in their size, resulted in a reduction in the overall synaptic surface area. These data suggest that, compensatory mechanisms notwithstanding, brain aging is linked to a certain degree of structural disorganization at both the synaptic and the mitochondrial levels. Moreover, the data support our view[2,4] that senescence is accompanied by a progressive impairment in the ability of mitochondria to counteract their oxy-radical-inflicted losses through the process of organellar replication.

Another prediction of our hypothesis is that aging must result in a certain degree of biochemical impairment of the mitochondria in all types of differentiated cells. Although there are some contradictory findings, the data reviewed elsewhere[2-8] show that aging in this cell type is indeed accompanied by a variety of biochemical changes. These include the above-summarized mtDNA deletions, a decrease in mtDNA transcription and in the levels of mtRNA, GSH, cytochrome aa_3, and cytochrome c mRNA. There is also an impairment in calcium homeostasis and a decreased activity of the enzymes that catalyze oxidative phosphorylation.

The recent study by Paradies et al.[41] on both respiratory and lipid components of the mitochondrial membranes deserves attention, since it deals with cytochrome c oxidase, the terminal enzyme complex of the mitochondrial electron transport chain that is responsible for most oxygen consumption in differentiated mammalian cells. The study shows a senescent decrease in the maximal activity of this enzyme complex in mitochondria isolated from rat heart, which according to the authors may be due to the age-related decrease in the mitochondrial phospholipid, cardiolipin, a normal concentration of which is required to support the catalytic work of cytochrome oxidase.

Data on the effects of aging on brain mitochondria are especially relevant to our hypothesis, since this organ contains the highly differentiated and extremely oxygen-dependent nerve cells.

The subject of age-dependent changes in CNS mitochondria abounds in conflicting data, probably because of technical problems, including the fact that usually the organelles are obtained from tissue samples which contain, side by side, aging fixed postmitotic cells (i.e., neurons) and relatively nonaging cells (i.e., glia). Nevertheless, it seems well established by electron microscopic research that neurons suffer senescent changes in the amount and structure of their mitochondrial populations, with transformation of many mitochondria into the age pigment, lipofuscin, through a process of lysosomal digestion.[42]

The mitochondrial theory of aging is also supported by a recent study by Bowling et al.,[43] showing an impairment in the activity of electron transport chain enzymes from primate neocortex, especially in the respiratory complexes I and IV. This finding is consistent with injury to mtDNA, as this genome encodes seven subunits of complex I and three subunits of complex IV. Nevertheless, as pointed out by the authors, pathogenetic mechanisms unrelated to mitochondrial genetic injury could be responsible for the especial age-related sensitivity of those complexes, since complex I is very sensitive to attack by the hydroxyl radical, complex IV is affected by hydrogen peroxide, and both complexes are influenced by the lipid environment.

A comparative study on synaptic and nonsynaptic mitochondria from rat brain showed age-dependent changes only in the last.[44] Senescence resulted in a loss of cytochromes $c+c_1$ and in a decreased activity of cytochrome c oxidase, with the decline being very striking when malate or glutamate were utilized as substrate. This study also showed that, under conditions of high metabolic demand or low oxygen tension, the rate of oxygen reduction by cytochrome oxidase is decreased up to 50% in aged rats. The authors conclude that in hypoxemia caused by low blood pressure or transient circulatory changes, respiration and ATP synthesis in the synaptic mitochondria from old animals may suffer a striking decline.

Our own research on synaptic mitochondria isolated from mouse brain has shown that aging is accompanied by a significant decrease in the respiratory activity of complex IV and V.[45] Since complex V (ATP synthase) is the key enzyme of energy metabolism, this age-related change may impair an energy-dependent process as important as neurotransmission, thus contributing to the senescent decline in memory and other CNS functions. Further work from our laboratory[46] has tested the hypothesis that brain aging may be linked to oxygen stress, by determination of the lipid peroxide and glutathione levels in synaptic mitochondria. Our data show that old mice have lower lipid peroxide and higher glutathione levels in their mitochondria as compared to young animals. Therefore we conclude that, although oxygen stress may indeed occur, the senescent decrease in cytochrome oxidase activity (and thereby in O_2 utilization) results in a decline in the release of oxy-radicals in the respiratory chain, with a concomitant decrease in lipid peroxide accumulation and a sparing effect on the antioxidant GSH.

Brain senescence is not only linked to changes in mitochondrial respiration and bioenergetics, since other age-related dysfunctions such as a decrease in the synthesis of mtRNA[47] and DNA[48] and in the mitochondrial uptake of calcium ions[49,50] have been found.

Our hypothesis also predicts an age-related decline in ATP production, which is in agreement with the finding that mitochondria isolated from organs of aged animals show a decreased ADP/ATP exchange across the inner membrane and a fall in the endogenous pool of adenine nucleotides at the expense of ATP.[51] These changes are accompanied by a decreased ATPase activity and a raised oligomycin-sensitive proton conduction in brain and heart mitochondria from aged rats, with concomitant dissipation of the electrochemical proton gradient linked to the electron transport chain and decreased ATP production.[52]

In addition, research by Corbisier and Remacle[53] has provided quite strong evidence for an age-related bioenergetic failure in mitochondria in human WI fibroblasts. When these cells were microinjected with mitochondria isolated from the cells of old animals or with uncoupled mitochondria from young animals, an appreciable amount of fibroblasts suffered a process of degeneration. This seemed to be due to energy failure, since cellular degeneration was prevented by supplementing the culture medium with the easily metabolized energy substrate DC(–)-β-hydroxybutyrate sodium salt.

Whatever the specific mechanisms involved at the mitochondrial genome and membrane levels, it seems that aging is accompanied by a decline in the mitochondrial production of energy by oxidative phosphorylation. This may lead not only to a general loss of vigor but also to specific functional loss in organs such as brain, heart, skeletal muscle, kidney, liver, pancreas, and testis, which depend on a high rate of oxygen utilization. As pointed out by Wallace,[54] if the ATP production falls below certain levels this age-related decline in mitochondrial performance may contribute to the pathogenesis of ischemic heart disease. Moreover, according to Bowling et al.[43] "age-dependent reductions in mitochondrial functions could contribute to the delayed onset and age dependent increase in the incidence of various disorders affecting human brain."

IV. CONCLUSIONS

Our hypothesis, that integrates concepts from the "somatic mutation" and "free radical" theories of aging and is compatible with the ideas of Minot and Pearl on the relation of aging with cell differentiation and metabolic rate, is in agreement with many of the biochemical and functional manifestations of senescence at every level of biological organization. This is not surprising since a mitochondrial-bioenergetic decline must have far-ranging effects on cells and physiological systems.

Our hypothesis is also compatible with the mosaic appearance of energy deficient and atrophic cells in the tissues of aged animals and humans, since this reflects the degree of mitochondrial dysfunction suffered by the various cells composing a tissue.[11] Moreover, the diverse manifestations of aging shown by different organs and the large differences in life span between animal species can also be explained as the outcome of both the rate of mitochondria-damaging oxygen radical release and the mitochondrial resistance to oxidative injury in the diverse cell types. This depends on many factors including the number of mitochondria per cell, rate of organellar replication and of turnover of their genetic and structural components, size and coding capacity of their genomes, and levels of intramitochondrial antioxidant enzymes.

As pointed out elsewhere,[6] the *mitochondrial damage-energy loss* concept of aging explains not only where in the organism the senescent involution may start but also why aging made its appearance in the biosphere. Thus, we view aging as the unprogrammed but unavoidable result of mitochondrial oxidative phosphorylation in fixed postmitotic cells. These cells are in double jeopardy because of the high levels of oxygen utilization required to support their specialized physiological work and the loss of the mitochondrial regeneration process associated with the organellar division which accompanies mitosis.

In summary, we propose that although the evolutionary acquisition of mitochondria by previously anaerobic cells (with a striking increase in ATP production from oxidative phosphorylation as compared to that obtained from glycolysis) made possible the appearance of differentiated cells and metazoans, it also resulted in cell aging and concomitant organism death as the result of energy exhaustion because of oxygen stress-related disorganization of the ATP-producing organelles. Morover, if senescence and its associated degenerative diseases are linked to mitochondrial dysfunction and energy loss, future preventive geriatrics may benefit from pharmacologically induced preservation of mitochondrial biogenesis and stimulation of energy production in aging cells.

ACKNOWLEDGMENTS

The author thanks Ms. Margarita Blasco for her help in the preparation of the manuscript. This work was supported by Grant FIS 94/1348.

REFERENCES

1. Medvedev, Z. A., An attempt at a rational classification of theories of aging, *Biol. Rev.*, 66, 375, 1990.
2. Miquel, J., Economos, A. C., Fleming, J. E., and Johnson, J. E., Jr., Mitochondrial role in cell aging, *Exp. Gerontol.*, 15, 575, 1980.
3. Miquel, J., Oro, J., Bensch, K. G., and Johnson, J. E., Jr., Lipofuscin: fine structural and biochemical studies, in *Free Radicals in Biology*, Vol. 3, Pryor, W., Ed., Academic Press, New York, 1977, 133.

4. Miquel, J. and Fleming, J. E., Theoretical and experimental support for an "oxygen radical-mitochondrial injury" hypothesis of aging, in *Free Radicals, Aging and Degenerative Diseases*, Johnson, J. E., Jr., Walford, R., Harman, D., and Miquel, J., Eds., Alan R. Liss, New York, 1986, 57.

5. Fleming, J. E., Miquel, J., Cottrell, S. F., Yengoyan, L. S., and Economos, A. C. Is cell aging caused by respiration-dependent injury to the mitochondrial genome?, *Gerontology*, 28, 44, 1982.

6. Miquel, J., An integrated theory of aging as the result of mitochondrial DNA mutation in differentiated cells, *Arch. Gerontol. Geriatr.*, 12, 99, 1991.

7. Miquel, J., An update on the mitochondrial-DNA mutation hypothesis of cell aging, *Mutat. Res.*, 275, 209, 1992.

8. Miquel, J. and Blasco, M., Aging as a mitochondrial-energy deficiency disease, *Facts Res. Gerontol.*, 8, 28, 1994.

9. Harman, D., The biologic clock: the mitochondria?, *J. Am. Geriatr. Soc.*, 20, 145, 1972.

10. Richter, C., Do mitochondrial DNA fragments promote cancer and aging?, *FEBS Lett.*, 241, 1, 1988.

11. Linnane, A. W., Marzuki, S., Ozawa, T., and Tanaka, M., Mitochondrial DNA mutations as an important contributor to ageing and degenerative diseases, *Lancet*, i, 642, 1989.

12. Miquel, J. and Fleming, J. E., A two-step hypothesis on the mechanisms of *in vitro* cell aging: cell differentiation followed by intrinsic mitochondrial mutagenesis, *Exp. Gerontol.*, 19, 31, 1984.

13. Wallace, D. C., Mitochondrial genetics: a paradigm for aging and degenerative diseases, *Science*, 256, 628, 1992.

14. Muller-Hocker, J., Mitochondria and ageing-enzyme-immunohistochemical and *in situ* hybridization studies, *Bull. Mol. Biol. Med.*, 18, 25, 1993.

15. Bittles, A. H., Evidence for and against the causal involvement of mitochondrial DNA mutation in mammalian ageing, *Mutat. Res.*, 275, 217, 1992.

16. Miquel, J., Johnson, J. E., and Cervos-Navarro, J., Comparison of CNS aging in humans and experimental animals, in *Brain Aging: Neuropathology and Neuropharmacology*, Cervos-Navarro, J. and Sarkander, H.-I., Eds., Raven Press, New York, 1983.

17. Miquel, J., Economos, A. C., Bensch, K. G., Atlan, H. and Johnson, J. E., Jr., Review of cell aging in *Drosophila* and mouse, *Age*, 2, 78, 1979.

18. Weissman, A., *Essays Upon Heredity and Kindred Biological Problems*, Oxford University-Clarendon Press, New York, 1891.

19. Minot, C. S., The problem of age, growth and death, *Popular Science Monthly*, 71, 509, 1907.

20. Sun, A. S., Aggarwal, B. B., and Packer, L., Enzyme levels of normal human cells aging in culture, *Arch. Biochem. Biophys.*, 170, 1, 1975.

21. Chance, B., Sies, H., and Boveris, A., Hydroperoxide metabolism in mammalian organs, *Physiol. Rev.*, 59, 257, 1979.

22. Nohl, H., Hegner, D., and Summer, K. H., The mechanism of toxic action of hyperbaric oxygenation on the mitochondria of rat heart cells, *Biochem. Pharmacol.*, 30, 1753, 1981.

23. Pearl, R., *The Rate of Living*, University of London Press, U.K., 1928.

24. Shock, N. W., Some physiological aspects of aging in man, *Bull N.Y. Acad. Med.*, 32, 268, 1958.

25. Economos, A. C. and Miquel, J., Usefulness of stochastic analysis of body weight as a tool in experimental aging research, *Exp. Aging Res.*, 6, 417, 1980.

26. Miquel, J. and Blasco, M., A simple technique for evaluation of vitality loss in aging mice, by testing their muscular coordination and vigor, *Exp. Gerontol.*, 13, 389, 1978.

27. De la Fuente, M., Ferrandez, D., Muñoz, F., De Juan, E., and Miquel, J., Stimulation by the antioxidant thioproline of the lymphocyte functions of old mice, *Mech. Ageing Dev.*, 68, 27, 1993.

28. Miquel, J., Lundgren, P. R., and Binnard, R., Negative geotaxis and mating behavior in control and gamma-irradiated *Drosophila*, *Drosophila Inform. Serv.*, 48, 60, 1972.

29. Economos, A. C., Miquel, J., and Binnard, R., Quantitative analysis of mating behavior in aging male *Drosophila melanogaster*, *Mech. Ageing Dev.*, 10, 233, 1979.

30. Holmes, G. E., Bernstein, C., and Bernstein, H., Oxidative and other DNA damages as the basis of aging: a review, *Mutat. Res.*, 275, 305, 1992.

31. Alexander, P., The role of DNA lesions in processes leading to aging in mice, *Symp. Soc. Exp. Biol.*, 21, 29, 1967.

32. Asano, K. S., Amagase, S., Matsuura, E. T., and Yamagishi, H., Changes in the rat liver mitochondrial DNA upon aging, *Mech. Ageing Dev.*, 60, 275, 1991.

33. Cortopassi, G. A. and Arnheim, N., Detection of a specific mitochondrial DNA deletion in tissues of older humans, *Nucl. Acids Res.*, 18, 6927, 1990.

34. Hayakawa, M., Torii, K., Sugiyama, S., Tanaka, M., and Ozawa, T., Age-associated accumulation of 8-hydroxydeoxyguanosine in mitochondrial DNA of human diaphragm, *Biochem. Biophys. Res. Commun.*, 179, 1023, 1991.

35. Yen, T. C., Su, J. H., King, K. L., and Wei, Y. H., Ageing-associated 5kb deletion in human liver mitochondrial DNA, *Biochem. Biophys. Res. Commun.*, 178, 124, 1991.

36. Hattori, K., Tanaka, M., Sugiyama, S., Obayashi, T., Ito, Y., Satake, T., Hanaki, Y., Asai, J., Nagano, M., and Ozawa, Y., Age-dependent increase in deleted mitochondrial DNA in the human heart: possible contributory factor to presbycardia, *Am. Heart J.*, 121, 1735, 1991.

37. Byrne, E., Trounce, I., and Dennet, X., Mitochondrial theory of senescence: respiratory chain protein studies in human skeletal muscle, *Mech. Ageing Dev.*, 60, 295, 1991.

38. Linnane, A. W., Baumer, A., Maxwell, R. J., Preston, H., Zhang, C. F., and Mazuki, S., Mitochondrial gene mutation: the ageing process and degenerative diseases, *Biochem. Int.*, 22, 1067, 1990.

39. Kiessling, K. H., Pilstrom, I., Karlsson, J., and Piehl, K., Mitochondrial volume in skeletal muscle from young and old physically untrained and trained healthy men and from alcoholics, *Clin. Sci.*, 44, 547, 1973.

40. Bertoni-Freddari, C., Fattoretti, C., Casoli, P., Spagna, T., Meier-Ruge, C. and Ulrich, J., Morphological plasticity of synaptic mitochondria during aging, *Brain Res.*, 628, 193, 1991.

41. Paradies, G., Ruggiero, F. M., Petrosillo, G., and Quagliariello, E., Age dependent decrease in the cytochrome c oxidase activity and changes in phospholipids in rat-heart mitochondria, *Arch. Gerontol. Geriatr.*, 16, 263, 1993.

42. Miquel, J., Economos A. C., and Johnson, J. E., Jr., A systems analysis-thermodynamic view of cellular and organismic aging, in *Aging and Cell Function*, Johnson, J. E., Jr., Ed., Plenum Press, New York, 1984, 247.

43. Bowling, A. C., Mutisya, E. M., Walker, L. C., Price, D. L., Cork, L. C., and Flint Beal, M., Age-dependent impairment of mitochondrial function in primate brain, *J. Neurochem.*, 60, 1964, 1993.

44. Harmon, H. J., Nank, S., and Floyd, R. A., Age-dependent changes in rat brain mitochondria of synaptic and non-synaptic origins, *Mech. Ageing Dev.*, 38, 167, 1987.

45. Ferrandiz, M. L., Martinez, M., De Juan, E., Diez, A., Bustos, G., and Miquel, J., Impairment of mitochondrial oxidative phosphorylation in the brain of aged mice, *Brain Res.*, 644, 335, 1994.

46. Martinez, M., Ferrandiz, M. L., De Juan, E., and Miquel, J., Age related changes in glutathione and lipid peroxide content in synaptic mitochondria: relationship to cytochrome oxidase, *Neurosci. Lett.*, 170, 121, 1994.

47. Fernandez Silva, P., Petruzella, J., Fracasso, F., Gadaleta, M. N. and Cantatore, P., Reduced synthesis of mtRNA in isolated mitochondria of senescent rat brain, *Biochem. Biophys. Res. Commun.*, 176, 645, 1991.

48. Gadaleta, M. N., Petruzella, V., Renis, M., Fracasso, F., and Cantatore, P., Reduced transcription of mitochondrial DNA in the senescent rat. Tissue dependence and effect of acetyl-L-carnitine, *Eur. J. Biochem.*, 187, 501, 1990.

49. Vitorica, J. and Satrustegui, J., Involvement of mitochondria in the age dependent decrease in calcium uptake of rat brain synaptosomes, *Brain Res.*, 378, 36, 1986.

50. Michaelis, M. L., Foster, C. T., and Jagawicreme, C., Regulation of calcium levels in brain tissue from adult and aged rats, *Mech. Ageing Dev.*, 62, 291, 1992.

51. Foris, G. and Leovey, A., Age related changes in cAMP and cGMP levels during phagocytosis in human polymorphonuclear leukocytes, *Mech. Ageing Dev.*, 27, 233, 1980.

52. Guerrieri, F., Capozza, G., Kalous, M., Zanotti, F., Drahota, Z., and Papa, S., Age-dependent changes in the mitochondrial FoF_1 ATP synthase, *Arch. Gerontol. Geriatr.*, 14, 299, 1992.

53. Corbisier, P. and Remacle, J., Involvement of mitochondria in cell degeneration, *Eur. J. Cell Biol.*, 57, 173, 1990.

54. Wallace, D. C., Mitochondrial genetics: a paradigm for aging and degenerative disease?, *Science*, 256, 628, 1992.

II
THE FLOW OF INFORMATION

Chapter 6

MODIFICATIONS OF THE CELL SURFACE LEADING TO CELL ELIMINATION

Hans U. Lutz

CONTENTS

0-8493-4786-6/95/$0.00+$.50

I. POSSIBLE ROUTES IN CELL ELIMINATION (AN INTRODUCTION)

Multicellular organisms that live longer than some of their tissue cells eliminate senescent cells and replace them by the progeny of stem cells (for reviews see References 1 and 2). This phenomenon is called tissue homeostasis, since it maintains tissue functions. Many organisms eliminate some cells long before they have reached a state of senescence or functional impairment. This type of cell elimination is initiated by apoptosis or programmed cell death (for reviews see References 3 and 4). Apoptosis occurs in genetically susceptible cells,[5,6] is triggered by either a lack or the presence of a cytokine,[7] by hormones,[8] antibodies,[9,10] oxidative stress,[11] or other stimuli, and serves important purposes in development. It initiates clearance of larval cells in metamorphosis from insects to amphibia, of primordial tissue in ontogeny of mammals, and it provides immune tolerance by eliminating certain autoreactive T cells.[4,12] Higher organisms can further kill cells of their own body by lytic principles, like the complement system,[13] perforin from cytotoxic cells,[14] and tumor necrosis factors (TNF).[15]

Although these lytic principles are activated in conjunction with specificity-providing antibodies and cells, respectively, they also lyse innocent bystander cells once the lytic substances are set free. In brief, cell elimination is initiated by several means: cellular senescence, apoptosis, and lytic principles, while completion of the various modes of elimination seems to operate exclusively by phagocytosis. As phagocytes do not randomly engulf particles and soluble protein complexes, disposal of the cellular waste calls for recognition mechanisms. These mechanisms include soluble mediators and/or a steadily increasing number of phagocytic receptors which directly recognize modifications on target cell surfaces. While the *in vitro* specificity of many receptors is known, their *in vivo* functional relevance is yet unclarified. Thus, a similar uncertainty exists about the crucial surface modifications.

We know little about the chemical modifications on apoptotic cells which ultimately result in the clearance of apoptotic blebs and apoptotic bodies. *In vitro* experiments suggested that apoptotic cells are cleared by binding to either the vitronectin,[16] the scavenger receptor,[17] or the phosphatidylserine receptor[18] on macrophages. However, it remains unclear what makes these receptors bind to the apoptotic and not the original cell. So far, apoptotic cells have been considered as a whole, despite the formation of blebs of which many are released and apoptotic bodies which differ from each other both in their contents and their surface properties, as has recently been exemplified on keratinocytes by showing that apoptosis is accompanied by a reorganization of cellular proteins, either into apoptotic blebs or apoptotic bodies.[19] Hence, recognition mechanisms for blebs and bodies may differ.

Likewise, we do not know how the protein complexes which are released from lysed cells are specifically detected and cleared by phagocytes. More is known about modifications on senescent as well as oxidatively stressed erythrocytes which are selectively recognized by phagocytes and eliminated. The tissue homeostatic mechanisms operating in the elimination of erythrocytes may serve as a paradigm for other types of cell eliminations, since cellular modifications can best be studied on anucleated erythrocytes. The suggested congruence is not unlikely, since apoptotic blebs, for example, have much in common with erythrocytes, as they represent particles surrounded by a plasma membrane lacking a nucleus. Hence, the idea of this review is to discuss recent work on membrane modifications on senescent and oxidatively stressed erythrocytes, since oxidative stress is a major determinant of cellular aging.[20,21] The discussion on modes of recognition and elimination will be focused primarily on erythrocytes, and where available on apoptotic cells, with special emphasis of the effectiveness of these processes under physiological conditions.

II. MODIFICATIONS ON AGING CELLS

A. What Properties are Characteristic for Senescent Erythrocytes?

1. Predominant Clearance of Senescent Erythrocytes by Phagocytes

Mammalian erythrocytes, so far, are the best model system to study cell aging, since cellular aging phenomena are not perturbed by ongoing protein synthesis. Erythrocytes reach a species-characteristic life span[22] before being eliminated as senescent cells, except in some species (e.g., rabbit, porcine, and even mice), where a portion of cells is randomly cleared.[1] Senescent mammalian erythrocytes are eliminated from the circulation by phagocytes of the reticuloendothelial system. Undoubtedly, the best evidence for this claim was given by Morrison's group,[23] who have used Ganzoni's sequential hypertransfusion protocol on mice to suppress erythropoiesis over 8 weeks. Erythrocytes from hypertransfused animals were indeed senescent, with a half life of 0.9 days as compared to one of 15.3 days for a normal, tagged red cell population.[23] Peritoneal macrophages[24] and a macrophage cell line (IC-21)[23] engulfed hypertransfused erythrocytes up to fivefold better than unseparated erythrocytes from normal mice. Unequivocal data were also achieved by biotinylating erythrocytes, reinjecting them into an animal, and collecting the aged cells on immobilized avidin. This approach allowed Dale and collaborators[25,26] to show that biotinylated erythrocytes had exactly the same *in vivo* survival as ^{14}C-cyanate-labeled erythrocytes in rabbits. When biotinylated cells were also ^{14}C-cyanate labeled, the biotinylated cells recovered after 60 days retained more than 90% of the label, while the unfractionated erythrocyte population contained only a few percent.

2. Physiological and Biochemical Markers of Senescent Erythrocytes

The hypertransfusion experiments and the survival studies with biotinylated cells further allowed the researchers to define the modifications that characterize membranes of senescent erythrocytes. This information was of utmost relevance, since none of these methods could be applied on humans. Instead, density separation of erythrocytes is used on human blood and yields young cells in the light fraction and senescent cells in the densest fraction.[1,2,27] The relationship between erythrocyte age and density has, however, been challenged,[27,28] primarily because some density-separation techniques were in fact not efficient.[29] However, Stractan-,[30] Percoll-,[31] and self-forming Percoll-gradients[32,33] yield dense erythrocytes that show various signs of a progressive deterioration, a single exponential decrease in glutamate-oxalacetate transaminase and pyruvate kinase activity per gram of hemoglobin[30] have lost up to 50% of complement receptor 1[32,34,35] and decay-accelerating factor.[32] Likewise, light erythrocytes had a half life of 28 days, while the densest 1.5 to 3.5% of all cells had one of less than a day.[36] Hence, density separation can effectively enrich young and senescent erythrocytes.

Human erythrocytes of increasing density were progressively more dehydrated and less deformable, with the densest cells having a maximal deformability of 62% of that of unseparated cells, but being almost nondeformable at physiological osmolalities.[32] The same results were obtained with human erythrocytes separated on Stractan gradients[37] and on biotinylated rabbit erythrocytes aged *in vivo*.[38] Moreover, membranes of *in vivo*-aged erythrocytes from hypertransfused mice[39] and from biotinylated rabbit erythrocytes,[40] as well as density-separated human erythrocytes,[32,41] revealed a marked increase in the content of band 4.1a and a concomitant decrease in band 4.1b. This alteration represents the most obvious one on stained SDS PAGE from membranes of young and old erythrocytes in almost all species studied, and the actual ratio correlates with the life span.[42]

The change in band 4.1 with erythrocyte age is indeed a protein modification, since the two proteins generated the same peptide maps[43] and only band 4.1b, but not band 4.1a incorporated [^{35}S]methionine in pulse chase experiments for up to 3 h.[42] The two bands differ by deamidation of two asparagine residues, of which only the one of Asn 502 appeared responsible for the conformational change of band 4.1b to 4.1a, resulting in an apparent shift of 2 kDa on SDS PAGE.[44]

B. Spontaneous Chemical Modifications on Integral Membrane Proteins and Ectoproteins

1. Deamidation

Deamidation of asparaginyl residues is a common, spontaneous, nonenzymatic "aging" process which preferentially occurs in small peptides and in random coil domains of proteins: asparaginyl residues initially form succinimides with the nearest nitrogen atom of the peptide chain, whereby the amide group is lost from the asparaginyl residue.[45] A subsequent, spontaneous hydrolysis of the succinimidyl ring yields aspartyl or isoaspartyl residues.[46] Thus, asparaginyl residues spontaneously become charged L-aspartyl residues and even L-isoaspartyl residues, with a distorted structure of the peptide chain. Moreover a small percentage of the unstable succinimide rings will racemize in C2 of the original asparaginyl residues, whereby also D-aspartyl and D-isoaspartyl residues are generated following hydrolysis of the ring. Membrane proteins from senescent human erythrocytes indeed revealed upon hydrolysis D-aspartic and D-isoaspartic acids, with a D/L aspartic acid ratio increasing from 0.03 to 0.065 for integral membrane proteins, but very little for cytoskeletal proteins and none for cytosolic proteins.[47]

Lowensen and Clarke[48] simulated the damage that might occur by this process during the life span of an erythrocyte and found that a protein of 100 kDa would then contain, instead of 39, only 33 asparaginyl, but 6 L-isoaspartyl and about 0.6 D-aspartyl and D-isoaspartyl residues.[48] An L-isoaspartyl residue not only introduces a negative charge, where an uncharged asparaginyl was located, but also distorts the secondary structure of a protein. A total of six such changes per protein molecule could impair its function considerably. In any case, the damage would be more extensive than actually measured on senescent erythrocytes.[47] The reason for this discrepancy is most likely due to a cellular repair system, by which L-isoaspartyl and D-aspartyl residues are converted to L-aspartyl residues.[49] Erythrocytes and most other cells contain type II protein carboxy methyltransferase, which catalyzes a methyl esterification primarily of L-isoaspartyl and D-aspartyl residues.[49] Since the carboxymethylated residues more readily form a succinimide than the free acids, the methylated residues can revert spontaneously to normal L-aspartyl residues. Repeated cycles of succinimide formation, hydrolysis, and carboxymethylation will eventually correct most of the damage, but not deamidation. This is true for cytoplasmic and cytoskeletal proteins, but less for integral membrane proteins and not for their exoplasmic domains, since the repair enzyme is localized intracellularly. In accordance with this conclusion, methylation of intact, density-separated erythrocytes with L-[methyl-^{3}H]methionine labeled primarily cytoskeletal proteins rather than integral membrane proteins.[50] In contrast to this, when isolated membranes were incubated with exogenous carboxy methyltransferase, integral membrane proteins were predominantly labeled.[51] Thus, we have to expect that exoplasmic, not well-structured domains of integral membrane proteins, ectoproteins, and extracellular proteins suffer the most from this nonenzymatic aging process that leads to the structurally impaired L-isoaspartyl residues. On the other hand, most integral membrane proteins whose three-dimensional structure is established or deduced from their sequence rarely have random coils on their exoplasmic, but quite often on their cytoplasmic phase. Nevertheless, it is at least conceivable that deamidation not only introduces charges, but also significant structural alterations in exoplasmic domains of membrane proteins which might become neoantigens on aged cells. So far, there is no direct evidence for the existence of such a neoantigen. However, in extracellular β-amyloid deposits of patients with Alzheimer's disease both D-aspartyl- and L-isoaspartyl residues are abundant and probably involved in aggregate formation.[52]

2. Glycation

Reducing carbohydrates contain in their open structure aldehyde groups which can form Schiff bases with the N-terminal amino groups of proteins or the ε–amino group of lysyl residues.[53] The Schiff base rearranges to a ketoamine, the Amadori product, known from glycated hemoglobin A_{1c}.[54] The ketoamine eventually forms irreversible adducts, the so-called "advanced glycosylation endproducts". The Amadori product is similarly reducible by sodium borohydride as carbonyl groups generated by oxidative damage (see Section II.E). In fact, some authors presented evidence for glycation to be partially mediated by sugar autooxidation.[55] In autooxidation aldoses transiently form an aldimine with a protein. Instead of generating an enolamine, which is the tautomeric form of the Amadori product, the aldimine takes up water by forming a 1-amino-1,2-diol, which dissociates from the protein yielding a 1-oxo-2-hydroxy-derivative. This modified sugar molecule is oxidized by a metal ion-catalyzed reaction to the 1,2-dioxo-derivative, which subsequently reacts with protein amino groups by generating a 1-amino-1-hydroxy-2-oxo-derivative.[55] *In vitro* experiments with high concentrations of sugars have shown that nonenzymatic glycation can affect enzyme activity,[56] transport protein function,[57] and the organization of extracellular matrix proteins.[53] One of the advanced glycation endproducts is [2-furoyl-4-(5)-2-furanyl-1-imidazole]-hexanoic acid.[53] Artificial coupling of this glycation endproduct to human erythrocytes rendered them susceptible to *in vitro* phagocytosis by human macrophages derived from peripheral monocytes.[58] Ingestion of the modified erythrocytes was inhibited by albumin that was similarly derivatized. Likewise, erythrocytes incubated for 2 days with 100 mM glucose or glucose-6-phosphate were also phagocytosed, suggesting that glycation endproducts were directly recognized by a specific macrophage receptor for advanced glycation endproducts which appeared to differ from the macrophage scavenger receptor.[17] It is unclear whether the macrophages recognized the modified proteins as such or some newly generated protein-protein cross-links, whose formation appears to accompany generation of protein-bound aldehydes. The findings do not exclude the possibility that the macrophages recognized ATP-depleted erythrocytes, since the authors did not prevent ATP-depletion during modification with the advanced glycation endproduct. Thus, the rapid *in vivo* clearance of similarly glycated erythrocytes[59] does not conclusively demonstrate that the erythrocytes were eliminated because of the introduced modification. Unfortunately, phagocytosis of glycated erythrocytes was not studied by adding various serum constituents as potential competitors. Thus, the physiological relevance of this mode of recognition has yet to be established.

C. Membrane Loss with Aging

Aging erythrocytes lose water and surface, as is evident from a 30 to 35% lowered MCV,[60] and an 8 to 10% lower lipid content.[61,62] They further lose glycosyl-phosphatidylinositol-anchored (GPI-anchored) ectoproteins, like acetylcholinesterase,[62,63] decay accelerating factor (DAF),[32] and even integral membrane proteins like the complement receptor 1 (CR1).[34,35] This loss of membrane must occur without lysis and most probably occurs by vesiculation. Vesiculation is not a random process, since senescent erythrocytes have lost up to 50% of CR1 and DAF[32,34,35,64] but only 8 to 10% of their lipids. This comparison implies that some membrane proteins drastically redistribute in the plane of the membrane during aging. It seems conceivable that GPI-anchored proteins can easily reorganize, since the lateral mobility of their lipid anchor is expected to be high. Reorganization of CR1 is less likely, as this integral membrane protein protrudes the membrane once and thus has a reduced lateral mobility. On the other hand, an unproportionally high loss of CR1 to vesicles was possible if vesicles budded at sites where CR1 occurs in clusters. A significant portion of CR1 molecules indeed exists as small clusters on erythrocytes,[65] but functional studies suggest that the release of vesicles did not change the binding efficiency for C3b-coated immune complexes and thus the proportion of clustered vs. unclustered CR1.[66] The membrane loss from aging erythrocytes has much in common with the spontaneous release of cytoskeleton-free vesicles from ATP-depleted erythrocytes[67,68] and erythrocytes stored under blood bank conditions.[69,70] These hemoglobin-containing vesicles are enriched two- to threefold in acetylcholinesterase,[67,71] DAF,[66,71] and also in CR1,[66] and thus have a composition which could account for a preferential loss of these components from *in vivo* aged erythrocytes. Thus, membrane loss from aging erythrocytes may proceed by a selective vesiculation from areas that are enriched in GPI-anchored proteins and CR1, but containing slightly lower proportions of the major integral membrane proteins (band 3 and glycophorin) than the original erythrocytes.[67] In support of this conclusion, young erythrocytes release more vesicles during ATP-depletion than senescent cells[72] and vesicles were detected in phagocytes from animals treated with phenylhydrazine.[73] Membrane loss from aging erythrocytes further explains why senescent erythrocytes contain less sialic acid per cell, but yet the same amount of sialic acid per glycophorin.[33]

When *in vivo* aging erythrocytes preferentially lose CR1, they become functionally impaired, since they then have a lowered capacity to clear immune complexes.[74] In addition, a 50% loss of DAF renders human erythrocytes considerably more sensitive to complement deposition, because erythrocytes lack membrane cofactor protein (MCP) and exclusively have DAF to protect them from C3-convertases.[75] Complement-mediated lysis of senescent erythrocytes by heterologous serum was in fact two to three times higher than that of young cells.[64] On the other hand, the release of membrane in the form of vesicles could also constitute a means for the cell to escape elimination, since band 3 protein in vesicles from ATP-depleted erythrocytes formed clusters, based on cross-linking data, and the vesicles bound four times more autologous IgG than young erythrocytes.[76] The ability to form such vesicles is in fact used by erythrocytes *in vitro* to escape a complement lysis.[77]

D. Exposure of Phosphatidylserine (PS) on the Outer Monolayer

Phosphatidylserine is almost exclusively located in the inner membrane leaflet of mature erythrocytes.[78] This asymmetry is also found in most other cells, but less pronounced than in erythrocytes. Asymmetry is maintained by the ATP-requiring aminophospholipid translocase.[79] Impairment of the enzyme or deprivation of energy will slow down PS uptake and eventually destroy PS asymmetry, since the spontaneous, partially protein-mediated flip from the in- to the outside[80] continues to operate. Thus, ATP-depleted erythrocytes expose PS on the outer monolayer.[81] Quite recently, Schroit's group has demonstrated that the PS content in the outer monolayer of the densest erythrocytes was 104 ng/10^7 erythrocytes, about twice as high than that of the youngest cells, when determined by the sensitive prothrombinase activation.[82] Earlier measurements with spin-labeled phospholipids revealed a 50% lower initial rate of PS translocation in senescent erythrocytes, which was due to a functional impairment of the aminophospholipid translocase.[83] Exoplasmic exposure of PS was also found on apoptotic cells obtained by irradiation,[18] and an even higher increase of three- to sevenfold has been claimed for a tumorigenic epidermal keratinocyte line.[84] Phagocytosis of the apoptotic cells was inhibited by PS-containing liposomes, when measured on thioglycolate-elicited peritoneal macrophages, and by peptides containing arginyl-glycyl-aspartyl residues (one letter code: the RGD domain), when assayed on bone marrow-derived macrophages.[18] It is true that the occurrence of PS on dense erythrocytes correlates with accelerated *in vivo* clearance and rosetting,[82] but the erythrocyte surface content of IgG and C3 fragments also correlates with these properties.[85] Thus, a correlation alone can not yield a causal connection.

Mature erythrocytes derivatized with PS containing a fluorescent probe were indeed rapidly cleared from the circulation, while erythrocytes modified with similarly labeled phosphatidylcholine molecules were not.[86] Likewise, liposomes similarly derivatized with PS were also rapidly cleared from the circulation, suggesting that PS is recognized by the reticuloendothelial system,[87] presumably by a PS receptor, as suggested elsewhere.[18] Others carried out *in vitro* phagocytosis assays with liposomes mimicking the inner and outer monolayer of erythrocytes. Macrophages ingested primarily the multilamellar liposomes containing the inner phospholipids and the extent of phagocytosis was greatly stimulated by serum in which the complement system was active.[88] Hence, it is equally possible that clearance of PS liposomes is mediated by naturally occurring antibodies to phospholipids along with complement. Antiphospholipid antibodies with a preferred reactivity to negatively charged phospholipids have been found, not only in sera from patients with systemic lupus erythematosus,[89,90] but also in normal sera, and had an anticoagulant activity, as if they reacted with phospholipids that have a procoagulant activity.[91,92] These latter findings were obtained following a heat treatment of sera. Whether the heat treatment in fact "unmasked these antibodies"[92] or simply aggregated specific IgG molecules with other IgG molecules in sera and thereby enhanced the opsonic potential,[93] remains to be shown .

E. Oxidative Damage, Membrane Protein Topology, and Opsonization

1. Membrane Protein Topology on Aging Erythrocytes

The preferential loss of CR1 from aging erythrocytes suggests significant topologic alterations have occured. Direct evidence for topologic changes has been reported for band 3 protein and glycophorin, the most abundant erythrocyte membrane proteins. Casey and Reithmeier[94] used a rapid size exclusion HPLC method to characterize detergent-extracted band 3 protein and found that extracts from senescent erythrocytes contained 56% of band 3 protein in oligomers larger than dimers, while corresponding extracts from young cells contained only 22%, respectively. This suggests that band 3 oligomerization increases with erythrocyte age. A similar conclusion was drawn from studying lateral and rotational mobility of band 3 protein on intact, eosin maleimide-tagged erythrocytes under deoxygenation: the fraction of laterally mobile band 3 protein decreased with cell age by about 50%.[95] These oligomers were not cross-linked by SS bonds, since rehydration of the osmotically shrunken, dense cells restored the lateral mobility to that found in unseparated cells. The arrangement of band 3 protein was earlier studied by cross-linking. Bivalent, impermeant, and rapidly reacting succinimidyl derivatives generated primarily intramolecular and less intermolecular cross-links between monomers, suggesting that band 3 proteins existed as dimers in erythrocyte membranes .[96,97] More recent work, using anion transport inhibitors to prevent intramonomeric cross-links, revealed covalently linked dimers, either noncovalently associated as a SDS-resistant tetramer or not.[98] The conditions used in these cross-linking studies, namely incubation with bis(sulfosuccinimidyl)suberate for 1 h at 37°C could, however, not differentiate between preexisting oligomers and diffusion-induced ones. More than 10 years ago we addressed the same question by using the equally reactive dithiobis(succinimidyl propionate) as a cross-linker on erythrocytes which had been modified with labeled arylalkyldiamine or aniline following galactose oxidase treatment of the carbohydrates.[99] This approach was designed to provide additional free amino-groups for cross-linking exoplasmic domains of glycoproteins and to specifically monitor exoplasmic cross-links within 15 min at 4°C. Band 3 cross-linking on arylalkyldiamine-treated erythrocytes reached only 1.5% for young and 1.9% for senescent cells (different at a confidence level of 0.06). This stringent use of a cross-linking agent yielded results which differ from those obtained by measuring the dynamics of band 3 protein,[95] and from data obtained by cross-linking for 1 h at 37°C.[98] On the other hand, the minute increase in cross-linked band 3 proteins on senescent erythrocytes at high stringency[99] yet corresponds to ≤4000 molecules per cell. Thus, two types of topologic changes might occur among integral membrane proteins on aging erythrocytes. Both the portion of dynamically associated band 3 protein and of fixed band 3 aggregates increase with cell age, with the fixed aggregates being generated presumably by oxidative damage.

2. Oxidative Damage to Lipid and Protein

Mixed function oxidases in metal-catalyzed reactions are the primary cause of oxidative protein damage.[21] Hydroxyl radicals generated by this pathway oxidize arginine, proline, and lysine residues involved in metal coordination to semialdehydes, implying that proteins, like hemoglobin, are particularly vulnerable. Hydroxyl radicals, generated by ionization, damage proteins more randomly by generating methionine sulfoxide, tyrosine-tyrosine cross-links, and SS cross-links involving cysteines. Lipid peroxidation yields malondialdehyde and 4-hydroxynonenal,[21] which modifies proteins by forming adducts with amino acid residues containing nucleophiles. Senescent erythrocytes indeed contain increased amounts of carbonyl-modified proteins,[100] methionine sulfoxide,[101,102] and have a sevenfold higher content of malondialdehyde phospholipid adducts.[103] Dityrosine is produced in hemoglobin when erythrocytes are exposed to H_2O_2.[104]

Oxidized proteins and oxidized lipids are preferentially degraded[105] as part of a repair mechanism or cellular homeostasis. Hydroperoxylinoleoyl-containing phosphatidylcholine in lipid monolayers extends their surface area and is preferentially hydrolyzed by phospholipase A_2.[106] The occurrence of dityrosine in hemoglobin seems to trigger a selective proteolysis of modified hemoglobin by an endogenous protease called macroxyproteinase.[104] Others immunoprecipitated the macroxyproteinase and claimed that this had no effect on a selective proteolysis of oxidized hemoglobin which yet was degraded by a metalloinsulinase.[107] As the degrading enzymes also lose activity as the cell ages, modified forms of proteins tend to accumulate late in the life span. Selective degradation of modified proteins serves the purpose of repair by "*de novo* synthesis" in cells having an ongoing protein synthesis. Erythrocytes no longer synthesize proteins and therefore reveal oxidative damage in lipids, hemoglobin, and membrane proteins. Some of this accumulating damage induces changes in the surface protein topology and results in opsonization.

3. Topological Changes Associated with Oxidative Damage and Opsonization

The presence of small amounts of immobilized band 3 protein aggregates that differ from loosely associated proteins was best explained by a cytoplasmic fixation of these aggregates by SS bonded cysteines and/or intracellular binding of denatured hemoglobin or hemin.[108,109] There is ample evidence for fixation of such complexes in the course of hemoglobinopathies and oxidative stress induced by fava beans or chemicals in glucose-6-phosphate dehydrogenase-deficient subjects, where the oxidatively stressed erythrocytes are cleared prematurely by the normal clearance mechanisms rather than by induced antibodies.[110,111] The first evidence that high molecular weight material from senescent erythrocytes contained band 3 and was associated with autologous IgG came from immunoprecipitation experiments on extracts from surface-^{125}I-iodinated young and senescent erythrocytes.[112,113] Protein A precipitated IgG along with high molecular weight material containing band 3 protein from extracts of senescent and less from young erythrocytes. This observation suggested the possibility that naturally occurring anti-band 3 antibodies[114] might preferentially bind bivalently to oligomers of band 3 protein.

The fraction of high molecular weight protein aggregates has since been studied in great detail on unseparated erythrocytes from patients with hemoglobinopathies,[109,115-117] and density-separated normal[118] and artificially oxidized erythrocytes.[119,120] The high molecular weight material comprising 1.3% in sickle erythrocytes,[116] or 1.6% in β-thalassemic cells[117] of the total membrane protein contained primarily globin, band 3 protein, glycophorin, some minor cytoskeletal proteins, and 3/4 of the surface-associated IgG.[116] A similar composition was found for aggregates from senescent, normal erythrocytes which comprised only 0.09% of the total membrane protein, but being enriched 640-fold in surface IgG and containing roughly similar amounts of band 3, globin, and spectrin, after stripping most of the globin.[118] High molecular weight material from senescent erythrocytes which was purified by gelfiltration in SDS also contained covalently linked C3b-IgG complexes.[121] IgG liberated from these complexes by hydroxylamine bound primarily to band 3 on blots from erythrocyte membranes.[122]

The relevance of IgG associated with senescent erythrocytes was questioned on the basis that biotinylated erythrocytes recovered from the circulation revealed only a small, if any, increment for cell-associated IgG in rabbits.[123] The doubts are based on experiments that also have their drawbacks, namely: rabbits clear a significant portion of their erythrocytes randomly.[1] This may have increased the number of opsonized cells not having reached their life span, whereby the increment in bound antibodies from young to senescent became smaller. Secondly, the plasma of certain animals may contain naturally occurring antibodies to biotin, as was found for 10% of normal human subjects.[124] Both the partial random clearance and the possible existence of biotin-reactive autoantibodies could cover up an age-dependent increase of IgG, but does not interfere with the potential of the method to isolate really senescent cells at the end of the life span. In fact, biotinylated dog erythrocytes recovered at the end of their life span were indeed three- to fourfold enriched in cell-associated IgG as compared to the whole-cell population at the day of collection.[125]

Erythrocyte-associated IgG eluted from normal senescent,[126] sickle cells, and erythrocytes with unstable hemoglobins, e.g., Hb Köln, bound primarily to band 3 protein on blots,[115] suggesting that the majority of cell-associated IgG represented naturally occurring anti-band 3 antibodies. Erythrocytes from vitamin E-deficient rats were oxidatively damaged because they lacked an important antioxidant. Their extent of phagocytosis was six times higher than that of control cells. Blots from their membranes which were incubated with an induced anti-band 3 antibody revealed band 3 breakdown products, but also a band 3 oligomer (Figure 1A in Reference 127) that went unnoticed by the authors. Erythrocytes oxidatively damaged by diamide and opsonized with serum were phagocytosed by adherent monocytes.[128] Phagocytosis of diamide-treated cells required opsonization by C3b, since complement inactivation abolished phagocytosis.[129] Naturally occurring anti-band 3 antibodies, affinity purified from pooled human IgG[114] and added to serum, further stimulated opsonization by C3b under conditions favoring the alternative complement pathway C3b deposition.[129] Binding of anti-band 3 antibodies to diamide-treated erythrocytes and to blotted proteins from their membranes increased with the extent of oligomers containing band 3 protein. Thus, oligomerization of band 3 protein appears to elicit a firm bivalent binding of anti-band 3 antibodies. Once bound firmly and in clusters, C3b deposition is initiated which elicits a selective phagocytosis of diamide-treated erythrocytes.

The observation that oligomerization of band 3 protein increases the number of firmly bound antibodies has since been further explored by using oxidative agents other than diamide[130] and by artificially generating clusters of integral membrane proteins.[119,120] A treatment of erythrocytes with 1 mM $ZnCl_2$, followed by a chemical cross-linking of the topologically altered protein organization, generated band 3 containing oligomers, and enhanced binding of autologous IgG and C3b from serum.[119] IgG purified from these opsonized cells bound on blots to band 3 protein and its oligomers.[120] Moreover, a cleavage of the cross-linked complexes with mercaptoethanol reversed the effect of clustering, lowered binding of IgG and C3b by 80%, and abolished phagocytosis.[119] Reversal of the oxidative damage by a reducing agent similarly lowered binding of naturally occurring anti-band 3 antibodies to erythrocytes.[130] These findings support the hypothesis[114] that binding of naturally occurring anti-band 3 antibodies requires an oligomerization of band 3 rather than the formation of a neoantigen.[131]

III. RECOGNITION AND INGESTION OF CELLS BY PHAGOCYTES

A. Recognition of Target Cells by Phagocytes

Senescent but not young erythrocytes are eliminated by phagocytes. Hence, the surface of senescent cells ought to differ in some respects from that of young cells in order to provide a means for a selective recognition. This question is intimately related to the tools that can sense the altered property on senescent erythrocytes and mediate the contact to the phagocyte. The most likely tools, but not the only ones, are antibodies in conjunction with complement opsonins. In order to better evaluate the role of other types of mediators and phagocytic receptors in the clearance of senescent erythrocytes and apoptotic cells, it is a necessity to differentiate between phagocytosis in serum-poor media and phagocytosis *in vivo*.

1. Antibodies and Complement

The most powerful mediators are antibodies. They specifically bind to target cells or soluble constituents and mediate contact with phagocytes via Fc receptors. In contrast to most other mediators, they can further enhance their effect by stimulating complement deposition to target cells.[132-135] Their ability to activate complement is in fact crucial, since physiological concentrations of monomeric IgG completely inhibited macrophage and neutrophil phagocytosis, when mediated by antibody alone.[136-138] On the other hand, physiological concentrations of IgG did not significantly inhibit internalization when target cells were opsonized with antibody and complement together.[137] Thus, a physiologically relevant and effective internalization requires participation of two independent receptors for Fc and C3b (CR1)[139-141] or for Fc and iC3b (CR3).[142]

2. Recognition Mediated by Naturally Occurring Antibodies and Complement

The possible involvement of antibodies in tissue homeostatic processes is difficult to comprehend, since our understanding of antibodies originates from what we have learned from induced antibodies against non-self. Hence it appeared quite logical that most investigators searched for a neoantigen in small amounts on aging erythrocytes and assumed that the immune system might have generated a high affinity antibody against this neoantigen. In the meantime, the knowledge about autoreactive naturally occurring antibodies has increased exponentially and has opened a somewhat different view on a potential role of antibodies in tissue homeostasis.[143-145]

Naturally occurring antibodies are secreted by certain B cells as autoantibodies which are compatible with normal life, mainly because they are either directed to normally not exposed self antigens[146,147] or, when directed to exposed self antigens, they have a low affinity and occur in concentrations lower than their association constant.[144,145,148] Naturally occurring antibodies are exact or almost exact copies of germ line Ig information.[149-151] Hence the set of naturally occurring antibodies and their specificity are inherited and conserved in evolution.[152] Some of their properties appeared atypical for antibodies: many of them are polyspecific,[153,154] primarily those of the IgM class. Polyspecificity may represent one way to overcome a weak affinity, since it allows for bi- or multivalent binding once the two different antigens are encountered in a complex.

Many naturally occurring IgG antibodies are reasonably specific,[155] but only bind firmly to their oligomeric antigen.[114] Note the difference between a high affinity and a low affinity antibody — a high affinity antibody can bind monovalently and before it dissociates it can recruit a diffusing antigen and thereby patch surface antigens. A weakly binding naturally occurring antibody, however, is not able to patch antigens, since it dissociates rapidly. Hence, bivalent binding of naturally occurring antibodies to cell surfaces requires the cell to provide antigen oligomers. Once a weakly binding naturally occurring antibody interacts with clustered antigen, it remains firmly bound, since its dissociation is 100 to 1000 times lower when bound bivalently.[156] Firm binding alone does not represent a sufficient signal to trigger phagocytosis, because the number of bound opsonins remains too low.[2] Thus, firmly bound naturally occurring antibodies at concentrations below their association constant remain nonfunctional, unless these antibodies can enhance opsonization otherwise. Naturally occurring anti-band 3 antibodies appear to mediate phagocytosis of oxidatively stressed, *in vitro* aged, and senescent erythrocytes (for reviews see References 1, 2, 131, 148, and 157). These antibodies have a weak affinity for C3 at a site independent of the antigen binding region.[155] This affinity exceeds that of other IgG[158] for C3 by about a 100-fold and conveys functional potency by attracting nascent C3b such that anti-band 3 antibodies preferentially form C3b-IgG complexes.[122] C3b-IgG complexes can nucleate an alternative C3 convertase,[159] whereby they stimulate alternative complement pathway C3b deposition. C3b deposition, however, is limited by the number of proteins that protect from complement deposition.[2] As the protecting proteins DAF[75] and CR1[160] decrease with cell age,[32,34,35] the chances for a C3b deposition to greatly exceed the number of bound antibodies increase. C3b-anti-band 3 complexes bound bivalently via their Fab portions to oligomerized band 3 protein can yet serve as the best opsonins, since antigen-bound C3b-IgG complexes induce recognition by Fc receptors and complement receptors simultaneously and phagocytosis mediated in this way is not inhibited by fluid phase IgG.[137] Evidence obtained with artificially generated C3b-anti-band 3 complexes further suggests that once such a complex is either generated in the fluid phase or dissociates from the membrane it no longer can interact bivalently with erythrocytes, presumably because the bulky C3b prevents a bivalent binding.[161]

3. Effective Phagocytosis by Other Receptors also Depends on the Involvement of Two Receptors

Antibodies alone and other mediators make contact between a target cell and one type of receptor on phagocytes. Fibronectin, for example, associates with a target cell and via the RGD domain with its receptor on phagocytes.[162,163] Recognition of target cells by the phagocytic receptors for mannose,[164,165] oxidized low density lipoproteins,[166,167] vitronectin,[16] and even for PS,[18] also seems to involve only one type of receptor, at least when studied *in vitro* in media not containing physiological concentrations of immunoglobulins and albumin. Such *in vitro* assays help to characterize receptor-target cell interactions and even the involvement of different receptors on differently prepared macrophages.[18] However, the results can not be extrapolated to the *in vivo* situation.

Considering the limited efficacy of specific antibodies and Fc receptors alone in mediating phagocytosis at physiological IgG and albumin concentrations, target cell interactions with these and other types of receptors should be studied under conditions approaching physiological situations. This is not trivial, since high concentrations of serum tend to remove phagocytes from their support. Some groups tried to study the effect of serum components by coating the plates with appropriate proteins, for example with whole human IgG[168] or anti-albumin antibodies. Immobilized IgG, for example, inhibited phagocytosis of target cells recognized by the mannose receptor, implying that Fc receptors also were required for an efficient uptake of target cells that might interact primarily with the mannose receptor.[169] A similar observation was made on neutrophils ingesting either concanavalin-treated erythrocytes or unopsonized *E. coli*:[170] while both target cells bound to neutrophils via the mannose receptor, internalization was mediated by the Fc receptor, since aggregated IgG or a monoclonal antibody to a particular epitope of the FcR inhibited internalization. These findings imply that the target cells were also bound by two independent receptors which strengthened their interaction.

The use of pairs of receptors for efficient internalization is not restricted to mannose and Fc receptors. Efficient phagocytosis of unopsonized yeast cells required a concomitant binding to mannose and β-glucan receptor,[171] that of a virulent strain of mycobacteria, the mannose, and complement receptors.[172] Hence, it is quite possible that efficient recognition and ingestion requires binding of a target cell by two independent phagocytic receptors.

B. Recognition and Elimination of Senescent and Oxidatively Stressed Erythrocytes as well as Apoptotic Cells

1. Recognition by Fc Receptors and a Second Receptor

Phagocytosis of *in vitro* aged or oxidatively stressed erythrocytes was stimulated by opsonization with serum,[119,128,173] whole IgG, or eluates from senescent erythrocytes,[174,175] and by serum supplemented with purified naturally occurring anti-band 3 antibodies.[121,129,130] Opsonization of oxidatively stressed and senescent erythrocytes was accompanied by C3b deposition.[119,121,129,176] Correspondingly, phagocytosis was partially inhibited by blocking Fc receptors,[173,177] CR1,[178,179] and CR3[178] on phagocytes. These results suggest that oxidatively damaged as well as senescent erythrocytes are recognized by naturally occurring antibodies involving primarily anti-band 3 antibodies which mediate a C3b deposition, and thereby facilitate a simultaneous binding of the target cell to Fc and complement receptors on phagocytes.

A recent report claims that oxidatively stressed erythrocytes were recognized directly by the mouse macrophage receptor for oxidized low density lipoproteins.[180] These *in vitro* experiments, using human erythrocytes and mouse peritoneal macrophages, appeared to render much of what has been published meaningless. In reality, the report brings no new insight, since the receptor for oxidized low density lipoproteins is nothing else than an Fc receptor, the mouse FcRII, as reported by others.[166] While the latter group demonstrated that an anti-FcRII antibody blocked the uptake of oxidized lipoproteins, the former group did not study whether a pretreatment with an anti-FcRII antibody or addition of aggregated IgG inhibited phagocytosis of senescent erythrocytes. In fact, there was plenty of IgG around in their assays, since erythrocytes were washed only three times in PBS before being oxidized with $CuSO_4$ and ascorbate by a method described elsewhere.[181] Small amounts of naturally occurring antibodies present in the surrounding fluid, or even loosely associated with erythrocytes, do play a very important role as has been nicely demonstrated by Horn et al.[177] These authors also studied phagocytosis of oxidatively stressed human erythrocytes by thioglycollate-induced peritoneal macrophages from mice. They depleted the blood first from leukocytes (another source of IgG) and washed erythrocytes six times and then treated them with phenylhydrazine. Thus, the surrounding fluid did not contain significant amounts of IgG. Nevertheless, phagocytosis was inhibited to 50% by adding aggregated IgG or by blocking FcRII, and to 90% by simultaneously adding galactose and aggregated IgG. The data imply that small amounts of cell-associated IgG (naturally occurring antibodies) may redistribute on oxidatively stressed erythrocytes and become firmly bound upon applying an oxidative stress. The cell-associated IgG molecules amounted to less than 50 molecules per cell, a number similar to the increment of bound anti-band 3 antibodies obtained by a diamide treatment of erythrocytes,[129] and to the number of IgG molecules associated with erythrocytes from patients with glucose-6-phosphate dehydrogenase deficiency.[177] In this case, the number of surface IgG molecules correlated well with the extent of *in vitro* phagocytosis and the degree of anemia.[177]

The question remains, however, why galactose partially inhibited phagocytosis of oxidatively stressed erythrocytes,[177] and of senescent erythrocytes.[182,183] Liver, but not splenic macrophages, appear to have a galactose-binding protein which in fact represents membrane-bound C-reactive protein.[184,185] Another possibility is that certain Fc receptors have a lectin-like property. This was suggested for rat and human macrophages, on the basis that IgG antibodies carrying either terminal galactose or mannose residues in the Fc domain were at least twofold more effective in inducing IgG-dependent phagocytosis of erythrocytes than those differently glycosylated.[186,187] The same group could also verify this effect *in vivo*, where 1 mg mannan or 40 mg of a protein containing α1-6 mannosyl residues inhibited Fc receptor-dependent phagocytosis in the spleen and prolonged the half lives of injected red cells twofold.[169] Thus, the carbohydrate side chains in the CH2 domain of the Fc portions of IgG molecules appear to be important for interactions with Fc receptors. In fact, the complete absence of carbohydrate on Asn 297 in this domain even alters the three-dimensional structure of IgG antibody molecules and thereby lowers their affinity for FcRI by 115-fold.[188,189] The relative effect of carbohydrate and protein structure illustrate that IgG interactions with Fc receptors, nevertheless, are primarily protein mediated.

While minute amounts of erythrocyte-associated IgG molecules have a mediator function for the selective recognition of oxidatively stressed erythrocytes,[129,177] others claim that less than 10% of phagocytosis was inhibited by preincubating erythrocytes with protein G.[179] Instead, they report a 50 to 60% inhibition by agents which interfere with CR1 and galactose.

2. Recognition by Receptors Other than FcR and CR

Phagocytosis of oxidatively stressed erythrocytes was enhanced by cultivating thioglycollate-induced macrophages on immobilized fibronectin in the absence of serum.[190] The enhancing effect was abolished by adding an RGD-containing peptide, implying that fibronectin either bound to the fibronectin receptor [163] or to CR3 that also has a RGD-inhibitable binding site.[191] The finding does not mean that oxidatively stressed erythrocytes were recognized by fibronectin. Fibronectin had to be immobilized by coating the plate. In this form it most likely aggregated fibronectin receptors on the macrophage surface, whereby the phagocytic potential was activated. This phenomenon was observed with intact macrophages as well as with trypsinized macrophages, implying that recognition of oxidatively stressed erythrocytes could yet be mediated by tiny amounts of erythrocyte-associated naturally occurring antibodies and Fc receptors that withstand a mild trypsinization.

Plasma fibronectin is unlikely to mediate a selective recognition of either oxidatively stressed or senescent erythrocytes. It seems, however, to act as an enhancer of opsonization induced by antibodies and C3b during a massive transfusion reaction with incompatible erythrocytes *in vivo*.[192] Fibronectin has three separate binding sites for immunoglobulins, of which only one is effective under physiological conditions.[193] Hence, fibronectin may serve as a secondary opsonin during dramatic episodes of antibody-mediated opsonization.

The activating effect of immobilized fibronectin on the phagocytic properties of macrophages is a general phenomenon for ligands. If a potential ligand is offered in coated form, the immobilized ligand interacts multivalently with its receptors on the phagocyte and induces their clustering. This is best established for Fc receptors — their aggregation signals a cytoplasmic tyrosine phosphorylation within the tyrosine-containing activation motif.[194,195] This, in turn, activates the phagocytic potential. The same is observed with macrophages binding to immobilized C3b molecules: interaction with immobilized C3b enhanced phagocytosis of IgG-antibody-containing erythrocytes two- to threefold, although the target cells did not contain C3b.[196] Vitronectin or complement component S[197] elicited a similar stimulation of phagocytosis of antibody-coated erythrocytes.[198]

In attempts to overcome the cell-detaching effect of serum many investigators coated the plate with a potential ligand to study whether it can inhibit phagocytosis. If a potential ligand does not inhibit, when offered in coated form, the result is not conclusive since the immobilized ligand could have stimulated the adherent macrophage. Hence, the selective recognition of senescent neutrophils and lymphocytes (apoptotic cells) by the vitronectin receptor[16] remains a nice *in vitro* study, with little value *in vivo*. Important serum components that might interfere with the vitronectin receptor-mediated recognition were tested in their coated form: collagen, fibrinogen, and albumin did not inhibit. A first step towards physiology, where albumin exists at 50 mg/ml, was taken with 100 µg/ml of fluid phase albumin, which also did not inhibit. The same group has since studied phagocytosis of apoptotic neutrophils *in vivo* and under more physiological conditions, with the conclusion that phagocytosis by mesangial cells of senescent neutrophils required 1 to 10% serum, which stimulated ingestion fivefold.[199]

IV. CONCLUSIONS

"Much is to be learned about *the nature and in-vivo specificity* of ligand binding by the vitronectin receptor"[200] and all the other mediators and receptors in cell elimination. The selective recognition of senescent cells cannot be compared with the binding of a hormone to its receptor, since cell elimination is in all cases a cooperative phenomenon mediated by several weakly interacting components rather than one high affinity binding event. The scientific approach to unravel the mechanisms of recognition requires *in vitro* experiments — simplified model systems which will rarely simulate the complexity under which these processes occur *in vivo*. Nevertheless, the relevance of the described processes needs to be verified by approaching physiological conditions. The current trend is to elucidate the initiation phase of apoptosis, the triggers of cellular senescence, and questions regarding the mode of a selective recognition and cell elimination have less room. This review combines recently acquired knowledge on the modifications on aging cells, the recognition and selective elimination of senescent erythrocytes, with the scarce information on the mediators and receptors which help phagocytes to eliminate apoptotic cells. Particularly, the evidence for the role of naturally occurring antibodies in the elimination of senescent and oxidatively stressed erythrocytes offers conceptually new routes of recognition which have not been investigated on apoptotic cell elimination. Likewise, the *in vivo* effect of affinity purified or monoclonal naturally occurring antibodies will be studied. It is further expected that transfection of phagocytic receptors[160,164,166] will allow the setup of *in vitro* experiments with a limited number of expressed receptors under conditions mimicking the composition of body fluids. Detailed research on the selective recognition of apoptotic blebs is at its onset with promising findings regarding topological changes of membrane proteins[19,201] and the involvement of oxidative stress in mediating apoptosis.[11]

ACKNOWLEDGMENTS

I thank Dr. Emiliana Jelezarova for helpful discussions and reading the manuscript. The author acknowledges support from the Swiss National Science Foundation Grant 31-32383.91 and from the Union Bank of Switzerland on behalf of a client.

REFERENCES

1. Clark, M. R., Senescence of red blood cells: progress and problems, *Physiol. Rev.*, 68, 503, 1988.
2. Lutz, H. U., Erythrocyte clearance, in *Blood Cell Biochemistry, Vol. 1, Erythroid Cells*, Harris, J. R., Ed., Plenum Press, New York, 1990, 81.
3. McConkey, D. J., Orrenius, S., and Jondal, M., Cellular signalling in programmed cell death (apoptosis), *Immunol. Today*, 11, 120, 1991.
4. Cohen, J. J., Programmed cell death in the immune system, *Adv. Immunol.*, 50, 55, 1991.
5. Bissonnette, R. P., Echeverri, F., Mahboubi, A., and Green, D. R., Apoptotic cell death induced by c-myc is inhibited by bcl-2, *Nature*, 359, 552, 1992.
6. Lagasse, E. and Weissman, I. L., Bcl-2 inhibits apoptosis of neutrophils but not their engulfment by macrophages, *J. Exp. Med.*, 179, 1047, 1994.
7. Xie, K. P., Huang, S. Y., Dong, Z. Y., and Fidler, I. J., Cytokine-induced apoptosis in transformed murine fibroblasts involves synthesis of endogenous nitric oxide, *Int. J. Oncol.*, 3, 1043, 1993.
8. Iwata, M., Hanaoka, S., and Sato, K., Rescue of thymocytes and T cell hybridomas from glucocorticoid-induced apoptosis by stimulation via the T cell receptor/CD3 complex: a possible in vitro model for positive selection of the T cell repertoire, *Eur. J. Immunol.*, 21, 643, 1991.
9. Shi, Y. F., Bissonnette, R. P., Parfrey, N., Szalay, M., Kubo, R. T., and Green, D. R., In vivo administration of monoclonal antibodies to the CD3 T cell receptor complex induces cell death (apoptosis) in immature thymocytes, *J. Immunol.*, 146, 3340, 1991.
10. Debatin, K. M., Goldman, C. K., Waldmann, T. A., and Krammer, P. H., APO-1-induced apoptosis of leukemia cells from patients with adult T- cell leukemia, *Blood*, 81, 2972, 1993.
11. Buttke, T. M. and Sandstrom, P. A., Oxidative stress as a mediator of apoptosis, *Immunol. Today*, 15, 7, 1994.
12. MacDonald, H. R., Schneider, R., Lees, R. K., Howe, R. C., Acha-Orbea, H., Festenstein, H., Zinkernagel, R. M., and Hengartner, H., T-cell receptor Vβ use predicts reactivity and tolerance to Mls-endcoded antigens, *Nature*, 332, 40, 1988.
13. Ross, G. D., *Immunobiology of the Complement System*, Academic Press, Orlando, FL, 1986.

14. Lichtenheld, M. G., Olsen, K. J., Lu, P., Lowrey, D. M., Hameed, A., Hengartner, H., and Podack, E. R., Structure and function of human perforin, *Nature*, 335, 448, 1988.
15. Clark, W., Ostergaard, H., Gorman, K., and Torbett, B., Molecular mechanism of CTL-mediated lysis: a cellular perspective, *Immunol. Rev.*, 103, 37, 1988.
16. Savil, J., Dransfield, I., Hogg, N., and Haslett, C., Vitronectin receptor-mediated phagocytosis of cells undergoing apoptosis, *Nature*, 343, 170, 1990.
17. Kodama, T., Freeman, M., Rohrer, L., Zabrecky, J., Matsudaira, P., and Krieger, M., Type I macrophage scavenger receptor contains α-helical and collagen-like coiled coils, *Nature*, 343, 531, 1990.
18. Fadok, V. A., Savill, J. S., Haslett, C., Bratton, D. L., Doherty, D. E., Campbell, P. A., and Henson, P. M., Different populations of macrophages use either the vitronectin receptor or the phosphatidylserine receptor to recognize and remove apoptotic cells, *J. Immunol.*, 149, 4029, 1992.
19. Casciola-Rosen, L. A., Anhalt, G., and Rosen, A., Autoantigens targeted in systemic lupus erythematosus are clustered in two populations of surface structures on apoptotic keratinocytes, *J. Exp. Med.*, 179, 1317, 1994.
20. Ames, B. N. and Shigenaga, M. K., Oxidants are a major contributor to aging, *Ann. N.Y. Acad. Sci.*, 663, 85, 1992.
21. Stadtman, E. R., Protein oxidation and aging, *Science*, 257, 1220, 1992.
22. Kurata, M., Suzuki, M., and Agar, N. S., Antioxidant systems and erythrocyte life-span in mammals, *Comp. Biochem. Physiol. [B].*, 106, 477, 1993.
23. Walker, W. S., Singer, J. A., Morrison, M., and Jackson, C. W., Preferential phagocytosis of in vivo aged murine red blood cells by a macrophage-like cell line, *Br. J. Haematol.*, 58, 259, 1984.
24. Singer, J. A., Jennings, L. K., Jackson, C. W., Dockter, M. E., Morrison, M., and Walker, W. S., Erythrocyte homeostasis: antibody-mediated recognition of the senescent state by macrophages, *Proc. Natl. Acad. Sci. U.S.A.*, 83, 5498, 1986.
25. Suzuki, T. and Dale, G. L., Biotinylated erythrocytes: in vivo survival and in vitro recovery, *Blood*, 70, 791, 1987.
26. Suzuki, T. and Dale, G. L., Senescent erythrocytes: isolation of in vivo aged cells and their biochemical characteristics, *Proc. Natl. Acad. Sci. U.S.A.*, 85, 1, 1988.
27. Clark, M. R. and Shohet, S. B., Red cell senescence, *Clin. Haematol.*, 14, 223, 1985.
28. Beutler, E., The relationship of red cell enzymes to red cell life-span, *Blood Cells*, 14, 69, 1988.
29. Murphy, J. R., Influence of temperature and method of centrifugation on the separation of erythrocytes, *J. Lab. Clin. Med.*, 82, 334, 1973.
30. Piomelli, S. and Seaman, C., Mechanism of red blood cell aging — relationship of cell density and cell age, *Am. J. Hematol.*, 42, 46, 1993.
31. Vettore, L., DeMatteis, M. C., and Zampini, P., A new density gradient system for the separation of human red blood cells, *Am. J. Hematol.*, 8, 291, 1980.
32. Lutz, H. U., Stammler, P., Fasler, S., Ingold, M., and Fehr, J., Density separation of human red blood cells on self forming Percoll® gradients: correlation with cell age, *Biochim. Biophys. Acta*, 1116, 1, 1992.
33. Lutz, H. U. and Fehr, J., Total sialic acid content of glycophorins during senescence of human red blood cells, *J. Biol. Chem.*, 254, 11177, 1979.
34. Ripoche, J. and Sim, R. B., Loss of complement receptor type 1 (CR1) on ageing of erythrocytes. Studies of proteolytic release of the receptor, *Biochem. J.*, 235, 815, 1986.
35. Moldenhauer, F., Botto, M., and Walport, M. J., The rate of loss of CR1 from ageing erythrocytes in vivo in normal subjects and SLE patients: no correlation with structural or numerical polymorphisms, *Clin. Exp. Immunol.*, 72, 74, 1988.

36. ten Brinke, M. and de Regt, J., ^{51}Cr-half life time of heavy and light human erythrocytes, *Scand. J. Haematol.*, 7, 336, 1970.

37. Clark, M. R., Mohandas, N., and Shohet, S. B., Osmotic gradient ektacytometry: comprehensive characterization of red cell volume and surface maintenance, *Blood*, 61, 899, 1983.

38. Waugh, R. E., Narla, M., Jackson, C. W., Mueller, T. J., Suzuki, T., and Dale, G. L., Rheologic properties of senescent erythrocytes. Loss of surface area and volume with red blood cell age, *Blood*, 79, 1351, 1992.

39. Mueller, T., Jackson, C. W., Dockter, M. E., and Morrison, M., Membrane skeletal alterations during *in vivo* mouse red cell aging, *J. Clin. Invest.*, 79, 492, 1987.

40. Suzuki, T. and Dale, G. L., Membrane proteins in senescent erythrocytes, *Biochem. J.*, 257, 37, 1989.

41. Sauberman, N., Fortier, N. L., Fairbanks, G., and O'Conner, R. J., Red cell membrane in hemolytic disease: studies on variables affecting electrophoretic analylsis, *Biochim. Biophys. Acta*, 556, 292, 1979.

42. Inaba, M. and Maede, Y., Correlation between protein 4.1a/4.1b ratio and erythrocyte life span, *Biochim. Biophys. Acta*, 944, 256, 1988.

43. Goodman, S. R., Shiffer, K., Coleman, D. B., and Whitfield, C. F., Erythrocyte membrane skeletal protein 4.1: a brief review, in *The Red Cell: Sixth Ann Arbor Conference*, Alan R. Liss, New York, 1984, 415.

44. Inaba, M., Gupta, K. C., Kuwabara, M., Takahashi, T., Benz, E. J., and Maede, Y., Deamidation of human erythrocyte protein-4.1 — possible role in aging, *Blood*, 79, 3355, 1992.

45. Geiger, T. and Clarke, S., Deamidation, isomerization, and racemization at asparaginyl and aspartyl residues in peptides, *J. Biol. Chem.*, 262, 785, 1987.

46. Stephenson, R. C. and Clarke, S., Succinimide formation from aspartyl and asparaginyl peptides as a model for the spontaneous degradation of proteins, *J. Biol. Chem.*, 264, 6164, 1989.

47. Brunauer, L. S. and Clarke, S., Age-dependent accumulation of protein residues which can be hydrolyzed to D-aspartic acid in human erythrocytes, *J. Biol. Chem.*, 261, 12538, 1986.

48. Lowenson, J. D. and Clarke, S., Spontaneous degradation and enzymatic repair of aspartyl and asparaginyl residues in aging red cell proteins analyzed by computer simulation, *Gerontology*, 37, 128, 1991.

49. McFadden, P. N. and Clarke, S., Conversion of isoaspartyl peptides to normal peptides: implications for the cellular repair of damaged proteins, *Proc. Natl. Acad. Sci. U.S.A.*, 84, 2595, 1987.

50. Barber, J. R. and Clarke, S., Membrane protein carboxyl methylation increases with human erythrocyte age, *J. Biol. Chem.*, 258, 1189, 1983.

51. O'Connor, C. M. and Clarke, S., Methylation of erythrocyte membrane proteins at extracellular and intracellular D-aspartyl sites in vitro, *J. Biol. Chem.*, 258, 8485, 1983.

52. Lowenson, J. D., Roher, A. E., and Clarke, S., Protein aging — extracellular amyloid formation and intracellular repair, *Trend. Cardiovasc. Med.*, 4, 3, 1994.

53. Lee, A. T. and Cerami, A., Role of glycation in aging, *Ann. N.Y. Acad. Sci.*, 663, 63, 1992.

54. Bunn, H. F., Non-enzymatic glycosylation of proteins: a form of molecular aging, *Schweiz. Med. Wochenschr.*, 111, 1503, 1981.

55. Wolff, S. P. and Dean, R. T., Glucose autoxidation and protein modification. The potential role of 'autoxidative glycosylation' in diabetes, *Biochem. J.*, 245, 243, 1987.

56. Blakytny, R. and Harding, J. J., Glycation (non-enzymic glycosylation) inactivates glutathione reductase, *Biochem. J.*, 288, 303, 1992.

57. Bilan, P. J. and Klip, A., Glycation of the human erythrocyte glucose transporter in vitro and its functional consequences, *Biochem. J.*, 268, 661, 1990.

58. Vlassara, H., Valinsky, J., Brownlee, M., Cerami, C., Nishimoto, S., and Cerami, A., Advanced glycosylation endproducts on erythrocyte cell surface induce receptor-mediated phagocytosis by macrophages, *J. Exp. Med.*, 166, 539, 1987.

59. Vlassara, H., Moldawer, L., and Chan, B., Macrophage monocyte receptor for nonenzymatically glycosylated proteins is upregulated by cachectin tumor necrosis factor, *J. Clin. Invest.*, 84, 1813, 1989.

60. Mohandas, N., Kim, Y. R., Tycko, D. H., Orlik, J., Wyatt, J., and Groner, W., Accurate and independent measurement of volume and hemoglobin concentration of individual red cells by laser light scattering, *Blood*, 68, 509, 1986.

61. Winterbourn, C. C. and Batt, R. D., Lipid composition of human red cells of different ages, *Biochim. Biophys. Acta*, 202, 1, 1970.

62. Cohen, N. S., Ekholm, J. E., Luthra, M. G., and Hanahan, D. J., Biochemical characterization of density-separated human erythrocytes, *Biochim. Biophys. Acta*, 419, 229, 1976.

63. Galbraith, D. G. and Watts, D. C., Human erythrocyte acetylcholinesterase in relation to cell age, *Biochem. J.*, 195, 221, 1981.

64. Fishelson, Z. and Marikovsky, Y., Reduced CR1 expression on aged human erythrocytes. Immuno-electron microscopic and functional analysis, *Mech. Ageing Dev.*, 72, 25, 1993.

65. Paccaud, J.-P., Carpentier, J.-L., and Schifferli, J. A., Direct evidence for the clustered nature of complement receptors type 1 in the erythrocyte membrane, *J. Immunol.*, 141, 3889, 1988.

66. Pascual, M., Lutz, H. U., Steiger, G., Stammler, P., and Schifferli, J. A., Release of vesicles enriched in complement receptor-1 from human erythrocytes, *J. Immunol.*, 151, 397, 1993.

67. Lutz, H. U., Liu, S.-C., and Palek, J., Release of spectrin-free vesicles from human erythrocytes during ATP depletion, *J. Cell Biol.*, 73, 548, 1977.

68. Mueller, H., Schmidt, U., and Lutz, H. U., On the mechanism of vesicle release from ATP-depleted human red blood cells, *Biochim. Biophys. Acta*, 649, 462, 1981.

69. Rumsby, M. G., Trotter, J., Allan, D., and Michell, R. H., Recovery of membrane micro-vesicles from human erythrocytes stored for transfusion: a mechanism for the erythrocyte discocyte-to-spherocyte shape transformation, *Trans. Biochem. Soc.*, 5, 126, 1977.

70. Greenwalt, T. J., Bryan, D. J., and Dumaswala, U. J., Erythrocyte membrane vesiculation and changes in membrane composition during storage in citrate-phosphate-dextrose-adenine-1, *Vox Sang.*, 47, 261, 1984.

71. Bütikofer, P., Kuypers, F. A., Xu, C. M., Chiu, D. T. Y., and Lubin, B., Enrichment of 2 glycosyl-phosphatidylinositol-anchored proteins, acetylcholinesterase and decay accelerating factor, in vesicles released from human red blood cells, *Blood*, 74, 1481, 1989.

72. Snyder, L. M., Fairbanks, G., Trainor, J., Fortier, N. L., Jacobs, J. B., and Leb, L., Properties and characterization of vesicles released by young and old human red cells, *Br. J. Haematol.*, 54, 513, 1985.

73. Zimmermann, N., Pätzold, L., Halbhuber, K.-J., and Linss, W., Evidence for erythrocyte -microvesiculation in vivo, *Anat. Anz. Jena*, 158, 117, 1985.

74. Kinoshita, T., Complement receptors and regulation of humoral immune response, *Complement Today*, 1, 46, 1993.

75. Morgan, B. P. and Meri, S., Membrane proteins that protect against complement lysis, *Springer Semin. Immunopathol.*, 15, 369, 1994.
76. Mueller, H. and Lutz, H. U., Binding of autologous IgG to human red blood cells before and after ATP-depletion. Selective exposure of binding sites (autoantigens) on spectrin-free vesicles, *Biochim. Biophys. Acta*, 729, 249, 1983.
77. Iida, K., Whitlow, M. B., and Nussenzweig, V., Membrane vesiculation protects erythrocytes from the destruction of complement, *J. Immunol.*, 147, 2638, 1991.
78. Devaux, P. F., Protein involvement in transmembrane lipid asymmetry, *Annu. Rev. Biophys. Biomol. Struc.*, 21, 417, 1992.
79. Morrot, G., Hervé, P., Zachowski, A., Fellmann, P., and Devaux, F., Aminophospholipid translocase of human erythrocytes: phospholipid substrate specificity and effect of cholesterol, *Biochemistry*, 28, 3456, 1989.
80. Vondenhof, A., Oslender, A., Deuticke, B., and Haest, C. W. M., Band 3, an accidental flippase for anionic phospholipids, *Biochemistry*, 33, 4517, 1994.
81. Middelkoop, E., Van der Hoek, E. E., Bevers, E. M., Comfurius, P., Slotboom, A. J., Op den Kamp, J. A. F., Zwaal, R. F. A., and Roelofsen, B., Involvement of ATP-dependent aminophospholipid translocation in maintaining phospholipid asymmetry in diamide-treated human erythrocytes, *Biochim. Biophys. Acta*, 981, 151, 1989.
82. Connor, J., Pak, C. C., and Schroit, A. J., Exposure of phosphatidylserine in the outer leaflet of human red blood cells — relationship to cell density, cell age, and clearance by mononuclear cells, *J. Biol. Chem.*, 269, 2399, 1994.
83. Herrmann, A. and Devaux, P. F., Alteration of the aminophospholipid translocase activity during in vivo and artificial aging of human erythrocytes, *Biochim. Biophys. Acta*, 1027, 41, 1990.
84. Utsugi, T., Schroit, A. J., Connor, J., Bucana, C. D., and Fidler, I. J., Elevated expression of phosphatidylserine in the outer membrane leaflet of human tumor cells and recognition by activated human blood monocytes, *Cancer Res.*, 51, 3062, 1991.
85. Szymanski, I. O., Odgren, P. R., and Valeri, C. R., Relationship between the third component of human complement (C3) bound to stored preserved erythrocytes and their viability *in vivo*, *Vox Sang.*, 49, 34, 1985.
86. Schroit, A. J., Madsen, J. W., and Tanaka, Y., In vivo recognition and clearance of red blood cells containing phosphatidylserine in their plasma membranes, *J. Biol. Chem.*, 260, 5131, 1985.
87. Allen, T. M., Williamson, P., and Schlegel, R. A., Phosphatidylserine as a determinant of reticuloendothelial recognition of liposome models of the erythrocyte surface, *Proc. Natl. Acad. Sci. U.S.A.*, 85, 8067, 1988.
88. Symes, M. A. and Patel, H. M., Phagocytosis of liposomes that mimic lipid composition of senescent and sickle erythrocytes, *Biochem. Soc. Trans.*, 20, 327S, 1992.
89. Arvieux, J., Roussel, B., Ponard, D., and Colomb, M. G., Reactivity patterns of anti-phospholipid antibodies in systemic lupus erythematosus sera in relation to erythrocyte binding and complement activation, *Clin. Exp. Immunol.*, 84, 466, 1991.
90. Sthoeger, Z., Sthoeger, D., Green, L., and Geltner, D., The role of anticardiolipin autoantibodies in the pathogenesis of autoimmune hemolytic anemia in systemic lupus erythematosus, *J. Rheumatol.*, 20, 2058, 1993.
91. Ismail, R. and Cheng, H. M., Anticoagulant activity of heat-unmasked antiphospholipid autoantibody in normal human plasma, *Thromb. Res.*, 73, 143, 1994.

92. Cheng, H. M., Differential binding of antiphospholipid autoantibody in normal and autoimmune sera to prothrombin/phospholipid antigen complex, *Blood*, 83, 1157, 1994.

93. Lutz, H. U., Stammler, P., and Nater, M., Heat-treated serum contains instead of monomeric, immune-complex-like IgG aggregates that carry inactivated C3. The pro and contra heat treatment of serum, *Br. J. Haematol.*, 87(Suppl. 1), 112, 1994.

94. Casey, J. R. and Reithmeier, R. A. F., Analysis of the oligomeric state of band-3, the anion transport protein of the human erythrocyte membrane, by size exclusion high performance liquid chromatography — oligomeric stability and origin of heterogeneity, *J. Biol. Chem.*, 266, 15726, 1991.

95. Corbett, J. D. and Golan, D. E., Band-3 and glycophorin are progressively aggregated in density-fractionated sickle and normal red blood cells. Evidence from rotational and lateral mobility studies, *J. Clin. Invest.*, 91, 208, 1993.

96. Staros, J. V. and Kakkad, B. P., Cross-linking and chymotryptic digestion of the extracytoplasmic domain of the anion exchange channel in intact human erythrocytes, *J. Membrane Biol.*, 74, 247, 1983.

97. Jennings, M. L. and Nicknish, J. S., Localization of a site of intermolecular cross-linking in human red blood cell band 3 protein, *J. Biol. Chem.*, 260, 5472, 1985.

98. Salhany, J. M., Sloan, R. L., and Cordes, K. A., In situ cross-linking of human erythrocyte band-3 by bis(sulfosuccinimidyl)suberate. Evidence for ligand modulation of 2 alternate quaternary forms — covalent band-3 dimers and noncovalent tetramers formed by the association of 2 covalent dimers, *J. Biol. Chem.*, 265, 17688, 1990.

99. Schweizer, E., Angst, W., and Lutz, H. U., Glycoprotein topology on intact human red blood cells reevaluated by cross-linking following amino-group supplementation, *Biochemistry*, 21, 6807, 1982.

100. Oliver, C. N., Ahn, B.-W., Moerman, E. J., Goldstein, S., and Stadtman, E. R., Age-related changes in oxidized proteins, *J. Biol. Chem.*, 262, 5488, 1987.

101. Seppi, C., Castellana, M. A., Minetti, G., Piccinini, G., Balduini, C., and Brovelli, A., Evidence for membrane protein oxidation during in vivo aging of human erythrocytes, *Mech. Ageing Dev.*, 57, 247, 1991.

102. Castellana, M. A., Piccinini, G., Minetti, G., Seppi, C., Balduini, C., and Brovelli, A., Oxidation of membrane proteins and functional activity of band-3 in human red cell senescence, *Arch. Gerontol. Geriatr.*, (Suppl.)3, 101, 1992.

103. Jain, S. K., Evidence for membrane lipid peroxidation during the in vivo aging of human erythrocytes, *Biochim. Biophys. Acta*, 937, 205, 1988.

104. Giulivi, C. and Davies, K. J. A., Dityrosine and tyrosine oxidation products are endogenous markers for the selective proteolysis of oxidatively modified red blood cell hemoglobin by (the 19-S) proteasome, *J. Biol. Chem.*, 268, 8752, 1993.

105. Davies, K. J. A., Protein modification by oxidants and the role of proteolytic enzymes, *Biochem. Soc. Trans.*, 21, 346, 1993.

106. Vandenberg, J. J. M., Denkamp, J. A. F. O., Lubin, B. H., and Kuypers, F. A., Conformational changes in oxidized phospholipids and their preferential hydrolysis by phospholipase-A(2). A monolayer study, *Biochemistry*, 32, 4962, 1993.

107. Fagan, J. M. and Waxman, L., The ATP-independent pathway in red blood cells that degrades oxidant-damaged hemoglobin, *J. Biol. Chem.*, 267, 23015, 1992.

108. Waugh, S. M. and Low, P. S., Hemichrome binding to band 3: nucleation of Heinz bodies on the erythrocyte membrane, *Biochemistry*, 24, 34, 1985.

109. Waugh, S. M., Willardson, B. M., Kannan, R., Labotka, R. J., and Low, P. S., Heinz bodies induce clustering of band 3, glycophorin, and ankyrin in sickle cell erythrocytes, *J. Clin. Invest.*, 78, 1155, 1986.

110. Chiu, D. and Lubin, B., Oxidative hemoglobin denaturation and RBC destruction: the effect of heme on red cell membranes, *Semin. Hematol.*, 26, 128, 1989.

111. Arese, P. and De Flora, A., Pathophysiology of hemolysis in glucose-6-phosphate dehydrogenase deficiency, *Semin. Hematol.*, 27, 1, 1990.

112. Lutz, H. U., Elimination alter Erythrozyten aus der Zirkulation: Freilegung eines zellalter-spezifischen Antigens auf alternden Erythrozyten, *Schweiz. Med. Wochenschr.*, 111, 1507, 1981.

113. Lutz, H. U. and Stringaro-Wipf, G., Senescent red cell-bound IgG is attached to band 3 protein, *Biomed. Biochim. Acta*, 42, 117, 1983.

114. Lutz, H. U., Flepp, R., and Stringaro-Wipf, G., Naturally occurring autoantibodies to exoplasmic and cryptic regions of band 3 protein of human red blood cells, *J. Immunol.*, 133, 2610, 1984.

115. Schlüter, K. and Drenckhahn, D., Co-clustering of denatured hemoglobin with band 3: its role in binding of autoantibodies against band 3 to abnormal and aged erythrocytes, *Proc. Natl. Acad. Sci. U.S.A.*, 83, 6137, 1986.

116. Kannan, R., Labotka, R., and Low, P. S., Isolation and characterization of the hemichrome-stabilized membrane protein aggregates from sickle erythrocytes, *J. Biol. Chem.*, 263, 13766, 1988.

117. Yuan, J., Kannan, R., Shinar, E., Rachmilewitz, E. A., and Low, P. S., Isolation, characterization, and immunoprecipitation studies of immune complexes from membranes of beta-thalassemic erythrocytes, *Blood*, 79, 3007, 1992.

118. Kannan, R., Yuan, J., and Low, P. S., Isolation and partial characterization of antibody-enriched and globin-enriched complexes from membranes of dense human erythrocytes, *Biochem. J.*, 278, 57, 1991.

119. Turrini, F., Arese, P., Yuan, J., and Low, P. S., Clustering of integral membrane proteins of the human erythrocyte membrane stimulates autologous IgG binding, complement deposition, and phagocytosis, *J. Biol. Chem.*, 266, 23611, 1991.

120. Turrini, F., Mannu, F., Arese, P., Yuan, J., and Low, P. S., Characterization of the autologous antibodies that opsonize erythrocytes with clustered integral membrane proteins, *Blood*, 81, 3146, 1993.

121. Lutz, H. U., Fasler, S., Stammler, P., Bussolino, F., and Arese, P., Naturally occurring anti-band 3 antibodies and complement in phagocytosis of oxidatively-stressed and in clearance of senescent red cells, *Blood Cells*, 14, 175, 1988.

122. Lutz, H. U., Stammler, P., and Fasler, S., Preferential formation of C3b-IgG complexes in vitro and *in vivo* from nascent C3b and naturally occurring anti-band 3 antibodies, *J. Biol. Chem.*, 268, 17418, 1993.

123. Dale, G. L. and Daniels, R. B., Quantitation of immunoglobulin associated with senescent erythrocytes from the rabbit, *Blood*, 77, 1096, 1991.

124. Dale, G. L., Gaddy, P., and Pikul, F. J., Antibodies against biotinylated proteins are present in normal human serum, *J. Lab. Clin. Med.*, 123, 365, 1994.

125. Christian, J. A., Rebar, A. H., Boon, G. D., and Low, P. S., Senescence of canine biotinylated erythrocytes — increased autologous immunoglobulin binding occurs on erythrocytes aged in vivo for 104 to 110 days, *Blood*, 82, 3469, 1993.

126. Kay, M. M. B., Goodman, S. R., Sorensen, K., Whitfield, C. F., Wong, P., Zaki, L., and Rudloff, V., Senescent cell antigen is immunologically related to band 3, *Proc. Natl. Acad. Sci. U.S.A.*, 80, 1631, 1983.

127. Kay, M. M. B., Bosman, G. J. C. G. M., Shapiro, S. S., Bendich, A., and Bassel, P. S., Oxidation as a possible mechanism of cellular aging. Vitamin E deficiency causes premature aging and IgG binding to erythrocytes, *Proc. Natl. Acad. Sci. U.S.A.*, 83, 2463, 1986.

128. Bussolino, F., Turrini, F., and Arese, P., Measurement of phagocytosis utilizing ^{14}C-cyanate-labelled human red cells and monocytes, *Br. J. Haematol.*, 66, 271, 1987.

129. Lutz, H. U., Bussolino, F., Flepp, R., Fasler, S., Stammler, P., Kazatchkine, M. D., and Arese, P., Naturally occurring anti-band 3 antibodies and complement together mediate phagocytosis of oxidatively stressed human red blood cells, *Proc. Natl. Acad. Sci. U.S.A.*, 84, 7368, 1987.

130. Beppu, M., Mizukami, A., Nagoya, M., and Kikugawa, K., Binding of anti-band 3 autoantibody to oxidatively damaged erythrocytes, *J. Biol. Chem.*, 265, 3226, 1990.

131. Kay, M. M. B., Marchalonis, J. J., Schluter, S. F., and Bosman, G., Human erythrocyte aging: Cellular and molecular biology, *Transf. Med. Rev.*, 3, 173, 1991.

132. Mollison, P. L., Crome, P., Hughes-Jones, N. C., and Rochna, E., Rate of removal from the circulation of red cells sensitized with different amounts of antibody, *Br. J. Haematol.*, 11, 461, 1965.

133. Schreiber, A. D. and Frank, M. M., Role of antibody and complement in the immune clearance and destruction of erythrocytes. I. In vivo effects of IgG and IgM complement-fixing sites, *J. Clin. Invest.*, 51, 575, 1972.

134. Schreiber, A. D., Frank, M. M., Role of antibody and complement in the immune clearance and destruction of erythrocytes. II. Molecular nature of IgG and IgM complement-fixing sites and effects of their interaction with serum, *J. Clin. Invest.*, 51, 583, 1972.

135. Wiener, E., The ability of IgG subclasses to cause the elimination of targets in vivo and to mediate their destruction by phagocytosis/cytolysis in vitro, in *The Human IgG Subclasses*, Shakib, F., Ed., Pergamon Press, Oxford, 1990, 135.

136. Kurlander, R. J. and Rosse, W. F., Monocyte-mediated destruction in the presence of serum of red cells coated with antibody, *Blood*, 54, 1131, 1979.

137. Fries, L. F., Siwik, S. A., Malbran, A., and Frank, M. M., Phagocytosis of target particles bearing C3b-IgG covalent complexes by human monocytes and polymorphonuclear leukocytes, *Immunology.*, 62, 45, 1987.

138. Malbran, A., Frank, M. M., and Fries, L. F., Interactions of monomeric IgG bearing covalently bound C3b with polymorphonuclear leukocytes, *Immunology.*, 61, 15, 1987.

139. Ehlenberger, A. G. and Nussenzweig, V., The role of membrane receptors for C3b and C3d in phagocytosis, *J. Exp. Med.*, 145, 357, 1977.

140. Law, S. K. A., C3 receptors on macrophages, *J. Cell Sci.*, 9, 67, 1988.

141. Schifferli, J. A., Ng, Y. C., and Peters, D. K., The role of complement and its receptor in the elimination of immune complexes, *New Engl. J. Med.*, 315, 488, 1986.

142. Ross, G. D. and Vetvicka, V., CR3 (CD11b, CD18) — a phagocyte and NK cell membrane receptor with multiple ligand specificities and functions, *Clin. Exp. Immunol.*, 92, 181, 1993.

143. Varela, F. J. and Coutinho, A., Second generation immune networks, *Immunol. Today*, 12, 159, 1991.

144. Avrameas, S. and Ternynck, T., The natural autoantibodies system — between hypotheses and facts, *Mol. Immunol.*, 30, 1133, 1993.

145. Avrameas, S., Natural autoantibodies. From horror autotoxicus to *gnothi seauton*, *Immunol. Today*, 12, 154, 1991.

146. Guilbert, B., Dighiero, G., and Avrameas, S., Naturally occurring antibodies against nine common antigens in human sera, *J. Immunol.*, 128, 2779, 1982.

147. Lutz, H. U. and Wipf, G., Naturally occurring autoantibodies to skeletal proteins from human red blood cells, *J. Immunol.*, 128, 1695, 1982.

148. Lutz, H. U., Naturally occurring anti-band 3 antibodies, *Transf. Med. Rev.*, 6, 201, 1992.

149. Huang, C. C. and Stollar, B. D., A majority of Ig H-Chain cDNA of normal human adult blood lymphocytes resembles cDNA for fetal Ig and natural autoantibodies, *J. Immunol.*, 151, 5290, 1993.

150. Sanz, I., Casali, P., Thomas, J. W., Notkins, A. L., and Capra, J. D., Nucleotide sequences of eight human natural autoantibody V_H regions reveals apparent restricted use of V_H families, *J. Immunol.*, 142, 4054, 1989.

151. Baccala, R., Quang, T. V., Gilbert, M., Ternynck, T., and Avrameas, S., Two murine natural polyreactive autoantibodies are encoded by nonmutated germline genes, *Proc. Natl. Acad. Sci. U.S.A.*, 86, 4624, 1989.

152. Kaveri, S. V., Kang, C. Y., and Kohler, H., Natural mouse and human antibodies bind to a peptide derived from a germline V_H chain — evidence for evolutionary conserved self-binding locus, *J. Immunol.*, 145, 4207, 1990.

153. Guigou, V., Guilbert, B., Moinier, D., Tonnelle, C., Boubli, L., Avrameas, S., Fougereau, M., and Fumoux, F., Ig repertoire of human polyspecific antibodies and B-cell ontogeny, *J. Immunol.*, 146, 1368, 1991.

154. Turman, M. A., Casali, P., Notkins, A. L., Bach, F. H., and Platt, J. L., Polyreactivity and antigen specificity of human xenoreactive monoclonal and serum natural antibodies, *Transplantation*, 52, 710, 1991.

155. Lutz, H. U., Nater, M., and Stammler, P., Naturally occurring anti-band 3 antibodies have a unique affinity for C3, *Immunology*, 80, 191, 1993.

156. Vos, Q., Klasen, E. A., and Haaijman, J. J., The effect of divalent and univalent binding on antibody titration curves in solid-phase ELISA, *J. Immunol. Meth.*, 103, 47, 1987.

157. Garratty, G., Effect of cell-bound proteins on the in vivo survival of circulating blood cells, *Gerontology*, 37, 68, 1991.

158. Kulics, J., Rajnavölgyi, E., Füst, G., and Gergely, J., Interaction of C3 and C3b with immunoglobulin G, *Mol. Immunol.*, 20, 805, 1983.

159. Fries, L. F., Gaither, T. A., Hammer, C. H., and Frank, M. M., C3b covalently bound to IgG demonstrates a reduced rate of inactivation by factors H and I, *J. Exp. Med.*, 160, 1640, 1984.

160. Makrides, S. C., Scesney, S. M., Ford, P. J., Evans, K. S., Carson, G. R., and Marsh, H. C., Cell surface expression of the C3b/C4b receptor (CR1) protects Chinese hamster ovary cells from lysis by human complement, *J. Biol. Chem.*, 267, 24754, 1992.

161. Lutz, H. U., Stammler, P., Koch, D., and Taylor, R. P., Opsonic potential of C3b-anti-band 3 complexes when generated on senescent and oxidatively stressed red cells or in fluid phase, in *Red Cell Aging*, Magnani, M., Ed., Plenum Press, New York, 1991, 367.

162. Ruoslahti, E., Integrins as receptors for extracellular matrix, in *Cell Biology of Extracellular Matrix*, Hay, E. D., Ed., Plenum Press, New York, 1991, 343.

163. Brown, E. J. and Goodwin, J. L., Fibronectin receptors of phagocytes. Characterization of the Arg-Gly-Asp binding proteins of human monocytes and polymorphonuclear leukocytes, *J. Exp. Med.*, 167, 777, 1988.

164. Ezekowitz, R. A. B., Sastry, K., Bailly, P., and Warner, A., Molecular characterization of the human macrophage mannose receptor — demonstration of multiple carbohydrate recognition-like domains and phagocytosis of yeasts in Cos-1 cells, *J. Exp. Med.*, 172, 1785, 1990.

165. Super, M. and Ezekowitz, R. A. B., The role of mannose-binding proteins in host defense, *Infect. Agent. Dis.*, 1, 194, 1992.

166. Stanton, L. W., White, R. T., Bryant, C. M., Protter, A. A., and Endemann, G., A macrophage Fc receptor for IgG is also a receptor for oxidized low density lipoprotein, *J. Biol. Chem.*, 267, 22446, 1992.

167. Endemann, G., Stanton, L. W., Madden, K. S., Bryant, C. M., White, R. T., and Protter, A. A., CD36 is a receptor for oxidized low density lipoprotein, *J. Biol. Chem.*, 268, 11811, 1993.

168. Speert, D. P., Wright, S. D., Silverstein, S. C., and Mah, B., Functional characterization of macrophage receptors for in vitro phagocytosis of unopsonized *Pseudomonas aeruginosa*, *J. Clin. Invest.*, 82, 872, 1988.

169. Malaise, M. G., Hoyoux, C., Franchimont, P., Foidart, J. B., and Mahieu, P. R., Effects of mannose and mannose derivatives on the clearance of IgG antibody-coated erythrocytes in the rat, *Immunology*, 68, 126, 1989.

170. Salmon, J. E., Kapur, S., and Kimberly, R. P., Opsonin-independent ligation of Fc gamma receptors. The 3G8-bearing receptors on neutrophils mediate the phagocytosis of concanavalin A-treated erythrocytes and nonopsonized *Escherichia coli*, *J. Exp. Med.*, 166, 1798, 1987.

171. Giaimis, J., Lombard, Y., Fonteneau, P., Muller, C. D., Levy, R., Makayakumba, M., Lazdins, J., and Poindron, P., Both mannose and beta-glucan receptors are involved in phagocytosis of unopsonized, heat-killed *Saccharomyces cerevisiae* by murine macrophages, *J. Leukocyte Biol.*, 54, 564, 1993.

172. Schlesinger, L. S., Macrophage phagocytosis of virulent but not attenuated strains of Mycobacterium-Tuberculosis is mediated by mannose receptors in addition to complement receptors, *J. Immunol.*, 150, 2920, 1993.

173. Hebbel, R. P. and Miller, W. J., Phagocytosis of sickle erythrocytes: immunologic and oxidative determinants of hemolytic anemia, *Blood*, 64, 733, 1984.

174. Kay, M. M. B., Mechanism of removal of senescent cells by human macrophages in situ, *Proc. Natl. Acad. Sci. U.S.A.*, 72, 3521, 1975.

175. Kay, M. M. B., Role of physiologic autoantibody in the removal of senescent human red cells, *J. Supramol. Struct.*, 9, 555, 1978.

176. Freedman, J., Membrane-bound immunoglobulins and complement components on young and old red cells, *Transfusion*, 24, 477, 1984.

177. Horn, S., Bashan, N., and Gopas, J., Phagocytosis of phenylhydrazine oxidized and G-6-PD-deficient red blood cells. The role of cell-bound immunoglobulins, *Blood*, 78, 1818, 1991.

178. Gattegno, L., Saffar, L., and Vaysse, J., Inhibition by monoclonal anticomplement receptor type 1 on interactions between senescent human red blood cells and monocytic-macrophagic cells, *J. Leucocyte Biol.*, 45, 422, 1989.

179. Shapiro, S., Kohn, D., and Gershon, H., A role for complement as the major opsonin in the sequestration of erythrocytes from elderly and young donors, *Br. J. Haematol.*, 83, 648, 1993.

180. Sambrano, G. R., Parthasarathy, S., and Steinberg, D., Recognition of oxidatively damaged erythrocytes by a macrophage receptor with specificity for oxidized low density lipoprotein, *Proc. Natl. Acad. Sci. U.S.A.*, 91, 3265, 1994.

181. Shinar, E., Rachmilewitz, E. A., Shifter, A., Rahamim, E., and Saltman, P., Oxidative damage to human red cells induced by copper and iron complexes in the presence of ascorbate, *Biochim. Biophys. Acta*, 1014, 66, 1989.

182. Gattegno, L., Prigent, M. J., Saffar, L., Baldier, D., Vaysse, J., and Lefloch, A., Carbohydrate specificity and opsonin dependency of the interaction between human senescent red cells and autologous monocytes, *Glycoconjugate J.*, 3, 379, 1986.

183. Vaysse, J., Gattegno, L., Bladier, D., and Aminoff, D., Adhesion and erythrophagocytosis of human senescent erythrocytes by autologous monocytes and their inhibition by β-galactosyl derivatives, *Proc. Natl. Acad. Sci. U.S.A.*, 83, 1339, 1986.

184. Kempka, G., Roos, P. H, and Kolb-Bachofen, V., A membrane-associated form of C-reactive protein is the galactose-specific particle receptor on rat liver macrophages, *J. Immunol.*, 144, 1004, 1990.

185. Ballou, S. P. and Cleveland, R. P., Binding of human C-reactive protein to monocytes. Analysis by flow cytometry, *Clin. Exp. Immunol.*, 84, 329, 1991.

186. Malaise, M. G., Hoyoux, C., Franchimont, P., and Mahieu, P. R., Evidence for a role of accessible galactosyl or mannosyl residues of Fc domain in the in vivo clearance of IgG antibody-coated autologous erythrocytes in the rat, *Clin. Immunol. Immunopathol.*, 54, 469, 1990.

187. Malaise, M. G., Franchimont, P., and Mahieu, P. R., The ability of normal human monocytes to phagocytose IgG-coated red blood cells is related to the number of accessible galactosyl and mannosyl residues in the Fc domain of the anti-red blood cell IgG antibody molecules, *J. Immunol. Methods*, 119, 231, 1989.

188. Lund, J., Tanaka, T., Takahashi, N., Sarmay, G., Arata, Y., and Jefferis, R., A protein structural change in aglycosylated IgG3 correlates with loss of huFcγRI and huFcγRII binding and/or activation, *Mol. Immunol.*, 27, 1145, 1990.

189. Matsuda, H., Nakamura, S., Ichikawa, Y., Kozai, K., Takano, R., Nose, M., Endo, S., Nishimura, Y., and Arata, Y., Proton nuclear magnetic resonance studies of the structure of the Fc fragment of human immunoglobulin G1: comparison of native and recombinant proteins, *Mol. Immunol.*, 27, 571, 1990.

190. Beppu, M., Masa, H., Hora, M., and Kikugawa, K., Augmentation of macrophage recognition of oxidatively damaged erythrocytes by substratum-bound fibronectin and macrophage surface fibronectin, *FEBS Lett.*, 295, 135, 1991.

191. Wright, S. D., Reddy, P. A., Jong, M. T. C., and Erickson, B. W., C3bi receptor (complement receptor type 3) recognizes a region of complement protein C3 containing the sequence arg-gly-asp, *Proc. Natl. Acad. Sci. U.S.A.*, 84, 1965, 1987.

192. Hathaway, T. K. and Adams, J. L., Plasma fibronectin: a third opsonic protein involved in immune clearance and destruction of erythrocytes after infusion of incompatible blood, *Transplant. Proc.*, 20, 1096, 1988.

193. Rostagno, A. A., Frangione, B., and Gold, L., Biochemical studies on the interaction of fibronectin with Ig, *J. Immunol.*, 146, 2687, 1991.

194. Greenberg, S., Chang, P., and Silverstein, S. C., Tyrosine phosphorylation is required for Fc-Receptor mediated phagocytosis in mouse macrophages, *J. Exp. Med.*, 177, 529, 1993.

195. Daeron, M., Malbec, O., Bonnerot, C., Latour, S., Segal, D. M., and Fridman, W. H., Tyrosine-containing activation motif-dependent phagocytosis in mast cells, *J. Immunol.*, 152, 783, 1994.

196. Waytes, A. T., Malbran, A., Bobak, D. A., and Fries, L. F., Pre-ligation of CR1 enhances IgG-dependent phagocytosis by cultured human monocytes, *J. Immunol.*, 146, 2694, 1991.

197. Mollnes, T. E. and Lachmann, P. J., Regulation of complement, *Scand. J. Immunol.*, 27, 127, 1988.

198. Kumpel, B. M., Wiener, E., Urbaniak, S. J., and Bradley, B. A., Human monoclonal anti-D antibodies. II. The relationship between IgG subclass, Gm allotype and Fc mediated function, *Br. J. Haematol.*, 71, 415, 1989.

199. Savill, J., Smith, J., Sarraf, C., Ren, Y., Abbott, F., and Rees, A., Glomerular mesangial cells and inflammatory macrophages ingest neutrophils undergoing apoptosis, *Kidney Int.*, 42, 924, 1992.

200. Horton, M., Vitronectin receptor — tissue specific expression or adaptation to culture, *Int. J. Exp. Pathol.*, 71, 741, 1990.

201. Malorni, W. and Donelli, G., Cell death — general features and morphological aspects, *Ann. N.Y. Acad. Sci.*, 663, 218, 1992.

Chapter **7**

PROTEIN KINASE C SIGNAL TRANSMISSION DURING AGING

Fiorenzo Battaini, Stefano Govoni, and Marco Trabucchi

CONTENTS

0-8493-4786-6/95/$0.00+$.50
© 1995 by CRC Press, Inc.

I.   INTRODUCTION

It is becoming increasingly clear that senescence affects intracellular brain signal transduction at a number of different levels, from receptor availability and coupling with effector systems, to production of second messengers and activation of protein kinases.[1,2] Intercellular communication may also be affected by aging, as a consequence of changes in neurotransmitter release and uptake, resulting in modifications of cell function and, at a more integrated level, cognitive and neurological impairments. Current research, therefore, is focused at investigating the molecular mechanisms of neurotransmission as possible targets for intervention to ameliorate the functional decay that occurs during aging and to prevent cell degeneration. Protein phosphorylation represents the common final pathway in the actions of various neurotransmitters and is also an important regulatory feedback mechanism for all the steps involved in production of intracellular second messengers. A number of protein kinases exist in the central nervous system, with a variety of different activators (cyclic nucleotides, calcium ions, diacylglycerol, arachidonic acid).[3] Depending on the substrate protein phosphorylated, cell responses can range from short-term events, like modification of ion channel function, to mid-term actions such as changes in receptor availability and/or affinity, to long term changes such as in synaptic efficacy and gene expression.[4]

II.   FOCUSING ON PKC

Among the kinases, protein kinase C (PKC) has recently received intense scrutiny. This kinase is stimulated by an intramembrane increase in diacylglycerol (DAG) levels, derived from hydrolysis of phospholipids (phosphatidylinositol 4,5-bisphosphate by phospholipase C, and phosphatidylcholine by phospholipase D), and by interaction with phosphatidylserine (PS) present in the membrane compartment.[5]

In addition, agonists that induce turnover of inositol phospholipids (PITR) often induce release of arachidonic acid from phospholipid degradation by phospholipase A_2. Arachidonic acid and other cis unsaturated fatty acids (oleic, linoleic, linolenic) stimulate PKC synergistically with activation by diacylglycerol.[5]

PKC is composed of various different isoforms distinguished on the basis of primary structure of the polypeptide chain. Molecular cloning studies initially described four cDNA clones encoding the α, βI, βII, and γ isoforms. βI and βII isoforms are derived from a single RNA transcript, through alternative splicing and the encoded proteins differ in a 50 amino acid residue of the polypeptide carboxy-terminal. In humans the genes are located on distinct chromosomes. These isoforms require free calcium ions (Ca^{2+}) for full activation (in addition to DAG and PS) and are referred to as "classical" and/or Ca^{2+}-dependent PKCs. Another group of cDNA clones encode, up to the time of writing, eight additional subspecies, referred to as new and atypical PKCs (also known as Ca^{2+}-independent). The novel PKCs are represented by the δ, ε, η, θ, and μ isoforms, being independent of Ca^{2+} and dependent only on DAG and PS for activation. PKC ζ, λ, and ι are referred to as "atypical" because they are not activated by either Ca^{2+} or DAG.[6,7] In addition to PS, the activators for atypical PKCs might be free fatty acids and phosphatidylinositol 3,4,5-trisphosphate.[8] Brain tissues express most of the PKC isoforms.[6,7,9] The different isoforms show closely related but different structures.

The polypeptide sequence of PKCs is composed of two subunits: one regulatory, at the N-terminal and the other catalytic, at the carboxy-terminal.[5,6] The former has binding sites for DAG, PS, and Ca^{2+}, while the latter has the ATP and the substrate binding sites (see Figure 1). The regulatory subunit inhibits the catalytic domain through a sequence termed the pseudosubstrate site. In the presence of the specific activators (lipids, DAG, Ca^{2+}, depending on the isoforms) a conformational change occurs exposing the catalytic domain and increasing the association of the whole polypeptide with the membrane compartment containing phosphatidylserine. Exposure of the catalytic site permits binding of substrates to PKC and their subsequent phosphorylation. Phorbol esters, such as phorbol 12,13-dibutyrate (PdBu) and phorbol 12-myristate 13-acetate (PMA) bind and activate PKC.

III. PKC AND BRAIN FUNCTION

At the brain level, PKC is highly expressed and experimental data support its involvement in the regulation of neuronal activity.[9] Physiological substrates for PKC include ion channels and pumps and also proteins regulating gene expression. The most studied and characterized *in vivo* substrates for PKC are protein B-50 (otherwise called GAP-43, F1, neuromodulin) involved in the control of PITR, neurite outgrowth, neurotransmitter release, and potentiation of synaptic strength;[10-13] protein P87 (also called MARCKS) involved in cytoskeleton/neurotransmitter vesicle interactions;[14] and protein p17 (called neurogranin) involved in the postsynaptic control of long-term neuronal excitability.[15,16]

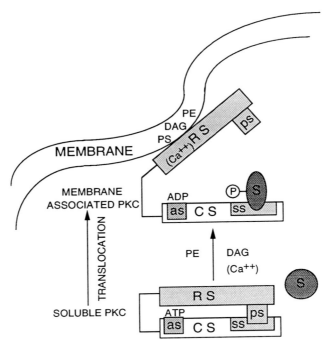

Figure 1

Scheme of PKC structure and activation. Soluble PKC is maintained in an inactive conformation by interaction of the regulatory subunit (RS) with the catalytic subunit (CS) through the pseudosubstrate sequence (ps) with the substrate binding site (ss). An increase in intracellular free calcium ions (Ca^{2+}) and in membrane diacylglycerol (DAG) favors interaction of the enzyme with the membrane compartment, thereby changing conformation and exposing the ss. Binding of the substrate protein (S) to the ss leads to its phosphorylation by ATP associated with the ATP binding site (as). Phorbol esters (PE) induce the association of soluble PKC with the membrane compartment.

IV. PKC IN SYNAPTIC PLASTICITY, LEARNING, AND MEMORY

Increasing evidence indicates that PKC plays a role in learning and memory processes. In *in vitro* electrophysiological correlates of memory such as in long term synaptic potentiation (LTP), PKC translocation and phosphorylation of endogenous proteins is augmented.[13,17,18] Associative learning in different invertebrate and vertebrate animal models (*Drosophila*,[19] *Aplysia*,[20] *Hermissenda*,[21] and rabbits[22]) is related to changes in PKC at a neuronal level. Animals with different spatial learning capabilities express brain PKC activity proportional to the performance of the animal.[23] Behavioral training of rodents (spatial discrimination) is related to changes in brain PKC labeling with phorbol esters[24] and activity.[25] Moreover, experience-dependent synaptic plasticity is associated with modifications in PKC activity at a central level.[26,27] In addition, on one hand behavioral evidence demonstrates that PKC activators[28] or inhibitors[29] facilitate or inhibit, respectively, spatial memory performance in rodents, while on the other hand pharmacological evidence indicates that drugs known to improve cognitive performance in animal models of memory deterioration are able to induce *in vivo* and *in vitro* brain PKC translocation.[30-32] Recent data have also documented that rats with chemically induced cognitive impairment present changes in PKC-dependent phosphorylation of the endogenous PKC substrate, protein B-50.[33]

A physiological model of cognitive deterioration is represented by the aging process. It is in fact well established that aging is associated with modifications in cognitive function.[34]

V. PHYSIOLOGICAL AGING AND PKC

Various observations indicate that PKC might be a target for the aging process. In fact, in addition to the observation that several neurotransmitters acting through PKC activation (such as acetylcholine, serotonin, excitatory amino acids, and peptides) are modified centrally as a consequence of aging,[35,36] the receptors and the production of second messengers, such as DAG and Ca^{2+} (specific activators of PKC), are also reported to change with age.[37-40]

Various studies have focused attention on the effects of aging on PKC in different strains of rodents. Early studies on aged mice demonstrated that whole-brain PKC activity in soluble and particulate fractions did not change as a consequence of aging; the only relevant age-related change in PKC was observed in splenic tissues, where particulate PKC was decreased in 24-month-old rats when compared to young (2-month-old) rats.[41] In aged Fisher 344 rats, PKC activity does not change in hippocampal structures[42] but activity is decreased in both soluble and particulate fractions of cortical structures.[43] Moreover, in this strain of rats, enzyme function, evaluated either as translocation to the membrane fraction in response to stimulation with phorbol ester[43] or with neurotransmitters coupled to PKC activation,[44] is impaired in aged rats when compared with adult and young animals.[42]

In the Sprague-Dawley strain, the direction of age-related changes in brain PKC levels and activity can differ according to the area investigated (i.e., decrease in cortex and increase in hippocampus).[45] Moreover, phosphorylation of endogenous substrates, such as protein B-50, is decreased in hippocampus under depolarized conditions.[46] In the case of the gerbil brain, opposite changes in PKC labeling by tritiated phorbol esters have also been reported in different brain regions, in particular, a decrease occurred in cortical structures, namely in the frontal cortex whereas an increase occurred in hippocampal structures, in particular, in the dentate gyrus.[47] Similar age-related modifications in phorbol ester binding to PKC have been reported in Fisher 344 rats.[48]

The reduction of PKC labeling in cortical structures may indicate either a defect in the turnover of the kinase or a modification in the characteristics of binding to the regulatory domain of PKC. The increase in PKC in hippocampal structures may represent a compensatory process for reduced synaptic excitability during aging, as indicated by electro-physiological measurements[49] possibly linked to altered intracellular Ca^{2+} handling.[50-52] It remains to be determined whether such an increase is the result of enhanced arborization of the dendritic tree where most PKC binding sites are localized[53] — a phenomenon observed in areas like the hippocampus that show neuronal loss during aging[54] — or is the consequence of the process of gliosis that occurs in the aging brain. Some lines of evidence indicate that PKC isoforms (α and β) are overexpressed in reactive glial cells.[55]

Fordyce and Wehner[56] have extended their previous studies on brain PKC in different strains of young mice with variable spatial learning capabilities[23] to aged mice and found that the age-related decline in spatial learning performance is related to a decline in hippocampal PKC activity.[56]

PKC has also been investigated during physiological aging in humans. PKC levels, assessed as labeled [^{3}H]-PdBu binding, decrease with age in prefrontal cortex structures.[57] In erythrocytes the age-dependent increase in intracellular Ca^{2+} levels is associated with PKC redistribution to cell membrane fractions.[58] In neutrophils from aged patients, PKC levels remain unmodified in respect to young controls, but enzyme activity is decreased in the soluble compartment.[59] Moreover, indirect evidence points to a defective PKC system in the T cell response of aged patients[60] and in platelets from donors of various ages; the levels of membrane PKC are also positively correlated with age.[61]

VI. STRAIN AND SUBSTRATE-DEPENDENT CHANGES IN PKC DURING AGING

We extended our previous studies on brain PKC in aged Sprague-Dawley rats[45,62,63] to the Wistar strain. This strain of rats has been extensively investigated during aging using behavioral, neurochemical, and electrophysiological approaches.[64-66]

Analysis of PKC activity using histone as an exogenous substrate indicate that no changes in kinase activity were present in soluble and membrane fractions prepared from young (3 month), adult (8 month) and aged (28 month) rat cortical, hippocampal, and cerebellar structures. Accordingly, enzyme levels, assessed as capacity and affinity of [³H]-PdBu binding to PKC, indicated that there were no changes in binding parameter as a function of age in the same fractions utilized to assess kinase activity.[67]

On the other hand, the utilization of a relevant endogenous substrate for PKC, purified protein B-50, enabled us to detect changes in kinase activity during aging. B-50 phosphorylation was decreased in the cortex in both adult and aged rats when compared with young animal, while as regards PKC from the hippocampus, B-50 phosphorylation steadily increases with aging, being significantly different in aged rats when compared with the young counterpart.[68] These data indicate that the *in vitro* use of a relevant endogenous substrate for PKC permits identification of age-related changes in brain PKC activity that otherwise could remain undetected.

VII. PKC ISOFORMS IN THE AGING BRAIN

In light of the reported specificity in B-50 phosphorylation by the various PKC isoforms[69,70] it was important to investigate eventual age-related changes in PKC isoform expression that might explain the substrate-dependent changes in PKC activity during aging.

The data on classical PKC α, β, and γ indicate that the mRNA for the various isoforms presents developmental changes (decrease for the α and β mRNA) evident in adult animals in the cortex, but aged animals express similar mRNA levels to the adult animals. PKC γ mRNA remains constant throughout all ages in cortex, hippocampus, and cerebellum.[68]

The possibility of hippocampal subfield changes during aging was investigated with *in situ* hybridization studies. The mRNA for PKC α, β, and γ did not show age-related changes in hippocampal subfields (CA_{1-3}) or in the dentate gyrus. Also, other regions important for memory processing, such as the amygdala, did not show age-dependent changes.[71] These data suggested that the reported changes in PKC levels during aging might be either strain specific and/or at a level of protein expression. To answer this question, we also evaluated the expression of the isoforms PKC α, βI, βII, and γ during aging, using specific polyclonal antisera.[72] Western blot data indicated that PKC α, βI, and βII did not show changes with aging in both soluble and particulate fractions from cortical and cerebellar structures. The only age-related change was observed in the hippocampal expression of PKC γ at a membrane level, that was increased by roughly 40% with respect to both adult and young animals. The decrease in message observed in Northern blots is not coupled to a decrease in the respective protein codified — indicating a lack of parallelism between message and protein expressed and, therefore, suggesting a modification in protein turnover. A similar situation to possible modified protein turnover is observed in the hippocampus, where the PKC γ expressed is modified in spite of no parallel change in mRNA levels. Changes in PKC protein turnover not coupled to parallel changes in mRNA levels have been reported previously in other systems.[73] One possible explanation for the increase in PKC γ protein in the hippocampus of aged rats could be that it is correlated with the already-mentioned phenomenon of dendritic sprouting occurring with aging;[54] PKC γ has been demonstrated to be preferentially located at a postsynaptic level,[74] where the dendritic tree is highly represented, and in aged rat hippocampus calcium ions are particularly abundant in dendrites[75] indicating a possible modification in the distribution of PKC γ at a membrane level. We are now investigating the calcium-independent PKCs with a view to their proposed role in the late phase of LTP.[76,77] Preliminary data on Ca^{2+}-independent PKC activity, utilizing as substrate the peptide $[Ser^{25}]$ PKC_{19-31}[6] and on PKC δ, ε, and ζ immunodetection,[72] indicate that no significant age-related changes are present on these isoforms during aging (Battaini et al., unpublished).

VIII. ENZYME TRANSLOCATION AS THE KEY AGE-RELATED DEFECT IN BRAIN PKC

Translocation is a term denoting those changes in intracellular location of PKC that occur upon exposure of tissues or cells to specific PKC activators, such as hormones or transmitters coupled to receptor-dependent PITR or, bypassing receptor activation, with phorbol esters such as PMA; it refers to the induced association of PKC with the membrane and is considered to be an index of PKC activation (see Figure 1).

Kinase C activity is assessed *in vitro* under optimal conditions for activators (Ca^{2+}, DAG, and PS for the calcium-dependent isoforms and DAG and PS for the calcium-independent isoforms) and represents the amount of enzyme present in soluble or particulate fractions under static conditions. On the other hand, it is known that aging might modify the different PKC activators such as (1) calcium ion availability[37,78] and the mechanisms of transport from extracellular[79] and intracellular sites,[80] (2) DAG production,[39,81] and (3) membrane PS levels.[46]

We decided, then, to search for age-dependent changes in PKC translocation during aging. Experiments on cross-chopped brain slices of young, adult, and aged rats activated *in vitro* for a short period with phorbol esters (PMA 160 nM for 15 min) show that the ability of PKC to translocate, as indicated by an increase in particulate activity coupled to a decrease in soluble activity, is maintained in young and adult rats but is lost in aged rats in both cortex and hippocampus.[82] This loss of enzyme translocation in aged animals is important from a functional point of view because it might blunt physiologic PKC activation. Because in the adopted experimental conditions we bypassed receptor activation, and the consequent production of DAG *in vitro*, this observation suggests impaired PKC function in aged rats irrespective of neurotransmitter levels, receptor availability, and second messenger production. Investigating this issue further, Pisano and co-workers studied receptor-mediated brain PKC translocation in aged Fisher 344 rats in response to transmitters activating PKC, and found that both serotonin and carbachol-induced PKC translocation was deficient in aged rats.[44] Moreover, in this strain of rats, the calcium ionophore (A 23187)-mediated PKC translocation is also impaired in aged cortex.[83]

It is clear from these data that brain PKC presents age-related modifications that are dependent on the strain of rats utilized. This is not surprising, because several experimental results with other neurochemical and behavioral parameters support this contention.[84]

It is known that aging is associated, in addition to a decline in cognitive function, with a decreased capability to adapt to stress.[85] One interesting model is represented by the Wistar Kyoto (WKY) normotensive strain of rats. Among different strains of rats investigated, the WKY strain has a short life span and is more reactive to stressors.[85]

We decided to investigate brain PKC in aging WKY rats because of its proposed involvement in various aspects of the stress response.[86-88] Figure 2 shows an analysis of the levels of membrane-bound PKC as autoradiographic binding of [^{3}H]-PdBu to horizontal brain sections in adult (6 months), middle aged (12 months) and aged (24 months) WKY rats. The levels of PKC do not change with aging in hippocampal structures such as CA subfields and dentate gyrus, or in basal ganglia, cortex (frontal, parietal, and entorhinal), and cerebellum.

As a further control, we investigated PKC activity and translocation in cortex and hippocampus during aging (Figure 3). As with the data on the Wistar strain, enzyme activity (utilizing histone as substrate) did not change in the WKY strain as a consequence of aging, while PKC translocation, in response to short-term exposure of the tissue slices to phorbol esters, was impaired in aged WKY rats in both cortex and hippocampus. These data are in agreement with those previously reported for the Wistar strain and underscore an impaired activation of the PKC system in aged WKY rats, in spite of unmodified enzyme levels and activity under basal conditions. It is possible that stressful conditions may unmask changes in PKC activity undetected under basal conditions.

The data presented here indicate that, during aging, brain PKC displays strain and substrate-dependent changes in phosphorylating activity when assayed under optimal conditions of *in vitro* enzyme activation.

On the other hand, enzyme translocation upon PMA challenge is the only component of the PKC system that exhibits a reproducible age-

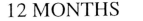

6 MONTHS   12 MONTHS   24 MONTHS

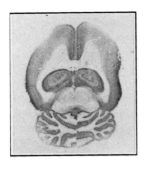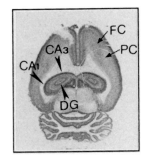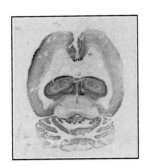

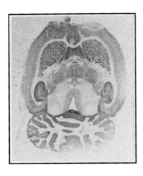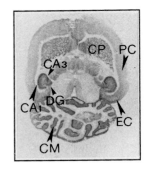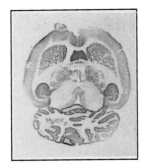

Figure 2

Binding of [³H]-PdBu in horizontal brain sections of WKY rats of different ages. Sections (12 μm) were thaw-mounted on gelatin-coated slides and kept at –80°C until use (within 1 month) and binding performed as detailed previously.[47] Specific binding appears black. (FC) Frontal cortex; (PC) parietal cortex; (EC) entorhinal cortex; (CA$_1$) Fields; (CA$_3$) Ammon's horn; (DG) dentate gyrus; (CP) caudate putamen; (CM) cerebellum molecular layer. The binding values (means ± SD from 3 to 4 rats) in 6-month-old rats were: FC 109 ± 13, PC 40 ± 12, EC 98 ± 10, CA$_1$ 101 ± 16, CA$_3$ 93 ± 11, DG 93 ± 24, CP 61 ± 14, and CM 101 ± 9. Such values were similar in 12- and 24-month-old rats. Binding is expressed as nCi/mg tissue (Amerham ³H microscales).

related impairment among the different strains used.[43,44,67,82] The impaired PKC translocation in aged rats might also be important in organization of neuronal architecture, because PMA-induced phosphorylation of cytoskeletal proteins (such as α-tubulin, microtubule-associated proteins, and TAU proteins) observed in adult rats are completely absent in aged animals.[44] From a functional point of view, the blunted enzyme translocation during aging may lead to an increased proportion of soluble vs. membrane-bound PKC upon physiological activation in aged animals. No data are currently available on the function of the enzyme in the two compartments in vertebrates, but data from invertebrates (*Hermissenda*

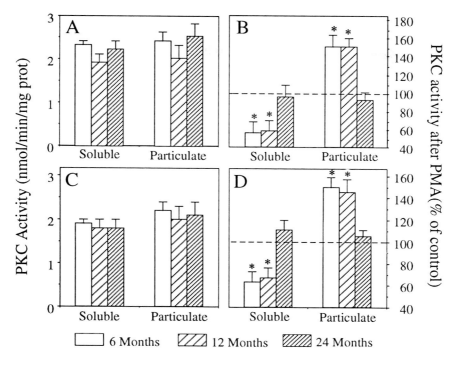

Figure 3

PKC activity (A,C) and translocation (B,D) from cortex (A,B) and hippocampus (C,D) in WKY rats of different ages. Values are expressed as means ± S.E. of three different experiments with samples in triplicate. Slices were exposed for 15 min to either solvent dimethylsulfoxide 0.01% or PMA 160 nM. Fractions were prepared and PKC activity assayed as described;[31] * p <0.05, Student's t test.

crassicornis) have demonstrated a common target for neuronal PKC on K^+ channel modulation. Membrane PKC inhibits, while soluble PKC activates, an outward K^+ current, thus stimulating or inhibiting cellular excitability, respectively.[89] If the same regulation is operant in the vertebrate brain, the higher proportion of soluble PKC (derived from an impaired translocation during aging in response to various stimuli) would increase K^+ fluxes, thus decreasing neuronal excitability through a hyperpolarization effect.

This interpretation is consistent with data from the literature showing a facilitation of transmitter (serotonin) release by PKC activation with phorbol esters in cortical structures from 6- and 12-month-old rats, in which PKC translocation is operant, while the reported inhibition of transmitter release induced by phorbol esters in 24-month-old rats[43] could be due to an imbalance in the soluble vs. particulate PKC, thereby causing K^+ channel stimulation. Electrophysiological data indicate that neuronal excitability is decreased in aged vertebrate hippocampus, probably because of an increase in a K[+] outward current through a calcium-dependent K[+] channel.[49] Recent studies have demonstrated that in classically conditioned animals PKC translocation is more efficient than in unconditioned animals,[90] direct evidence of the importance of functional PKC (enzyme translocation) in memory formation.

This notion might also have pharmacological relevance in light of recent data showing that certain cognition-enhancing drugs induce brain PKC translocation *in vivo* and *in vitro*.[30-32] The capacity to employ drugs to interfere with the process that is specifically affected in aged animals is a possibility that has theoretical application but that has not yet been investigated and warrants further analysis.

Impaired PKC translocation could be related to different expression of PKC isoforms in aged animals. It is known, in fact, that PKC γ is much less sensitive to short-term phorbol ester-induced translocation when compared to α and β isoforms,[91] so that a higher proportion of PKC γ in aged animals could make the system less sensitive to PMA-induced translocation. This interpretation, however, is not completely supported by our data. While this could be the case in the hippocampus of aged rats, where PKC γ is increased in membranes, the same cannot be said of cortical structures, where PKC translocation is impaired but expression of the γ isoform is not changed in either the soluble or particulate fractions from aged animals. We are thus inclined to speculate that age-related changes in brain membrane composition,[92] rather than a modification in a particular PKC isoform, are responsible for the impaired PKC translocation.

Recent data have investigated the importance of PKC isoforms in various models of learning and memory. Because of its unique distribution at a neuronal level, PKC γ has received particular attention.

Data in monkeys have demonstrated that in areas important for visual processing, PKC γ follows an increased gradient (up to 10 times in expression of the immunoreactive protein) in parallel with the elaboration of visual input. Such a gradient, on the other hand, is not evident with the α and β isoforms that are expressed constantly throughout visual processing in cortical pathways.[93] These data point to the importance of PKC γ in visual information memory. Accordingly, evidence in rodents exists correlating different kinds of learning with specific translocation of the PKC γ isoform in various brain areas.[94,95] A different approach was taken by Tonegawa's group. They generated a mouse mutant lacking PKC γ and investigated the importance of this PKC isoform in synaptic plasticity and learning paradigms. Their results indicate that PKC γ is a regulatory component for long-term synaptic changes[96] and that mild changes in learning are dependent on the expression of this isoform.[97] In addition, data from the Routtenberg laboratory have pointed to the importance of PKC γ in the process of stabilization of synapses after LTP induction.[98] Our data showing that PKC γ is increased in aged rats at a hippocampal level could be reconciled with the possibility that the increase in PKC γ in aged rats might be detrimental for physiologic enzyme translocation. Analysis of specific isoform translocation could clarify this point and is one focus of our current experiments.

It is interesting to recall that in the hippocampus PKC controls neuronal excitability, through either inhibition of calcium-dependent afterhyperpolarization[99] or potentiation of excitatory aminoacid-induced calcium fluxes.[100] The unexpected observation of an increase in B-50 phosphorylation and PKC γ expression in this area of aged rats, also in the light of previous data showing a direct involvement in a variety of processes related to neuronal plasticity and memory phenomena,[12,13,18,94-97] could be regarded as a compensatory process expressed in aged animals aimed at restoring age-related decreases in neuronal excitability.[49,65] On the other hand, it may represent an age-related physiological expression of a decreased input of inhibitory synapses to hippocampal structures.[101]

It is known that a general population of aged animals can be subdivided, using specific learning paradigms, into good and bad learners.[102] Analysis of PKC activity in the brain of aged good and bad learners could define more easily detected differences in kinase activity correlated with learning capabilities.

To summarize our data on age-related changes in brain PKC, evidence has been provided that:

1. Histone-directed PKC activity, as a result of its dependence on the strain investigated, cannot be considered a consistent measure describing age-related changes in brain PKC; although it is possible that in more strict conditions, such as after selecting aged good and bad learners, this measure would also be affected;

2. PKC translocation upon phorbol ester challenge, however, is a consistent age-dependent change because this process is equally affected (impaired) in different strain of animals; this observation has importance because enzyme translocation is a prerequisite for physiologic PKC activation and pharmacologic strategies aimed at antagonizing age-related deficits could be targeted at this aspect of PKC function;

3. The selective modifications in PKC γ isoform which occur in the hippocampus indicate that during aging compensatory changes indices of active neural responsiveness aimed at antagonizing the age-related deficits are still possible, although the inability of the kinase to translocate may blunt this compensatory response.

The reported data suggest that age-related events are not simply the expression of a general decline in neuronal function, but rather reflect cell- and transmitter-selective modifications occurring at particular molecular steps of neurotransmission, from receptor availability to protein phosphorylation. Presumably, the pacemakers that determine the timing of age-related processes are the integrated result of intrinsic and extrinsic influences. Within this context, the changes of PKC so far described in the senescent brain, that at a more integrated level underly modified cognitive and behavioral functions, can be regarded as associated with unsuccessful aging, since differences between behaviorally competent and impaired old animals have been demonstrated. This poses the problem of identification of the neurochemical abnormalities that may be associated with pathological manifestations of aging, such as in neurodegenerative disorders. In particular, the focus of the following sections will be on the involvement of PKC in the etiology or expression of Alzheimer's disease (AD).

IX. PKC IN PATHOLOGICAL AGING: ALZHEIMER'S DISEASE

A variety of observations have demonstrated an involvement of PKC in AD. The enzyme levels (measured as phorbol ester binding to tissue homogenate) and activity (assessed as phosphorylation of exogenous histone) and endogenous (protein P86, possibly MARCKS) substrates are decreased in AD frontal cortex patients.[103] Autoradiographic studies on [³H]-PdBu binding to brain sections, on the other hand, have not detected changes in AD brain.[104] An interesting observation by Masliah et al. also concerns the selective presence of PKC βII isoform in membranous structures of fine neuronal processes apposed to the amyloid of diffuse plaques.[105] The data suggest that alterations in PKC-dependent phosphorylation may be involved in the early stage of amyloid deposit formation and could therefore represent an early biochemical marker in AD pathophysiology. The finding that the levels of particulate PKC βII and the PKC-dependent phosphorylation of the P86 protein are reduced, not only in the cortex of AD patients but also in nondemented subjects with cortical diffuse plaques,[106] is consistent with this view (although other factors may contribute to the maturation of diffuse plaques into neuritic plaques).

X. ALZHEIMER'S DISEASE-RELATED CHANGES IN PKC SPECIFIC SUBSTRATES

An important aspect of this pathology concerns the phenomena of synaptogenesis and sprouting, aimed at remodeling those regions particularly vulnerable to neurodegenerative processes. There is evidence that, while the overall levels of the PKC substrate GAP-43 (the already mentioned protein B-50) are decreased in the neocortex,[107] an increase is observed in the hippocampus, the region most affected by neuronal loss and compensatory extension of the dendritic tree associated with AD. In addition, GAP-43 immunoreactivity has also been found in neuritic plaques. These findings may reflect a role for GAP-43 phosphorylation in the mechanisms of synaptic plasticity as well as in the processes of aberrant sprouting in neuritic plaques.[108]

XI. CHANGES OF PKC IN PERIPHERAL TISSUES OF AD PATIENTS

It is important to underline that a decrease in PKC content and activity has also been reported in fibroblasts from AD patients,[109-112] suggesting that alterations in this kinase system at a central level are not merely the consequence of neuronal degeneration and death, but rather represent causative events. These observations raise the question of identification of biochemical markers in accessible peripheral tissues for the study of pathogenetic mechanisms and possibly diagnosis of CNS pathologies.

Several studies support speculation that Alzheimer's disease is not limited to the brain, although the expression is prominent in neuronal tissue.[113] In particular, abnormalities occur in a number of accessible nonneuronal tissues, including skin fibroblasts. A number of metabolic/biochemical processes have been found to be abnormal in cultured skin fibroblasts derived from AD patients, including alterations in calcium content and mobilization, mitochondrial function, choline transport, adhesiveness, expression of Alzheimer antigens, protein kinase activity, and ion channel expression.[113-118] Some of the described alterations (for example, the appearance of protein typical of plaques and tangles or the changes in kinase activity) may be useful in probing cellular mechanisms of the diseased brain, since they occur both in fibroblasts and in neuronal tissue. The observation that PKC is altered both in fibroblasts and in the brain of AD patients underscores the possibility that the study of this family of enzymes may represent a useful approach in investigations of the cellular pathophysiology of AD.

The mechanisms responsible for abnormal protein kinase activity in AD are unknown. Genetic mutations leading to an altered synthesis of amyloid precursor protein (APP) have been demonstrated to represent one pathogenetic factor in a subpopulation of patients with hereditary AD; it cannot be excluded that other genetic defects, as well as environmental conditions yet unidentified, may cause the pathological accumulation of amyloid both in familial and in sporadic AD. As an example, it has been shown that the presence of two copies of the gene for ApoE4, which codes for one of the three major forms of the lipoprotein found in humans, is associated with an increased overall risk of AD.[119] The link has been also observed when analyzing the expressed protein in plasma samples.[120,121] It has been proposed that ApoE may function as a pathological chaperone,[122] binding β-amyloid and favoring its deposition. This observation once again supports the concept of AD as a systemic disease and the importance of the search for accessible biochemical markers.

The picture emerging from current research is that pathological aging is associated with profound modifications in protein phosphorylation, which might be involved in the onset and development of neurodegenerative processes, including formation of plaques and tangles, and may provide a target for new therapeutic opportunities[123] aimed not only at partial recovery of lost functions and/or delaying loss of function but also at preventing neurodegeneration. On this issue, it has recently been demonstrated that compounds which activate the PKC system can modulate APP release in various cell lines,[124,125] in human fibroblasts,[126] and in primary cultures of rat hippocampus and cerebral cortex.[127]

ACKNOWLEDGMENTS

The authors thank Dr. T. Schuurman for providing Wistar rats, Dr. P.N.E. De Graan for the gift of purified protein B-50, and Dr. W.C. Wetsel for the antisera to PKCs. The normotensive Wistar Kyoto (WKY) rats were provided as part of a contract with the National Program of Pharmacological Research (Rif. 1139/191-07-8603) by the Italian Consortium for Technologies and Drugs for the Cerebral Aging (CITFI) for the Italian Ministry of University and Scientific and Technological Research. We thank Mrs. L. Fusar Imperatore for expert secretarial assistance.

REFERENCES

1. Roth, G. S. and Hess, G. D., Changes in the mechanisms of hormone and neurotransmitter action during aging: current status of the role of receptor and post receptor alterations, *Mech. Ageing Dev.*, 20, 175, 1982.
2. Magnoni, M. S., Govoni, S., Battaini, F., and Trabucchi, M., The aging brain: protein phosphorylation as a target of changes in neuronal function, *Life Sci.*, 48, 373, 1991.
3. Hemmings, H. C., Jr., Nairn, A. C., McGuiness, T. L., Huganir, R. L., and Greengard, P., Role of protein phosphorylation in neuronal signal transduction, *FASEB J.*, 3, 1583, 1989.
4. Walaas, S. I. and Greengard, P., Protein phosphorylation and neuronal function, *Pharm. Rev.*, 43, 299, 1991.

5. Nishizuka, Y., Intracellular signaling by hydrolysis of phospholipids and activation of protein kinase C, *Science*, 258, 607, 1992.
6. Hug, H. and Sarre, T. F., Protein kinase C isoenzymes: divergence in signal transduction?, *Biochem. J.*, 291, 329, 1993.
7. Dekker, L. V. and Parker, P. J., Protein kinase C — a question of specificity, *TIBS*, 19, 73, 1994.
8. Nakanishi, H., Brewer, K. A., and Exton, J. H., Activation of the ζ isozyme of protein kinase C by phosphatidylinositol 3,4,5-trisphosphate, *J. Biol. Chem.*, 268, 13, 1993.
9. Nishizuka, Y., The molecular heterogeneity of protein kinase C and its implications of cellular regulation, *Nature*, 334, 661, 1988.
10. Skene, J. H. P., Axonal growth-associated proteins, *Annu. Rev. Neurosci.*, 12, 127, 1989.
11. De Graan, P. N. E., Oestreicher, A. B., Schotman, P., and Schrama, L. H., Protein kinase C substrate B-50 (GAP-43) and neurotransmitter release, *Progr. Brain Res.*, 89, 187, 1991.
12. Akers, R. F. and Routtenberg, A., Calcium-promoted translocation of protein kinase C to synaptic membranes: relation to the phosphorylation of an endogenous substrate (protein F1) involved in synaptic plasticity, *J. Neurosci.*, 7, 3976, 1987.
13. Gianotti, C., Nunzi, M. G., Gispen, W. H., and Corradetti, R., Phosphorylation of the presynaptic protein B-50 is increased in electrically induced long-term potentiation, *Neuron*, 8, 843, 1992.
14. Stumpo, D. J., Graff, J. M., Albert, K. A., Greengard, P., and Blackshear, P. J., Molecular cloning characterization, expression of a cDNA encoding the "80- to 87-kDa" myristoylated alanine-rich C kinase substrate: a major cellular substrate for protein kinase C, *Proc. Natl. Acad. Sci. U.S.A.*, 86, 4012, 1989.
15. Baudier, J., Deloulme, J. C., Van Dorsselaer, A., Black, D., and Matthes, H. W. D., Purification and characterization of a brain-specific protein kinase C substrate, neurogranin (p17), *J. Biol. Chem.*, 266, 229, 1991.
16. Klann, E., Chen, S. J., and Sweatt, J. D., Increased phosphorylation of a 17-kDa protein kinase C substrate (p17) in LTP, *J. Neurochem.*, 58, 1576, 1992.
17. Akers, R. F., Lovinger, D. M., Colley, P. A., Linden, D. J., and Routtenberg, A., Translocation of protein kinase C activity may mediate hippocampal long-term potentiation, *Science*, 231, 587, 1986.
18. Leahy, J. C., Luo, Y., Kent, C. S., Meiri, K. F., and Vallano, M. L., Demonstration of presynaptic protein kinase C activation following long-term potentiation in rat hippocampal slices, *Neuroscience*, 52, 563, 1993.
19. Choi, K. W., Smith, R. F., Buratowski, R. M., and Quinn, W. G., Deficient protein kinase C activity in *turnip*, a *Drosophila* learning mutant, *J. Biol. Chem.*, 266, 15999, 1991.
20. Sacktor, T. C. and Schwartz, J. H., Sensitizing stimuli cause translocation of protein kinase C in Aplysia sensory neurons, *Proc. Natl. Acad. Sci. U.S.A.*, 87, 2036, 1990.
21. Etcheberrigaray, R., Matzel, L. D., Lederhendler, I. I., and Alkon, D. L., Classical conditioning and protein kinase C activation regulate the same single potassium channel in Hermissenda crassicornis photoreceptors, *Proc. Natl. Acad. Sci. U.S.A.*, 89, 7184, 1992.
22. Bank, B., DeWeer, A., Kuzirian, A. M., Rasmussen, H., and Alkon, D. L., Classical conditioning induces long-term translocation of protein kinase C in rabbit hippocampal CA1 cells, *Proc. Natl. Acad. Sci. U.S.A.*, 85, 1988, 1988.
23. Wehner, J. M., Sleight, S., and Upchurch, M., Hippocampal protein kinase C activity is reduced in poor spatial learners, *Brain Res.*, 523, 181, 1990.

24. Olds, J. L., Golski, S., McPhie, D. L., Olton, D., Mishkin, M., and Alkon, D. L., Discrimination learning tasks alters the distribution of protein kinase C in the hippocampus of rats, *J. Neurosci.*, 10, 3707, 1990.

25. Nogues, X., Micheau, J., and Jaffard, R., Protein kinase C activity in the hippocampus following spatial learning tasks in mice, *Hippocampus*, 4, 71, 1994.

26. Elkabes, S., Cherry, J. A., Schoups, A. A., and Black, I. B., Regulation of protein kinase C activity by sensory deprivation in the olfactory and visual systems, *J. Neurochem.*, 60, 1835, 1993.

27. Paylor, R., Morrison, S. K., Rudy, J. W., Waltrip, L. T., and Wehner, J. M., Brief exposure to an enriched environment improves performance on the Morris water task and increases hippocampal cytosolic protein kinase C activity in young rats, *Behav. Brain Res.*, 52, 49, 1992.

28. Paylor, R., Rudy, J. W., and Wehner, J. M., Acute phorbol ester treatment improves spatial learning performance in rats, *Behav. Brain Res.*, 45, 189, 1991.

29. Mathis, C., Lehmann, J., and Ungerer, A., The selective protein kinase C inhibitor, NPC 15437, induces specific deficits in memory retention in mice, *Eur. J. Pharm.*, 220, 107, 1992.

30. Govoni, S., Lucchi, L., Battaini, F., and Trabucchi, M., Protein kinase C increase in rat brain cortical membranes may be promoted by cognition enhancing drugs, *Life Sci.*, 50, PL125, 1992.

31. Lucchi, L., Pascale, A., Battaini, F., Govoni, S., and Trabucchi, M., Cognition stimulating drugs modulate protein kinase C activity in cerebral cortex and hippocampus of adult rats, *Life Sci.*, 53, 1821, 1993.

32. Govoni, S., Battaini, F., Lucchi, L., Pascale, A., and Trabucchi, M., PKC translocation in rat brain cortex is promoted in vivo and in vitro by α-glycerylphosphorylcholine, a cognition-enhancing drugs, *Ann. N.Y. Acad. Sci.*, 695, 307, 1993.

33. Di Luca, M., Cimino, M., De Graan, P. N. E., Oestreicher, A. B., Gispen, W. H., and Cattabeni, F., Microencephaly reduces the phosphorylation of the PKC substrate B-50(GAP-43) in rat cortex and hippocampus, *Brain Res.*, 538, 95, 1991.

34. Ingram, D. K., Bartus, R. T., Olton, D. S., Kachaturian, Z. S., Experimental models of age-related memory dysfunction and neurodegeneration, *Neurobiol. Aging*, 9, 443, 1988.

35. Finch, C. E., Neurotransmitters, genetics, and aging, in *Modification of Cell to Cell Signals during Normal and Pathological Aging*, Govoni, S. and Battaini, F., Eds., Springer Verlag, Berlin, 1987, 63.

36. Wang, Z. P., Man, S. Y., and Tang, F., Age-related changes in the content of neuropeptides in the rat brain and pituitary, *Neurobiol. Aging*, 14, 529, 1993.

37. Gibson, G. E. and Peterson, C., Calcium and the aging nervous system, *Neurobiol. Aging*, 8, 329, 1987.

38. Battaini, F., Trabucchi, M., Chikvaidze, V., and Govoni, S., Effect of aging on brain voltage-dependent calcium channels, in *Calcium Antagonists Pharmacology and Clinical Research*, Godfraind, T., Govoni, S., Paoletti, R., and Vanhoutte, P. M., Eds., Kluwer Academic, Norwell, MA, 1993, 231.

39. Crews, F. T., Gonzales, R. A., Palovcik, R., Phillips, M. I., Theiss, C., and Raizada, M., Changes in receptor stimulated phosphoinositide hydrolysis in brain during ethanol administration, aging, and other pathological conditions, *Psychopharmacol. Bull.*, 22, 775, 1986.

40. Nalepa, I., Pintor, A., Fortuna, S., Vetulani, J., and Michalek, H., Increased responsiveness of the cerebral cortical phosphatidylinositol system to noradrenaline and carbachol in senescent rats, *Neurosci. Lett.*, 107, 195, 1989.

41. Blumenthal, E. J. and Malkinson, A. M., Age-dependent changes in murine protein kinase and protease enzymes, *Mech. Aging Dev.*, 46, 201, 1988.

42. Barnes, C. A., Mizumori, S. J. Z., Lovinger, D. M., Sheu, F. S., Murakami, K., Chan, S. Y., Linden, D. J., Nelson, R. B., and Routtenberg, A., Selective decline in protein F1 phosphorylation in hippocampus of senescent rats, *Neurobiol. Aging*, 9, 393, 1988.

43. Friedman, E. and Wang, H. Y., Effect of age on brain cortical protein kinase C and its mediation of 5-hydroxytryptamine release, *J. Neurochem.*, 52, 187, 1989.

44. Pisano, M. R., Wang, H. Y., and Friedman, E., Protein kinase activity changes in the aging brain, *Biomed. Environ. Sci.*, 4, 173, 1991.

45. Battaini, F., Del Vesco, R., Govoni, S., and Trabucchi, M., Regulation of phorbol ester binding and protein kinase C activity in aged rat brain, *Neurobiol. Aging*, 11, 563, 1990.

46. Gianotti, C., Porta, A., De Graan, P. N. E., Oestreicher, A. B., and Nunzi, M. G., B-50/GAP-43 phosphorylation in hippocampal slices from aged rats: effects of phosphatidylserine administration, *Neurobiol. Aging*, 14, 401, 1993.

47. Hara, H., Onodera, H., Kato, H., and Kogure, K., Effects of aging on signal transmission and transduction systems in the gerbil brain: morphological and autoradiographic study, *Neuroscience*, 46, 475, 1992.

48. Yurko, K. A., Pisano, M. R., Yadin, E., and Friedman, E., Age-related changes in ^3H phorbol binding and protein kinase C immunoreactivity in Fisher-344 rat brain, *Soc. Neurosci. Abstr.*, 17, 603, 1991.

49. Landfield, P. W., Thibault, O., Mazzanti, M. L., Porter, N. M., and Kerr, D. S., Mechanisms of neuronal death in brain aging and Alzheimer's disease: role of endocrine-mediated calcium dyshomeostasis, *J. Neurobiol.*, 23, 1247, 1992.

50. Leslie, S. W., Chandler, L. J., Barr, E., and Ferrar, R. P., Reduced calcium uptake by rat brain mitochondria and synaptosomes in response to aging, *Brain Res.*, 329, 177, 1985.

51. Giovannelli, L. and Pepeu, G., Effect of age on K^+ induced cytosolic calcium changes in rat cortical synaptosomes, *J. Neurochem.*, 53, 392, 1989.

52. Martinez-Serrano, A., Blanco, P., and Satrustegui, J., Calcium binding to the cytosol and calcium extrusion mechanisms in intact synaptosomes and their alteration with aging, *J. Biol. Chem.*, 267, 4672, 1992.

53. Worley, P. F., Baraban, J. M., and Snyder, S. H., Heterogeneous localization of protein kinase C in rat brain: autoradiographic analysis of phorbol ester receptor binding, *J. Neurosci.*, 6, 199, 1986.

54. Flood, D. G., Critical issues in the analysis of dendritic extent in aging humans, primates, and rodents, *Neurobiol. Aging*, 14, 649, 1993.

55. Clark, E. A., Leach, K. L., Trojanowski, A., and Lee, V. M. Y., Characterization and differential distribution of the three major human protein kinase isozymes (α, β, γ) of the CNS in normal and Alzheimer's disease brains, *Lab. Invest.*, 64, 35, 1991.

56. Fordyce, D. E. and Wehner, J. M., Effect of aging on spatial learning and hippocampal protein kinase C in mice, *Neurobiol. Aging*, 14, 309, 1993.

57. Nishino, N., Kitamura, N., Nakai, T., Hashimoto, T., and Tanaka, C., Phorbol ester binding sites in human brain: characterization, regional distribution, age-correlation, and alterations in Parkinson's disease, *J. Mol. Neurosci.*, 1, 19, 1989.

58. Ramachandran, M. and Abraham, E. C., Age-dependent variation in the cytosol/membrane distribution of red cell protein kinase C, *Am. J. Hematol.*, 31, 69, 1989.

59. Indelicato, S. R., Udupa Kodetthoor, B., Balazovich, K. J., Boxer, L. A., and Lipschitz, D. A., Effect of age on phorbol-ester stimulation of human neutrophils, *J. Gerontol.*, 45, B75, 1990.

60. Chopra, R., Nagel, J., and Adler, W., Decreased response of T cell from elderly individuals to phytohemagglutinin (PHA) stimulation can be augmented by phorbol myristate acetate (PMA) in conjunction with Ca-ionophore A23187, *Gerontologist*, 47, 204A, 1987.

61. Matsushima, H., Shimohama, S., Yamaoka, Y., Kimura, J., Taniguchi, T., Hagiwara, M., and Hidaka, H., Alteration of human platelets protein kinase C with normal aging. *Mech. Ageing Dev.*, 69, 129, 1993.

62. Battaini, F., Govoni, S., Del Vesco, R., Moresco, R. M., and Trabucchi, M., Signal transduction in the aging brain: calcium channels and calcium-phospholipid-dependent kinases, in *Aging Brain and Dementia: New Trends in Diagnosis and Therapy*, Battistin, L. and Gerstenbrandt, F., Eds., Alan R. Liss, New York, 1989, 169.

63. Battaini, F., Del Vesco, R., Govoni, S., Lopez, C. M., and Trabucchi, M., Area-dependent modification in phorbol ester binding and phosphokinase C activity in aging rat brain, in *Protein Metabolism in Aging*, Segal, H. L., Rothstein, M., and Bergamini, E., Eds., Wiley-Liss, New York, 1990, 355.

64. Schuurman, T., Klein, H., Beneke, M., and Traber, J., Nimodipine and motor deficits in the aged rat, *Neurosci. Res. Commun.*, 1, 9, 1987.

65. Potier, B., Lamour, Y., and Dutar, P., Age-related alterations in the properties of hippocampal pyramidal neurons among rat strains, *Neurobiol. Aging*, 14, 17, 1993.

66. Scriabine, A., Schuurman, T., and Traber, J., Pharmacological basis for the use of nimodipine in CNS disorders, *FASEB J.*, 3, 1799, 1991.

67. Battaini, F., Govoni, S., Lucchi, L., Ladisa, V., Bergamaschi, S., and Trabucchi, M., Age-related changes in brain protein kinase C expression, activity, and translocation, *Drugs in Develop.*, 2, 275, 1993.

68. Battaini, F., Bergamaschi, S., Elkabes, S., Govoni, S., De Graan, P. N. E., Schuurman, T., and Trabucchi, M., Protein kinase C activity and isozyme mRNA expression in aging Wistar rat brain, *Biol. Psych.*, 29, 261, 1991.

69. Sheu, F. S., Marais, R. M., Parker, P. J., Bazan, N. G., and Routtenberg, A., Neuron-specific protein F1/GAP-43 shows substrate specificity for the beta sub-type of protein kinase C, *Biochem. Biophys. Res. Commun.*, 171, 1236, 1990.

70. Heemskerk, F. M. J., De Graan, P. N. E., and Huang, F. L., In vitro phosphory-lation of protein kinase C substrates by isozymes type I, II, and III, *Soc. Neurosci. Abstr.*, 17, 602, 1991.

71. Battaini, F., Lucchi, L., Bergamaschi, S., Ladisa, V., Trabucchi, M., and Govoni, S., Intracellular signalling in the aging brain. The role of protein kinase C and its calcium-dependent isoforms, *Ann. N.Y. Acad. Sci.*, 719, 271, 1994.

72. Wetsel, W. C., Khan, W. A., Merchenthaler, I., Rivera, H., Halpern, A. E., Phung, H. M., Negro-Vilar, A., and Hannun, Y. A., Tissue and cellular distribution of the extended family of protein kinase C isoenzymes, *J. Cell Biol.*, 117, 121, 1992.

73. Young, S., Parker, P. J., Ullrich, A., and Stabel, S., Down-regulation of protein kinase C is due to an increased rate of degradation, *Biochem. J.*, 244, 775, 1987.

74. Shearman, M. S., Shinomura, T., Oda, T., and Nishizuka, Y., Synaptosomal protein kinase C subspecies A. Dynamic changes in the hippocampus and cer-ebellar cortex concomitant with synaptogenesis, *J. Neurochem.*, 56, 1255, 1991.

75. Fifkova, E. and Cullen-Dockstader, K., Calcium distribution in dendritic spines of the dentate fascia varies with age, *Brain Res.*, 376, 357, 1986.

76. Klann, E., Chen, S.-J., and Sweatt, J. D., Mechanism of protein kinase C activation during the induction and maintenance of long-term potentiation probed using a selective peptide substrate, *Proc. Natl. Acad. Sci. U.S.A.*, 90, 8337, 1993.

77. Sacktor, T. C., Osten, P., Valsamis, H., Jiang, X., Naik, M. U., and Sublette, E., Persistent activation of the ζ isoform of protein kinase C in the maintenance of long-term potentiation, *Proc. Natl. Acad. Sci. U.S.A.*, 90, 8342, 1993.

78. Khachaturian, Z. S., The role of calcium regulation in brain aging: reexamination of a hypothesis, *Aging*, 1, 17, 1989.

79. Battaini, F., Govoni, S., Magnoni, M. S., and Trabucchi, M., Calcium ion homeostasis in the aging brain: regulation of voltage-dependent calcium channels, in *Ion Channels and Ion Pumps*, Foà, P. P. and Walsh, M. F., Eds., Springer-Verlag, New York, 1994, chap. 19.

80. Martini, A., Battaini, F., Govoni, S., and Volpe, P., Inositol 1,4,5-trisphosphate receptor and ryanodine receptor in the aging brain of Wistar rats, *Neurobiol. Aging*, 15, 203, 1994.

81. Tandon, P., Mundy, W. R., Ali, S. F., Nanry, K., Rogers, B. C., and Tilson, H. A., Age-dependent changes in receptor-stimulated phosphoinositide turnover in the rat hippocampus, *Pharmacol. Biochem. Behav.*, 38, 861, 1991.

82. Battaini, F., Elkabes, S., Bergamaschi, S., Ladisa, V., Lucchi, L., De Graan, P.N.E., Schuurman, T., Wetsel, W.C., Trabucchi, M., and Govoni, S., Protein kinase C activity, translocation and calcium-dependent isoenzymes in the aging rat brain, *Neurobiol. Aging*, 16, 137, 1995.

83. Meyer, E. M., Judkins, J. H., Momol, A. E., and Hardwick, E. D., Effect of peroxidation and aging on rat neocortical Ach-release and protein kinase C, *Neurobiol. Aging*, 15, 63, 1994.

84. Lorens, S. A., Hata, N., Handa, R. J., Van de Kar, L. D., Guschwan, M., Goral, J., Lee, J. M., Hamilton, M. E., Bethea, C. L., and Clancy, J., Jr., Neurochemical, endocrine and immunological responses to stress in young and old Fischer 344 male rats, *Neurobiol. Aging*, 11, 139, 1990.

85. Gilad, G. M., Rabey, J. M., Tizabi, Y., and Gilad, V. H., Age-dependent loss and compensatory changes of septohippocampal cholinergic neurons in two rat strains differing in longevity and response to stress, *Brain Res.*, 436, 311, 1987.

86. Battaini F., Del Vesco, R., Govoni, S., Lopez, C. M., and Trabucchi M., Stressful conditions and brain transducing mechanisms during aging, in *Stress and the Aging Brain*, Nappi, G. and Genazzani, A. R. Eds., Raven Press, New York, 1990, 83.

87. Yurko, K., Wang, H. Y., and Friedman, E., Immobilization stress induces translocation of protein kinase C (PKC), *Neurosci. Soc. Abstr.*, 12, 1179, 1990.

88. Rouge, P. J., Ritz, M. F., and Malviya, A. N., Impaired gene transcription and nuclear protein kinase C activation in the brain and liver of aged rats, *FEBS Lett.*, 334, 351, 1993.

89. Alkon, D. L., Naito, S., Kubota, M., Chen, C., Bank, B., Smallwood, J., Gallant, P., and Rasmussen, H., Regulation of *Hermissenda* K+ channels by cytoplasmic and membrane-associated C-kinase, *J. Neurochem.*, 51, 903, 1988.

90. Sunayashiki-Kusuzaki, K., Lester, D. S., Schreurs, B. G., and Alkon, D. L., Associative learning potentiates protein kinase C activation in synaptosomes of the rabbit hippocampus, *Proc. Natl. Acad. Sci. U.S.A.*, 90, 4286, 1993.

91. Oda, T., Shearman, M. S., and Nishizuka, Y., Synaptosomal protein kinase C subspecies. B. Down-regulation promoted by phorbol ester and its effect on evoked norephinephrine release, *J. Neurochem.*, 56, 1263, 1991.

92. Oestreicher, A. B., De Graan, P. N. E., and Gispen, W. H., Neuronal cell membranes and brain aging, *Progress in Brain Research*, 70, 239, 1986.

93. Huang, K. P., Huang, F. L., Nakabayashi, H., and Yoshida, Y., Roles of protein kinase C isozymes in cellular regulation, in *Advances in Experimental Medicine and Biology*, Vol. 255, Calcium protein signaling, Hidaka, H., Ed., Plenum Press, NY, 21, 1989.

94. Van der Zee, E. A., Compaan, J. C., de Boer, M., and Luiten, P. G. M., Changes in PKC γ immunoreactivity in mouse hippocampus induced by spatial discrimination learning, *J. Neurosci.*, 12, 4808, 1992.

95. Beldhuis, H. J. A., Everts, H. G. J., Van der Zee, E. A., Luiten, P. G. M., and Bohus, B., Amygdala kindling-induced seizures selectively impair spatial memory. I. Behavioral characteristics and effects on hippocampal neuronal protein kinase C isoforms, *Hippocampus*, 2, 397, 1992.

96. Abeliovich, A., Chen, C., Goda, Y., Silva, A. J., Stevens, C. F., and Tonegawa, S., Modified hippocampal long-term potentiation in PKCγ mutant mice, *Cell*, 75, 1253, 1993.

97. Abeliovich, A., Paylor, R., Chen, C., Kim, J. J., Wehner, J. M., and Tonegawa, S., PKCγ mutant mice exhibit mild deficits in spatial and contextual learning, *Cell*, 75, 1263, 1993.

98. Meberg, P. J., Barnes, C. A., McNaughton, B. L., and Routtenberg, A., Protein kinase C and F1/GAP-43 gene expression in hippocampus inversely related to synaptic enhancement lasting 3 days, *Proc. Natl. Acad. Sci. U.S.A.*, 90, 12050, 1993.

99. Baraban, J. M., Snyder, S. H., and Alger, B. F., Protein kinase C regulates ionic conductance in hippocampal pyramidal neurons: electrophysiological effects of phorbol esters, *Proc. Natl. Acad. Sci. U.S.A.*, 82, 2538, 1985.

100. Ben-Ari, Y., Aniksztejn, L., and Bregestovski, P., Protein kinase C modulation of NMDA currents: an important link for LTP inductions, *TINS*, 15, 333, 1992.

101. De Jong, G. I., Van der Zee, E. A., Bohus, B., and Luiten, P. G. M., Reversed alterations of hippocampal parvalbumin and protein kinase C γ immunoreactivity after stroke in spontaneously hypertensive stroke-prone rats, *Stroke*, 24, 2082, 1993.

102. Gallagher, M., Burwell, R. D., Kodsi, M. H., McKinney, M., Southerland, S., Vella-Rountree, L., and Lewis, M. H., Markers for biogenic amines in the aged rat brain: relationship to decline in spatial learning ability, *Neurobiol. Aging*, 11, 507, 1990.

103. Cole, G., Dobkins, K. R., Hansen, L. A., Terry, R. D., and Saitoh, T., Decreased levels of protein kinase C in Alzheimer brain, *Brain Res.*, 452, 165, 1988.

104. Horsburgh, K., Dewar, D., Graham, D. I., and McCulloch, J., Autoradiographic imaging of ³H-phorbol 12,13-dibutyrate binding to PKC in Alzheimer's disease, *J. Neurochem.*, 56, 1121, 1991.

105. Masliah, E., Cole, G. M., Hansen, L. A., Mallory, M., Albright, T., Terry, R. D., and Saitoh, T., Protein kinase C alteration is an early biochemical marker in Alzheimer's disease, *J. Neurosci.*, 11, 2759, 1991.

106. Masliah, E., Cole, G., Shimohama, S., Hansen, L., De Teresa, R., Terry, R. D., and Saitoh, T., Differential involvement of PKC isozymes in Alzheimer's disease, *J. Neurosci.*, 10, 2113, 1990.

107. Masliah, E., Mallory, M., Hansen, L., Alford, M., Albright, T., De Teresa, R., and Saitoh, T., Patterns of aberrant sprouting in Alzheimer's disease, *Neuron*, 6, 729, 1991.

108. Florez, J. C., Nelson, R. B., and Routtenberg, A., Contrasting patterns of protein phosphorylation in human normal and Alzheimer brain: focus on protein kinase C and protein F1/GAP43, *Exp. Neurol.*, 112, 264, 1991.

109. Bruel, A., Cherqui, G., Columelli, J. L., Margelin, D., Roudier, M., Sinet, P. M., Perignon, J. L., and Delabar, J., Reduced protein kinase C activity in sporadic Alzheimer's disease fibroblasts, *Neurosci. Lett.*, 133, 89, 1991.

110. Van Huynh, T., Cole, G., Katzman, R., Huang, K. P., and Saitoh, T., Reduced PKC immunoreactivity and altered protein phosphorylation in Alzheimer's disease fibroblasts, *Arch. Neurol.*, 46, 1195, 1989.

111. Govoni, S., Bergamaschi, S., Racchi, M., Battaini, F., Binetti, G., Bianchetti, A., and Trabucchi, M., Cytosol protein kinase C down regulation in fibroblasts from Alzheimer's disease patients, *Neurology*, 43, 2581, 1993.

112. Racchi, M., Wetsel, W. C., Govoni, S., Trabucchi, M., Battaini, F., Binetti, G., Bianchetti, A., and Bergamaschi, S., PKCα immunoreactivity is decreased in fibroblasts from AD patients, *Soc. Neurosci. Abstr.*, 19, 623, 1993.
113. Blass, J. P., Baker, A. C., Sheu, R. K. F., Blach, R. S., and Smith, A., Use of cultured skin fibroblasts in studies of Alzheimer's disease, in *Biological Markers of Alzheimer's Disease*, Boller, F., Katzman, R., Rascol, A., Signoret, J. L., and Christen, Y., Eds., Springer-Verlag, New York, 1989, 153.
114. Peterson, C., Ratan, R. R., Shelanski, M. L., and Goldman, J. E., Cytosolic free calcium and cell spreading decrease in fibroblasts from aged and Alzheimer's donors, *Proc. Natl. Acad. Sci. U.S.A.*, 83, 7999, 1986.
115. Mokrasch, L. C., Studies on choline transport enhancement into fibroblasts from normals and Alzheimer's donors, *Neurochem. Res.*, 16, 757, 1991.
116. Blass, J. P., Baker, A. C., Ko, L., Sheu, R. K. F., and Black, R. S., Expression of "Alzheimer antigens" in cultured skin fibroblasts, *Arch. Neurol.*, 48, 709, 1991.
117. Etcheberrigaray, R., Ito, E., Oka, K., Tofel-Grehl, B., Gibson, G. E., and Alkon, D. L., Potassium channel dysfunction in fibroblasts identifies patients with Alzheimer's disease, *Proc. Natl. Acad. Sci. U.S.A.*, 90, 8209, 1993.
118. McCoy, K. R., Mullins, R. D., Newcomb, T. G., Ng, G. M., Pavlinkova, G., Polinsky, R. J., Nee, L. E., and Sisken, J. E., Serum and bradykinin-induced calcium transients in familial Alzheimer's fibroblasts, *Neurobiol. Aging*, 14, 447, 1993.
119. Corder, E. H., Saunders, A. M., Strittmatter, W. L. J., Schmechel, D. E., Gaskell, P. C., Small, G. W., Roses, A. D., Haines, J. L., and Pericak-Vance, M. A., Gene dose of apolipoprotein E type 4 allele and the risk of Alzheimer's disease in late onset families, *Science*, 261, 921, 1993.
120. Frisoni, G., Bianchetti, A., Govoni, S., Trabucchi, M., Calabresi, L., Franceschini, G., Is apolipoprotein E ε4 allele uniquely associated with Alzheimer's disease?, *JAMA*, 1994.
121. Frisoni, G., Calabresi, L., Geroldi, C., Bianchetti, A., D'Acquarica, A. L., Govoni, S., Franceschini, G., and Trabucchi, M., Apolipoprotein E ε4 allele in Alzheimer's disease and vascular dementia, *Dementia*, 5, 240, 1994.
122. Wisniewski, T. and Frangione, B., Apolipoprotein E: a pathological chaperone protein in patients with cerebral and systemic amyloid, *Neurosci. Lett.*, 135, 235, 1992.
123. Gandy, S. and Greengard, P., Amyloidogenesis in Alzheimer's disease: some possible therapeutic opportunities, *TIPS*, 13, 108, 1992.
124. Buxbaum, J. D., Koo, E. H., and Greengard, P., Protein phosphorylation inhibits production of Alzheimer amyloid β/A4 peptide, *Proc. Natl. Acad.Sci. U.S.A.*, 90, 9195, 1993.
125. Hung, A. Y., Haas, C., Nitsch, R. M., Qiu, W. Q., Citron, M., Wurtman, R. J., Growdon, J. H., and Selkoe, D. J., Activation of protein kinase C inhibits cellular production of the amyloid β-protein, *J. Biol. Chem.*, 268, 22959, 1993.
126. Bergamaschi, S., Bianchetti, A., Binetti, G., Racchi, M., Battaini, F., Trabucchi, M., and Govoni, S., PKC regulates β-Amyloid precursor protein (APP) secretion in fibroblasts from control and Alzheimer's disease patients, *Soc. Neurosci.*, Abstr., 20, 849, 1994.
127. Racchi, M., Trabucchi, M., Battaini, F., Govoni, S., Parenti, M., and Cattaneo, E., Characterization of APP secretion from primary hippocampus and cortex cultures: role of potassium channel, cholinergic receptor, and protein kinase C modulation, *Soc. Neurosci. Abstr.*, 20, 849, 1994.

Chapter **8**

CHANGES IN TRANSMEMBRANE SIGNALING MECHANISMS DURING AGING — CELLULAR AND MOLECULAR ASPECTS

Atsushi Miyamoto and George S. Roth

CONTENTS

0-8493-4786-6/95/$0.00+$.50
© 1995 by CRC Press, Inc.

I. INTRODUCTION

Aging has been defined as a progressive loss of physiological capacity that culminates in death.[1] Although the field of aging research has many theories,[2] no single theory appears to account for most age-dependent changes. For example, at present few believe that there is a single gene controlling aging. Similarly, the concept that aging is the result of the accumulation of random errors in genes and proteins is no longer tenable. It is becoming increasingly evident that "aging" results from a number of sequential and/or parallel biochemical events regulated by different genes. However, it is not quite clear to what extent a particular genetic change is the cause or consequence of aging, because the reciprocal relationships between aging and gene expression are not well understood.

Most physiological functions do decline with age, but to different extents.[3,4] Many physiologic and biochemical processes are mediated via membrane receptors. Control of physiological functions by hormones and neurotransmitters represents a key mechanism by which homeostatic balance is maintained.[5,6] The past few years have yielded an explosion of new knowledge regarding cellular regulation by hormones and neurotransmitters that act via cell surface receptors embedded within the lipid bilayer.[7-11] Neurotransmitter receptors mediating the generation of intracellular responses may be grouped into two main categories: metabotropic types around the G-protein-coupled receptors; and ionotropic types around the three types of gated ion channels (Figure 1). Effector systems activated by G-protein-coupled receptors include adenylyl cyclase, which produces cAMP, and phosphatidylinositol-specific phospholipase C, which generates inositol 1,4,5-trisphosphate (IP_3), and diacylglycerol (DG).[12-14] These products act as second messengers, modulating the activities of protein kinases, and the intracellular free Ca^{2+} concentration. However, many ion channels are the target of various hormones and neurotransmitters.[15,16] Ion channels are distinguished from ion carriers by the high rates at which they transport ions once they are opened. The ion channels considered here are opened either by membrane potential or by specific ligands and are usually highly selective for a given ion species. These changes in transmembrane signal transduction may be related to the causes or results in the process of aging. Many recent reviews have addressed the problem of age changes in hormone and neurotransmitter responsiveness.[17-20] The current review focuses on aging-dependent changes in transmembrane signaling mechanisms and functional aspects around the metabotropic and the ionotropic types in cellular signal transduction.

(A) Metabotropic type

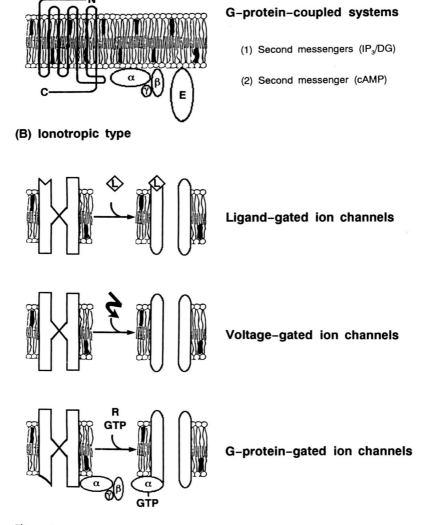

G–protein–coupled systems

(1) Second messengers (IP$_3$/DG)

(2) Second messenger (cAMP)

(B) Ionotropic type

Ligand–gated ion channels

Voltage–gated ion channels

G–protein–gated ion channels

Figure 1
Summary of the two major pathways for transmembrane receptors and signal transduction. (A) Metabotropic type: many agonists bind to 7-membrane-spanning receptors (N to C), which use a GTP-binding protein (αβγ) to activate effector (E) enzymes such as phospholipase C and adenylyl cyclase; (B) ionotropic type: three types of gated ion channels; L, ligand; R, receptor.

II. AGE-RELATED CHANGES IN METABOTROPIC TYPES AROUND G-PROTEIN-COUPLED SYSTEMS

Many physiologic responses are dependent on membrane receptor stimulation as the primary event in effecting the biochemical processes that result in the response. A large number of these biochemical processes have been shown to change with age. Thus, it is a logical hypothesis that many of the age-related changes would be explained, at least in part, by age-related changes in the membrane receptor signaling systems, and more particularly by changes in receptor protein interactions.

Some years ago, we proposed that changes in receptors during aging might constitute one mechanism by which responsiveness to hormones and neurotransmitters might be altered.[3,5,17-19] As previously reviewed, age-related changes in receptors have been closely linked to altered responsiveness in several cases. In the following years, numerous reports of age changes in receptors have appeared. Despite some disagreements between laboratories and specific model systems, it seems reasonable to conclude that receptor change constitutes one important class of alterations resulting in impaired hormone-neurotransmitter action during aging.

In theory, disruption of cellular signal transduction mechanisms may occur at the receptor recognition site; the coupling of receptors to the effector systems such as phospholipase C or adenylyl cyclase; and the intracellular actions of second messengers (Figure 1). In general, the term G-protein refers to the heterotrimeric (abg), plasma membrane-associated GTP-binding proteins which transduce signals from receptors to effector enzymes or ion channels. In contrast to the receptor level, the involvement of G-proteins and several different second messengers has not been thoroughly investigated in previous aging studies. In many situations in which receptor changes do not occur, or appear to be functionally unimportant during aging, postreceptor mechanisms have been examined. In our group, the most studied of the age-related impaired Ca^{2+} mobilization system has been the a_1-adrenoceptor-stimulated rat parotid cells.[21-26] Recently, we found that age-related impairments in a_1-adrenergic-stimulated secretory function are due to reduced IP_3 production and subsequent Ca^{2+} mobilization[21,23] GTPgS and NaF mediated IP_3 production is unaltered in the aging parotid, indicating that the decline in a_1-adrenoceptor-mediated Ca^{2+} mobilization is due to an uncoupling between the receptor and the G-proteins.[23,26] A number of laboratories have reported age-related shifts in the proportion of high and low affinity sites for various G-protein coupled receptors.[27,28] We have elucidated a new manifestation of this type of aging change — namely, a decreased ability of GTP to shift the receptor complex from the high to low affinity form.[23] This phenomenon has been observed for both a_1-adrenoceptors and muscarinic receptors of the rat corpus striatum.[29,30] Interestingly, a similar type of receptor-G-protein uncoupling (impairments in high to low affinity shifts) has been reported for muscarinic receptors in Alzheimer's disease patients,[31-33] D_1 dopamine receptors in Huntington's disease patients,[34] and b-adrenoceptor mutants.[35] Further work will be required to elucidate the mechanisms by which receptor-G-protein uncoupling during aging are modulated.

The phospholipase C enzyme is not the only effector system linked to cell surface receptors by G-proteins. During aging, there is a reduction in β-adrenergic responsiveness in the brain,[36,37] heart,[38-40] and blood vessels.[41-43] This is evidenced by reduced inotropic and chronotropic responses to β-receptor stimulation in the heart and by reduced β-receptor-stimulated vascular relaxation. Accumulation of cAMP in response to β-receptor agonists is decreased during aging in the brain, heart, and blood vessels, indicating that the site of the alteration is in close proximity to the receptor. There is some evidence for reductions in adenylyl cyclase activity and in responsiveness to cAMP, which may help to account for reduced β-receptor responsiveness in the heart. The reduced responsiveness is probably not attributable solely to alterations in adenylyl cyclase or cAMP responses. Complementation studies demonstrate a reduced ability of G-proteins extracted from aged heart to stimulate adenylyl cyclase, suggesting that alterations at the Gsα-protein expression contribute to the loss of β-receptor responses during aging.[44] Furthermore, there is an age-related decrease in cardiac β-receptor affinity for agonists and a reduction in the ability of guanine nucleotides to affect agonist affinity, which may be due to reduced receptor-G-protein interactions.[27,28] These studies strongly suggest that altered G-protein function may contribute to the reduction during aging in cardiac and vascular reactivity to β-adrenergic agonists.

III. AGE-RELATED CHANGES IN IONOTROPIC TYPES AROUND ION CHANNELS

Ligand-gated channels and voltage-gated channels comprise the two major classes of ion channels in excitable membranes.[45-47] Ligand-gated channels are sensitive to specific ligands; examples are nicotinic acetylcholine (nACh) receptors, γ-aminobutyric acid ($GABA_A$) receptors, N-methyl-D-aspartate (NMDA) receptors, (RS)-α-amino-3-hydroxy-5-methyl-4-isoxazolepropionic acid (AMPA) receptors, Ca^{2+}-activated K^+ channels, and nucleotide-gated channels. Voltage-gated channels are sensitive to changes in membrane potential; examples are Na^+, K^+, and Ca^{2+} channels. G-protein-gated ion channels[48,49] are sensitive to specific signal-transducing, membrane-associated G-proteins that act directly on ion channels, making them more likely to open. Direct G-protein gating has already been identified for K^+ channels[48] and for Ca^{2+} channels.[49]

Several approaches have been utilized to evaluate ionotropic types in the aging nervous system. A more common method for evaluating changes in ionotropic types during aging has been ligand binding. Previous studies on $GABA_A$ receptor pharmacology during aging have provided somewhat controversial results, depending on the rat strain or on the brain region tested.[50] Recently, Ruano et al.[51] reported that neither the affinity nor the density for $GABA_A$ receptor complex were modified during aging in cortical membranes from Wistar or Fischer rats. Many groups have reported a decline of nicotinic binding sites during aging.[52,53] The NMDA receptors are known to play an important role for neuronal plasticity and memory acquisition. Saransaari and Oja[54] reported that despite the unchanged affinity for NMDA subtype of the glutamate receptor, the density increased three times in aging mice.

A major function of G-protein-linked receptors in the heart is to regulate the ion channels that control the rate and force of cardiac contraction. Brown and Birnbaumer[48] have proposed that the channel may also be modulated directly by G-proteins in addition to the indirect mechanism of phosphorylation. Direct G-protein control of ion channels has assumed considerable recent significance. Calcium channels appear to be likely candidates, together with potassium channels, for such direct control.[49] Thus, the α-subunit of the Gs protein appears to directly gate cardiac L channels in addition to its indirect control through the cAMP cascade. Recently, it has been suggested that, as part of the $Gs\alpha$ subunit function, alterations of cardiac excitation and contraction coupling during aging may not only regulate adenylyl cyclase activity but also ion channels.[44] Other classes of calcium channels, including the N channel, although less well investigated, are likely to be regulated also through such G-protein interactions.

IV. IMPAIRED RESPONSIVENESS TO CALCIUM MOBILIZATION DURING AGING

The Ca^{2+}-mediated signaling system and regulation of Ca^{2+} homeostasis appear to be the final common pathway for such cellular changes. The "Ca^{2+} hypothesis of aging" proposed that cellular mechanisms which regulate the homeostasis of cytosolic free Ca^{2+} ion play a critical role in aging, and that altered $[Ca^{2+}]i$ might account for a number of age-related changes in neuronal and cellular function.[18,19] Table 1 lists of some of the calcium-dependent systems that have been reported to exhibit altered responsiveness during aging. A wide variety of stimuli, types of responses, and species are represented.

In addition, studies of membrane structure and function are essential to a better understanding of the mechanisms by which intracellular

TABLE 1.

Systems Exhibiting Impaired Stimulation of Calcium Mobilization
During Aging

Stimulus	Species	Tissue or cell	Response	Ref.
α_1-Adrenergic	Rat	Parotid	Electrolyte secretion	21,22,26
α_1-Adrenergic	Rat	Parotid	Glucose oxidation	69,70
α_1-Adrenergic	Rat	Aorta	Contraction	71,72
α_1-Adrenergic	Rat	Heart	Contraction	73
β-Adrenergic	Rat	Heart	Contraction	44,74
Cholinergic	Rat	Brain	Dopamine release	75
Depolarization	Rat	Heart	Contraction	76
Depolarization	Rat	Brain	ACh release	77,78
Depolarization	Mouse	Brain	ACh release	79
Depolarization	Rat	Brain	Serotonin release	80
Depolarization	Rat	Brain	Calcium current	81
Depolarization	Mouse	Brain (Cells)	Calcium mobilization	82
Depolarization	Mouse	Whole animal	Motor function	83
Depolarization	Rat	Whole animal	Maze learning	84
Serotonergic	Rat	Aorta	Contraction	71
Glucose	Rat	Pancreas	Insulin release	85
LHRH	Rat	Pituitary	LH release	61,62
Lectin	Rat	Lymphocyte	Mitogenesis	86,87
Lectin	Rat	Lymphocyte	Mitogenesis	88,89
Lectin	Rat	Lymphocyte	Mitogenesis	90,91
Compound 48/80	Rat	Mast cell	Histamine release	92
FMLP	Human	Neutrophil	Superoxide generation	93
TH	Human	Erythrocyte	Calcium ATPase	94
Low-density lipoprotein	Human	Polymorpho-nuclear leukocytes	Release of β-glucuronidase	95
Cytochalasin B	Human	Polymorpho-nuclear leukocytes	Release of β-glucuronidase	95
Ouabain	Guinea pig	Whole animal	Arrhythmogenic toxicity	96
Bay K8644	Rat	Aorta	Contraction	97
Phosphatidylserine	Rat	Brain	ACh release	98

messengers mediate neuromodulation. Critical issues for studies of brain aging concern questions of how and what cellular changes may lead to desensitization of calcium homeostasis within the cytosol and/or disruption of calcium-mediated signal transduction processes. A crucial challenge is to determine the mechanism(s) that produces such changes. At present, we do not know the precise details of the processes that regulate intracellular concentration of $[Ca^{2+}]i$ during aging. It is not clear whether $[Ca^{2+}]i$ changes are the result or the cause of other pathogenetic effects.

Little is known about how aging reduces the calcium-triggered release of ACh. It does not appear to involve a decrease in the synthesis or levels of ACh available for release, since the reductions in ACh release can occur without changes in these presynaptic parameters. Aging does not reduce the voltage-sensitive influx of Ca^{2+} in the cerebral cortex, which may account for the reduced ACh release, at least in part. Alternatively, aging has been shown to increase functional neuronal cytoplasmic calcium levels,[55,56] increase membrane-lipid peroxidation,[57] and reduce brain membrane fluidity[58-60] — each of which conceivably could alter the coupling between calcium uptake and transmitter release. To test the hypothesis that the coupling between intracellular Ca^{2+} and ion efflux, hormone, and neurotransmitter release was altered by aging, we examined the effects of the calcium ionophore A23187 in adult and old rats. A23187 directly elevates intracellular calcium levels, thereby bypassing any age-related difference in voltage-dependent calcium uptake. We previously reported that age differences in stimulated K^+ efflux and luteinizing hormone (LH) release could be partially abolished if α_1-adrenoceptors and LH-releasing hormone (LHRH) receptors, respectively, were bypassed and intracellular calcium concentrations raised artificially by the ionophore A23187.[21,61,62] Thus, selective impairments in calcium mobilization may be at least partially responsible for reduced K^+ efflux and LH release from parotid cells and pituicytes, respectively, of aged rats.

V. AGE-RELATED CHANGES IN TRANSMEMBRANE SIGNALING MECHANISMS AND MEMBRANE ENVIRONMENT

Changes in membrane properties during aging may occur in many physiological and pharmacological situations.[57] However, membrane-bound receptors are sensitive to the structural and physical properties of the lipids, with which they interact. This sensitivity may involve conformational changes that affect the binding sites of receptors or coupling. Other properties of receptors that may be affected include their lateral mobility within the membrane or their interactions with other membrane components such as G-proteins.[63] Any of these perturbations could produce a functional change in receptor-mediated responses.

There are several ways to modulate membrane environment, both *in vivo* and *in vitro*. Dietary manipulations such as starvation[64] and fatty acid[65] or cholesterol supplementation[66] may modify membrane lipid composition and thus influence function. In addition, aging may modify membrane structure.[26,60,67] It appears to reflect an alteration in the coupling of α_1-adrenoceptors-G-proteins-phospholipase C pathways and/or the loss of receptor density following alterations in the membrane environment during aging. In general, changes in membrane composition with aging cause membranes to become more rigid in rat cortex[60] and bladders.[68]

Since receptor and ion channel proteins are believed to be a membrane receptor embedded within the lipid bilayer, changes in membrane fluidity during aging have been proposed to modulate receptor/G-protein interactions and/or many ion channel activities.

VI. CONCLUSIONS AND FUTURE DIRECTIONS

It is clear that various membrane signal transduction mechanisms become altered during aging, resulting in functional changes. This review has defined several categories of such alterations and indicated our current level of knowledge regarding mechanisms and possible modulation. However, even more perceptive cell biological studies during aging will be needed to precisely define the transmembrane signaling mechanisms and functional aspects within living cells, as well as the mechanisms involved in regulation of membrane fluidity or composition during aging.

ACKNOWLEDGMENTS

The authors thank Hideyo Ohshika, M.D., Ph.D., Professor of Pharmacology, Sapporo Medical University School of Medicine, Japan, for comments and suggestions concerning this review. A.M. would like to dedicate this review to Dr. Hideyo Ohshika on the 10th anniversary of his career as a Professor. Research was supported in part by grants from the Ministry of Education, Science, and Culture, Japan (06670121) and the Hokkaido Geriatric Research Institute, Japan.

REFERENCES

1. Shock, N. W., The physiology of aging, *Soc. Am.*, 206, 100, 1962.
2. Warner, H. R., Butler, R. N., Sprott, R. L., and Schneider, E. L., *Modern Biological Theories of Aging*, Raven Press, New York, 1987, 1.
3. Roth, G. S. and Hess, G. D., Changes in the mechanisms of hormone and neurotransmitter action during aging. Current status of the role of receptor and postreceptor alterations, *Mech. Ageing Dev.*, 20, 175, 1982.
4. Dax, E. M., Age-related changes in membrane receptor interactions, *Endocrinol. Metabolism Clinics*, 16, 947, 1987.
5. Roth, G. S., Changes in hormone neurotransmitter action during aging, in *Homeostatic Function and Aging*, Davis, B. B. and Wood, W. G., Eds., Raven Press, New York, 1985, 41.
6. Williams, R. H., Ed., *Textbook of Endocrinology*, W. B. Saunders, Philadelphia, 1981.

7. Nishizuka, Y., The role of protein kinase C in cell surface signal transduction and tumour promotion, *Nature*, 308, 693, 1984.
8. Dohlman, H. G., Thorner, J., Caron, M. G., and Lefkowitz, R. J., Model systems for the study of seven-transmembrane-segment receptors, *Ann. Rev. Biochem.*, 60, 653, 1991.
9. Simon, M. I., Strathmann, M. P., and Gautam, N., Diversity of G proteins in signal transduction, *Science*, 252, 802, 1991.
10. Berridge, M. J., Inositol trisphosphate and calcium signalling, *Nature*, 361, 315, 1993.
11. Watson, S. and Girdlestone, D., Receptor and Ion Channel Nomenclature Supplement (5th Ed.) 1993, *Trends Pharmacol. Sci.*, 1994.
12. Gilman, A. G., G proteins: transducers of receptor-generated signals, *Ann. Rev. Biochem.*, 56, 615, 1987.
13. Minneman, K. P., α_1-Adrenergic receptor subtypes, inositol phosphates, and sources of cell Ca^{2+}, *Pharmacol. Rev.*, 40, 87, 1988.
14. Fain, J. N., Regulation of phosphoinositide-specific phospholipase, C, *Biochim. Biophys. Acta*, 1053, 81, 1990.
15. Hepler, J. R. and Gilman, A. G., G proteins, *Trends Biochem. Sci.*, 17, 383, 1992.
16. Spiegel, A. M., Shenker, A., and Weinstein, L. S., Receptor-effector coupling by G proteins. Implications for normal and abnormal signal transduction, *Endocrine Rev.*, 13, 536, 1992.
17. Roth, G. S., Calcium homeostasis and aging. Role in altered signal transduction, *Ann. N.Y. Acad. Sci.*, Khachaturian, Z. S., Cotman, C. W., and Pettegrew, J. W., Eds., The New York Academy of Sciences, New York, 1989, 68.
18. Roth, G. S., Changes in hormone action with age. Altered calcium mobilization and/or responsiveness impairs signal transduction, in *Endocrine Function and Aging*, Armbrecht, H. J., Coe, R. H., and Wongsurawat, N., Eds., Springer-Verlag, New York, 1989, 26.
19. Roth, G. S., Mechanisms of altered hormone-neurotransmitter action during aging. From receptors to calcium mobilization, in *Ann. Rev. Geront. Geriatrics.*, 1990, chap. 8.
20. Dice, J. F., Cellular and molecular mechanisms of aging, *Physiol. Rev.*, 73, 149, 1993.
21. Ito, H., Baum, B. J., Uchida, T., Hoopes, M. T., Bodner, L., and Roth, G. S., Modulation of rat parotid cell α-adrenergic responsiveness at a step subsequent to receptor activation, *J. Biol. Chem.*, 257, 9532, 1982.
22. Bodner, L., Hoopes, M. T., Gee, M., Ito, H., Roth, G. S., and Baum, B. J., Multiple transduction mechanisms are likely involved in calcium mediated exocrine secretory events in rat parotid cells, *J. Biol. Chem.*, 258, 2774, 1983.
23. Miyamoto, A., Villalobos-Molina, R., Kowatch, M. A., and Roth, G. S., Altered coupling of α_1-adrenergic receptor-G protein in rat parotid during aging, *Am. J. Physiol.*, 262, C1181, 1992.
24. Villalobos-Molina, R., Miyamoto, A., Kowatch, M. A., and Roth, G. S., α_1-Adrenoceptors in parotid cells. Age does not alter the ratio of α_{1A} and α_{1B} subtypes, *Eur. J. Pharmacol.*, 226, 129, 1992.
25. Miyamoto, A., Kowatch, M. A., and Roth, G. S., Similar effects of saponin treatment and aging on coupling of α_1-adrenergic receptor-G-protein, *Exp. Gerontol.*, 28, 349, 1993.
26. Miyamoto, A., Araiso, T., Koyama, T., and Ohshika, H., Adrenoceptor coupling mechanisms which regulate salivary secretion during aging, *Life Sci.*, 53, 1873, 1993.

27. Narayanan, N. and Derby, J. A., Alterations in the properties of β-adrenergic receptors of myocardial membranes in aging. Impairments in agonist-receptor interactions and guanine nucleotide regulation accompany diminished catecholamine responsiveness of adenylate cyclase, Mech. Ageing Dev., 19, 127, 1982.

28. Scarpace, P. J. and Abrass, I. B., β-Adrenergic agonist-mediated desensitization in senescent rats, Mech. Ageing Dev., 35, 255, 1986.

29. Yamagami, K., Joseph, J. A., and Roth, G. S., Decrement of muscarinic receptor-stimulated low-Km GTPase in striatum and hippocampus from the aged rat, Brain Res., 576, 327, 1992.

30. Villalobos-Molina, R., Joseph, J. A., and Roth, G. S., α_1-Adrenergic stimulation of low Km GTPase in rat striata is diminished with age, Brain Res., 590, 303, 1992.

31. Smith, C. J., Perry, E. K., Perry, R. H., Fairbairn, A. F., and Birdsall, N. J. M., Guanine nucleotide modulation of muscarinic cholinergic receptor binding in postmortem human brain — a preliminary study in Alzheimer's disease, Neurosci. Lett., 82, 227, 1987.

32. Warpman, U., Alafuzoff, I., and Nordberg, A., Coupling of muscarinic receptors to GTP proteins in postmortem human brain — alterations in Alzheimer's disease, Neurosci. Lett., 150, 39, 1993.

33. Cowburn, R. F., Vestling, M., Fowler, C. J., Ravid, R., Winblad, B., and O'Neill, C., Disrupted β_1-adrenoceptor-G protein coupling in the temporal cortex of patients with Alzheimer's disease, Neurosci. Lett., 155, 163, 1993.

34. Keyser, J. D., Backer, J.-P. D., Ebinger, G., and Vauquelin, G., Coupling of D_1 dopamine receptors to the guanine nucleotide binding protein Gs is deficient in Huntington's disease, Brain Res., 496, 327, 1989.

35. Fraser, C. M., Chung, F. Z., Wang, C. D., and Venter, J. C., Site-directed mutagenesis of human β-adrenergic receptors. Substitution of aspartic acid-130 by asparagine produces a receptor with high-affinity agonist binding that is uncoupled from adenylate cyclase, Proc. Natl. Acad. Sci. U.S.A., 85, 5478, 1988.

36. Mooradian, A. D. and Scarpace, P. J., 3,5,3'-L-Triiodothyronine regulation of β-adrenergic receptor density and adenylyl cyclase activity in synaptosomal membranes of aged rats, Neurosci. Lett., 161, 101, 1993.

37. Sugawa, M. and May, T., Age-related alteration in signal transduction. Involvement of the cAMP cascade, Brain Res., 618, 57, 1993.

38. Docherty, J. R., Cardiovascular responses in ageing. A review, Pharmacol. Rev., 42, 103, 1990.

39. Lakatta, E. G., Cardiovascular regulatory mechanisms in advanced age, Physiol. Rev., 73, 413, 1993.

40. Miyamoto, A., Kimura, H., Kawana, S., and Ohshika, H., Desensitization of the myocardial β-adrenergic receptor system in aged rats, in The Mechanism and New Approach on Drug Resistance of Cancer Cells, Miyazaki, T., Takaku, F., and Sakurada, K., Eds., Excerpta Medica, Amsterdam, 1993, 237.

41. Fleisch, J. H., Maling, H. M., and Brodie, B. B., β-Receptor activity in aorta. Variations with age and species, Cir. Res., XXVI, 151, 1970.

42. Hyland, L., Warnock, P., and Docherty, J. R., Age-related alterations in α_1 and β-adrenoceptors mediated responsiveness of rat aorta, Naunyn-Schmiedeberg's Arch. Pharmacol., 335, 50, 1987.

43. Crass, M. F., Borst, S. E., and Scarpace, P. J., β-Adrenergic responsiveness in cultured aorta smooth muscle cells. Effects of subculture and aging, Biochem. Pharmacol., 43, 1811, 1992.

44. Miyamoto, A., Kawana, S., Kimura, H., and Ohshika, H., Impaired expression of Gsα protein mRNA in rat ventricular myocardium with aging, *Eur. J. Pharmacol.*, 266, 147, 1994.

45. Olsen, R. W. and Tobin, A. J., Molecular biology of GABA_A receptors, *FASEB J.*, 4, 1469, 1990.

46. Wonnacott, S., Drasdo, A., Sanderson, E., and Rowell, P., Presynaptic nicotinic receptors and the modulation of transmitter release, in *The Biology of Nicotine Dependence*, Block, G. and Marsh, J., Eds., John Wiley & Sons, West Sussex, 1990, 87.

47. Trautwein, W. and Hescheler, J., Regulation of cardiac L-type calcium current by phosphorylation and G proteins, *Ann. Rev. Physiol.*, 52, 257, 1990.

48. Brown, A. M. and Birnbaumer, L., Direct G protein gating of ion channels, *Am. J. Physiol.*, 254, H401, 1988.

49. Brown, A. M., Regulation of heartbeat by G protein-coupled ion channels, *Am. J. Physiol.*, 259, H1621, 1990.

50. Miller, L. G., Lumpkin, M., Galpern, W. R., Greenblatt, D. J., and Shader, R. I., Modification of γ-aminobutyric acid_A receptor binding and function by N-ethoxy-carbonyl-2-ethoxy-1,2-dihydroquinoline in vitro and in vivo. Effects of aging, *J. Neurochem.*, 56, 1241, 1991.

51. Ruano, D., Machado, A., and Vitorica, J., Absence of modifications of the pharmacological properties of the GABA_A receptor complex during aging, as assessed in 3- and 24-month-old rat cerebral cortex, *Eur. J. Pharmacol.*, 246, 81, 1993.

52. Whitehouse, P. J., Martino, A. M., Antuono, P. G., Lowenstein, P. R., Coyle, J. T., Price, D. L., and Kellar, K. J., Nicotinic binding sites in Alzheimer's disease, *Brain Res.*, 371, 146, 1986.

53. Schulz, D. W., Kuchel, G. A., and Zigmond, R. E., Decline in response to nicotine in aged rat striatum. Correlation with a decrease in a subpopulation of nicotinic receptors, *J. Neurochem.*, 61, 2225, 1993.

54. Saransaari, P. and Oja, S. S., Strychnine-insensitive glycine binding to cerebral cortical membranes in developing and ageing mice, *Mech. Ageing Dev.*, 72, 57, 1993.

55. Landfield, P. W. and Pitler, T. A., Prolonged Ca^{2+}-dependent after hyperpolarizations in hippocampal neurons of aged rats, *Science*, 226, 1089, 1984.

56. Sugawa, M., Alterations of inositol phosphate turnover in striatum of aged rats, *Eur. J. Pharmacol.*, 247, 39, 1993.

57. Schroeder, F., Role of membrane lipid asymmetry in aging, *Neurobiol. Aging*, 5, 323, 1984.

58. Ando, S., Tanaka, Y., and Kon, K., Membrane aging of the brain synaptosomes with special reference to gangliosides, in *Gangliosides and Neuronal Plasticity*, Tettamanti, G., Ledeen, R. W., Sandhoff, K., Nagai, Y., and Toffano, G., Eds., Liviana Press, Padova, 1986, 105.

59. Henry, J. M. and Roth, G. S., Modulation of rat striatal membrane fluidity. Effects of age-related differences in dopamine receptor concentrations, *Life Sci.*, 39, 1223, 1986.

60. Miyamoto, A., Araiso, T., Koyama, T., and Ohshika, H., Membrane viscosity correlates with α_1-adrenergic signal transduction of the aged rat cerebral cortex, *J. Neurochem.*, 55, 70, 1990.

61. Chuknyiska, R. S., Blackman, M. R., and Roth, G. S., Ionophore A23187 partially reverses LH secretory defect of pituitary cells from old rats, *Am. J. Physiol.*, 253, E233, 1987.

62. Miyamoto, A., Maki, T., Blackman, M. R., and Roth, G. S., Age-related changes in the mechanisms of LHRH-stimulated LH release from pituitary cells in vitro, *Exp. Gerontol.*, 27, 211, 1992.

63. Conklin, B. R. and Bourne, H. R., Structural elements of Gα subunits that interact with Gβγ, receptors, and effectors, *Cell*, 73, 631, 1993.

64. Katz, M. S., Food restriction modulates β-adrenergic sensitive adenylate cyclase in rat liver during aging, *Am. J. Physiol.*, 254, E54, 1988.
65. Stubbs, C. D. and Smith, A. D., The modulation of mammalian membrane polyunsaturated fatty acid composition in relationship to membrane fluidity and function, *Biochim. Biophys. Acta*, 779, 89, 1984.
66. Murchie, E. J. and Patten, G. S., Dietary cholesterol influences cardiac β-adrenergic receptor adenylate cyclase activity in the marmoset monkey by changes in membrane cholesterol status, *Biochim. Biophys. Acta*, 942, 324, 1988.
67. Miyamoto, A. and Ohshika, H., Age-related changes in [^{3}H]prazosin binding and phosphoinositide hydrolysis in rat ventricular myocardium, *Gen. Pharmacol.*, 20, 647, 1989.
68. Wheeler, M. A., Pontari, M., Nishimoto, T., and Weiss, R. M., Changes in lipid composition and cholesterol- and ethanol-stimulated adenylate cyclase activity in aging Fischer rat bladders, *J. Pharmacol. Exp. Ther.*, 254, 277, 1990.
69. Ito, H., Hoopes, M. T., Roth, G. S., and Baum, B. J., Adrenergic and cholinergic mediated glucose oxidation by rat parotid gland acinar cells during aging, *Biochem. Biophys. Res. Commun.*, 98, 275, 1981.
70. Gee, M. V., Ishikawa, Y., Baum, B. J., and Roth, G. S., Impaired adrenergic stimulation of rat parotid cell glucose oxidation during aging. The role of calcium, *J. Gerontol.*, 41, 331, 1986.
71. Cohen, M. L. and Berkowitz, B. A., Vascular contraction. Effect of age and extracellular calcium, *Blood Vessels*, 67, 139, 1976.
72. Hyland, L., Warnock, P., and Docherty, J. R., Age-related alterations in α_1- and β-adrenoceptors mediated responsiveness of rat aorta, *Naunyn-Schmiedeberg's Arch. Pharmacol.*, 335, 50, 1987.
73. Kimball, K. A., Cornett, L. E., Seifen, E., and Kennedy, R. H., Aging: changes in cardiac α_1-adrenoceptor responsiveness and expression, *Eur. J. Pharmacol.*, 208, 231, 1991.
74. Guarnieri, T., Filburn, C. R., Zitnik, G., Roth, G. S., and Lakatta, E. G., Mechanisms of altered cardiac inotropic responsiveness during aging in the rat, *Am. J. Physiol.*, 239, H501, 1980.
75. Joseph, J. A., Dalton, T. K., Roth, G. S., and Hunt, W. A., Alterations in muscarinic control of striatal dopamine autoreceptors in senescence. A deficit at the ligand-muscarinic receptor interface?, *Brain Res.*, 454, 149, 1988.
76. Elfellah, M. S. and Shepherd, J. A., Effect of age on responsiveness of isolated rat atria to carbachol and on binding characteristics of atria muscarinic receptors, *J. Cardiovasc. Pharmacol.*, 8, 873, 1986.
77. Peterson, C. and Gibson, G. E., Aging and 3,4-diaminopyridine alter synaptosomal calcium uptake, *J. Biol. Chem.*, 258, 11482, 1983.
78. Meyer, E. M., Crews, F. T., Otero, D. H., and Larsen, K., Aging decreases the sensitivity of rat cortical synaptosomes to calcium ionophore-induced acetylcholine release, *J. Neurochem.*, 47, 1244, 1986.
79. Hartmann, H., Eckert, A., and Müller, W. E., Aging enhances the calcium sensitivity of central neurons of the mouse as an adaptive response to reduced free intracellular calcium, *Neurosci. Lett.*, 152, 181, 1993.
80. Friedman, E. and Wang, H.-Y., Effect of age on brain cortical protein kinase C and its mediation of 5-hydroxytryptamine release, *J. Neurochem.*, 52, 187, 1989.
81. Reynolds, J. N. and Carlen, P. L., Diminished calcium currents in aged hippocampus dentate gyrus granule neurons, *Brain Res.*, 479, 384, 1989.
82. Hartmann, H. and Müller, W. E., Age-related changes in receptor-mediated and depolarization-induced phosphatidylinositol turnover in mouse brain, *Brain Res.*, 622, 86, 1993.
83. Peterson, C. and Gibson, G. E., Amelioration of age-related neurochemical and behavioral deficits by 3,4-diaminopyridine, *Neurobiol. Aging*, 4, 25, 1983.

84. Davis, H. P., Idowu, A., and Gibson, G. E., Improvement of 8-arm maze performance in aged Fischer 344 rats with 3,4-diaminopyridine, *Exp. Aging Res.*, 9, 211, 1983.
85. Castro, M., Pedrosa, D., and Osuna, J. I., Impaired insulin release in aging rats. Metabolic and ionic events, *Experientia*, 49, 850, 1993.
86. Wu, W., Pahlavani, M., Richardson, A., and Cheung, H. T., Effect of maturation and age on lymphocyte proliferation induced by A23187 through an interleukin independent pathway, *J. Leukocyte Biol.*, 38, 531, 1985.
87. Segal, J., Studies on the age-related decline in the response of lymphoid cells to mitogens. Measurements of concanavalin A binding and stimulation of calcium and sugar uptake in thymocytes from rats of varying ages, *Mech. Ageing Dev.*, 33, 295, 1986.
88. Miller, R. A., Jacobson, B., Weil, G., and Simons, E. R., Diminished calcium influx in lectin-stimulated T cells from old mice, *J. Cell Physiol.*, 132, 337, 1987.
89. Proust, J. J., Filburn, C. R., Harrison, S. A., Buchholz, M. A., and Nordin, A. A., Age-related defect in signal transduction during lectin activation of murine T lymphocytes, *J. Immunol.*, 139, 1472, 1987.
90. Chopra, R., Nagel, J., and Adler, W., Decreased response of T cells from elderly individuals to phytohemagglutinin (PHA) stimulation can be augmented by phorbol myristate acetate (PMA) in conjunction with Ca^{2+}-ionophore A23187, *Gerontologist*, 27, 204A, 1987.
91. Grossman, A., Ledbetter, J. A., and Rabinovitch, P. S., Reduced proliferation in T-lymphocytes in aged humans is predominant in the CD8$^+$ subset, and is unrelated to defects in transmembrane signaling which are predominantly in the CD4$^+$ subset, *Exp. Cell Res.*, 180, 367, 1989.
92. Orida, N. and Feldman, J. D., Age related deficiency in calcium uptake by mast cells, *Fed. Proc.*, 41, 822, 1982.
93. Lipschitz, D. A., Udupa, K. B., and Boxer, L. A., Evidence that microenvironmental factors account for the age-related decline in neutrophil function, *Blood*, 70, 1131, 1987.
94. Davis, P. J., Davis, F. B., and Blas, S. D., Donor age-dependent decline in response of human red cell Ca^{2+}-ATPase activity to thyroid hormone in vitro, *J. Clin. Endocrinol. Metab.*, 64, 921, 1987.
95. Fülöp, T., Jr., Fóris, G., Wórum, I., Paragh, G., and Leövey, A., Age related variations of some polymorphonuclear leukocyte functions, *Mech. Ageing Dev.*, 29, 1, 1985.
96. Khatter, J. C., Navaratnam, S., and Agbanyo, M., Mechanisms of reduced digitalis tolerance with advancing age in the guinea pig, *Biochem. Pharmacol.*, 40, 997, 1990.
97. Wanstall, J. C. and O'Donnell, S. R., Age influences responses of rat isolated aorta and pulmonary artery to the calcium channel agonist, Bay K8644, and to potassium and calcium, *J. Cardiovasc. Pharmacol.*, 13, 709, 1989.
98. Pedata, F., Giovannelli, L., Spignoli, G., Giovannini, G., and Pepeu, G., Phosphatidylserine increases acetylcholine release from cortical slices in aged rats, *Neurobiol. Aging*, 6, 337, 1985.

Chapter 9

STRUCTURAL CHANGES MODIFYING THE INTRACELLULAR FLOW OF INFORMATION

A. Macieira-Coelho

CONTENTS

0-8493-4786-6/95/$0.00+$.50

I. STRUCTURE-RELATED FUNCTIONAL CHANGES DURING CELL AGING

One of the first changes described during senescence of proliferative cell compartments, was an increase in cell volume.[1] This was detected by measuring cell diameters with the aid of an ocular micrometer and was later confirmed with electronic counters[2-5] and with measurements of the cell area on microphotographic paper.[6-8]

Increases in cell volume were first found to be coupled with the decline in the probability of cycling of nonmammalian cells.[9] These studies were followed by the analysis of the relationship between cell volume and cell division in mammalian cells, with different methodologies. Tritiated thymidine labeling,[6] direct analysis by cinematography,[10] and comparison of cell volume with the population doubling time,[4] all led to the conclusion that larger cells have a decreased probability of entering the division cycle. With the increase in cell volumes, higher growth factor concentration and larger substratum areas became necessary for proliferation.[11]

In proliferative cell compartments, when the probability of dividing decreases significantly cell enlargement becomes very pronounced with striking changes in cell morphology (Figure 1). The cells become flat with few microvilli, show little ruffling activity, and are almost completely devoid of macropinocytosis.[12] Not only does the cytoplasm increase, but also the nuclear and nucleolar areas, and the pattern of increase is similar for the three areas;[8] these studies suggest modifications of the nuclear matrix where DNA is anchored. In the nucleus and the cytoplasm these spatial modifications are accompanied by significant changes at the supramolecular level.[13]

In the nucleus, a close relationship could be ascertained between the number of population doublings and the progressive reorganization taking place in the high order structure of chromatin.[13] Using an image processor, it was found that at the nuclear periphery where DNA synthesis-initiating sites are anchored, a progressive decrease in the density and an increase in the spacing of the chromatin fibers occurs at each doubling (Figure 2).

It is pertinent to the problem discussed herein that the pattern of evolution of the density and spacing of the chromatin fibers has analogies with that of the fraction of cells synthesizing DNA during a 24-h period, which is illustrated in Figure 3. Indeed the percentage of cells synthesizing DNA during the first 24 h after seeding them on a substratum, declines progressively through the cell population life span, like the density of the chromatin fibers. The spacing, however, increases significantly only during the last divisions, like the maximal percentage of cells synthesizing DNA during a 24-h period between seeding the cells on the substratum for attachment and the time when they reach resting phase.

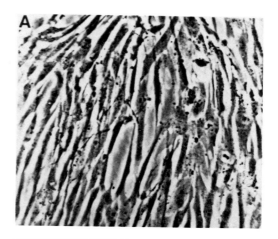

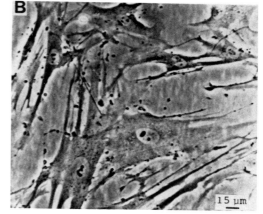

Figure 1
(A) Young human fibroblasts; (B) the same cells at the end of their proliferative life span. Cells assume different morphologies during serial proliferation that are between these two extremes.

These results emphasize the role of cell attachment and spreading on the initiation of DNA synthesis and its deregulation during cell senescence. They show that when cells have secreted the extracellular molecules and built up their attachment sites, they can enter division at the same rate during most of their proliferative life span. With senescence though, it takes longer to build up those sites and to attach and spread, so that the initiation of the division cycle is delayed after having inoculated the cells. This suggests that the delay in the organization of the cytoskeleton for cell attachment is associated with changes in the anchorage of chromatin and with the initiation of DNA synthesis. The data emphasizes the need of this flow of information running from the membrane to the nucleus in order to trigger DNA synthesis.

On the other hand, the profound disorganization of the chromatin (increase in spacing) at the end of the proliferative history of these cells (Figure 4), coincides with the striking changes in cell morphology (Figure 1) and cytoskeleton organization.

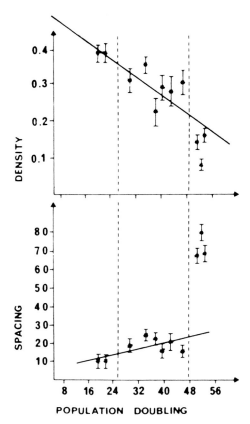

Figure 2
Plot of the values for the density and spacing of the 30-nm chromatin fibers, obtained with an image analyzer, found in human fibroblasts at different population doubling levels. The bars represent the 95% confidence limits; the vertical dashed lines indicate the approximate limits of Phases II, III, and IV.

Alterations of the cytoskeleton were first reported by Bowman and Daniel,[14] who observed that older cells lack prominent bundles of microfilaments and that this deficiency coincides with reduced motility and decreased ability to incorporate ³H-labeled thymidine. On the other hand, Wang and Gundersen[15] found an increased organization of microfilaments into bundles. From the results of Raes et al.,[16,17] what seems to take place is a more heterogeneous distribution of microfilaments in the slow-dividing cell; these authors could distinguish a cortical, an annular, and a central cytoplasmic area, each with a different organization of microfilaments. In contrast, in actively dividing cells these filaments run in parallel arrays along the axis of the cell. An increased actin concentration in old cells, mainly of one protein species homologous to muscle actin, has also been reported.[18] Intermediate filaments are also affected, since they present an unusual organization into large bundles.[19]

Another major change in the cytoplasm of slow-dividing cells is that reported by Raes et al.[16,17] and Van Gansen et al.[20] concerning the microtubules. Pertinent to the problem of the flow of information running from

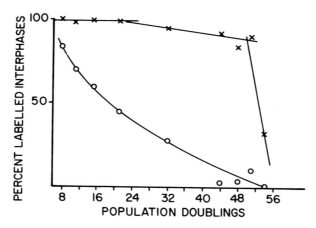

Figure 3
Percent labeled interphases found during the first 24 h after subcultivation when the cells build their attachment sites (o), and maximal percentage reached during a 24-h period thereafter (x), before the cell population reached resting phase. The measurements were performed at different population doubling levels.

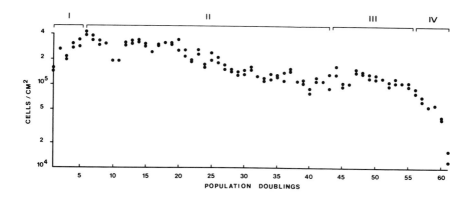

Figure 4
Proliferative life span of a human embryonic lung fibroblast population, expressed as the maximal cell densities recorded after each cell population doubling. Each dot corresponds to a cell count from a different culture vessel. Phase I concerns the first five doublings when the cell densities increase due to selection of the fibroblast population and elimination of other cell types. Phase II lasts from the 5th to approximately the 43rd doubling when close to 100% of the cells enter DNA synthesis during a 24-h period and the population doubling time is stable. Phase III lasts from the 43rd to around the 55th doubling, when close to 100% of the cells still synthesize DNA during a 24-h period but the population doubling time increases. Phase IV corresponds to the last three to five doublings, when the number of cells capable of synthesizing DNA during a 24-h period declines rapidly and the doubling time increases pronouncedly.

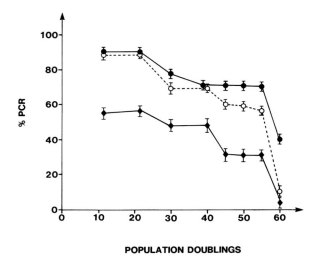

POPULATION DOUBLINGS

Figure 5
Contractile activity throughout the proliferative history of the same cell population
whose life span is plotted in Figure 4. The activity was measured in the absence (●)
and presence of 0.06 (○) and 0.12 (♦) mM of cystamine. Bars represent the 95%
confidence limits.

the membrane to the nucleus is the fact that this reorganization of the
microtubule network involves a loss of polarity, since the polymerization
wave of the microtubules becomes centrifugal instead of centripetal as in
the young cells.[17]

These rearrangements in the cytoskeletal network are certainly responsible for the loss of motility and contractility during cellular senescence. A decreased motility with *in vivo* cellular aging became apparent
when cell migration from explants was measured.[21] Migration from a
wound performed on a confluent human fibroblast monolayer has also
been shown to decrease in cultures from old donors.[22]

Cell contractility during senescence of proliferative compartments
was checked, evaluating the capacity of quiescent human fibroblasts to
retract a plasma clot through their proliferative life span (Figure 4). The
results showed (Figure 5) that the retraction was maximal early during the
cell population life span (Phase II), declined progressively during Phase
III, and declined in a more pronounced way during Phase IV. The same
pattern was observed in the presence of cystamine but was accentuated by
the drug. Cystamine oxidizes SH groups, thereby inhibiting *inter alia*
transglutaminase, an enzyme implicated in cell motile events.[23,24]

The same test was performed on quiescent and proliferating cells at
the 16th and 52nd population doubling level, in the absence and in the
presence of increasing concentrations of cystamine (Figure 6). The decline

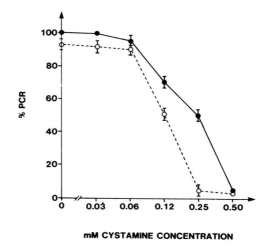

Figure 6
Contractile activity of the human embryonic lung fibroblasts at the 16th (top) and 52nd (bottom) population doubling level, in the presence of different concentrations of cystamine. Proliferating (●——●) and resting (○– – –○) cells. Bars represent the 95% confidence limits.

in the retractile activity of older cells was more manifest in the resting phase than in proliferating cells. The increased sensitivity of older cells to the inhibitory action of cystamine was more apparent at lower doses.

These experiments show that the contractile power of the cells is higher in proliferative cells when the turnover of cytoskeletal elements is higher than in the quiescent cells; it suggests that during cellular aging it takes longer to activate the contractile cell structures. These observations fit the conclusions described above concerning the longer time needed to build up the focal adhesion sites and to organize the cytoskeleton for cell attachment during cell senescence. When the cells are proliferating and the flexibility of the cytoskeleton is already engaged, the differences in the

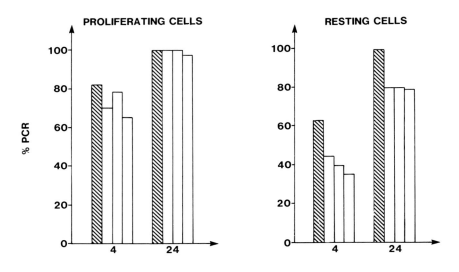

Figure 7
Contractile activity of embryonic (▨) and postnatal (□) human fibroblasts at 4 h and
24 h after suspending proliferating and resting cells in plasma. Each white column
corresponds to a fibroblast population from a different donor.

contractile power and in the capacity to cycle is less pronounced between
young and older cells.

Embryonic and postnatal skin fibroblasts were also compared in regard to their contractile capacity, both during proliferation and in the
resting phase (Figure 7). The decreased retractile activity of postnatal
fibroblasts was apparent only in the resting phase; it reiterates the finding
that the decreased contractile activity caused by cell senescence becomes
manifest when the cells are in a relaxed state.

Overall, the data support the idea of a coupling between changes in
cell attachment, cell shape, contractile activity, chromatin anchorage, and
the initiation of DNA synthesis.

II. CORRELATION BETWEEN CELL STRUCTURE
AND FUNCTION

What could be the nature of the information flowing through the cell,
coupling modifications in cell structure with functional changes? In order
to find an answer to this question, substrata suitable for the cultivation of
cells were developed whose physicochemical properties could be

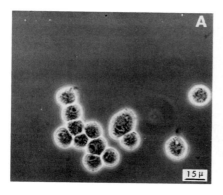
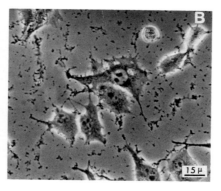

Figure 8
Mouse L cells on negatively (A) and positively (B) charged surfaces.

changed;[25,26] accordingly, cells assumed different shapes and changed phenotype, depending on the surface to which they attached.

A. Influence of Cell Structure on Cell Division

Tissue culture flasks were coated with a protein polymer made of bovine serum albumin (BSA) which was then covered with substances with different electric charges. It was found that mouse cells assumed different morphologies depending on the electric charge of the surface where they were seeded (Figure 8). The growth of the cells was related with their morphology (Figure 9). On the negatively charged surfaces covered with polyglutamic acid or heparin the cells became round, the density was lower, and the DNA synthetic activity was reduced. Higher growth rates were obtained when cells became spread and stretched on positively charged surfaces.

B. Influence of Cell Structure on Cell Differentiation

The effect of these substrata on cell differentiation was also tested.[27,28] It was found that differentiation of mouse myoblasts could be completed on negatively charged surfaces, but that it stopped when the cells were attached on the polymer covered with polylysine (Figure 10).

Scanning electron microscopy revealed striking differences between the myoblast seeded on a negatively charged or on a positively charged substratum (Figure 11). They concerned the cell surface which was smooth on the negatively charged substratum, contrary to that of cells

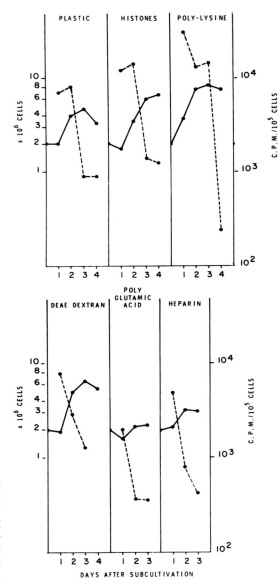

Figure 9
Growth of mouse L cells on a
plastic surface and on positively
(histones, polylysine, DEAE
dextran) and negatively
(polyglutamic acid, heparin)
charged surfaces. Cell counts (—)
and DNA synthesis (– – – –).

on polylysine where the surfaces was covered with blebs and villosities. Only the cells with smooth surfaces could fuse to form myotubes (Figure 11).

The measurement of the cloning efficiency of myogenic cells grown on negatively and positively charged surfaces revealed (Figure 12) that on the former the cloning efficiency fell to less than 10% on the 6th day after

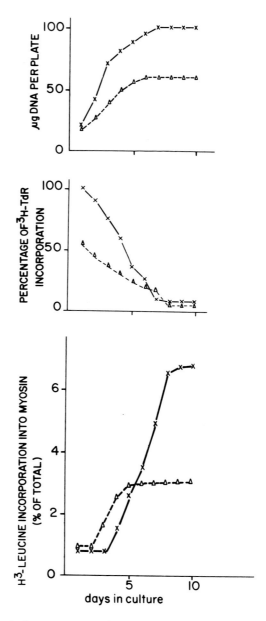

Figure 10
Growth and differentiation of rat
L6 myoblasts on negatively (x) and
positively (△) charged surfaces.

plating the cells, when differentiation was completed. On the polylysine-coated surface, however, on the 6th day after subcultivation 30 to 35% of the cells still had the potential to divide, judged by their cloning efficiency, although growth was arrested as revealed by the DNA synthesis curve and the amount of DNA per culture.

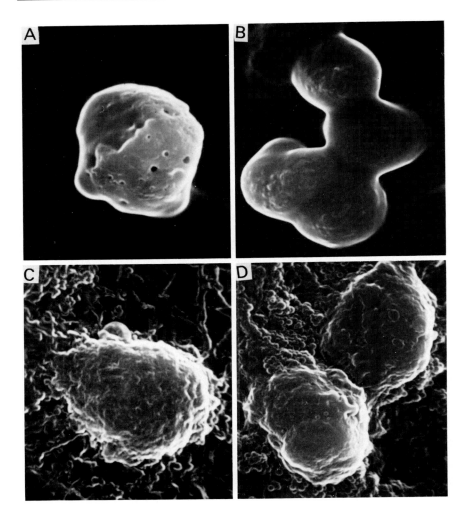

Figure 11
Scanning electron microscopy of rat L6 myoblasts on negatively (A and B) and positively (C and D) charged surfaces. On the left, individual cells; when the cells made contacts on the negatively charged surface (B) they fused forming myotubes; on positively charged surface (D) they did not fuse.

C. Influence of Cell Structure on the Cell Malignant Potential

Evidence was also obtained showing how cell malignancy can be influenced by cell shape.[29] When L1210 mouse leukemic cells were subcultivated on a BSA polymer treated with positively charged substances, a few cells eventually lost the rounded shape and spread out, assuming a fibroblastic shape (Figure 13). The fibroblastic cells progressively invaded the whole surface while the round cells were lost during

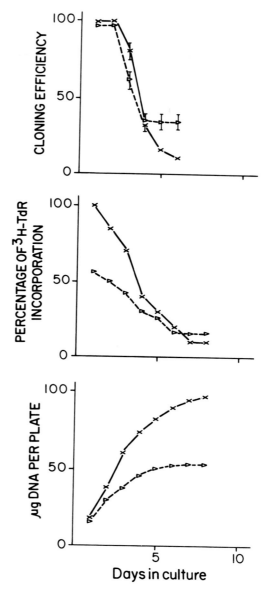

Figure 12
Cloning efficiency and growth of
rat L6 myoblasts on negatively
(x) and positively (▷) charged
surfaces.

trypsinization. These cells that acquired adhesive properties and became fibroblast-like, had lost the malignant potential (Figure 14). Indeed, 10^5 wild-type cells injected per mice killed all animals, while all animals survived when 10^8 revertant cells were injected.

The L1210 cells were serially passaged during a year. After this time, round cells grown in suspension could again be recovered and carried separately. This population had reacquired their malignant potential,

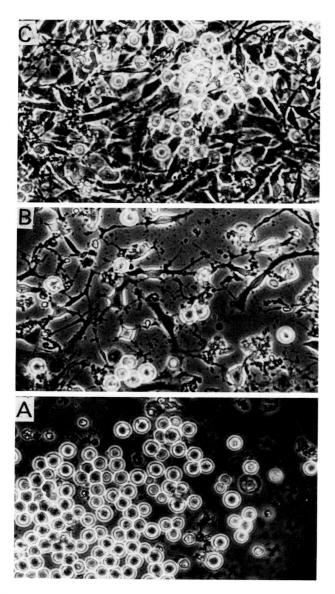

Figure 13
Attachment (A) and switch to a fibroblastic morphology (B and C) of L1210 mouse leukemic cells on a positively charged surface.

although not fully, since 10^6 cells per mouse took longer to kill the animals and one survived (Figure 15).

Overall, the results show that cell shape can be modified through the interaction of the membrane with the extracellular matrix, with subsequent

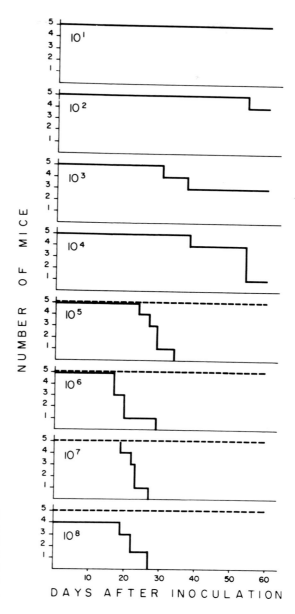

Figure 14
Survival of mice injected with the indicated amount of L1210 mouse leukemic cells that have grown in suspension *in vitro* (—) or that had become fibroblastic-like (– – –).

change in the cell phenotype. The regulation of cell differentiation and of the malignant potential through substratum-dependent modifications of cell morphology suggest that new structural constraints can influence gene expression in a stable fashion.

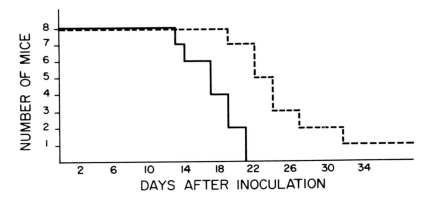

Figure 15
Survival of mice injected with 10^6 mouse L1210 leukemic wild-type cells that grow
in suspension (—) and with 10^6 cells that had reverted back to growth in suspension
after proliferating during a year as fibroblasts (– – –).

III. NATURE OF THE SIGNALS REGULATING THE STRUCTURE-DEPENDENT FLOW OF INFORMATION

Several facts brought out by the experiments described above suggest
that the substratum where cells were attached had no direct effect on cell
metabolism. Indeed, the changes in the morphology of the cells were
strictly dependent on the electric charge and had no relation with the
biological properties of the molecules determining the charge.[25,26] Different positively charged substances induced spreading, while neutral or
negatively charged ones caused rounding of the cells independently of
other properties.

Another finding suggesting no direct effect of the substratum on cell
metabolism was the fact that both the L and D- forms of the molecules used
to determine the charge of the supporting surface could equally modulate
the cell phenotypes.[26] Polymerized proteins used as substratum lost their
biological properties as promoters of growth and of transport across the
cell membrane.[26] Finally, nutrients bound to the substratum did not enter
the cell.[26]

If the coupling of the cell architecture with the cell phenotype is not
mediated primarily by a direct effect on cell metabolism, it means that the
first signals must be of a mechanical type. This led to the conclusion that
the network of structures extending from the periphery to the nuclear
cage, that constitute the cellular scaffolding, is first regulated by the way
its elements are connected, i.e., by its topology. The probability of triggering new topological constraints, and thus to switch functions, depends
upon conformational changes within this network.

In order to understand this relationship between the cell architecture
and the intracellular flow of information, it is important to recollect the

molecular organization of a mammalian cell. Mammalian DNA is a molecule more than 1 m long, confined in a sphere, the nucleus, with a diameter of about 5 μ. This implies an elaborate folding which is regulated *inter alia* by the structure of DNA, by DNA-bound proteins, by enzymes, and by anchorage of this make-up to a protein matrix. In addition, there are glycoproteins present whose role is yet to be determined; since these molecules are highly charged, it is reasonable to think that they must also function as regulators of chromatin conformation.

In general, at least three hierarchical levels of nuclear DNA organization resulting from DNA folding are accepted. The first level corresponds to the 10-nm "bead-on-a-string" chromatin fiber that results from the repeating unit formed by two superhelical turns of the DNA double helix around a histone core. The unit is called the nucleosome and the number of base pairs of the repeating structure is called the DNA repeat length.

The second level results from the folding of the 10-nm fiber into a 30-nm-wide solenoid with a helical pitch of 11 nm and 6 to 8 nucleosomes per turn. There is no complete agreement concerning the organization at this level.

Finally, the third level results from the further folding of the solenoid into supercoiled loops, each with approximately 10,000 bp of DNA, anchored at the periphery of the nucleus.

This elaborate organization of the DNA molecule is fundamental for gene expression; it is thermodynamically unstable and thus is in permanent movement and variance, the structural flexibility being crucial for its function.

The scaffold upon which chromatin is anchored plays a crucial role in its high order structure. There is indeed a protein framework called the nuclear matrix with which DNA is associated. The anchorage of DNA is crucial for its replication and for transcription, since nascent RNA is associated with the nuclear cage.

The nuclear lamina, a filamentous protein meshwork lining the nucleoplasmic surface of the nuclear envelope, provides an anchoring site at the nuclear periphery for chromatin.

The lamina is composed of proteins called lamins which seem to be intermediary structures between DNA-binding proteins and the cytoskeleton. Indeed, on the one hand the lamina is tightly bound to chromatin since it can be dissociated from chromatin only by a high-salt solution which also extracts the tightly bound histones in the nucleosome core.[30] On the other hand, lamins have a striking sequence homology with intermediate filaments, a component of the cytoskeleton.[31] Evidence in favor of the influence of intermediate filaments on chromatin conformation was recently reported.[32]

Thus, the anchorage of chromatin seems to be fulfilled with the preservation of the continuity with the cytoplasmic scaffold. This way, DNA is linked to the cytoskeleton through its anchorage to the nuclear cage, and via the former to the cell membrane and the extracellular matrix. This whole structure acts as an integrator, not only of space, but of function as well; it has to be seen as a tridimensional manifold where the information flows to a great extent through topological constraints. The experiments described above favor this view.

From a thermodynamic point of view, the initiation of information flowing from the cell periphery to the nucleus can be seen as a series of activation-energy barriers. The first energy barrier is the cytoplasmic membrane. To be activated, a conformational change has to take place originated by the binding of a ligand to a receptor or by changes in the binding of the membrane to the extracellular matrix. The new topological constraint activates phosporylation and dephosphorylation processes, ion pumps, and the flow of electrons. This way, free energy becomes available to activate the barrier and new topological constraints can be created along the pathway leading to the nucleus, where DNA will assume the conformational competence for gene expression.

This implies that conformational flexibility at the molecular and supramolecular levels is crucial for the transmission of information within the cell. Precisely, one of the striking events accompanying cell senescence is a modification of that flexibility; many of the functional changes underlying cellular aging can be explained through this mechanism.

In regard to DNA synthesis, the steric position of the initiating sites must be crucial for entrance into the S period. The alterations that occur during senescence in the cellular scaffold will slow down the conformational changes, and thus decrease the probability of the chromatin structure attaining the appropriate conformation and of DNA synthesis-initiating sites the appropriate steric position to enter the S period.

IV. CONCLUSION

Structure and function are interdependent in a cell through the flexibility of a network of structures that extend from the periphery to the nuclear cage and that constitute a cellular scaffolding. This network is regulated through molecules with the correct steric configuration. Cell behavior is to a great extent determined by the way this network of structures is connected, i.e., by its topology.

The curve plotted in Figure 4 illustrates some aspects of the evolution of a dividing cell compartment. During these phases the cell phenotype evolves and is expressed through changes in cell morphology, function, and in the response to molecular messengers[33] and to carcinogens.[34] The genome rearrangements taking place at each cell division seem to be the *primum movens* for the modifications occurring in the network of structures responsible for the integration of space and function within the cell, through variations in the synthesis of its components and of the energy-supplying systems.

Experimental evidence buttresses the view that the evolution of the potential for replication is coupled with the structural modifications originated during the history of a proliferative compartment. Replication is just one function among others; along with the alterations in replication, other functional changes become apparent through the cell population's proliferative history that are also related with the new constraints created by the structural-dependent changes in the flow of information.

REFERENCES

1. Simons, J. W., The use of frequency distributions of cell diameters to characterize cell populations in tissue culture, *Exp. Cell Res.*, 45, 336, 1967.
2. Macieira-Coelho, A. and Pontén, J., Analogy in growth between late passage human embryonic and early passage human adult fibroblasts, *J. Cell Biol.*, 43, 374, 1969.
3. Simons, J. E. and VandenBroeck, C., Comparison of ageing in vitro by means of cell size analysis using a Coulter counter, *Gerontologia*, 16, 340, 1970.
4. Mitsui, Y. and Schneider, E. L., Relationship between cell replication and volume in senescent human diploid fibroblasts, *Mech. Ageing Dev.*, 5, 45, 1976.
5. Whatley, S. A. and Hill, B. T., The relationship between DNA content, cell volume and growth potential in ageing human embryonic mesenchymal cells, *Cell Biol. Int. Rep.*, 3, 671, 1979.
6. Bowman, P. D., Meek, R. L., and Daniel, C. W., Aging of human fibroblasts in vitro, correlation between DNA synthetic ability and cell size, *Exp. Cell Res.*, 93, 184, 1975.
7. Greenberg, S. B., Grove, G. L., and Cristofalo, V. C., Cell size in aging monolayer cultures, *In Vitro*, 13, 297, 1977.
8. BeMiller, P. M. and Miller, J. E., Cytological changes in senescing WI-38 cells: a statistical analysis, *Mech. Ageing Dev.*, 10, 1, 1979.
9. Lima, L. and Macieira-Coelho, A., Parameters of aging in chicken embryo fibroblasts cultivated in vitro, *Exp. Cell Res.*, 70, 279, 1972.
10. Absher, P. M. and Absher, R. G., Clonal variation and aging of diploid fibroblasts. Cinematographic studies of cell pedigrees, *Exp. Cell Res.*, 103, 247 1976.
11. Collins, V. P., Arro, E., Blomquist, E., Brunk, U., Frederikson, B. A., and Westermark, B., Cell locomotion and proliferation in relation to available surface area, serum concentration and culture age, *Scann. Electr. Microsc.*, 111, 411, 1979.
12. Blomquist, E., Arro, E., Brunk, U., and Westermark, B., Plasma membrane motility of cultured human glia cells in phase II and III, *Act. Path. Micr. Scand. Sect. A*, 86, 257, 1978.
13. Macieira-Coelho, A., Chromatin reorganization during senescence of proliferating cells, *Mutat. Res.*, 256, 81, 1991.
14. Bowman, P. D. and Daniel, C. W., Aging of human fibroblasts in vitro, surface features and behaviour of aging WI-38 cells, *Mech. Ageing Dev.*, 4, 147, 1975.
15. Wang, E. and Gundersen, D., Increased organization of cytoskeleton accompanying the aging of human fibroblasts in vitro, *Exp. Cell Res.*, 154, 191, 1984.

16. Raes, M. and Remacle, J., Alteration of the microtubule organization in aging WI-38 fibroblasts. A comparative study with embryonic hamster lung fibroblasts, *Exp. Gerontol.*, 22, 47, 1978.

17. Raes, M., Genens, G., de Brabander, M., and Remacle, J., Microtubules and microfilaments in ageing hamster embryo fibroblasts in vitro, *Exp. Gerontol.*, 18, 241, 1983.

18. Anderson, P. J., Actin in young and senescent fibroblasts, *Biochem. J.*, 169, 169, 1978.

19. Wang, E., Are cross-bridging structures involved in the bundle formation of intermediate filaments and the decrease in locomotion that accompany cell aging?, *J. Cell Biol.*, 100, 1466, 1985.

20. Van Gansen, P., Siebertz, B., Capone, B., and Malherbe, L., Relationship between cytoplasmic-microtubular complex, DNA synthesis and cell morphology in mouse embryonic fibroblasts (effects of age, serum deprivation, aphidicolin, cytochalasin B and colchicine), *Biol. Cell.*, 52, 161, 1984.

21. Soukopova, M. and Holeckova, E., The latent period of explanted organs of new born adult and senile rats, *Exp. Cell Res.*, 33, 361, 1964.

22. Muggleton-Harris, A. L., Reisert, P. S., and Burgoff, R. L., In vitro characterization of response to stimulus (wounding) with regard to ageing in human skin fibroblasts, *Mech. Ageing Dev.*, 19, 37, 1982.

23. Alarcon, C., Valverde, I., and Malaisse, W. J., Transglutaminase and cellular motile events: retardation of proinsulin conversion by glycine methylester, *Biosci. Rep.*, E, 581, 1985.

24. Macieira-Coelho, A. and Azzarone, B., Correlation between contractility and proliferation in human fibroblasts, *J. Cell. Phys.*, 142, 610, 1990.

25. Macieira-Coelho, A. and Avrameas, S., Modulation of cell behavior in vitro by the substratum in fibroblastic and leukemic mouse cell lines, *Proc. Natl. Acad. Sc. U.S.A.*, 69, 2469, 1972.

26. Macieira-Coelho, A., Berumen, L., and Avrameas, S., Properties of protein polymers as substratum for cell growth in vitro, *J. Cell. Phys.*, 83, 379, 1974.

27. Wahrmann, J. P., Delain, D., Bournoutian, C., and Macieira-Coelho, A., Modulation of differentiation in vitro. I. Influence of the attachment surface on myogenesis, *In Vitro*, 17, 752, 1981.

28. Sénéchal, H., Wahrmann, J. P., Delain, D., and Macieira-Coelho, A., Modulation of differentiation in vitro. II. Influence of cell spreading and surface events on myogenesis, *In Vitro*, 20, 692, 1984.

29. Macieira-Coelho, A. and Avrameas, S., Protein polymers as a substratum for the modulation of cell proliferation in vitro, in *Tissue Culture: Methods and Applications*, Kruze, P. F., Jr. and Patterson, M. K., Eds., Academic Press, New York, 1973, Sect. VII.

30. Bouvier, D., Hubert, J., Seve, A. P., and Bouteille, M., Characterization of lamina-bound chromatin in the nuclear shell isolated from HeLa cells, *Exp. Cell Res.*, 156, 500, 1985.

31. Gerace, L., Structural proteins in the eukaryotic nucleus, *Nature*, 318, 508, 1985.

32. Hay, M. and Deboni, U., Chromatin motion in neuronal interphase nuclei — changes induced by disruption of intermediate filaments, *Cell Motil. Cytoskeleton*, 18, 63, 1991.

33. Macieira-Coelho, A., *Biology of Normal Proliferating Cells in Vitro. Relevance for in Vivo Aging*, S. Karger, New York, 1988, chap. 6.

34. Macieira-Coelho, A., Cancer and aging at the cellular level, in *Cancer and Aging*, Macieira-Coelho, A. and Nordenskjöld, B., Eds., CRC Press, Boca Raton, FL, chap. 1.

Chapter 10

THE AGING OF THE NEURONAL CYTOSKELETON

P. Klosen and Ph. van den Bosch de Aguilar

CONTENTS

0-8493-4786-6/95/$0.00+$.50
© 1995 by CRC Press, Inc.

I. INTRODUCTION

The shape of living cells is supported by an intricate inner scaffolding of fibers which make up the cytoskeleton. As early as the beginning of this century, silver impregnation techniques allowed histologists to visualize a network of filaments crisscrossing the cytoplasm and extending into cellular processes. Since then, electron microscopy and biochemical techniques have greatly increased our knowledge of the cytoskeleton. The neuronal cytoskeleton, like that of most mammalian cells, is composed of three biochemically, morphologically, and functionally distinct systems: microfilaments, intermediate filaments, and microtubules (Table 1). These interacting organelles do not restrict themselves to a static, "skeletal" function. They also act as cellular "muscles" and a cellular "vascular" system.

A. Microfilaments

Microfilaments have a diameter of 4 to 6 nm and are composed of actin. As actin is a highly conserved protein, a whole family of actin-associated proteins (AAPs) confers specialized functions to these actin

TABLE 1.

The Cytoskeleton

Filament system	Ø (nm)	Main protein	Cell type	Associated proteins
Microfilaments	4–6	Actin	All cells	Spectrin, filamin, gelsolin, myosin, tropomyosin, synapsin, etc.
Intermediate filaments	8–12	Vimentin	Mesenchyme, glia	
		Cytokeratins	Epithelia	
		Desmin	Muscle	
		GFAP	Glia	
		Neurofilament	Neurons	
		α-Internexin	Neurons	
		Peripherin	Neurons	
		Nestin	Neurons	
		Lamins	All cells (nuclei)	
Microtubules	25	α,β-Tubulin	All cells	MAPs, STOP, tau, kinesin, dynein, etc.

filaments according to the needs of individual cells.[1] The 42-kDa actin monomers (G-actin) polymerize into double-helical filaments (F-actin). This polymerization is dependent on ATP hydrolysis. Actin polymerization is a very dynamic process controlled mostly by actin-associated proteins such as profilin (G-actin sequestering) and gelsolin (filament nucleating). Other AAPs such as spectrin and myosin cross-link existing filaments into a network. Ankyrin and spectrin anchor actin filaments to the plasma membrane and to other cellular organelles. Myosin is the motor of cell motility by a sliding filament mechanism. Motility can also appear from transitions between the gel and the sol state of actin filaments interacting with other cytoskeletal filaments and the cell membrane. Through these mechanisms, actin filaments are involved in cell motility, adhesion, membrane stability, determination of cell shape, exocytosis, and cytokinesis.[2] Microfilaments, therefore, act simultaneously as the cell "skeleton and muscles".

As the organelle in charge of cell motility, microfilaments are involved in the migration of neurons from the neuroepithelium to their final location during development. Microfilament-based motility of filopodes and lamellipodes at the level of the growth cones also controls the migration of the axon towards its target. Exocytosis in the form of neurotransmitter secretion is another example of microfilament function in neurons.[3] Finally, as the major component of the plasma membrane-associated cytoskeleton, actin filaments are also responsible for the specific positioning of ion channels and receptors in the neuronal membrane.[4]

B. Intermediate Filaments

Neurofilaments, the neuronal intermediate filaments, are the molecular substrate of the silver impregnation techniques. Their name stems from their 10-nm-diameter size, intermediate between the 4- to 6-nm microfilaments and the 25-nm microtubules. They are composed of a family of proteins characterized by a tissue-specific expression and divided into six types (Table 2).[5,6] All types are characterized by a central alpha-helical domain of about 40 kDa. Unlike microfilaments and microtubules, the properties of intermediate filaments are determined by their amino- and carboxy-terminal domains, rather than by associated proteins. They form very stable filaments and most probably represent the cell's mechanical skeleton. Several neuronal intermediate filament proteins have been identified. The classical neurofilament triplet is composed by three type IV intermediate filament peptides of 68-kDa (NF-L), 160-kDa (NF-M), and 200-kDa (NF-H) molecular weight. A fourth type IV neuronal intermediate filament peptide of 66 kDa, α-internexin, has recently been identified.[7] Along with the type III vimentin intermediate filament peptide, these type IV intermediate filament peptides can be found in most neurons. The type

TABLE 2.

Intermediate Filament Types

Type	IF proteins	MW (kDa)
I	Acid keratins	40–56
II	Neutral-basic keratins	53–67
III	Vimentin	57
	Desmin	53–54
	GFAP	50
	Peripherin	57
IV	NF-L	68
	NF-M	160
	NF-H	200
	α-Internexin	66
V	Lamin A	70
	Lamin B	67
	Lamin C	60
VI	Nestin	240

III peripherin protein is expressed primarily in the peripheral nervous system. Finally, the recently described type VI nestin intermediate filament peptide is restricted to *neuro-*epithelial *st*em cells, from which its name derives.[8]

Being involved in the maintenance of cell shape, neuronal intermediate filaments are in charge of sustaining the specific interactions between neurons through their dendrites and axons. The mechanical strains that act upon axons running from the motoneuron cell body in the lumbar spinal cord down through the leg to muscles located in the calf illustrate the importance of such a mechanical support to neurons.

C. Microtubules

Microtubules, the third cytoskeletal component, are hollow tubes of 25 nm diameter formed by protofilaments composed of alpha and beta tubulin heterodimers. Like actin, the tubulins are highly conserved proteins and microtubule functionality is thus modulated by a family of associated proteins to adapt the microtubule cytoskeleton to the needs of different cell types. These proteins are called MAPs, for microtubule-associated proteins.[9-11] The diversity of both tubulin isoforms and MAPs is highest in the brain, illustrating the importance of microtubules in neurons. Three main functions are executed by MAPs: microtubule stabilization, microtubule cross-linking, and organelle transport along microtubules. Like actin filaments, microtubules are mostly unstable filaments whose polymerization is often characterized as a dynamic equilibrium controlled by the concentration of tubulin monomers, GTP and calcium, as well as MAPs like the tau protein. The recently discovered gamma-tubulin acts as microtubule nucleating protein.[12,13] This protein, whose concentration in individual cells is extremely low, is located in the microtubule organizing center (MTOC). The MTOC is an area normally located close to the nucleus from which microtubules irradiate throughout the cytoplasm. It is noteworthy that intermediate filaments also seem to irradiate from this area. However, the interaction of intermediate filaments with the MTOC has not been studied so far.

Microtubules are involved in the initial stages of neurite extension during development, as well as in the stabilization of dendrites and axons. However, the main function of microtubules in neurons, as well as in other cells, is to support intracellular transport.[14-16] Indeed, they serve as transport rails along which vesicular organelles like mitochondria and secretory vesicles are transported between different cellular compartments. The motors of this transport mechanism are kinesin and cytoplasmic dynein (termed MAP1c).[14,17] This role is particularly important in neurons due to the axons' incapacity of nonmitochondrial protein synthesis. Axonal transport is thus indispensable for the survival of axons, which may be up to 1 m in length in humans. These intracellular transports are probably also involved in the organization of the cytoplasm into several functional domains (dendrites, cell body, and axon). Furthermore, synaptic function depends on vesicles, enzymes, and neurotransmitters transported by anterograde axonal transport. Retrograde axonal transport carries neurotrophic factors from the target to the cell bodies. These neurotrophic factors are essential to neuronal survival and to maintain a functional phenotype.

Microfilaments, intermediate filaments, and microtubules collaborate in the tasks they execute in neurons. As already shown, there are many functional and physical interactions between these three systems. Some of their functions, like migration and the neurite extension, are executed only during development. However, most of the cytoskeletal tasks are essential to the adult, fully differentiated neuron. Aging of the cytoskeleton may impair these functions and thus compromise neuronal performance.

II. CYTOLOGICAL ALTERATIONS OF THE CYTOSKELETON IN AGING

Aging is of particular interest to neurobiologists because neurons are postmitotic cells and cannot be replaced if they degenerate. Changes occurring in neurons during aging are thus also likely to permanently influence their performance. Many neuronal "cytoskeletal" alterations have been described since the beginning of this century. They are filamentous inclusions that are thought to derive from the cytoskeleton. It should be noted that for some of these alterations a cytoskeletal origin has not been clearly demonstrated. Also many of these changes are associated with neurodegenerative diseases. In this chapter we will describe some of these cytoskeletal changes which do also occur spontaneously during aging, albeit at a much lower frequency than in pathological states.

A. The Neurofibrillary Tangle

The neurofibrillary tangle (NFT) is the hallmark alteration of Alzheimer's disease. Although mostly associated with this pathology, NFTs occur also in healthy aged humans.[18] NFTs are classically visualized by silver impregnations. They appear as flame-shaped, filamentous perikaryal inclusions that often displace the nucleus to the periphery of the cell. Extracellular NFTs, also called ghost tangles, are the remains of these neurons after they have degenerated. Ultrastructurally, NFTs are compact bundles of paired helical filaments or PHFs.[19] Two 8- to 10-nm filaments twisted with a periodicity of 80 nm make up these PHFs. The size of these filaments led to the premature conclusion that they are derived from neurofilaments. Although early studies with antineurofilament antisera and monoclonal antibodies seemed to confirm this view,[20-22] PHF turned out to be composed mainly of the MAP tau.[23-26] The PHF tau is ubiquitinated and abnormally phosphorylated.[27-29] PHFs can also be found in the dystrophic neurites surrounding senile plaques. Here, they often completely fill the neurites, which are also distended by the accumulation of vesicles and mitochondria. No normal microtubules can be found at this level of the dystrophic neurites, indicating a breakdown of axonal transport. The presence of β-amyloid precursor protein (β-APP) epitopes on NFTs has been a subject of controversy until recently.[30]

NFTs can be found in 81% of people autopsied between 60 and 70 years, and in 99% of those over 70 years old.[18] Senile plaques with PHFs in the surrounding neurites are also common in healthy aged humans. NFTs have also been described in aged bears.[31] These tangles were positive for MAP tau, NF-H, and PHF-related antigens (Alz-50). Senile plaques with neurites immunopositive for Alz-50 were also present in these aged bears. While NFTs have only been observed in these bears and humans, senile plaques have been detected in aged monkeys and dogs.[18,32] However, while NFTs and the neurites surrounding senile plaques in animals sometimes display a similar immunochemical profile to their human counterparts, they never contain PHFs similar to those observed in humans.

B. The Hirano Body

The Hirano body is an eosinophilic, usually rod-shaped inclusion originally described in Parkinson-dementia complex of Guam.[33] The Hirano body is commonly present in neurons of nondemented old individuals, but is found in increasing numbers in a variety of pathological conditions, including Alzheimer's disease.[34,35] Hirano bodies are normally located in the cell body and proximal dendrites in neurons. However, they can also be found in axons and glial cells.[36-39]

Upon ultrastructural examination, Hirano bodies appear as para-crystalline inclusions. They are made of sheets of 6- to 10-nm filaments with granular material between the sheets. This classical appearance is often characterized as "beads on a string". The exact tridimensional structure has been a matter of controversy for some time.[40-43] However, using high-voltage electron microscopy on thick sections, Galloway et al.[44] have shown that the "beads" could be transformed into filaments by changing the angle at which the section is observed. Therefore, Hirano bodies appear to be composed of stacked sheets of parallel filaments, with the orientation of the filaments changing by 90° from one sheet to the next one.

Hirano bodies are composed of F-actin and the actin-associated proteins α-actinin, vinculin, and tropomyosin.[44] Hippocampal Hirano bodies, at least, appear to contain epitopes recognized by antibodies directed against the human NF-M protein.[45] Only about 20% of Hirano bodies also react with antibodies to the MAP tau.[46] Recently, Munoz et al.[47] showed that Hirano bodies accumulate C-terminal sequences of the β-amyloid precursor protein (β-APP). Thus, it appears that the Hirano body probably originates from alterations in the metabolism of microfilament protein, and later modification of the Hirano body may add NF-M, MAP-tau, and β-APP sequences to this core structure. As these last three types of antigens have only been assayed in hippocampal Hirano bodies in aging and in Alzheimer's disease, it might be interesting to determine whether Hirano bodies in other locations, pathological conditions, and glial cells have a similar immunochemical profile.

C. The Lewy Body

The Lewy body is the hallmark lesion of Parkinson's disease. Again, as for the Alzheimer neurofibrillary tangles, Lewy bodies can also be found in old patients without neurological disturbances, although in smaller numbers than in neurological diseases. The Lewy body is composed of densely packed 8- to 10-nm filaments which, at the center of the inclusion, often form a homogeneous granular mass.

Immunocytochemistry allowed the identification of neurofilament antigens,[48-51] as well as ubiquitin, in Lewy bodies.[52] MAP tau and tropomyosin have only been found in Lewy body disease and not in Parkinson's.[53,54] The presence of other MAPs in the Lewy body remains to be clarified.[49,50,52,55]

D. Other Filamentous Inclusions

A variety of other filamentous inclusions have been observed sporadically in aging. They appear as "tangles" of normal neurofilaments, which can be very tightly packed and arranged in a paracrystal. Some of these filament crystals are associated with granular material in the granulofilamentous body. These inclusions can be located in the cell body or the axon. They are less frequent in the dendrites. The less densely packed inclusions appear to be continuous with the normal cytoskeleton and resemble the accumulations of neurofilaments observed in axonal spheroids in a variety of diseases, like amyotrophic lateral sclerosis,[56] motor neuron disease,[57] giant axonal neuropathy,[58] and intoxications by chemical agents (for review see Reference 59). When located in the axon, these inclusions are often called "spheroids". These spheroids are typical of motor neuron disease and hexacarbon intoxications, but are also observed in healthy patients.[57,60] In the cell body, these inclusions appear similar to Alzheimer neurofibrillary tangles. However, these "tangles" should not be confused with Alzheimer neurofibrillary tangles, as they do not contain paired helical filaments and are composed by morphologically normal neurofilaments.[56,61] Similar accumulations of intermediate filaments can be observed in nonneuronal cells like Mallory bodies in alcoholic liver disease (cytokeratins), desmin accumulations in congenital myopathies, and Rosenthal fibers in astrocytomas (GFAP and vimentin) (for review see Reference 62).

As has been suspected by their ultrastructural appearance, immunocytochemistry has shown the neuronal inclusions to be made up mainly of neurofilaments.[63-65] In motor neurons, they also contain the peripheral neurofilament protein, peripherin.[66] Their phosphorylation state is apparently normal for axonal neurofilaments.[60,65,67] However, they present these axonal phosphorylation characteristics also when located in the cell body.[60,65] Some of these neurofilament tangles are also immunoreactive for ubiquitin, but interestingly, the ubiquitin immunoreactive inclusions are not detected with antibodies to neurofilament or peripherin.[66,68-70] As these accumulations of neurofilaments can be induced by agents cross-linking neurofilaments (carbon disulfide, acrylamide, and iminodipropionitrile) or interfering with axonal transport mechanisms (colchicine, maytansine, aluminum, etc.), their presence in normal aging may be due either to exposure to low levels of environmental toxins or to breakdown of axonal transports in some neurons.

E. Granulovacuolar Bodies

Like all the previously described alterations, the granulovacuolar body is an inclusion frequently seen in diseases like Alzheimer, but which is also present in normal aging at a lower frequency.[71,72] The number of cells with granulovacuolar bodies and the number of granulovacuolar bodies per cell in the hippocampus correlates with the severity of dementia.[71,72] Unlike the previously described alterations, granulovacuolar bodies do not appear as filamentous inclusions. They are membrane-bound cytoplasmic vacuoles with an electron-lucent matrix and an electron-dense granular body. They are considered to be derived from cellular autophagic mechanisms.[18,73] Immunocytochemistry has shown tubulin,[74] neurofilaments,[75,76] MAP tau, [77,78] and ubiquitin[79] to be associated with the granule in the granulovacuolar body.

III. MOLECULAR ALTERATIONS OF THE CYTOSKELETON DURING AGING

In view of the many molecular data generated by the research on cytoskeletal alterations in neurodegenerative diseases, it is surprising to note that relatively few data are available on normal aging of the cytoskeleton. The brain, if not afflicted by one of these diseases, actually ages pretty well and neurons display a remarkable plasticity even in advanced ages. This neuronal plasticity involves sprouting responses and establishment of new connections, two processes involving the cytoskeleton. This observation may explain the paucity of molecular data on the aging of the neuronal cytoskeleton. However, a few studies managed to locate certain subtle alterations in neuronal cytoskeletal metabolism. Again, these studies often started from pathological observations.

A. Microtubule-Associated Protein Tau and the Alz-50 Epitope

As described in the previous section, the MAP tau is an essential component of Alzheimer neurofibrillary tangles and the paired helical filaments. It can also be found in some Hirano and Lewy bodies. Alz-50 is a monoclonal antibody raised against brain homogenates from patients with Alzheimer's disease.[80] This antibody stains neurons and neurites in various stages of Alzheimer's disease.[81,82] Alz-50 has been shown to recognize MAP tau on Western blots.[83,84] The epitope recognized by Alz-50 in tau has been localized in the N-terminal part of this protein.[85] This epitope is apparently not exposed in most neurons in normal brain tissue. It can, however, be detected in neurons in the areas affected by Alzheimer's disease before these neurons display neurofibrillary tangles.[81] Similarly, abnormally phosphorylated tau in the cell body precedes the formation of neurofibrillary tangles.[86]

These observations have led to the hypothesis that the Alz-50 epitope and abnormally phosphorylated tau without neurofibrillary tangles might be markers of early disorganization of the cytoskeleton and neuronal death in diseases and normal aging.[81,86,87] As the Alz-50 epitope can also be detected in certain neuronal subpopulations during development, some authors have even extended this hypothesis to programmed neuronal death in development.[87,88] However, several studies have shown that certain neuronal populations, particularly in the hypothalamus and the striatum, express the Alz-50 epitope in the absence of pathological alterations.[89-93] Thus, it appears that the presence of the Alz-50 epitope is not necessarily correlated with degenerative changes.

Recent studies by Benzing et al.[94,95] have shown that dystrophic neurites containing accumulated neurotransmitters precede the appearance of Alz-50 and paired helical filaments in senile plaques in both Alzheimer and healthy aged patients. With the exception of certain defined neuronal populations, the appearance of abnormal forms of MAP tau in both cell bodies and neurites thus seems to precede the formation of cytological alterations of the cytoskeleton, both in normal aging and disease.[81,86]

B. Ubiquitin

Just like MAP tau, ubiquitin appears as a common constituent of many cytological alterations of the cytoskeleton observed during aging and disease. Ubiquitin is a 76-residue protein which is found throughout the animal and plant kingdoms.[96] This protein can be covalently conjugated to other intracellular proteins, a process that induces the selective proteolytic degradation of these protein-ubiquitin conjugates. However, some ubiquitin-protein conjugates are relatively stable, indicating that ubiquitin is also involved in regulatory processes more selective and specific than the destruction of defective proteins.[97] In particular, ubiquitin seems to be associated with the microtubule network in certain cells.[98] Several MAPs have been identified as the proteins carrying the ubiquitin tag in these microtubules.[97,98] However, the principal proteins composing cytoskeletal alterations are not normally conjugated to ubiquitin.

Ubiquitin is also a common component of intermediate filament inclusion bodies.[68] A common hypothesis for this ubiquitination is that it is a reaction of the cell to these inclusions.[29,99,100] Somehow, these inclusions appear to avoid proteolysis after conjugation with ubiquitin. This may be due to a deficit in the ubiquitin proteolytic pathway or to an intrinsic resistance of these conjugates to proteolysis. A role of ubiquitin in the formation of these inclusions has also been postulated.[29] However, ubiquitin immunoreactivity is often associated with inclusions that cannot be detected with antibodies to the normal constituent proteins and which also often display abnormal filament diameters.[66,68-70] This may indicate that ubiquitination occurs after the formation of the inclusions. Particularly in Alzheimer neurofibrillary tangles, abnormal phosphorylation precedes ubiquitination of MAP tau.[101] Ubiquitin can also be observed in dystrophic neurites in inclusion bodies, which display no filamentous features.[102]

Although ubiquitin involvement in cytoskeletal alterations is thus mostly analyzed in terms of dysfunctional proteolytic degradation of these proteins, regulation mechanisms of the cytoskeleton by ubiquitination constitute an alternative explanation.[97] However, so far these regulatory mechanisms of the cytoskeleton by ubiquitin are not known well enough to propose a detailed hypothesis of action. Also, protease inhibition in animal models of aging (see below) seems to comfort the hypothesis of a dysfunction of the ubiquitin-initiated proteolytic pathway.[103-105]

C. Alterations of Microtubules and Axonal Transport

Microtubules are the tracks along which vesicular material is rapidly transported along the axon. Anterograde transport is achieved by ATP-dependent translocation of vesicles by kinesin, a protein which binds both microtubules and vesicles.[15,16] Upon binding to the microtubule, a conformational change of kinesin pushes the attached vesicle along the microtubule. After detaching from the microtubule, this cycle can be repeated. Retrograde transport is achieved in a similar fashion with the ATPase MAP1c or brain dynein.[16,106] It has been known for some time that a slowing of the rate of fast axonal transport can be observed in aging animals.[107-111] More recently, these biochemical observations have been confirmed by direct measurement of vesicular transport rates by video-enhanced-contrast microscopy.[112] These authors also showed that large vesicles are more affected by this reduction in transport rates than small vesicles. It is noteworthy that while this last study and most of the biochemical studies demonstrated a generalized reduction of fast axonal transport rates, we have been able to show that only the fast transported G4 form of acetylcholinesterase is slowed during aging.[111] The transport rate of the A12 acetylcholinesterase form, which is also rapidly transported, is not slowed. This observation, as well as the vesicle size dependence on transport rate reduction, shows that this reduction of fast axonal transport rates is more subtle and that further studies are necessary to assess even the simple kinetic parameters of the aging of axonal transport.

Similar to the reduction of fast axonal transport, slow axonal transport of cytoskeletal proteins is also slowed during aging.[113-115] As the mechanisms of this slow axonal transport are not yet fully understood,[116,117] the reasons for this reduced slow axonal transport remain unexplained so far. Considering the mechanism of fast axonal transport, it is evident that the reason for the reduced transport rates may be independent from the cytoskeleton. As this transport is ATP dependent, mitochondrial aging could lead to reduced levels of ATP. Also, the mechanisms by which kinesin or dynein bind to vesicles may be impaired at the level of these vesicles. However, a few subtle changes have been observed in the organization and composition of the axonal microtubule network. Hinds and McNelly[118] have described a reduction in the number of axonal microtubules in the olfactory bulb. This reduction could account for reduced transport rates. Microtubules assembled from brain extracts of old rats have a much greater tendency to form microtubules with 14 instead of the usual 13 protofilaments.[119] This altered microtubule assembly is connected at least partially to increased proteolytic degradation of MAPs. Several studies have shown an increase of the insoluble proportion of tubulin.[120-122] Furthermore, Fifkova and Morales[123] have been able to detect an increase in the acetylation of cold/Ca^{2+}-stable tubulin fraction. Interestingly, Tashiro and Komiya[115] showed a decrease in the transport rate and in the proportion of the insoluble form of tubulin. The loss of insoluble tubulin has been attributed to proteolytic degradation of severely retarded insoluble proteins. This study appears to contradict the results of the previous studies. However, the methods used to distinguish between insoluble and soluble tubulin are different. Further studies with standardized methods will be necessary to clarify these observations. So far, these molecular changes of tubulin have not been related to the functional changes observed in fast axonal transport.

IV. EXPERIMENTAL MODELS OF AGING

By definition, aging is a spontaneous phenomenon and should not need an experimental model to be studied. However, even in rodents, obtaining animals old enough to compare to human aging takes more time than most researchers would like. Also, one of the major problems is the distinction between so-called "normal" aging, which results from normal biological processes, and the various pathologies that can accompany aging, thus clouding its normal manifestations. Finally, environmental factors modulate the course of the "normal" aging process. "Experimental" models of aging often try to speed up the normal process or to analyze certain environmental or pathological factors influencing this process.

While there are some genetic models such as the senescence-accelerated mouse model,[124,125] most of these models have not been analyzed in terms of aging of the cytoskeleton. In this part of the review, we will describe three models that have generated data on the aging of the neurocytoskeleton. The first is our longitudinal study of the aging of the dorsal root ganglion in the Wistar Louvain rat. The two other are original experimental approaches.

A. Aging of the Dorsal Root Ganglion (DRG) in the Wistar Louvain Rat

We have used the Wistar Louvain strain to analyze the aging of the spinal ganglion and its microenvironment. The Wistar Louvain rat strain has been reared at the University of Louvain since about 1920. These rats show no specific pathology as compared to the other Wistar strains. However, their body weight is stable throughout their adult life. Also, they already display a 50% mortality rate at 24 months of age (33 to 36 for standard Wistar rats) and reach 90% mortality by 30 months of age (39 to 42 for standard Wistar rats). Interestingly, the mortality rates are comparable to those of normal Wistar rats when Wistar Louvain rats are reared in specific pathogen-free conditions.

Up to 24 months of age, no particular changes of the neurocytoskeleton are observed in DRG of Wistar Louvain rats. The only alteration observed was a progressive accumulation of lipofuscin.[126,127] However, after 24 months of age, many filamentous inclusions appear in the cell body and the nerve fibers. In nerve fibers, densely packed accumulations of normal neurofilaments resemble the spheroids described previously. Some Hirano bodies are also seen, but in Schwann cells. At the level of the cell body, these "cytoskeletal" changes affect mainly the large A-type neurons, which are characterized by an abundant perikaryal cytoskeleton. These inclusions are mostly nematosomes, granulofilamentous bodies, and Hirano bodies. Nematosomes are spherical inclusions that comprise numerous interwoven filamentous threads of electron-dense material. Although fibrillar in appearance, they are apparently not derived from the cytoskeleton. Granulofilamentous bodies are ovoid or spherical inclusions made by dense granules intermingled with filamentous deposits whose exact nature remains to be established. We also observed two more peculiar inclusions — tubular bodies and paired helical filament-like inclusions.[128] Tubular bodies are composed of closely packed tubular structures. While some of these inclusions clearly display tubules with a diameter comparable to microtubules, some sections of larger tubular bodies progressively change with orientation to the typical aspect of Hirano bodies. PHF-like inclusions are composed of regularly arranged filaments that resemble PHFs observed in normal human aging and in Alzheimer's disease. However, the half period of the PHF helix is only 40 nm, compared to the 80 nm observed in humans. Similar inclusions have been observed in human pinealomas.[129] At low magnification, these inclusions closely resemble Hirano bodies or tubular bodies, which has led us to postulate that these three types of inclusions are merely different materializations of the same cytoskeletal alteration.

We have been able to confirm all these alterations with an identical time-course in the mesencephalic nucleus of the trigeminal nerve (Mes V), which is embryologically and functionally a dorsal root ganglion that did not migrate into the peripheral nervous system.[130] This observation shows that aging in this particular neuronal type apparently is not influenced by the presence of the blood-brain barrier. It has been suggested that peripheral nervous system neurons should be more sensitive to aging because they are more exposed to environmental influences. Although we have no data on the conditions of the blood-brain barrier in our rats aged 24 months or more, one can assume that the presence of this barrier, at least in young animals, should have protected Mes V neurons and thus delayed the changes relative to those in DRG neurons. Furthermore, aging alterations of the cytoskeleton and other organelles appear with a similar time-course in the DRG and the Mes V in normal and specific pathogen-free-raised Wistar Louvain rats, although the latter display a longer life span.[131]

Immunocytochemical studies in the DRG and the Mes V have proven difficult, as both DRG and Mes V A type neurons are known to contain phosphorylated neurofilament epitopes in the cell body. These interfere with the detection of human PHF-specific epitopes.[132,133] The alterations described above appear almost exclusively in A-type neurons, which have a very prominent cytoskeleton[134] and present a spontaneous phosphorylation of neurofilaments in the cell body.[135-137] This neurofilament phosphorylation is normally restricted to axons, but occurs in the cell body in neurodegenerative diseases[138-140] and after axotomy.[141,142] The particular cytoskeleton of these neurons could predispose them to developing cytoskeletal alterations during aging.

B. "Mini-Brains" in Peripheral Nerve

While studying the differentiation of fetal brain tissue transplanted into predegenerated peripheral nerve, Doering and Aguayo[143] noted several changes in the cytoskeleton of long-term (6 to 12 months) transplants. Hirano bodies appeared in neurons that had up to then differentiated almost as normally as they would *in situ*. Furthermore, perikaryal immunolabeling for phosphorylated NF-H developed in the transplanted neurons.[143,144] Phosphorylation of neurofilaments is usually restricted to axons.[145,146] The presence of phosphorylated NF-H epitopes has been described in a variety of neurological diseases[138-140,147-149] and after axotomy, both in the peripheral[150-153] and the central nervous system.[141,142] In long-term transplants, loss of MAP2 immunoreactivity could also be detected.[154] This latter change is probably related to changes in dendritic morphology. Regression of dendrites has also been observed in aging and disease.[155,156]

In a more recent study, Doering [157] also described abnormal "curly" nerve fibers that were immunopositive for MAP tau.

Adrenal medulla cografts prevented abnormal cytoskeletal changes and degeneration in long-term substantia nigra grafts.[158] A similar result was obtained with cografts of hippocampus and septum.[157] These two studies illustrate the importance of adequate target interaction in the maintenance of a normal cytoskeletal phenotype. A dysregulation of these target interactions could thus be responsible for cytoskeletal alterations in aging and disease. Aging of neurons and their cytoskeleton could be influenced by the aging of their central and peripheral target structures.

C. Ubiquitin and Protease Inhibitors

Several observations led to the development of an aging model based on inhibition of normal proteolytic pathways. First, as described in the previous sections, ubiquitin is a common component of many cytoskeletal alterations. Although the presence of ubiquitin might not necessarily be linked to an attempt to degrade these inclusions, this hypothesis remains plausible. Second, one of the abnormally processed molecules in Alzheimer's disease is the Alzheimer amyloid precursor protein (APP). Several isoforms of this transmembrane protein are produced in the brain. Two isoforms, APP 751 and APP 770, contain an insert that is homologous to a Kunitz serine protease inhibitor.[159,160]

Leupeptin is a potent inhibitor of both lysosomial and cytoplasmic Ca^{2+}-activated neutral cysteine proteases (calpains).[161-163] Administration of this protease inhibitor led to an increase in ubiquitin immunoreactivity in cerebellar Purkinje cells.[104,105] These same cells also were immunopositive for MAP tau with antibodies generated against human formic acid denatured PHF.[103] Antibodies to NF-L and NF-H revealed an increased perikaryal immunoreactivity as well as large bulbous protrusions in the axons of Purkinje cells.[164,165] The administration of leupeptin also induced the formation of lipofuscin deposits similar to those observed in normal aging.[103]

These observations clearly establish that an inhibition of proteolytic processes can produce alterations of the cytoskeleton resembling those observed in aging and disease. Alterations of lysosomial cathepsins have also been described in Alzheimer's disease.[166,167]

V. CONCLUSIONS

The multiple vital functions of the neuronal cytoskeleton make it a prime target for alterations during aging and pathologies. The changes observed in aging and disease are mostly the same. However, these alterations affect a considerably higher number of neurons in diseases. In normal aging, only a very limited number of neurons display an abnormal cytoskeleton. Even at the molecular level, the changes that can be observed are only minor and mostly very subtle. Thus, neurons, and particularly their cytoskeleton, do actually age very well. They display a considerable amount of functional plasticity even in advanced age. This plasticity is reduced only in very old patients.[155,156] Interestingly, even in very old (over 24 months of age) Wistar Louvain rats, a strong spontaneous regeneration of nerve fibers can be observed in peripheral nerves.[131] Given their apparent handicap of being postmitotic, these observations show that many neurons conserve a remarkable potential to readapt to a changing environment.

Among the molecular changes that can be observed, ubiquitin and MAP tau should be analyzed further. Many cytoskeletal alterations can be associated with these two molecules. As the ubiquitin presence in many inclusions and the ubiquitin model of aging illustrate, many changes may be due to the dysregulation of cellular mechanisms of elimination of faulty proteins.

Thus far, experimental models do not allow us to choose among extrinsic or intrinsic factors for the control of neuronal aging. The cograft experiments of Doering and Tokiwa[158] and Doering[157] show that appropriate target connections are important to maintain a normal cytoskeleton. On the other hand, our observations on the aging of dorsal root ganglion and mesencephalic trigeminal neurons indicate that aging of these particular neurons apparently is not influenced by the presence or absence of a blood-brain barrier or by a normal or a specific pathogen-free environment. However, our observations could also indicate that the aging of the peripheral targets controls the aging of the innervating neurons. Target-derived trophic influences are also of prime importance in the maintenance of a normal phenotype in nonaged, adult neurons.[168-170] Further experiments will thus have to clarify the involvement of intrinsic and extrinsic factors in aging.

REFERENCES

1. Weber, K. and Osborn, M., The molecules of the cell matrix, *Sci. Am.*, 253, 92, 1985.
2. Darnell, J. E., Lodish, H., and Baltimore, D., *Molecular Cell Biology*, Scientific American Books, New York, 1990, chap. 22.
3. Cheek, T. R. and Burgoyne, R. D., Cytoskeleton in secretion and neurotransmitter release, in *The Neuronal Cytoskeleton*, Burgoyne, R. D., Ed., Wiley-Liss, New York, 1991, 309.

4. Baines A. J., Neuronal plasma membrane associated cytoskeleton, in *The Neuronal Cytoskeleton*, Burgoyne, R. D., Ed., Wiley-Liss, New York, 1991, 161.
5. Fliegner, K. H. and Liem, R. K. H., Cellular and molecular biology of neuronal intermediate filaments, *Int. Rev. Cytol.*, 131, 109, 1991.
6. Albers, K. and Fuchs, E., The molecular biology of intermediate filament proteins, *Int. Rev. Cytol.*, 134, 243, 1992.
7. Fliegner, K. H., Ching, G. Y., and Liem, R. K. H., The predicted amino acid sequence of alpha-internexin is that of a novel neuronal intermediate filament protein, *EMBO J.*, 9, 749, 1990.
8. Lendahl, U., Zimmerman, L. B., and McKay, R. D. G., CNS stem cells express a new class of intermediate filament protein, *Cell*, 60, 585, 1990.
9. Black, M. M. and Kurdyla, J. T., Microtubule-associated proteins of neurons, *J. Cell Biol.*, 97, 1020, 1983.
10. Wiche, G., High-Mr microtubule-associated proteins. Properties and functions, *Biochem. J.*, 259, 1, 1989.
11. Riederer, B. M., Some aspects of the neuronal cytoskeleton in development, *Eur. J. Morphol.*, 28, 347, 1990.
12. Oakley, C. E. and Oakley, B. R., Identification of gamma tubulin, a new member of the tubulin superfamily encoded by mipA gene of *Aspergillus nidulans*, *Nature*, 338, 662, 1989.
13. Joshi, H. C., Gamma-tubulin — the hub of cellular microtubule assemblies, *Bioessays*, 15, 637, 1993.
14. Vale, R. D., Intracellular transport using microtubule-based motors, *Annu. Rev. Cell Biol.*, 3, 347, 1987.
15. Sheetz, M. P., Steuer, E. R., and Schroer, T. A., The mechanism and regulation of fast axonal transport, *Trends Neurosci.*, 12, 474, 1989.
16. Allan, V. J., Vale, R. D., and Navone, F., Microtubule-based organelle transport in neurons, in *The Neuronal Cytoskeleton*, Burgoyne, R. D., Ed., Wiley-Liss, New York, 1991, 257.
17. Paschal, B. M. and Vallee, R. B., Retrograde transport by the microtubule-associated protein MAP1c, *Nature*, 330, 181, 1987.
18. Wisniewski, H. M. and Terry, R. D., Morphology of the aging brain, human and animal, *Prog. Brain Res.*, 40, 167, 1973.
19. Kidd, M., Paired helical filaments in electron microscopy of Alzheimer's disease, *Nature*, 197, 192, 1963.
20. Anderton, B. H., Breinburg, D., Downes, M. J., Green, P. J., Tomlinson, B. E., Ulrich, J., Wood, J. N., and Kahn, J., Monoclonal antibodies show that neurofibrillary tangles and neurofilaments share antigenic determinants, *Nature*, 298, 84, 1982.
21. Gambetti, P., Autilio-Gambetti, L., Perry, G., Shecket, G., and Crane, R. C., Antibodies to neurofibrillary tangles of Alzheimer's disease raised from human and animal neurofilament fractions, *Lab. Invest.*, 49, 430, 1983.
22. Rasool, C., Abraham, C., Anderton, B. H., Haugh, M. C., Kahn, J., and Selkoe, D. J., Immunoreactivity of NFT with anti-NF and anti-PHF antibodies, *Brain Res.*, 310, 249, 1984.
23. Brion, J. P., Passareiro, H., Nunez, J., and Flament-Durand, J., Mise en évidence immunologique de la protéine tau au niveau des lésions de dégénérescence neurofibrillaire de la maladie d'Alzheimer, *Archives de Biologie (Bruxelles)*, 95, 229, 1985.
24. Delacourte, A. and Defossez, A., Alzheimer's disease: Tau proteins, the promoting factors of microtubule assembly, are major components of paired helical filaments, *J. Neurol. Sci.*, 76, 173, 1986.

25. Grundke-Iqbal, I., Iqbal, K., Quinlan, M., Tung, Y.-C., Zaidi, M. S., and Wisniewski, H. M., Microtubule-associated protein tau — a component of Alzheimer paired helical filaments, *J. Biol. Chem.,* 261, 6084, 1986.

26. Kosik, K. S., Joachim, C. L., and Selkoe, D. J., The microtubule-associated protein tau is a major antigenic component of paired helical filaments in Alzheimer's disease, *Proc. Natl. Acad. Sci. U.S.A.,* 83, 4044, 1986.

27. Grundke-Iqbal, I., Iqbal, K., Tung, Y.-C., Quinlan, M., Wisniewski, H. M., and Binder, L. I., Abnormal phosphorylation of the microtubule-associated protein tau in Alzheimer cytoskeletal pathology, *Proc. Natl. Acad. Sci. U.S.A.,* 83, 4913, 1986.

28. Mori, H., Kondo, J. and Ihara, Y., Ubiquitin is a component of paired helical filaments in Alzheimer's disease, *Science,* 235, 1641, 1987.

29. Perry, G., Manetto, V., and Mulvihill, P., Ubiquitin in Alzheimer and other neurodegenerative diseases, in *Alterations in the Neuronal Cytoskeleton in Alzheimer Disease,* Perry, G., Ed., Plenum Press, New York, 1987, 53.

30. Perry, G., Richey, P. L., Siedlak, S. L., Smith, M. A., Mulvihill, P., Dewitt, D. A., Barnett, J., Greenberg, B. D., and Kalaria, R. N., Immunocytochemical evidence that the beta-protein precursor is an integral component of neurofibrillary tangles of Alzheimer's disease, *Am. J. Pathol.,* 143, 1586, 1993.

31. Cork, L. C., Powers, R. E., Selkoe, D. J., Davies, P. D., Geyer, J. J., and Price, D. L., Neurofibrillary tangles and senile plaques in aged bears, *J. Neuropathol. Exp. Neurol.,* 47, 629, 1988.

32. Struble, R. G., Price, D. L., Jr., Cork, L. C., and Price, D. L., Senile plaques in cortex of aged normal monkeys, *Brain Res.,* 361, 267, 1985.

33. Hirano, A. N., Malamud, N., Elizan, T. S., and Kurland, L. T., Amyotrophic lateral sclerosis and Parkinson-dementia complex on Guam, *Arch. Neurol.,* 15, 35, 1966.

34. Ogata, J., Budzilovich, C. N., and Cravioto, H., A study of rod-like structures Hirano bodies in 240 normal and pathological brains, *Acta Neuropathol.,* 21, 61, 1972.

35. Gibson, P. H. and Tomlinson, B. E., Numbers of Hirano bodies in the hippocampus of normal and demented people with Alzheimer's disease, *J. Neurol. Sci.,* 33, 199, 1977.

36. Ramsey, H. J., Altered synaptic terminals in cortex near tumor, *Am. J. Pathol.,* 51, 1093, 1967.

37. Field, E. J., Mathews, J. D., and Raine, C. S., Electron microscopic observations on the cerebellar cortex in kuru, *J. Neurol. Sci.,* 8, 209, 1969.

38. Okamoto, K., Hirai, S., and Hirano, A., Hirano bodies in myelinated fibers of hepatic encephalopathy, *Acta Neuropathol.,* 58, 307, 1982.

39. Hirano, A. and Dembitzer, H. M., Eosinophilic rod-like structures in myelinated fibers of hamster spinal roots, *Neuropathol. Appl. Neurol.,* 2, 225, 1976.

40. Hirano, A., Dembitzer, H. M., Kurland, L. T., and Zimmerman, H. M., The fine structure of some intraganglionic alterations. Neurofibrillary tangles, granulo-vacuolar bodies and rod-like structures as seen in Guam amyotrophic lateral sclerosis and parkinsonism-dementia complex, *J. Neuropathol. Exp. Neurol.,* 27, 167, 1968.

41. Field, E. J. and Narang, H. K., An electron-microscopic study of scrapie in the rat: further observations on inclusion bodies and virus-like particles, *J. Neurol. Sci.,* 33, 199, 1972.

42. O'Brien, L., Shelley, K., Towfighi, J., and McPherson, A., Crystalline ribosomes are present in brains from senile humans, *Proc. Natl. Acad. Sci. U.S.A.,* 77, 2260, 1980.

43. Mori, H., Tomonaga, M., Baba, N., and Kanaya, K., The structure analysis of Hirano bodies by digital processing of electron micrographs, *Acta Neuropathol.*, 71, 32, 1986.

44. Galloway, P. G., Perry, G., and Gambetti, P., Hirano body filaments contain actin and actin-associated proteins, *J. Neuropathol. Exp. Neurol.*, 46, 185, 1987.

45. Schmidt, M. L., Lee, V. M. Y., and Trojanowski, J. Q., Analysis of epitopes shared by Hirano bodies and neurofilament proteins in normal and Alzheimer's disease hippocampus, *Lab. Invest.*, 60, 513, 1989.

46. Galloway, P. G., Perry, G., Kosik, K. S., and Gambetti, P., Hirano bodies contain tau protein, *Brain Res.*, 403, 377, 1987.

47. Munoz, D. G., Wang, D., and Greenberg, B. D., Hirano bodies accumulate C-terminal sequences of beta-amyloid precursor protein (beta-APP) epitopes, *J. Neuropathol. Exp. Neurol.*, 52, 14, 1993.

48. Goldman, J. E. and Yen, S.-H., Lewy bodies of Parkinson's disease contain neurofilament antigens, *Science*, 213, 1521, 1983.

49. Bancher, C., Lassman, H., Budka, H., Jellinger, K., Grundke-Iqbal, I., Iqbal, K., Wiche, G., Seitelberger, F., and Wisniewski, H. M., An antigenic profile of Lewy bodies: immunocytochemical indication for protein phosphorylation and ubiquitination, *J. Neuropathol. Exp. Neurol.*, 48, 81, 1989.

50. Galloway, P. G., Grundke-Iqbal, I., Iqbal, K., and Perry, G., Lewy bodies contain epitopes both shared and distinct from Alzheimer neurofibrillary tangles, *J. Neuropathol. Exp. Neurol.*, 47, 654, 1989.

51. Pollanen, M. S., Bergeron, C., and Weyer, L., Detergent-insoluble cortical Lewy body fibrils share epitopes with neurofilament and tau, *J. Neurochem.*, 58, 1953, 1992.

52. Kuzuhara, S., Mori, H., Izumiyama, N., Yoshimura, M., and Ihara, Y., Lewy bodies are ubiquitinated. A light and electron microscopic immunohistochemical study, *Acta Neuropathol.*, 75, 345, 1988.

53. Galloway, P. G., Bergeron, C., and Perry, G., The presence of tau distinguishes Lewy bodies of diffuse Lewy body disease from those in Parkinson's disease, *Neurosci. Lett.*, 100, 6, 1989.

54. Galloway, P. G. and Perry, G., Tropomyosin distinguishes Lewy bodies of Parkinson's disease from other neurofibrillary pathology, *Brain Res.*, 541, 347, 1991.

55. Fukuda, T., Tanaka, J., Watabe, K., Numoto, R. T., and Minamitani, M., Immunohistochemistry of neuronal inclusions in the cerebral cortex and brain-stem in Lewy body disease, *Acta Pathol. Jpn.*, 43, 545, 1993.

56. Hirano, A., Donnenfeld, H., Saski, S., and Nakano, I., Fine structural observations of neurofilamentous changes in amyotrophic lateral sclerosis, *J. Neuropathol. Exp. Neurol.*, 43, 461, 1984.

57. Leigh, P. N., Dodson, A., Swash, M., Brion, J.-P., and Anderton, B. H., Cytoskeletal abnormalities in motor neuron disease, *Brain*, 112, 521, 1989.

58. Prineas, J. W., Ouvier, R. A., Wright, R. G., Walsh, J. C., and McLeod, J. G., Giant axonal neuropathy: a generalized disorder of cytoplasmic microfilament formation, *J. Neuropathol. Exp. Neurol.*, 35, 458, 1976.

59. Sayre, L. M., Autilio-Gambetti, L., and Gambetti, P., Pathogenesis of experimental giant neurofilamentous axonopathies. A unified hypothesis based on chemical modification of neurofilaments, *Brain Res. Rev.*, 10, 69, 1985.

60. Schmidt, M. L., Carden, M. J., Lee, V. M. Y., and Trojanowski, J. Q., Phosphate dependent and independent neurofilament epitopes in the axonal swellings of patients with motor neuron disease and controls, *Lab. Invest.*, 56, 282, 1987.

61. Wisniewski, H. M., Shek, J. W., Gruca, S., and Stuman, J. A., Aluminium-induced neurofibrillary changes in axons and dendrites, *Acta Neuropathol.*, 63, 190, 1984.

62. Kunze, D. and Rustow, B., Pathobiochemical aspects of cytoskeleton components, *Eur. J. Clin. Chem. Clin. Biochem.*, 31, 477, 1993.

63. Selkoe, D. J., Liem, R. K. H., Shelanski, M. L., and Yen, S. H., Biochemical and immunological characterization of neurofilament in experimental neurofibrillary degeneration induced by aluminium, *Brain Res.*, 163, 235, 1979.

64. Ghetti, B. and Gambetti, P., Comparative immunocytochemical characterization of neurofibrillary tangles in experimental maytansine and aluminium encephalopathies, *Brain Res.*, 277, 388, 1983.

65. Troncoso, J. C., Sternberger, N. H., Sternberger, L. A., Hoffman, P. N., and Price, D. L., Immunocytochemical studies of neurofilament antigens in the neurofibrillary pathology induced by aluminium, *Brain Res.*, 364, 295, 1986.

66. Migheli, A., Pezzulo, T., Attanasio, A., and Schiffer, D., Peripherin immunoreactive structures in amyotrophic lateral sclerosis, *Lab. Invest.*, 68, 185, 1993.

67. Carden, M. J., Goldstein, M. E., Bruce, J., Cooper, H. S., and Schlaepfer, W. W., Studies of neurofilaments that accumulate in proximal axons of rats intoxicated with β, β′-iminodipropionitrile (IDPN), *Neurochem. Pathol.*, 7, 189, 1987.

68. Lowe, J., Blanchard, A., Morrell, K., Lennox, G., Reynolds, L., Billett, M., Landon, M., and Mayer, R. J., Ubiquitin is a common factor in intermediate filament inclusion bodies of diverse type in man, including those of Parkinson's disease and Alzheimer's disease, as well as Rosenthal fibers in cerebellar astrocytomas, cytoplasmic bodies in muscle and Mallory bodies in alcoholic liver disease, *J. Pathol.*, 155, 9, 1988.

69. Migheli, A., Autilio-Gambetti, L., Gambetti, P., Mocellini, C., Vigliani, M. C., and Schiffer, D., Ubiquitinated filamentous inclusions in spinal cord of patients with motor neuron disease, *Neurosci. Lett.*, 114, 5, 1990.

70. Schiffer, D., Autilio-Gambetti, L., Chiò, A., Gambetti, P., Giordana, M. T., Gullotta, F., Migheli, A., and Vigliani, M. C., Ubiquitin in motor neuron disease. Study at the light and electron microscope, *J. Neuropathol. Exp. Neurol.*, 50, 463, 1991.

71. Ball, M. J., Topographic distribution of neurofibrillary tangles and granulovacuolar degeneration in hippocampal cortex of aging and demented patients. A quantitative study, *Acta Neuropathol.*, 42, 73, 1978.

72. Ball, M. J., Granulovacuolar degeneration, in *Alzheimer's Disease: The Standard Reference*, Reisberg, B., Ed., The Free Press, New York, 1983, 62.

73. Okamoto, K., Hirai, S., Iizuka, T., Yanagisawa, T., and Watanabe, M., Reexamination of granulovacuolar degeneration, *Acta Neuropathol.*, 82, 340, 1991.

74. Price, D. L., Altschuler, R. J., Struble, R. G, Casanova, M. F., Cork, L. C., and Murphy, D. B., Sequestration of tubulin in neurons in Alzheimer's disease, *Brain Res.*, 385, 305, 1986.

75. Kahn, J., Anderton, B. H., Probst, U., Ulrich, J., and Esiri, M. M., Immunohistochemical study of granulovacuolar degeneration using monoclonal antibodies to neurofilament, *J. Neurol. Neurosurg. Psychiatry*, 48, 924, 1985.

76. Dickson, D. W., Ksiezak-Reding, H., Davies, P., and Yen, S.-H., A monoclonal antibody that recognizes a phosphorylated epitope in Alzheimer neurofibrillary tangles, neurofilaments and tau proteins immunostains granulovacuolar degeneration, *Acta Neuropathol.*, 73, 254, 1987.

77. Bondareff, W., Wischik, C. M., Novak, M., and Roth, M., Sequestration of tau by granulovacuolar degeneration in Alzheimer's disease, *Am. J. Pathol.*, 139, 641, 1991.

78. Dickson, D. W., Liu, W. K., Kress, Y., Ku, J., Dejesus, O., and Yen, S. H. C., Phosphorylated tau immunoreactivity of granulovacuolar bodies (GVB) of Alzheimer's disease — localization of 2 amino terminal tau epitopes in GVB, *Acta Neuropathol.*, 85, 463, 1993.

79. Love, S., Saitoh, T., Quijada, S., Cole, G. M., and Terry, R. D., Alz-50, ubiquitin and tau immunoreactivity of neurofibrillary tangles, Pick bodies and Lewy bodies, *J. Neuropathol. Exp. Neurol.*, 47, 393, 1988.

80. Wolozin, B., Pruchnicki, A., Dickson, D., and Davies, P., A neuronal antigen in the brains of Alzheimer patients, *Science*, 232, 648, 1986.

81. Hyman, B. T., Van Hoesen, G. W., Wolozin, B. L., Davies, P., Kromer, L. J., and Damasio, A. R., Alz-50 antibody recognizes Alzheimer-related neuronal changes, *Ann. Neurol.*, 23, 371, 1988.

82. Brady, D. R. and Mufson, E. J., Alz-50 immunoreactive neuropil differentiates hippocampal complex subfields in Alzheimer's disease, *J. Comp. Neurol.*, 305, 489, 1991.

83. Ksiezak-Reding, H., Davies, P., and Yen, S., Alz-50, a monoclonal antibody to Alzheimer's disease antigen, cross-reacts with tau proteins from bovine and normal human brain, *J. Biol. Chem.*, 263, 7943, 1988.

84. Goedert, M., Spillantini, G., and Jakes, R., Localization of the Alz-50 epitope in recombinant human microtubule-associated protein tau, *Neurosci. Lett.*, 129, 149, 1991.

85. Ksiezak-Reding, H., Chien, C.-H., Lee, V. M.-Y., and Yen, S.-H., Mapping of the Alz 50 epitope in microtubule-associated proteins tau, *J. Neurosci. Res.*, 25, 412, 1990.

86. Bancher, C., Brunner, C., Lassmann, H., Budka, H., Jellinger, K., Wiche, G., Seitelberger, F., Grundke-Iqbal, I., Iqbal, K., and Wisniewski, H. M., Accumulation of abnormally phosphorylated tau precedes the formation of neurofibrillary tangles in Alzheimer's disease, *Brain Res.*, 477, 90, 1989.

87. Wolozin, B. L., Scicutella, A., and Davies, P., Reexpression of a developmentally regulated antigen in Down syndrome and Alzheimer disease, *Proc. Natl. Acad. Sci. U.S.A.*, 85, 6202, 1988.

88. Al-Ghoul, W. M. and Miller, M. W., Transient expression of Alz-50 immunoreactivity in developing neocortex: a marker for naturally occuring neuronal death?, *Brain Res.*, 481, 361, 1989.

89. Valverde, F., Lopez-Mascaraque, L., and De Carlos, J. A., Distribution and morphology of Alz-50-immunoreactive cells in the developing visual cortex of kittens, *J. Neurocytol.*, 19, 662, 1990.

90. Byne, W., Mattiace, L., Kress, Y., and Davies, P., Alz-50 immunoreactivity in the hypothalamus of the normal and Alzheimer human and the rat, *J. Comp. Neurol.*, 306, 602, 1991.

91. Swaab, D. F., Eikelenboom, P., Grundke-Iqbal, I., Iqbal, K., Kremer, H. P. H., Ravid, R., and Van de Nes, J. A. P., Cytoskeletal alterations in the hypothalamus during aging and in Alzheimer's disease are not necessarily a marker for impending cell death, in *Alzheimer's Disease: Basic Mechanisms, Diagnosis and Therapeutic Strategies*, Iqbal, K., McLachlan, D. R. C., Winblad, B. and Wisniewski, H. M., Eds., John Wiley & Sons, New York, 1991, 181.

92. Nelson, P. T., Marton, L., and Saper, C. B., Alz-50 immunohistochemistry in the normal sheep striatum: a light and electron microscope study, *Brain Res.*, 600, 285, 1993.

93. Rye, D. B., Leverenz, J., Greenberg, S. G., Davies, P., and Saper, C. B., The distribution of Alz-50 immunoreactivity in the normal human brain, *Neuroscience*, 56, 109, 1993.

94. Benzing, W. C., Brady, D. R., Mufson, E. J., and Armstrong, D. M., Evidence that transmitter-containing dystrophic neurites precede those containing paired helical filaments within senile plaques in the entorhinal cortex of nondemented elderly and Alzheimer's disease patients, *Brain Res.*, 619, 55, 1993.

95. Benzing, W. C., Ikonomovic, M. D., Brady, D. R., Mufson, E. J., and Armstrong, D. M., Evidence that transmitter-containing dystrophic neurites precede paired helical filament and Alz-50 formation within senile plaques in the amygdala of nondemented elderly and patients with Alzheimer's disease, *J. Comp. Neurol.*, 334, 176, 1993.

96. Rechsteiner, M., Ubiquitin mediated pathways for intracellular proteolysis, *Annu. Rev. Cell Biol.*, 3, 1, 1987.

97. Fried, V. A. and Smith, H. T., Ubiquitin: a multifunctional regulatory protein associated with the cytoskeleton, *Prog. Clin. Biol. Res.*, 317, 733, 1989.

98. Murti, K. G., Smith, H. T., and Fried, V. A., Ubiquitin is a component of the microtubule network, *Proc. Natl. Acad. Sci. U.S.A.*, 85, 3019, 1988.

99. Gallo, J. M. and Anderton, B. H., Ubiquitous variations in nerves, *Nature*, 337, 687, 1989.

100. Papolla, M. A., Omar, R., and Saran, B., The normal brain: abnormal ubiquitinilated deposits highlight an age-related protein change, *Am. J. Pathol.*, 135, 585, 1989.

101. Bancher, C., Grundke-Iqbal, I., Iqbal, K., Fried, V. A., Smith, H. T., and Wisniewski, H. M., Abnormal phosphorylation of tau precedes ubiquitination in neurofibrillary pathology of Alzheimer disease, *Brain Res.*, 539, 11, 1991.

102. Migheli, A., Attanasio, A., Pezzulo, T., Gullotta, F., Giordana, M. T., and Schiffer, D., Age-related ubiquitin deposits in dystrophic neurites: an immunoelectron microscopic study, *Neuropathol. Appl. Neurol.*, 18, 3, 1992.

103. Ivy, G. O., Kitani, K., and Ihara, Y., Anomalous accumulation of tau and ubiquitin immunoreactivities in rat brain caused by protease inhibition and by normal aging: a clue to PHF pathogenesis?, *Brain Res.*, 498, 360, 1989.

104. Ivy, G. O., Ihara, Y., and Kitani, K., The protease inhibitor leupeptin induces several signs of aging in brain, retina and internal organs of young rats, *Arch. Gerontol. Geriatr.*, 12, 119, 1991.

105. Ivy, G. O., Protease inhibition causes some manifestations of aging and Alzheimer's disease in rodent and primate brain, *Ann. N.Y. Acad. Sci.*, 674, 89, 1992.

106. Vallee, R. B., Shpetner, H. S., and Paschal, B. M., The role of dynein in retrograde axonal transport, *Trends Neurosci.*, 12, 66, 1989.

107. Geinisman, Y., Bondareff, W., and Telser, A., Diminished axonal transport of glycoproteins in senescent rat brain, *Mech. Ageing Dev.*, 6, 363, 1977.

108. McMartin, D. and O'Connor, J. A., Effect of age on axoplasmic transport of cholinesterase in rat sciatic nerves, *Mech. Ageing Dev.*, 10, 241, 1979.

109. Stromska, D. P. and Ochs, S., Axoplasmic transport in aged rats, *Exp. Neurol.*, 77, 215, 1982.

110. Alberghina, M., Viola, M., Moschella, F., and Giuffrida, A. M., Axonal transport of glycerophospholipids in regenerating sciatic nerve of the rat during aging, *J. Neurosci. Res.*, 9, 393, 1983.

111. Goemaere-Vanneste, J., Couraud, J.-Y., Hassig, R., Di Giamberardino, L., and van den Bosch de Aguilar, Ph., Reduced axonal transport of the G4 molecular form of acetylcholinesterase in rat sciatic nerve during aging, *J. Neurochem.*, 51, 1746, 1988.

112. Viancour, T. A. and Kreiter, N. A., Vesicular fast axonal transport rates in young and old rat axons, *Brain Res.*, 628, 209, 1993.

113. Black, M. M. and Lasek, R. J., Slowing of the rate of axonal regeneration during growth and maturation, *Exp. Neurol.*, 63, 108, 1979.

114. McQuarrie, I. G., Brady, S. T., and Lasek, R. J., Retardation in the slow axonal transport of cytoskeletal elements during maturation and ageing, *Neurobiol. Aging*, 10, 359, 1989.

115. Tashiro, T. and Komiya, Y., Maturation and aging of the axonal cytoskeleton: biochemical analysis of transported tubulin, *J. Neurosci. Res.*, 30, 192, 1991.

116. Weisenberg, R. C., Flynn, J., Gao, B., Awodi, S., Skee, F., Goodman, S. R., and Riederer, B. M., Microtubule gelation-contraction. Essential components and relation to slow axonal transport, *Science*, 238, 1119, 1987.

117. Nixon, R. A., Axonal transport of cytoskeletal proteins, in *The Neuronal Cytoskeleton*, Burgoyne, R. D., Ed., Wiley-Liss, New York, 1991, 283.

118. Hinds, J. and McNelly, N., Aging in the olfactory bulb. Quantitative changes in mitral cell organelles and somato-dendritic synapses, *J. Comp. Neurol.*, 184, 811, 1979.

119. Qian, A., Himes, R. H., and Burton, P. R., Differences in protofilament number in microtubules assembled in extracts from young and old rat brains, *J. Cell Biol.*, 109, 24a, 1989.

120. Brady, S. T., Increases in cold-insoluble axonal tubulin during aging, *Soc. Neurosci. Abstr.*, 10, 273, 1984.

121. May, P. C. and Finch, C. E., Altered tubulin distribution in the hypothalamus of aging female C57BL/6J mice, *Neurobiol. Aging*, 6, 305, 1985.

122. Yan, S. B., Hwang, S., Rustau, T. D., and Frey, W. H., Human brain tubulin purification. Decrease in soluble tubulin with age, *Neurochem. Res.*, 10, 1, 1985.

123. Fifkova, E. and Morales, M., Aging and the neurocytoskeleton, *Exp. Gerontol.*, 26, 125, 1992.

124. Takeda, T., Hosokawa, M., Takeshita, S., Irino, M., Higuchi, K., Matsushita, T., Tomita, Y., Yasuhira, K., Hanamoto, H., Shimizu, K., Ishii, M., and Yamamuro, T., A new murine model of accelerated senescence, *Mech. Ageing Dev.*, 17, 183, 1981.

125. Takeda, T., Hosokawa, M., and Higuchi, K., Senescence-accelerated mouse SAM. A novel murine model of accelerated senescence, *J. Am. Geriatr. Soc.*, 39, 911, 1991.

126. van den Bosch de Aguilar, P. and Vanneste, J., Etude ultrastructurale des neurones ganglionaires spinaux au cours du vieillissement chez le rat, *Acta Anat.*, 110, 59, 1981.

127. Goemaere-Vanneste, J. and van den Bosch de Aguilar, Ph., Etude des fibres nerveuses périphériques au cours du vieillissement chez le rat, *La Cellule*, 74, 265, 1987.

128. van den Bosch de Aguilar, P. and Goemaere-Vanneste, J., Paired helical filaments in spinal ganglion neurons of elderly rats, *Virchows Arch. B*, 47, 217, 1984.

129. Hassoun, J., Devictor, B., Gambarelli, D., Peragut, J. C., and Toga, M., Paired twisted filaments: a new ultrastructural marker of human pinealomas, *Acta Neuropathol.*, 65, 163, 1984.

130. Klosen, P. and van den Bosch de Aguilar, Ph., Paired helical filament-like inclusions and Hirano bodies in the mesencephalic nucleus of the trigeminal nerve in the aged rat, *Virchows Arch. B*, 63, 91, 1993.

131. van den Bosch de Aguilar, Ph., Goemaere-Vanneste, J., Klosen, P., and Terao, E., Ageing changes of spinal ganglion neurons, in *Development and Involution of Neurones*, Fujisawa, K. and Morimatsu, Y., Eds., Japan Scientific Societies Press, Tokyo, 1992, 109.

132. Ksiezak-Reding, H., Dickson, D. W., Davies, P., and Yen, S. H., Recognition of tau epitopes by anti-neurofilament antibodies that bind to Alzheimer neurofibrillary tangles, *Proc. Natl. Acad. Sci. U.S.A.*, 84, 3410, 1987.

133. Nukina, N., Kosik, K. S., and Selkoe, D. J., Recognition of Alzheimer paired helical filaments by monoclonal neurofilament antibodies is due to cross-reaction with tau protein, *Proc. Natl. Acad. Sci. U.S.A.*, 84, 3415, 1987.

134. Lieberman, A. R., Sensory ganglia, in *The Peripheral Nerve*, Landon, D. N., Ed., Chapman and Hall, London, 1976, 188.

135. Lawson, S. N., Harper, A. A., Harper, E. I., Garson, J. A., and Anderton, B. H., A monoclonal antibody against neurofilament protein specifically labels a subpopulation of rat sensory neurons, *J. Comp. Neurol.*, 228, 263, 1984.

136. Poltorak, M. and Freed, W. J., Normal neuronal cell bodies of the nucleus tractus mesencephalici nervi trigemini react with antibodies against phosphorylated epitopes on neurofilaments, *Exp. Neurol.*, 97, 735, 1987.

137. Klosen, P., Goemaere-Vanneste, J., Terao, E., and van den Bosch de Aguilar, Ph., Approche expérimentale des manifestations de la démence sénile, *Acta Neurol. Belg.*, 89, 294, 1989.

138. Dickson, D. W., Yen, S.-M., Suzuki, K. I., Davies, P., and Garcia, J. H., Ballooned neurons in select neurodegenerative disease contain phosphorylated neurofilament epitopes, *Acta Neuropathol.*, 71, 216, 1986.

139. Munoz, D. G., Greene, C., Perl, D. P., and Selkoe, D. J., Accumulation of phosphorylated neurofilaments in anterior horn motoneurons of amyotrophic lateral sclerosis patients, *J. Neuropathol. Exp. Neurol.*, 47, 9, 1988.

140. Cork, L. C., Troncoso, J. C., Klavano, G. G., Johnson, E. S., Sternberger, L. A., Sternberger, N. H., and Price, D. L., Neurofilamentous abnormalities in motor neurons in spontaneously occuring animal disorders, *J. Neuropathol. Exp. Neurol.*, 47, 420, 1988.

141. Koliatsos, V. E., Applegate, M. D., Kitt, C. A., Walker, L. C., De Long, M. R., and Price, D. L., Aberrant phosphorylation of neurofilaments accompanies transmitter-related changes in rat septal neurons following transection of the fimbria-fornix, *Brain Res.*, 482, 205, 1989.

142. Klosen, P., Anderton, B. H., Brion, J.-P. and van den Bosch de Aguilar, Ph., Perikaryal neurofilament phosphorylation in axotomized and 6-OH-dopamine-lesioned CNS neurons, *Brain Res.*, 526, 259, 1990.

143. Doering L. C. and Aguayo, A. J., Hirano bodies and other cytoskeletal abnormalities develop in fetal rat CNS grafts isolated for long periods in peripheral nerve, *Brain Res.*, 401, 178, 1987.

144. Doering, L. C., Nilsson, O. G., and Aguayo, A. J., Abnormal perikaryal immunoreactivity to the phosphorylated heavy neurofilament unit in intracerebral basal forebrain transplants, *Exp. Neurol.*, 111, 1, 1991.

145. Nixon, R. A., Brown, B. A., and Marotta, C. A., Posttranslational modification of a neurofilament protein during axonal transport. Implications for regional specialization of CNS axons, *J. Cell Biol.*, 94, 150, 1982.

146. Sternberger, L. A. and Sternberger, N. H., Monoclonal antibodies distinguish phosphorylated and non-phosphorylated forms of neurofilaments *in situ*, *Proc. Natl. Acad. Sci. U.S.A.*, 80, 6126, 1983.

147. Manetto, V., Sternberger, N. H., Perry, G., Sternberger, L. A., and Gambetti, P., Phosphorylation of neurofilaments is altered in amyotrophic lateral sclerosis, *J. Neuropathol. Exp. Neurol.*, 47, 642, 1988.

148. Nakazato, Y., Hirato, J., Ishida, Y., Hoshi, S., Hasegawa, M., and Fukuda, T., Swollen cortical neurons in Creutzfeldt-Jakob disease contain a phosphorylated neurofilament epitope, *J. Neuropathol. Exp. Neurol.*, 49, 197, 1990.

149. Itoh, T., Sobue, G., Ken, E., Mitsuma, T., Takahashi, A., and Trojanowski, J. Q., Phosphorylated high molecular weight neurofilament protein in the peripheral motor, sensory and sympathetic neuronal perikarya. System-dependent normal variations and changes in amyotrophic lateral sclerosis and multiple system atrophy, *Acta Neuropathol.*, 83, 240, 1992.

150. Moss, T. H. and Lewkowicz, S. J., The axon reaction in motor and sensory neurones of mice studied by a monoclonal antibody marker of neurofilament protein, *J. Neurol. Sci.*, 60, 267, 1983.

151. Goldstein, M. E., Cooper, H. S., Bruce, J., Carden, M. J., Lee, V. M. Y., and Schlaepfer, W. W., Phosphorylation of neurofilament proteins and chromatolysis following transection of rat sciatic nerve, *J. Neurosci.*, 7, 1586, 1987.

152. Rosenfeld, J., Dorman, M. E., Griffin, J. W., Sternberger, L. A., Sternberger, N. H., and Price, D. L., Distribution of neurofilament antigens after axonal injury, *J. Neuropathol. Exp. Neurol.*, 46, 269, 1987.

153. Shaw, G., Winialski, D., and Reier, P., The effect of axotomy and deafferentation on phosphorylation dependent antigenicity of neurofilaments in rat superior cervical ganglion neurons, *Brain Res.*, 460, 227, 1988.

154. Doering, L. C., Transplantation of fetal CNS tissue into the peripheral nervous system. A model to study aberrant changes in the neuronal cytoskeleton, *J. Neural Trans. Plast.*, 2, 193, 1991.

155. Flood, D. G., Buell, S. J., Defiore, C. H., Horwitz, G. J., and Coleman, P. D., Age-related dendritic growth in dentate gyrus in human brain is followed by regression in the oldest old, *Brain Res.*, 345, 366, 1985.

156. Coleman, P. D. and Flood, D. G., Neuron numbers and dendritic extent in normal aging and Alzheimer's disease, *Neurobiol. Aging*, 8, 521, 1987.

157. Doering, L. C., Appropriate target interactions prevent abnormal cytoskeletal changes in neurons. A study with intra-sciatic grafts of the septum and the hippocampus, *J. Neurosci.*, 12, 3399, 1992.

158. Doering, L. C. and Tokiwa, M. A., Adrenal medulla and substantia nigra co-grafts in peripheral nerve. Chromaffin cells survive for long time periods and prevent degeneration of nigral neurons, *Brain Res.*, 551, 267, 1991.

159. Tanzi, R. E., McClatchey, A. J., Lampert, E. D., Villa-Komaroff, L., Gusella, J. F., and Neve, R. E., Protease inhibitor domain encoded by an amyloid precursor mRNA associated with Alzheimer's disease, *Nature*, 331, 528, 1988.

160. Ponte, P., Gonzales-DeWhitt, P., Schilling, J., Miller, J., Hsu, D., Greenberg, B., Davis, K., Wallace, W., Lieberburg, I., Fuller, F., and Cordell, B., A new A4 amyloid mRNA contains a domain homologous to serine proteinase inhibitors, *Nature*, 331, 525, 1988.

161. Aoyagi, T., Miyata, S., Nanbo, M., Kojima, F., Matusuzaki, M., Ishizuka, M., Takeuchi, T., and Umezawa, H., Biological activities of leupeptins, *J. Antibiot.*, 22, 558, 1969.

162. Toyo-oka, T., Shimazu, T., and Masaki, T., Inhibition of proteolytic activity of calcium activated neutral protease by leupeptin and antipain, *Biochem. Biophys. Res. Commun.*, 82, 484, 1978.

163. Barrett, A. J., The many forms and functions of cellular proteinases, *Fed. Proc.*, 39, 9, 1980.

164. Ivy, G. O., A proteinase inhibitor model of aging: implications for decreased neuronal plasticity, in *Neural Plasticity, Learning and Memory*, Milgram N. W., MacLeod C., and Petit T., Eds., Alan R. Liss, New York, 1987, 125.

165. Ivy, G. O., Decreased neural plasticity in aging and certain pathological conditions: possible roles of protein turnover, in *Neural Plasticity: A Lifespan Approach*, Petit, T. and Ivy, G., Eds., Alan R. Liss, New York, 1988, 351.

166. Cataldo, A. M. and Nixon, R. A., Enzymatically active lysosomial proteases are associated with amyloid deposits in Alzheimer brain, *Proc. Natl. Acad. Sci. U.S.A.*, 87, 3861, 1990.

167. Cataldo, A. M., Paskevich, P. A., Kominami, E., and Nixon, R. A., Lysosomal hydrolases of different classes are abnormally distributed in brains of patients with Alzheimer disease, *Proc. Natl. Acad. Sci. U.S.A.*, 88, 10998, 1991.

168. Svendsen, C. N., Cooper, J. D., and Sofroniew, M. V., Trophic factor effects on septal cholinergic neurons, *Ann. N.Y. Acad. Sci.*, 640, 91, 1991.

169. Sauer, H., Fischer, W., Nikkhah, G., Wiegand, S. J., Brundin, P., Lindsay, R. M., and Bjorklund, A., Brain-derived neurotrophic factor enhances function rather than survival of intrastriatal dopamine cell-rich grafts, *Brain Res.*, 626, 37, 1993.

170. Patterson, P. H., Cytokines and the function of the mature nervous system, *C. R. Acad. Sci. III Vie*, 316, 1150, 1993.

Chapter **11**

Transport of mRNA into the Cytoplasm

Werner E. G. Müller, Paul S. Agutter
and Heinz C. Schröder

CONTENTS

0-8493-4786-6/95/$0.00+$.50
© 1995 by CRC Press, Inc.

I. SUMMARY

Transport of mRNA from the nucleus to the cytoplasm is an ATP-dependent process, which occurs strictly vectorially. Because the mRNA is structurally bound during transport, mRNA transport may be considered as a "solid-state" process consisting of (1) mRNA release from the nuclear matrix, (2) mRNA translocation through the nuclear pore, and (3) cytoskeletal binding. The following components involved in the translocation step have been identified and purified:

1. The nuclear envelope (NE) nucleoside triphosphatase (NTPase) which is stimulated by the 3′poly(A) tail of mRNA,
2. The poly(A)-recognizing mRNA carrier,
3. The NE protein kinase, and
4. The NE phosphoprotein phosphatase.

In addition, it was found that a RNA helicase activity is present in NE, which may be implicated in regulation of transport of mRNA containing double-stranded RNA segments. Besides poly(A), other structural RNA elements such as AU-rich sequences or RNA-stem-loop structures may provide additional "signals" involved in modulating nuclear export of specific mRNA. The amount of mRNA transported from nuclei markedly decreases with age. Evidence is presented that this age-related change may be caused by an impairment of polyadenylation of mRNA, hnRNA processing, release of mRNA from the nuclear matrix, and translocation of mRNA from the nuclear to cytoplasmic compartment (decreased activities of NE NTPase, protein kinase, and phosphatase; reduced poly(A)-binding affinity of mRNA carrier).

II. INTRODUCTION

The exchange of macromolecules between the nucleus and the cytoplasm occurs across the NE pore complexes. The pore complexes have an octagonal symmetry. They consist of two ring-like and eight spoke-like components; concentric and transverse fibrils, which are connected with these components, form two basket-like structures, which may be involved in the mechanism of transport and/or may provide a closing mechanism of the pore (Figure 1).[1] There is a tight association between pore complexes, the nuclear lamina, and the nuclear matrix. The transport of mRNA ribonucleoprotein complexes (mRNPs) (diameter approximately 20 nm) across the nuclear pore (effective inner diameter 9 nm) cannot be explained by simple diffusion. The translocation of mRNPs through the pore complex is an energy-dependent step, which is mediated by a nucleoside triphosphatase (NTPase) (EC 3.6.1.15) which is localized in the NE.[2,3] The activity of this enzyme is stimulated by the polyadenylic acid [poly(A)] sequence, which is present at the 3'-terminus of most mRNAs.[4] For stimulation of the enzyme a minimal chain length of 15 to 20 adenylate residues is required. The passage of mRNA through the pore complex may be accompanied by changes in the three-dimensional structure of the mRNP complex.

The transport from the nucleus to the cytoplasm consists of three steps (for a review see References 5 and 6):

1. Release of mRNA from the intranuclear binding site (nuclear matrix),
2. Translocation of mRNA through a nuclear pore complex,
3. Association of the transported mRNA with the cytoplasmic cytoskeleton.

III. RELEASE OF mRNA FROM THE NUCLEAR MATRIX

In the nucleus, the nuclear matrix is assumed to provide a platform at which the assembly of spliceosomes and the posttranscriptional maturation

Cytoplasm

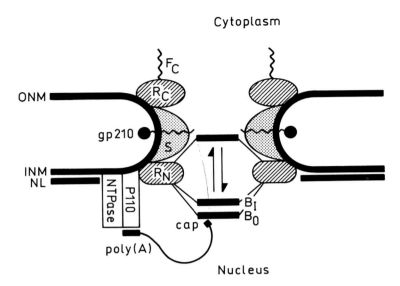

Figure 1

Scheme of a nuclear pore complex. The pore complexes consist of two ring-like structures which face the cytoplasmic (R_C) and the nuclear compartment (R_N), respectively, as well as eight spoke-like components (S), which point to the center of the pore. Two basket-like elements ("inner nuclear basket", B_I, and "outer nuclear basket", B_O) could build up a closure mechanism: (ONM) outer nuclear membrane; (INM) inner nuclear membrane; (NL) nuclear lamina. The exact localization of the NTPase and the mRNA carrier is uncertain.

("processing") of mRNA occur (for a review, see Reference 7). A major component of the matrix is DNA topoisomerase II.[8] Both the DNA and the hnRNA are found to be associated with the matrix. After completion of processing the mature mRNA is released from the matrix. We could demonstrate that this step requires the presence of ATP; thereby the mature mRNA is selectively released, while the immature mRNA precursors remain bound to the matrix.[9] At present the details of hnRNA attachment to the matrix are unclear. From our studies in HIV-infected cells the viral Tat protein may act as a linker between the TAR RNA stem loop of HIV mRNA and the nuclear matrix.[10] An attractive assumption is that the binding of hnRNA to the matrix occurs via the introns; the excision of the last intron might result in release of the mature mRNA, which is then transported through a nuclear pore into the cytoplasm. However, there is some evidence that the C group proteins of the ribonucleosome core are matrix-bound,[11] and these proteins are normally associated with exon sequences.[12]

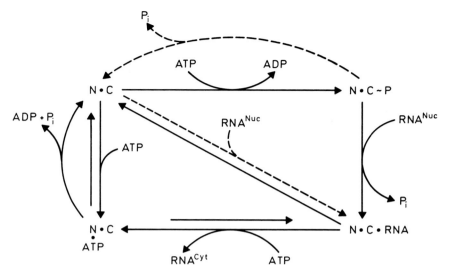

Figure 2
Scheme of poly(A)$^+$mRNA translocation across the nuclear envelope: (N) NTPase; (C) mRNA carrier; (RNA^{Nuc}) nuclear RNA; (RNA^{Cyt}) cytoplasmic RNA.

IV. TRANSLOCATION OF mRNA THROUGH THE NUCLEAR PORE

In recent years the following components involved in the translocation of polyadenylated mRNA [poly(A)$^+$mRNA] have been identified and purified (for reviews, see References 5, 6, and 13):

- Energy-delivering NTPase
- Poly(A)-recognizing mRNA carrier (= p106–110)
- Protein kinase, and
- Phosphoprotein phosphatase.

The poly(A) binding affinity of the mRNA carrier is modulated via phosphorylation/dephosphorylation by a NE-associated protein kinase[14-16] and phosphoprotein phosphatase.[15,16] Based on these facts, a tentative model for the transport of poly(A)$^+$mRNA has been postulated[6,17,18] (Figure 2). However, not all mRNAs are polyadenylated (e.g., most histone-mRNAs are poly(A)$^-$mRNAs). Evidence has been presented that transport of poly(A)$^-$mRNAs is mechanistically distinct from that of poly(A)$^+$mRNAs.[19]

In the following, a steady-state kinetic model for the transport of fully spliced mRNA is presented. In this model, it is assumed that only fully spliced mRNA is exported out of the nucleus. The sequence of events occurring during mRNA transport can be formulated as follows:

$$S_n + R \underset{k_{-1}}{\overset{k_{+1}}{\rightleftharpoons}} C_n \xrightarrow{k_{+2}} C_c \xrightarrow{k_{+3}} S_c + R \tag{1}$$

where S_n = nuclear RNA, S_c = cytoplasmic RNA, R = NE receptor, C_n = complex on nuclear face, C_c = complex on cytoplasmic face, and k_{+1}, k_{-1}, k_{+2}, and k_{+3} = rate constants.

Under steady-state conditions, we may write

$$\frac{dC_c}{d_t} = \frac{dC_n}{d_t} = 0 \tag{2}$$

i.e.,

$$k_{+2} \cdot C_n - k_{+3} \cdot C_c = 0 \tag{3}$$

therefore,

$$C_c = \frac{k_{+2}}{k_{+3}} C_n \tag{4}$$

$$v = k_{+3} \cdot C_c = k_{+2} \cdot C_n \tag{5}$$

and

$$k_{+1} \cdot S_n \cdot R - \left(k_{-1} + k_{+2}\right) \cdot C_n = 0 \tag{6}$$

and therefore,

$$C_n = \frac{k_{+1} \cdot S_n \cdot R}{k_{-1} + k_{+2}} \tag{7}$$

$$v = \frac{k_{+1} \cdot k_{+2} \cdot S_n \cdot R}{k_{-1} + k_{+2}} \tag{8}$$

The total number of NE receptors is

$$R_t = R + C_n + C_c$$

$$= R\left[1 + \frac{k_{+1} \cdot S_n}{k_{-1} + k_{+2}} \cdot \left[1 + \frac{k_{+2}}{k_{+3}}\right]\right] \tag{9}$$

therefore,

$$v = \frac{k_{+1} \cdot k_{+2} \cdot S_n \cdot R_t}{k_{-1} + k_{+2} + k_{+1} \cdot S_n \cdot \left[1 + \frac{k_{+2}}{k_{+3}}\right]}$$

$$= \frac{v_{max} \cdot S_n}{\left[\dfrac{k_{-1} \cdot k_{+3} + k_{+2} \cdot k_{+3}}{k_{+1} \cdot k_{+2}}\right] + S_n \cdot \left[1 + \dfrac{k_{+3}}{k_{+2}}\right]} \tag{10}$$

Since translocation is much faster than binding, i.e., $k_{+2} \gg k_{+1}$, and since $K_d \approx 10^{-7}\ M$, i.e., $k_{+1} \gg k_{-1}$, and assuming that $k_{+3} \approx k_{-1}$, and consequently $k_{+2} \gg k_{+3}$, it follows that

$$\left[1 + \frac{k_{+3}}{k_{+2}}\right] \approx 1 \tag{11}$$

Therefore,

$$v = \frac{v_{max} \cdot S_n}{K_m + S_n} \quad \text{where} \quad K_m = \frac{k_{-1} \cdot k_{+3} + k_{+2} \cdot k_{+3}}{k_{+1} \cdot k_{+2}} \tag{12}$$

i.e.,

$$K_m = \frac{k_{+3} \cdot (k_{-1} + k_{+2})}{k_{+1} \cdot k_{+2}} \approx \frac{k_{+3}}{k_{+1}} \quad \text{since } k_{+2} \gg k_{-1}$$

$$\approx \frac{k_{-1}}{k_{+1}} \approx K_d \approx 10^{-7}\ M \tag{13}$$

Summing up, under the assumptions that (1) k_{-1} and k_{+3} have a similar order of magnitude (since both rate constants describe the dissociation of the RNA-receptor complex), and (2) $k_{+2} \gg k_{+3}$ [since (a) k_{+2} refers to the ATP-dependent translocation step, which is faster than the binding, (b) k_{+1} describes the binding, and (c) $k_{+1} \approx 10^7 \cdot k_{-1}$], it follows that $K_m \approx k_{+3}/k_{+1} \approx$

k_{-1}/k_{+1}. This accords with the experimental results showing a K_m of about 10^{-7} M.[5,15,16,19]

V. ASSOCIATION OF mRNA WITH THE CYTOSKELETON

In the cytoplasm the mRNA is also associated with structural elements, the nature of which, however, is not fully clear. Involvement of actin filaments[15] and of the intermediate filament system have been discussed.[20] Based on the fact that glycoproteins exist both at the nuclear pores and in the cytoplasm as well as at the intranuclear sites of transcription and posttranscriptional processing,[21-23] nuclear lectins which interact with specific glycoproteins such as CBP67 or CBP35 (see below) could act as carrier molecules, which channel mRNP complexes through the nuclear pores from the nucleus into the cytoplasm. This transport may occur along "tracks" for specific mRNPs, which have been visualized intranuclearly by *in situ* hybridization.[24]

Association of mRNA with the cytoskeleton has been reviewed by Jones and Kirlpatrick.[25]

VI. COMPONENTS REQUIRED FOR DIFFERENTIAL mRNA TRANSPORT

A. Involvement of a RNA Helicase in mRNA Transport

Besides "poly(A)", RNA stem-loop structures, which are present at the 5'- and 3'-terminal untranslated regions of a number of mRNAs, can represent further recognition signals for the mRNA translocation system. These double-stranded RNA regions can serve as binding sites for regulatory proteins (e.g., in the case of ferritin-, poliovirus-, and HIV-1 mRNA) or they can increase the stability of the mRNAs (e.g., in the case of histone mRNAs). The double-stranded parts within the RNA stem loops are unwound by a NE-associated RNA helicase.[26] The helicase activity can be determined by measuring the unwinding of *in vitro* synthesized, partially double-stranded RNA substrates.[26] We showed that the enzyme in the NE really represents a helicase and not a RNA-modifying/unwinding activity; the unwound single-stranded RNAs can be rehybridized to form the double-stranded RNA substrate. Therefore the helicase is functionally distinct from RNA-modifying enzymes, which cause unwinding of double-stranded RNAs by transition of adenosine to inosine residues.[27]

Our studies revealed no identity of the NE RNA helicase with the nuclear protein p68 described by Ford et al.[28] The latter protein represents a RNA-dependent ATPase,[29] which, as shown by Hirling et al.[30] also possesses a helicase activity. P68 is a member of the "DEAD family" of RNA helicase-like proteins,[31] among which is also the initiation factor eIF4A.[32] Sequence analyses of a number of splicing factors in yeast suggest that a number of RNA-dependent ATPases are involved in the assembly of spliceosomes.[33] Notably, an ATP-dependent RNA helicase seems to be involved in the release of spliced mRNA from the spliceosomes in yeast.[34]

B. Modulation of Transport by Regulatory Proteins

Selective transport of a specific mRNA (or mRNA family) requires the existence of additional factors, which are able to recognize these mRNAs and facilitate their transport through the nuclear pore. Consequently, these mRNAs must be provided with specific recognition sequences. Two examples are described in the following: (1) the RRE element of HIV mRNAs,[35] and (2) the pentanucleotide AUUUA, which is present either singly or in multiple reiterations in mRNAs for lymphokines, cytokines, oncogene products, and some transcriptional activators.[36-39]

1. Rev Protein

HIV-1 encodes multiple regulatory proteins acting in *trans*. While the *trans*-activator protein Tat enhances the expression of both structural and regulatory genes of HIV-1, the protein encoded by the HIV-1-*rev* gene increases only the expression of the viral structural proteins.[40] From a series of studies, Rev most likely facilitates the export of the corresponding mRNAs from the nucleus into the cytoplasm (reviewed in Reference 41). Rev acts through binding to a target sequence within the HIV-*env* RNA, which is called RRE (= Rev-responsive element) (Figure 3). The RRE possesses a complex secondary structure. We showed that Rev protein interacts with the mRNA-transport system at the level of the NTPase-mediated translocation through the nuclear pore.[42] Rev is able to selectively channel RRE-containing RNA through the pore complex by direct interaction with the mRNA carrier/NTPase system (Figure 3). These studies showed for the first time that a nucleotide sequence within the coding region of a mRNA (here: RRE) serves as a signal for selective nucleocytoplasmic transport after association with a specific protein (Rev).

To investigate the interaction of Rev protein with the mRNA-translocation machinery different *in vitro* model systems were used which have proved to be suitable for the study of mRNA transport (for a review, see Reference 43). For transport studies "resealed NE vesicles" are used, in which either RRE-containing or RRE-free RNA has been entrapped. This *in vitro* model system, which has been introduced by Fasold's group,[44-46] allows translocation of RNA through the pore complex to be investigated

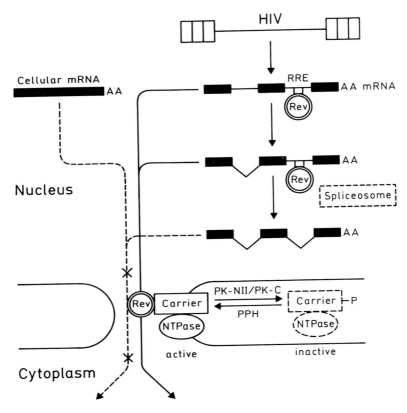

Figure 3

Effect of the HIV-1 Rev protein on mRNA transport. In the absence of Rev, formation of spliceosome complexes with HIV transcripts at the nuclear matrix can occur,
resulting in the nuclear export of fully spliced HIV mRNA. In the presence of Rev,
the viral RNA is covered by this protein, initiated by the binding of a single Rev
molecule to a high-affinity target sequence (Rev-responsive element, RRE), and
subsequent polymerization of additional Rev molecules along the whole RNA.[135]
This process may block spliceosome assembly, thus permitting transport of the
unspliced or incompletely spliced HIV RNA to the cytoplasm. In addition, Rev is
able to directly interact with the nucleocytoplasmic (mRNA-carrier/NTPase) translocation system (inhibition of transport of RRE⁻mRNA and promotion of transport
of RRE⁺mRNA). (PK) Protein kinase; (PPH) phosphoprotein phosphatase.

independently of the binding and release of RNA from the nuclear matrix
(where, e.g., splicing occurs). Using this system, we showed that in the
presence of Rev RRE-containing RNA is transported much faster than
RRE-free RNA.[42]

In the following, a steady-state kinetic model for the transport of both
spliced mRNAs (e.g., fully spliced 2-kb and incompletely spliced 4-kb
HIV-1 mRNA) and unspliced mRNA (e.g., 9-kb HIV-1 mRNA) is presented. The nomenclature is based on the following scheme:

U_n = steady-state concentration of pre-mRNA in the nucleus;

S_n = steady-state concentration of mRNA in the nucleus;

k_{und} = degradation rate constant of U_n;

k_{snd} = degradation rate constant of S_n;

k_{sp} = rate constant of splicing;

k_{ut} = rate constant for the nucleocytoplasmic transport of U_n;

k_{st} = rate constant for the nucleocytoplasmic transport of S_n;

U_c = steady-state concentration of pre-mRNA in the cytoplasm;

S_c = steady-state concentration of mRNA in the cytoplasm;

k_{ucd} = degradation rate constant of U_c;

k_{scd} = degradation rate constant of S_c.

Assuming that there is a constant rate of transcription, i.e., $k_T > 0$, we may write:

$$\frac{dU_c}{dt} = k_{ut} \cdot U_n - k_{ucd} \cdot U_c = 0 \quad \text{(steady - state conditions)} \tag{14}$$

Therefore,

$$U_c = \frac{k_{ut}}{k_{ucd}} \cdot U_n \tag{15}$$

$$\frac{dS_c}{dt} = k_{st} \cdot S_n - k_{scd} \cdot S_c = 0 \quad \text{(steady - state conditions)} \tag{16}$$

Therefore,

$$S_c = \frac{k_{st}}{k_{scd}} \cdot S_n \tag{17}$$

$$\frac{dU_n}{dt} = k_T - \left(k_{sp} + k_{ut} + k_{und}\right) \cdot U_n \tag{18}$$

At steady-state:

$$U_n = \frac{k_T}{k_{sp} + k_{ut} + k_{und}} \tag{19}$$

$$\frac{dS_n}{dt} = k_{sp} \cdot U_n - \left(k_{scd} + k_{st}\right) \cdot S_n = 0 \tag{20}$$

$$S_n = \frac{k_{sp}}{k_{snd} + k_{st}} \cdot U_n \tag{21}$$

Therefore,

$$\frac{S_n}{U_n} = \frac{k_{sp}}{k_{snd} + k_{st}} \approx \frac{k_{sp}}{k_{st}} \tag{22}$$

(since k_{snd} is usually $\ll k_{st}$).

$$S_c = \frac{k_{st}}{k_{scd}} \cdot S_n \approx \frac{k_{sp} \cdot k_{st}}{k_{st} \cdot k_{scd}} \cdot U_n \approx \frac{k_{sp}}{k_{scd}} \cdot U_n \tag{23}$$

Therefore,

$$\frac{S_c}{U_c} = \frac{k_{sp} \cdot k_{ucd}}{k_{ut} \cdot k_{scd}} \tag{24}$$

If $k_{ucd} = k_{scd}$, i.e., the pre-mRNA and mRNA have similar stabilities in the cytoplasm, it follows that

$$S_c / U_c = k_{sp} / k_{ut} \tag{25}$$

This model implies: (1) The ratio of spliced mRNA (2-kb HIV-1 mRNA and 4-kb HIV-1 mRNA) to unspliced pre-mRNA (9-kb HIV-1 mRNA) in the cytoplasm is equal to the ratio of the rate of splicing to the rate of transport of unspliced pre-mRNA (9-kb HIV-1 mRNA); and (2) the ratio of spliced mRNA (2-kb HIV-1 mRNA and 4-kb HIV-1 mRNA) to unspliced pre-mRNA (9-kb HIV-1 mRNA) in whole cells is also equal to the ratio of the rate of splicing to the rate of transport of unspliced pre-mRNA, if these two groups of mRNAs have similar stabilities in the cytoplasm.

The conclusions are

1. If the transport rate (k_{ut}) is much greater than the splicing rate (k_{sp}), then most of the cytoplasmic HIV-1 mRNA will not be spliced.
2. If the splicing rate is greater than the transport rate, then most of the HIV-1 mRNA will be spliced.
3. If the rate of splicing of HIV-1 mRNA in two different cell systems is the same, then the relative rates of nucleocytoplasmic transport of HIV-1 mRNA will determine the relative extent of splicing in the two systems.

2. AU Binding Protein

In addition, AU-rich elements occurring in the 3′-terminal nontranslated region of some cytokine- (e.g., tumor-necrosis factor, interleukin) and

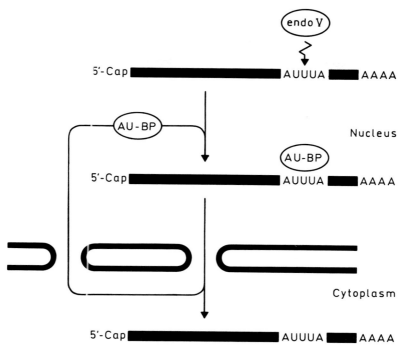

Figure 4

Regulation of nucleocytoplasmic transport of mRNA by AU-binding protein (AU-BP). In the nucleus AU-rich mRNA can be cleaved by the nuclear matrix-associated endoribonuclease V (endo V). The AU-binding protein prevents cleavage by binding to the AUUUA element and facilitates the transport of AU-rich mRNA through the pore complex. The AU binding protein can be transported back into the nucleus. Age-dependent changes of such cytosolic proteins can influence mRNA transport.

oncogene-mRNAs (e.g., *fos*, *myc*, and *sis*) may serve as recognition sequences for binding proteins. We demonstrated that the AU-specific endoribonuclease V[47] degrades AU-rich mRNA in unstimulated macrophages.[48] This degradation is prevented by a cytosolic protein (adenosine-uridine binding factor, AU binding protein[49,50]), which binds to the AUUUA motif of these mRNAs and thereby prolongs their half lives.[51] We could show that this protein is also able to selectively increase transport of AU-rich RNAs after binding to AUUUA. A hypothetical scheme of the mode of action of AU binding protein is shown in Figure 4.

3. CBP35 and CBP67

At present, little is known about the function of nuclear lectins (carbohydrate-binding proteins, CBPs),[23,52-54] although it has been shown that a number of nuclear proteins are glycoproteins, which could interact with these lectins. Examples include certain transcriptional factors, DNA polymerase α, and poly(A) polymerase (reviewed in Reference 22). Glycoproteins are also associated with the nuclear pore complexes and the nuclear matrix.[21,55] Earlier studies showed that nuclear lectins are predominantly localized in those nuclear regions that contain RNP complexes[23,52,54,56] and where transcription and splicing occur. The expression and intracellular distribution of nuclear CBPs depend on the physiological state of cells (for a review, see References 57 and 58). Evidence has been presented that at least some nuclear lectins are associated with hnRNP complexes to be exported into the cytoplasm.[52,53,59]

Two nuclear lectins, CBP35 and CBP67, have been characterized in more detail.[23,53,60] The nuclear carbohydrate-binding protein with a molecular mass of 35 kDa, CBP35, specifically binds to β-galactoside residues[61] and was identified as a protein of the hnRNP complex.[52,62] CBP35 consists of two domains, an amino-terminal portion that is homologous to certain regions of proteins of the hnRNP complex and a carboxyl-terminal portion that is homologous to β-galactoside-specific lectins. We succeeded in purifying a glucose-binding protein (CBP67) from nuclei of rat liver.[53] This nuclear lectin is present in RNP particles in the cell nucleus, but not in polysomal RNPs. Therefore, we researched on the potential function of this lectin during nucleocytoplasmic transport of mRNA. For these investigations we used closed NE vesicles containing entrapped nuclear RNP complexes as a system to study nuclear RNP export. We found that the efflux of nuclear RNPs from NE vesicles is inhibited by glucose-containing (neo)glycoproteins and that CBP67 binds to a specific receptor (ligand) in the NE, an 80-kDa polypeptide.[53] We concluded that CBP67 allows directed intranuclear transport of mRNPs to the nuclear pore. More recently, an additional glucose-binding protein with M_r 70,000 (CBP70) has been isolated in association with CBP35 from nuclei of the human tumoral cell line HL60.[63]

4. Insulin and Epidermal Growth Factor

Insulin and epidermal growth factor (EGF) modulate the rate of transport of poly(A)+mRNA by a direct interaction with the nucleocytoplasmic translocation system.[64] According to our results, the ratio between the rates of transport of high- and low-abundance mRNAs is decreased and increased, respectively, by insulin and EGF.

Insulin was found to stimulate the NE phosphoprotein phosphatase activity, which in turn dephosphorylates the NE poly(A) binding site (mRNA carrier). Hence, the NE NTPase activity is increased (because its activity is inversely correlated with the phosphorylation of p106-110). The enhancement of NTPase activity seems to be caused by an increase in the number of active enzyme molecules and not by an increase in affinity of the enzyme to its substrate (ATP or GTP). This conclusion was drawn from the finding that only v_{max} was enhanced in the presence of insulin, while the apparent K_m (for ATP) remained unchanged. In contrast, EGF does not affect the phosphoprotein phosphatase but stimulates the protein kinase, and thus inhibits the NTPase via phosphorylation of the carrier. The effect of insulin (and of EGF) is not due to a posttranslational modification of the NTPase protein itself, but seems to be due to an insulin-induced decrease (EGF-induced increase) in the extent of phosphorylation of the poly(A) binding mRNA carrier. This change in the phosphorylation state of the carrier results, in turn, in a stimulation in the case of insulin, or an inhibition in the case of EGF, of the NTPase through a coupling within the intact NE structure. This conclusion is based on the following findings:

1. The NTPase is not a phosphoprotein.[64]
2. Only the structure-bound and not the purified NTPase is modulated by the 3'poly(A) sequence of mRNA, because this sequence binds to the mRNA carrier and not to the NTPase.[3,16]
3. The purified NTPase does not show any response to insulin (or EGF), while the poly(A) binding affinity of the mRNA carrier embedded in the NE is significantly changed by these proteins.[64]

5. Transport-Stimulatory Proteins

The cytoplasm contains proteins that stimulate mRNA transport (for reviews see Reference 6). We have purified two mRNA transport stimulatory proteins [M_r 58 kDa (p58) and 31 kDa (p31)] from rat liver polysomes to apparent homogeneity.[18] Both proteins show particular affinities for poly(A). p31 increases the affinity of the poly(A) binding site in phosphorylated NE. Poly(A) binding stimulates the phosphatase activity and inhibits the kinase activity in the NE; in consequence poly(A) stimulates the NTPase. The capacity of poly(A) to inhibit the kinase and to stimulate the phosphatase is enhanced in the presence of p31; without poly(A), p31 has no effect on these enzymes. It is assumed that p31 promotes the rate of translocation of low-abundance mRNAs through the nuclear pore complex.[18] The other protein, p58, promotes the binding of poly(A) to unphosphorylated NE, but not to phosphorylated NE. It inhibits the kinase that downregulates the NTPase even in the absence of poly(A).

VII. AGE-DEPENDENT CHANGES IN NUCLEOCYTOPLASMIC TRANSPORT OF mRNA AND THEIR CAUSES

The amount of mRNA transported from nuclei per unit time is markedly reduced during aging.[65-69] The following causes are taken into consideration:

- Decrease in mRNA synthesis,
- Decrease in polyadenylation of mRNA,
- Impairment of hnRNA processing,
- Impairment of release of mRNA from the nuclear matrix, and
- Impairment of translocation of mRNA through the nuclear pore complex.

A. Changes at the Level of Transcription

Age-dependent alterations of transcription are summarized in the following review articles.[70-72] The rate of synthesis of both total RNA and polyadenylated RNA significantly decreases during aging.[73,74] Likewise the endogenous nucleotide pool decreases age-dependently.[75] The *in situ* activities of the enzymes involved in RNA synthesis are also reduced in old animals;[76] both free and bound RNA polymerases I and II from rat liver become more active after birth and then decline with increasing age.[77] Isolated nuclei from the livers and muscles of 30-month-old mice show a markedly reduced RNA synthesis compared to young adult animals.[78,79] Although the age-dependent decrease in RNA polymerase activities could often not be confirmed when an exogenous template was added to the soluble enzymes,[80] a number of studies showed that the matrix function of the chromatin from different organs displayed a decrease with increasing age after addition of exogenous RNA polymerase.[79,81-83]

B. Changes at the Posttranscriptional Level

After transcription, where a "coarse control" of gene expression occurs, a "fine control" of the information to be expressed occurs during posttranscriptional processing. Studies during the past few years have shown that a number of changes in processing occurs with time, which are considered to be age-related (reviewed in References 84 to 86). The importance of the posttranscriptional steps is also evident from the fact that only a small fraction of the originally synthesized sequences reaches the cytoplasm: thus the hnRNA in the nucleus has a 45-fold higher sequence complexity than the cytoplasmic mRNA.[87]

1. Polyadenylation

Most eukaryotic mRNAs (exception: replication-dependent histone mRNAs) contain a poly(A) sequence with a chain length of 200 to 250 AMP residues at their 3'-termini.[88,89] During aging of an individual mRNA molecule, a reduction of the initial poly(A) size to less than 50 nucleotides takes place, resulting in a heterogeneous poly(A) length distribution of the overall mRNA population within the cell.[90]

One function of the poly(A) sequence may be to stabilize the mRNA and thereby to determine the half-life of this macromolecule.[91] There is a linear relationship of the log of newly synthesized poly(A) size to the log of mRNA half-life.[92] Stabilization of mRNA requires a minimal poly(A) length of 21 AMP units. There is also a positive correlation between the length of the poly(A) sequence and the complexity of the species from which the RNA has been isolated.[92]

The synthesis of the 3'-terminal poly(A) segment of hnRNA and mRNA is catalyzed by poly(A) polymerases (EC 2.7.7.19).[93,94] Poly(A) degradation is catalyzed by two enzymes: endoribonuclease IV (EC 3.1.26.6)[95] and poly(A)-specific 2',3'-exoribonuclease (EC 3.1.13.4).[96] The activities of these enzymes can be modulated by phosphorylation[97] or interaction with cytoskeletal protein.[98] Age-dependence studies on quail oviduct revealed that the activity of 2',3'-exoribonuclease in old animals is three- to fourfold higher than in mature animals.[99] On the other hand, the changes in activities of poly(A) polymerase and endoribonuclease IV in the course of aging were found to be negligible. The conclusion drawn from these data, that the poly(A) segment of mRNA is shorter in senescent animals compared to adult ones, is supported by analytical results.[100] Determinations of the sizes of the poly(A) sequences of mRNAs from oviducts of mature and old quails revealed that the length of the poly(A) segment is shortened from an average value of 130 AMP units (adult animal group) to an average value of 70 AMP units (senescent animal group) (Figure 5A); similar results were obtained for liver and heart (Figure 5B and C). Further, the relative amounts of low-molecular-weight oligo(A) fragments formed *in vivo* in oviducts of mature and old animals have been shown to gradually decrease with aging of the animals;[101] the percentage of oligo(A)$_{2-6}$ sequences in the mature animal group was found to be six times higher than that of the old animal group. This result may be explained by the fact that due to the higher activity of poly(A) exoribonuclease, oligo(A) fragments, once formed, are rapidly degraded in organs of older animals.

The 2',3'-exoribonuclease is able to degrade 2',5'-oligoadenylates (2-5As) as well as poly(A), and age-related changes in the activity of this enzyme have been shown to be one causative factor in the age-dependent reduction in efficiency of the antiviral 2',5'-oligoadenylate synthetase/ribonuclease L-system.[102]

2. Splicing

Age-dependent changes also occur in the course of splicing. We demonstrated that distinct high-molecular-weight ovalbumin RNA precursors are accumulated in the old hen oviduct as compared with mature animals, suggesting that RNA splicing is impaired with age.[103] Northern blot analysis of the RNA from oviducts of hens of different age revealed that the

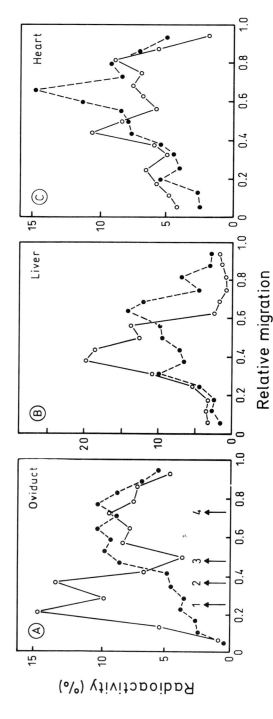

Figure 5

Age-dependent change in distribution of poly(A) chain lengths of mRNA from different organs of quails. Total RNA was isolated from oviduct (A), liver (B), and heart (C) of mature (○) and senescent (●) female quails. After labeling with [³H]dimethyl sulfate, radioactivity-labeled poly(A) was isolated by oligo(dT)-chromatography. Poly(A) was size-separated by polyacrylamide gel electrophoresis. The distribution of radioactivity in the gel is expressed as percentage total radioactivity per gel. The arrows mark the positions of the following markers: 1, poly(A)$_{160}$; 2, poly(A)$_{120}$; 3, poly(A)$_{90}$; 4, poly(A)$_{44}$.

Figure 6
Northern blot analysis of ovalbumin sequence containing RNAs in total RNA and poly(A)⁺RNA from oviducts of hens of different ages. Panel A: total RNA from oviducts of mature, egg-laying (lane a) and old, nonegg-laying hens (lane b) (3.2 to 3.3 μg of RNA each). Panels B and C: poly(A)⁺RNA from oviducts of mature (lanes a and b, 3.0 and 1.5 μg of RNA, respectively), and old animals (lane c, 3.0 μg of RNA). In panels A and B, autoradiograms were exposed for 48 h and, in panel C, for 192 h. The kb values on the right refer to the length of the ovalbumin sequence containing RNAs.

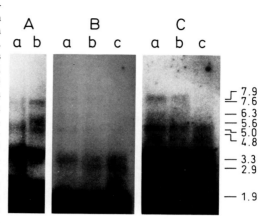

largest ovalbumin RNA precursor band (7.9 kb) was most intense if total RNA from old hen oviduct was checked (Figure 6, lane Ab) as compared with that from mature animals (lane Aa). Interestingly, poly(A) was not detectable in those ovalbumin mRNA precursors, which are enriched in old animals.[104] Thus, the 7.9-kb ovalbumin RNA precursor was invisible in the poly(A)⁺RNA fraction from old hen oviduct (Figure 6, lane Bc), even after overexposure (lane Cc). On the other hand, the 7.9-kb band was readily detected in the poly(A)⁺RNA from mature hen oviduct (Figure 6, lanes Ba and Bb and lanes Ca and Cb). These results suggest that age-dependent impairment of ovalbumin mRNA processing might be caused by altered polyadenylation of distinct RNA precursors.

3. Formation of Ribonucleoprotein Complex

The hnRNA is bound to a specific set of proteins to form hnRNP particles with sedimentation coefficients of 200 to 300 S.[105] The poly(A) sequence is also protected against attack by endoribonuclease IV through specific poly(A)-binding proteins.[106-111] By selective radiolabeling of the protein components in the polysomal poly(A)-RNP from L5178y mouse lymphoma cells with [³H]dansyl chloride, two protein species of M_r 77,000 (p77) and M_r 54,000 (p54) have been identified by Bernd et al.[109] A quantitative analysis revealed that the poly(A)-RNP complex is composed of 3.7 molecules of p54 and 1.9 molecules of p77 per 155 AMP residues. Digestion experiments with ribonuclease A indicated that p54 covers 15 to 20 AMP residues and p77 a sequence of 40 to 45 nucleotides on the poly(A)$_{155}$ stretch of L5178y cell poly(A)-RNP. Using different approaches,

Adams et al.[107] reported that a 45-nucleotide tract is covered by the poly(A)-associated proteins, while Baer and Kornberg[112] found fragments of 22 AMP units. Van Eekelen et al.[114] demonstrated that p73 was associated with poly(A) in HeLa cell cytoplasm, but not in the nucleus. It was shown that a different protein, p63, is the major poly(A)-associated protein in the nucleus.[114]

In the course of aging, a drop in the number of the poly(A)-associated protein molecules from approximately 4.7 molecules (mature oviduct) to 1.9 molecules (old oviduct) could be detected.[108] Thus the poly(A) sequence ceases to be sufficiently protected against the attack of poly(A) nucleases. The protective functions of the poly(A) segment in polysomal poly(A)$^+$mRNP and isolated poly(A)-RNP complex (p77 and p54) towards attack by endoribonuclease IV and poly(A)-specific 2′,3′-exoribonuclease determined by us in an earlier study.[106] It was found that the exoribonuclease hydrolyzes the poly(A) segment in poly(A)$^+$mRNP and poly(A)-RNP irrespective of the presence of poly(A)-associated proteins. In contrast, these proteins protect the poly(A) segment almost completely from nucleolytic attack of the endoribonuclease IV; after removal of these proteins by treatment with 1 M urea the poly(A) segment is highly susceptible to degradation by endoribonuclease IV.

C. Changes at the Level of Release of mRNA from the Nuclear Matrix

Aging is associated with increased levels of messengers for proteins normally not expressed in the given cell type, e.g., globin mRNAs appear in old mouse brain.[115] This phenomenon has been termed "relaxation" of gene expression. However, in the example described no synthesis of globin has been observed in the cytoplasm, most likely due to posttranscriptional control mechanisms.

Moreover, release of immature mRNA from the nuclear matrix and nuclear export of immature mRNA occurs in cells of old animals. Normally, only mature mRNA is transported out of the nucleus. Thereby, the selectivity of nucleocytoplasmic transport for mature mRNA species seems to be due to the selectivity of the ATP-induced release of mature mRNA from the nuclear matrix.[9] In the presence of superoxide radicals, the level of which is thought to increase with age, the selection mechanism for mature mRNA at the level of nuclear matrix attachment is disturbed.[116,117] Aging may therefore be partially caused by a superoxide radical-induced release of immature mRNA from its intranuclear binding site, resulting in the appearance of immature messengers in the cytoplasm and a subsequent disturbance of mRNA translation.

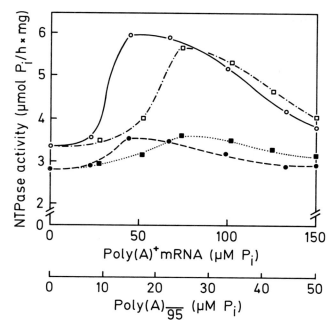

Figure 7
Age-dependence of stimulation of NE NTPase by the poly(A) sequence of mRNA. The NTPase activity was determined in NE from the livers of mature (o,□) and old (●,■) rats in the presence of different concentrations of poly(A)⁺mRNA (o,●) and poly(A)₉₅ (□,■). Poly(A)₉₅ was obtained from poly(A)-RNP complex.

D. Changes at the Level of Translocation of mRNA Through the Nuclear Pore

1. NTPase

We showed that the activity of the NE NTPase in quail oviduct drastically changes during development and aging.[118] In the course of maturation the activity of the enzyme strongly increases. During aging, the high level of NTPase reached in mature or (estrogen) hormone-treated immature quail oviduct is reduced to 50%.[118] There is a correlation between the extent of oviduct-specific ovalbumin synthesis and the level of NTPase activity.[118]

2. Stimulation of NTPase by Poly(A)

Likewise, the capacity of the NE NTPase to be stimulated by poly(A) displays drastic changes during development.[100,118,120] In rat livers, the NTPase is stimulated by poly(A) to about 170% in mature animals, while the enzyme from old animals is enhanced only to about 115%.[100] Poly(A)-

containing mRNA enhances the enzyme activity in "mature" rat liver to 177%, while the activity in "old" liver increases only to 126%; similar results have been obtained with the isolated poly(A) segment of poly(A)⁺mRNA (Figure 7).

3.   Protein Kinase and Phosphoprotein Phosphatase

Moreover, the activities of protein kinases and phosphoprotein phosphatase in the NE, which are involved in regulating the poly(A)-binding affinity of the mRNA carrier protein,[6] markedly change during development.[14,121] In immature quail oviduct these enzyme activities strongly increase in response to diethylstilbestrol and progesterone treatment.[121] A similar increase is observed during maturation. After the initial burst, the activity of the protein kinase increases slightly during aging, while the phosphoprotein phosphatase activity remains constant. The kinase is strongly inhibited by poly(A), while the activity of the phosphatase is stimulated by poly(A).[14] The affinity of the carrier for poly(A) is enhanced by phosphorylation and reduced by dephosphorylation.

4.   Poly(A)-Recognizing mRNA Carrier

This protein, which has a polypeptide molecular mass of 106 to 110 kDa and has been localized at the nucleoplasmic face of the NE,[122,123] has been identified and purified by us.[16] The mRNA carrier is a phosphoprotein. Both the protein kinase in the NE and the NE phosphoprotein phosphatase modulate the poly(A) binding affinity of the carrier protein: binding of poly(A) or poly(A)⁺mRNA to the carrier is enhanced by protein kinase-dependent phosphorylation; dephosphorylation of this protein by the phosphoprotein phosphatase results in a lower poly(A) binding affinity.[100] The poly(A)⁺mRNA carrier is also phosphorylated by Ca^{2+}-activated and phospholipid-dependent protein kinase (protein kinase C).[15,16] We demonstrated that protein kinase C reversibly binds to the NE. Binding of protein kinase C results in an inhibition of ATP-dependent efflux of mRNA from isolated nuclei, a decrease of NTPase activity, and an increase of poly(A)⁺mRNA binding to isolated NE (nuclear pore complex-laminae).[16]

Pore-complex laminae (obtained by treatment of NE with Triton X-100™) contain apparently only one class of mRNA binding sites with a high affinity for poly(A).[15,18] It was found that phosphorylation of isolated NE by endogenous NI- and NII-protein kinases results in a significant increase in the poly(A) binding affinity without alteration of the total number of poly(A) binding sites.[100] Scatchard plot analysis revealed that the number of poly(A) binding sites in unphosphorylated NE from old animals is significantly reduced, compared with those from mature animals.[100] This result was not replicated when phosphorylated NE was studied. The extent of phosphorylation of the poly(A)-recognizing carrier

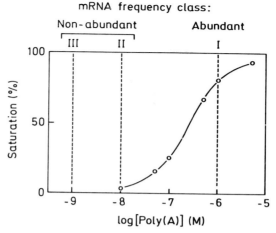

Figure 8
Binding of poly(A) to rat liver pore-complex laminae. NE were demembranated by treatment with Triton X-100® and the resulting pore-complex laminae were incubated with increasing concentrations of [³H]poly(A). The estimated intracellular concentrations of abundant mRNA (mRNA frequency class I) and nonabundant mRNA (less abundant class II mRNAs and scarce class III mRNAs)[124] are indicated by dotted lines.

protein, p106-110, changes drastically during development. In untreated animals (oviducts from untreated, immature quails), no phosphorylation of this protein is observed. During aging, the phosphorylation of p106-110 strongly increases.[121]

Changes in the poly(A) binding affinity of the NE mRNA translocation system may be important for regulation of the nucleo-cytoplasmic ratio between high-abundance and low-abundance mRNAs. At the estimated intracellular concentrations of high-abundance mRNAs (approximately 1 μM)[124] the pore-complex laminae are nearly saturated by poly(A), while in the range of the estimated intracellular concentrations of low-abundance mRNAs [less than one-hundredth (mRNA frequency class II) or one-thousandth (mRNA frequency class III)[124] of that of high-abundance mRNAs] poly(A) saturation amounted to less than 5% (Figure 8). Therefore, transport of high-abundance mRNAs should not be significantly enhanced by increasing the poly(A)-binding affinity of the carrier, in contrast to transport of low-abundance mRNAs. For example, transport of low-abundance cytokine mRNAs has been shown to be prone to modulation by transport-stimulatory proteins such as AUBF; binding of this factor to the recurrent AUUUA motifs in these RNAs strongly increases the affinity of this RNA to pore-complex laminae.[51] The total number of binding sites was not changed by AUBF.

The relationship between cytoplasmic mRNA abundance and nuclear mRNA content seems to be as follows. Suppose we represent the availability of mature mRNA in the nucleus by the symbol S_n (if the RNA were freely diffusible then S_n would be the intranuclear concentration of mRNA.) Suppose further that we represent the total number of binding sites in the pore complexes of a nucleus by R_t, the number of occupied receptors by C, and the number of free receptors by R. If collisions between mRNA and the free receptors were random (as assumed in solution chemistry), then, given a sufficiently long time, we would have:

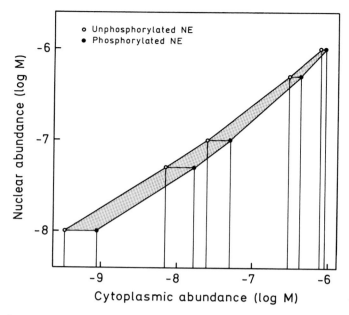

Figure 9

Amplification of mRNA abundance differences by the NE mRNA translocation system. Shown is a graph of the estimated values of cytoplasmic abundance [calculated according to the equation $(C/R_t) \cdot S_n$] as a function of nuclear abundance.

$$K_d = \frac{S_n \cdot R}{C} = \frac{S_n \cdot (R_t - C)}{C} \tag{26}$$

i.e.,

$$\frac{C}{R_t} = \frac{S_n}{K_d + S_n} \tag{27}$$

If we assume $K_d = 10^{-7} M$ for phosphorylated receptors and $3.0 \times 10^{-2} M$ for unphosphorylated receptors,[5] and furthermore that the cytoplasmic abundance becomes equal, after a long enough time, to $(C/R_t) \cdot S_n$, then we have the results shown in Figure 9. In effect, while the nuclear abundance changes over two orders of magnitude, the cytoplasmic abundance changes over three orders; thus the translocation system (even in this simplified model) can be seen to act as an amplifier of abundance differences. Note that if the receptor is unphosphorylated then the amplification is greater (Figure 9).

This amplification mechanism seems to be impaired during senescence. According to our data the number of poly(A) binding sites in unphosphorylated rat liver NE, being more potent in amplifying abundance differences than the phosphorylated ones, significantly decreased from 0.65 nmol poly(A) phosphate per milligram of NE protein (mature animals) to 0.49 nmol poly(A) phosphate per milligram (old animals).[100] No significant age-related difference existed in the number of binding sites in phosphorylated NE; they amounted to 0.71 (mature rats) and 0.72 nmol poly(A) phosphate per milligram of NE protein (old rats).[100]

5. Transport-Stimulatory Proteins

We showed that the efficiency of cytoplasmic transport-stimulatory proteins strongly decreases with age.[120] Similar results were obtained when the transport-stimulating activity of cytosolic extracts from animals of different age classes was studied.[69]

E. Transcription and Transport of Specific mRNAs

Different age-dependent alterations have been described for transcription and transport of certain specific mRNAs, which are partially opposed to the changes of total RNA synthesis and total RNA transport during aging; e.g., there is a marked increase in the amount of albumin mRNA sequences in rat liver between the 12th and 24th month of age.[125] On the other hand, the amount of translatable cytochrome P450-LM2 mRNA in rabbit liver decreases with age.[126] Despite the increase in cytoplasmic concentration of albumin mRNA, no age-dependent changes were found either in the rate of transcription of the albumin gene or the amount of albumin RNA sequences in nuclei from rat liver; this result may indicate that the turnover of this mRNA declines with increasing age.[127] Studies of transcription of the alpha 2u-globulin-gene family in rat liver revealed that their activation occurs during puberty and their shut-off with age is correlated with the association and dissociation of the corresponding gene domain with the nuclear matrix.[128] Studies of the age-dependent changes in expression of the cytochrome P-450 (b+e)-gene in rat after treatment with phenobarbital revealed that the cytoplasmic RNA appeared earlier in old animals, although stimulation of transcription by phenobarbital was higher in young animals.[129] This result may indicate a faster transport of transcripts from the nuclei of old animals.

F. Age-Dependent Alterations of mRNA Transport in the Brain

A highly complex population of mRNA molecules that are not polyadenylated [poly(A)⁻mRNA] exists in the brain of adult animals.[130] Thus, the mRNA from adult rat brain contains, in contrast to that from rat liver, about 50% poly(A)⁻mRNAs. The brain-specific poly(A)⁻mRNAs,

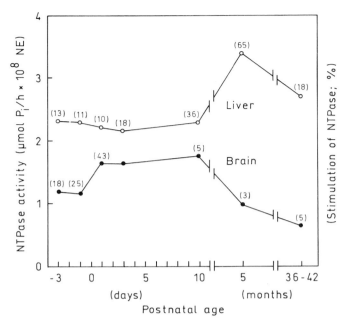

Figure 10
Age-dependent changes of NTPase activity and its stimulation by poly(A) in NE
from rat brain (●) and liver (○). The NTPase activity was determined in the absence
or presence of 90 μM poly(A).

characterized by a high sequence complexity,[131] appear postnatally in
addition to the poly(A)+mRNAs.[130] It is noteworthy that the brain NTPase
activity decreases postnatally as soon as the poly(A)⁻mRNA emerges (in
contrast to rat liver, where the NTPase strongly increases after birth)
(Figure 10).[120] The brain specific poly(A)⁻mRNA sequences can be detected in the nuclei several days before their appearance in the cytoplasm.[130] This lag phase is also observed when the stimulation of the brain
NTPase by poly(A) is measured: the poly(A) stimulation of the brain
enzyme is mostly lost exactly when the poly(A)⁻mRNA appears in the
cytoplasm.[120]

G. RNP-CBP35·CBP67 Interaction During Stress Response and Aging

Recently we demonstrated that under stress conditions the β-galactoside-specific lectin, CBP35, becomes associated to CBP67, which specifically binds to an α-D-glucose-conjugated support.[132] Because CBP35 itself
does not bind to glucose, binding of this lectin to the glucose-affinity
matrix requires a complex formation with CBP67.

In the experiment shown in Figure 11, nuclear glucose-binding proteins were extracted (1) from the livers of rats exposed to transient stress,

Figure 11

Binding of CBP67 and CBP35 to α-D-glucopyranoside-agarose affinity matrix. Nuclear extracts were prepared from the livers of unstressed (lane a) and stressed (immobilization stress for 2 h) mature rats (lane b) and applied to α-D-glucopyranoside-agarose matrix. Proteins retained were eluted with 1 M NaCl and analyzed by SDS-polyacrylamide gel electrophoresis (7.5% gel). Lane M, molecular weight markers. (A) Gel stained with Coomassie brilliant blue; (B) Western-blot detection of CBP35 with anti-CBP35 antibodies. Arrow, CPB35. Molecular weight markers are given as $M_r \times 10^{-3}$.

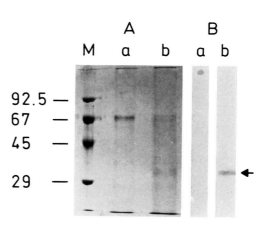

and (2) the livers of unstressed rats and were bound to immobilized α-D-glucose in the presence of divalent cations. Analysis of the proteins retained on the affinity matrix from extracts of unstressed rats by SDS gel electrophoresis revealed only one major protein band (67 kDa; = CBP67) (Figure 11A, lane a). However, nuclear extracts from the livers of rats which were transiently exposed to stress contained an additional major polypeptide band of 35 kDa, which bound to the glucose affinity column (Figure 11A, lane b). Western-blotting experiments revealed that the 35-kDa band was recognized by anti-CBP35 antibodies (Figure 11B, lane b). No immunostaining of a 35-kDa band was visible in the protein retained on the glucose matrix from unstressed animals (Figure 11B, lane a).

In the mature animals, association of CBP35 with CBP67 was even detectable several days after stress treatment. Hence, CBP35 may represent a long-term biomarker for stress exposure. Interestingly, the association of CBP35 to CBP67 was not seen in nuclear extracts from old animals after stress treatment.

At present, the physiological significance both of CBP35·CBP67 and CBP35·CBP70 interaction is unclear, but based on previous results[53,57-59] it can be hypothesized that CBP35·CBP67 may play an important role in spliceosome assembly, as previously proposed for CBP35·CBP70 association,[63] at the nuclear matrix[7] and/or nucleocytoplasmic transport. Evidence has been presented that CBP67, which is present in nuclear RNP particles but not in polysomal complexes, may have a role in nuclear export of mRNP, by directing mRNPs to the nuclear pores.[53] CBP35, on the other hand, has been shown to remain complexed with RNP in the cytoplasm[59] and seems to be cotransported with the mRNA in the form of a RNP complex.[60] It is still unclear how the carrier, p106, interacts with the

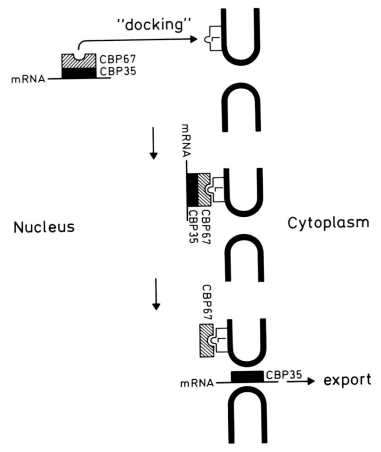

Figure 12
Hypothetic model of function of CBP35·CBP67 complex during nucleocytoplasmic mRNA transport. The mRNA is bound to the amino-terminal domain of CBP35. The carboxyl-terminal, β-galactoside-binding domain of CBP35 is associated with CBP67. The glucose-specific lectin, CBP67, targets the mRNA to the nuclear pore through binding to its NE ligand (L). Loosening of the CBP35·CBP67 association then allows the NTPase-driven and mRNA-carrier-mediated transport of the mRNA into the cytoplasm. CBP35 remains associated with the mRNA during transport.

specific NE ligand of CBP67.[53] A hypothetical scheme of the putative role of CBP35·CBP67 interaction in mRNA transport is shown in Figure 12.

The mechanism which leads to stress-induced CBP35·CBP67 complex formation is not known. Future studies are directed to find out whether this event is caused by a stress-induced enhancement of the plasma glucocorticoid or adrenalin levels. An increase with age in both resting and stress-induced plasma glucocorticoids has been reported by several authors (reviewed in Reference 133) although it is not clear if this is a general phenomenon.[134] Because the liver can be considered as part of the neu-roendocrine network under control of the hypothalamus-pituitary-adrenal axis,[133] elucidation of the mechanism(s) controlling CBP35·CBP67 interaction and its consequences for gene expression may also shed some light on the neuroendocrine hypothesis of aging.

VIII. CONCLUSIONS

In summary, the following factors may contribute to the observed age-dependent impairment of mRNA transport from the nucleus to the cytoplasm:

1. A decreased NTPase activity,
2. A reduced affinity of the poly(A)-binding site (= mRNA carrier) to the poly(A) sequence of mRNA, and
3. A low ability of the NTPase to be stimulated by poly(A).

With age, the functioning of the mRNA translocation system might additionally be reduced due to the occurrence of shortened poly(A) tails, through which the mRNAs cannot efficiently bind to the carrier, and to a decreased efficiency of cytoplasmic transport stimulatory proteins.

REFERENCES

1. Aebi, U., Pante, N., and Jarnik, M., Structure and function of the pore complex, a supramolecular machine mediating molecular trafficking across the nuclear envelope, *Verh. Dtsch. Zool. Ges.*, 85.2, 285, 1992.
2. Agutter, P. S., AcArdle, H. J., and McCaldin, B., Evidence for involvement of nuclear envelope nucleoside triphosphatase in nucleocytoplasmic translocation of ribonucleoprotein, *Nature*, 263, 165, 1976.
3. Schröder, H. C., Rottmann, M., Bachmann, M., and Müller, W. E. G., Purification and characterization of the major nucleoside triphosphatase from rat liver nuclear envelopes, *J. Biol. Chem.*, 261, 663, 1986.
4. Bernd, A., Schröder, H. C., Zahn, R. K., and Müller, W. E. G., Modulation of the nuclear-envelope nucleoside triphosphatase by poly(A)-rich mRNA and by microtubule-protein, *Eur. J. Biochem.*, 129, 43, 1982.
5. Agutter, P. S., *Between Nucleus and Cytoplasm*, Chapman and Hall, London, 1991.
6. Schröder, H. C., Bachmann, M., Diehl-Seifert, B., and Müller, W. E. G., Transport of mRNA from nucleus to cytoplasm, *Prog. Nucl. Acid Res. Molec. Biol.*, 34, 89, 1987.
7. Verheijen, R., van Venrooij, W., and Ramaekers, F., The nuclear matrix: structure and composition, *J. Cell Sci.*, 90, 11, 1988.

8. Schröder, H. C., Steffen, R., Wenger, R., Ugarkovic, D., and Müller, W. E. G., Age-dependent increase of DNA topoisomerase II activity in quail oviduct; modulation of the nuclear matrix-associated enzyme activity by protein phosphorylation and poly(ADP-ribosyl)ation, *Mutat. Res.*, 219, 283, 1989.

9. Schröder, H. C., Trölltsch, D., Friese, U., Bachmann, M., and Müller, W. E. G., Mature mRNA is selectively released from the nuclear matrix by an ATP/dATP-dependent mechanism sensitive to topoisomerase inhibitors, *J. Biol. Chem.*, 262, 8917, 1987.

10. Müller, W. E. G., Okamoto, T., Reuter, P., Ugarkovic, D., and Schröder, H. C., Functional characterization of Tat protein from human immunodeficiency virus. Evidence that Tat links viral RNAs to nuclear matrix, *J. Biol. Chem.*, 265, 3803, 1990.

11. Van Eekelen, C. A. G. and van Venrooij, W. J., hnRNA and its attachment to a nuclear matrix, *J. Cell. Biol.*, 88, 554, 1981.

12. Dreyfuss, G., Matunis, M. J., Piñol-Roma, S., and Burd, C. G., hnRNP Proteins and the biogenesis of mRNA, *Annu. Rev. Biochem.*, 62, 289, 1993.

13. Miller, M., Park, M. K., and Hanover, J. A., Nuclear pore complex: structure, function, and regulation, *Physiol. Rev.*, 71, 909, 1991.

14. Bachmann, M., Bernd, A., Schröder, H. C., Zahn, R. K., and Müller, W. E. G., The role of protein phosphokinase and protein phosphatase during the nuclear envelope nucleoside triphosphatase reaction, *Biochim. Biophys. Acta*, 773, 308, 1984.

15. Schröder, H. C., Diehl-Seifert, B., Rottmann, M., Messer, R., Bryson, B. A., Agutter, P. S., and Müller, W. E. G., Functional dissection of nuclear envelope mRNA translocation system. Effects of phorbol ester and a monoclonal antibody recognizing cytoskeletal structures, *Arch. Biochem. Biophys.*, 261, 394, 1988.

16. Schröder, H. C., Rottmann, M., Wenger, R., Bachmann, M., Dorn, A., and Müller, W. E. G., Studies on protein kinases involved in regulation of nucleocytoplasmic mRNA transport, *Biochem. J.*, 252, 777, 1988.

17. Prochnow, D., Schröder, H. C., Benson, M. A., Agutter, P. S., Fasold, H., and Müller, W. E. G., Effects of associated proteins on messenger RNA export from resealed nuclear envelope ghosts, *Eur. J. Biochem.*, submitted.

18. Schröder, H. C., Rottmann, M., Bachmann, M., Müller, W. E. G., McDonald, A. R., and Agutter, P. S., Messenger RNA transport stimulating proteins from rat liver cytosol. Purification and interactions with the nuclear envelope mRNA translocation system, *Eur. J. Biochem.*, 159, 51, 1986.

19. Schröder, H. C., Friese, U., Bachmann, M., Zaubitzer, T., and Müller, W. E. G., Energy requirement and kinetics of transport of poly(A)-free histone mRNA compared to poly(A)-rich mRNA from isolated L-cell nuclei, *Eur. J. Biochem.*, 181, 149, 1989.

20. Bachmann, M., Mayet, W. J., Schröder, H. C., Pfeifer, K., Meyer zum Büschenfelde, K.-H., and Müller, W. E. G., Association of La and Ro antigen with intracellular structures in HEp-2 carcinoma cells, *Proc. Natl. Acad. Sci. U.S.A.*, 83, 7770, 1986.

21. Hart, G. W., Haltiwanger, R. S., and Kelly, W. G., Glycosylation in the nucleus and cytoplasm, *Ann. Rev. Biochem.*, 58, 841, 1989.

22. Hubert, J., Sève, A. P., Facy, P., and Monsigny, M., Are nuclear lectins and nuclear glycoproteins involved in the modulation of nuclear functions?, *Cell Differ. Dev.*, 27, 69, 1989.

23. Sève, A. P., Hubert, J., Bouvier, D., Bourgeois, C., Midoux, P., Roche, A. C., and Monsigny, M., Analysis of sugar-binding sites in mammalian cells nuclei by quantitative flow microfluorometry, *Proc. Natl. Acad. Sci. U.S.A.*, 83, 5997, 1986.

24. Lawrence, J. B., Singer, R. H., and Marselle, L. M., Highly localized tracks of specific transcripts within interphase nuclei visualized by in situ hybridization, *Cell*, 57, 493, 1989.

25. Jones, N. L. and Kirlpatrick, B. A., The effects of human cytomegalovirus infection on cytoskeleton-associated polysomes, *Eur. J. Cell. Biol.*, 46, 31, 1988.
26. Schröder, H. C., Ugarkovic, D., Langen, P., Bachmann, M., Dorn, A., Kuchino, Y., and Müller, W. E. G., Evidence for involvement of a nuclear-envelope-associated RNA helicase activity in nucleocytoplasmic RNA transport, *J. Cell Physiol.*, 145, 136, 1990.
27. Wagner, R. W., Smith, J. E., Cooperman, B. S., and Nishikura, K., A double-stranded RNA unwinding activity introduces structural alterations by means of adenosine to inosine conversions in mammalian cells and *Xenopus* eggs, *Proc. Natl. Acad. Sci. U.S.A.*, 86, 2647, 1989.
28. Ford, M. J., Anton, I. A., and Lane, D. P., Nuclear protein with sequence homology to translation initiation factor eIF-4A. *Nature*, 332, 736, 1988.
29. Iggo, R. D. and Lane, D. P., Nuclear protein p68 is an RNA-dependent ATPase, *EMBO J.*, 8, 1827, 1989.
30. Hirling, H., Scheffner, M., Restle, T., and Stahl, H., RNA helicase activity associated with the human p68 protein, *Nature*, 339, 562, 1989.
31. Wassarman, D. A. and Steitz, J. A., Alive with DEAD proteins, *Nature*, 349, 463, 1991.
32. Ray, B. K., Lawson, T. G., Kramer, J. C., Cladaras, M. H., Grifo, J. A., Abramson, R. D., Merrick, W. C., and Thach, R. E., ATP-dependent unwinding of messenger RNA structure by eukaryotic initiation factors, *J. Biol. Chem.*, 260, 7651, 1985.
33. Schwer, B. and Guthrie, C., PRP16 is an RNA-dependent ATPase that interacts transiently with the spliceosome, *Nature*, 349, 494, 1991.
34. Company, M., Arenas, J., and Abelson, J., Requirement of the RNA helicase-like protein PRP22 for release of messenger RNA from spliceosomes, *Nature*, 349, 487, 1991.
35. Rosen, C. A., Regulation of HIV gene expression by RNA-protein interactions, *Trends Genet.*, 7, 9, 1991.
36. Brawerman, G., mRNA decay: finding the right targets, *Cell*, 57, 9, 1989.
37. Caput, D., Beutler, B., Hartog, K., Thayer, R., Brown-Shimer, S., and Cerami, A., Identification of a common nucleotide sequence in the 3′ untranslated region of mRNA molecules specifying inflammatory mediators, *Proc. Natl. Acad. Sci. U.S.A.*, 83, 1670, 1986.
38. Peppel, K., Vinci, J. M., and Baglioni, C., The AU-rich sequences in the 3′ untranslated region mediate the increased turnover of interferon mRNA induced by glucocorticoids, *J. Exp. Med.*, 173, 349, 1991.
39. Ryseck, R.-P., Hirai, S. I., Yaniv, M., and Bravo, R., Transcriptional activation of c-jun during the G_0/G_1 transition in mouse fibroblasts, *Nature*, 334, 535, 1988.
40. Pavlakis, G. N. and Felber, B. K., Regulation of expression of human immunodeficiency virus, *The New Biologist*, 2, 20, 1990.
41. Rosen, C. A. and Pavlakis, G. N., Tat and Rev: positive regulators of HIV gene expression, *AIDS*, 4, 499, 1990.
42. Pfeifer, K., Weiler, B. E., Ugarkovic, D., Bachmann, M., Schröder, H. C., and Müller, W. E. G., Evidence for a direct interaction of Rev protein with nuclear envelope mRNA-translocation system, *Eur. J. Biochem.*, 199, 53, 1991.
43. Schröder, H. C., Bachmann, M., and Müller, W. E. G., *Methods for Investigating Nucleo-Cytoplasmic Transport of RNA. A Laboratory Manual*, Gustav Fischer, New York, 1989.
44. Riedel, N. and Fasold, H., Preparation and characterization of nuclear envelope vesicles from rat liver nuclei, *Biochem. J.*, 241, 203, 1987.
45. Riedel, N. and Fasold, H., Nuclear envelope vesicles as a model system to study nucleocytoplasmic transport, *Biochem. J.*, 241, 213, 1987.

46. Riedel, N., Bachmann, M., Prochnow, D., Richter, H. P., and Fasold, H., Permeability measurements with closed vesicles from rat liver nuclear envelopes, *Proc. Natl. Acad. Sci. U.S.A.*, 84, 3540, 1987.

47. Schröder, H. C., Dose, K., Zahn, R. K., and Müller, W. E. G., Isolation and characterization of the novel polyadenylate- and polyuridylate-degrading endoribonuclease V from calf thymus, *J. Biol. Chem.*, 255, 5108, 1980.

48. Jochum, C., Voth, R., Rossol, S., Meyer zum Büschenfelde, K.-H., Hess, G., Will, H., Schröder, H. C., Steffen, R., and Müller, W. E. G., Immunosuppressive function of hepatitis B antigens *in vitro*. Role of the endoribonuclease V as one potential *trans* inactivator for cytokines in macrophages and human hepatoma cells, *J. Virol.*, 64, 1956, 1990.

49. Gillis, P. and Malter, J. S., The adenosine-uridine binding factor recognizes the AU-rich elements of cytokine, lymphokine, and oncogene mRNAs, *J. Biol. Chem.*, 266, 3172, 1991.

50. Malter, J. S., Identification of an AUUUA-specific messenger RNA binding protein, *Science*, 246, 664, 1989.

51. Müller, W. E. G., Slor, H., Pfeifer, K., Hühn, P., Bek, A., Orsulic, S., Ushijima, H., and Schröder, H. C., Association of AUUUA-binding protein with A+U-rich mRNA during nucleocytoplasmic transport, *J. Mol. Biol.*, 226, 721, 1992.

52. Laing, J.G. and Wang, J. L., Identification of carbohydrate binding protein 35 in heterogeneous nuclear ribonucleoprotein complex, *Biochemistry*, 27, 5329, 1988.

53. Schröder, H. C., Facy, P., Monsigny, M., Pfeifer, K., Bek, A., and Müller, W. E. G., Purification of a glucose-binding protein from rat liver nuclei: evidence for a role in targeting of nuclear mRNP to nuclear pore complex, *Eur. J. Biochem.*, 205, 1017, 1992.

54. Facy, P., Sève, A. P., Hubert, M., Monsigny, M., and Hubert, J., Analysis of nuclear sugar-binding components in undifferentiated and in vitro differentiated human promyelocytic leukemia cells (HL60), *Exp. Cell Res.*, 190, 151, 1990.

55. Hanover, J. A., Cohen, C. K., Willingham, M. C., and Park, M. K., O-linked N-acetylglucosamine is attached to proteins of the nuclear pore: evidence for cytoplasmic glycosylation, *J. Biol. Chem.*, 262, 9887, 1987.

56. Bourgeois, C. A., Sève, A. P., Monsigny, M., and Hubert, J., Detection of sugar-binding sites in the fibrillar and the granular components of the nucleolus: an experimental study in cultured mammalian cells, *Exp. Cell. Res.*, 172, 365, 1987.

57. Hubert, J., Sève, A. P., Facy, P., and Monsigny, M., Are nuclear lectins and nuclear glycoproteins involved in the modulation of nuclear functions?, *Cell Different. Dev.*, 27, 69, 1989.

58. Wang, J. L., Laing, J. G., and Anderson, R. L., Lectins in the cell nucleus, *Glycobiology*, 1, 243, 1991.

59. Wang, J. L., Werner, E. A., Laing, J. G., and Patterson, R. J., Nuclear and cytoplasmic localization of a lectin-ribonucleoprotein complex, *Biochem. Soc. Transact.*, 20, 269, 1992.

60. Agrwal, N., Wang, J. L., and Voss, P. G., Carbohydrate-binding protein 35. Levels of transcription and mRNA accumulation in quiescent and proliferating cells, *J. Biol. Chem.*, 264, 17236, 1989.

61. Roff, C. F. and Wang, J. L., Endogenous lectins from cultured cells, *J. Biol. Chem.*, 258, 10657, 1983.

62. Jia, S. and Wang, J. L., Carbohydrate-binding protein 35. Complementary DNA sequence reveals homology with proteins of the heterogeneous nuclear RNP, *J. Biol. Chem.*, 263, 6009, 1988.

63. Sève, A. P., Felin, M., Doyennette-Moyne, M. A., Sahraoui, T., Aubery, M., and Hubert, J., Evidence for a lactose-mediated association between two nuclear carbohydrate-binding proteins, *Glycobiology*, 3, 23, 1993.

64. Schröder, H. C., Wenger, R., Ugarkovic, D., Friese, K., Bachmann, M., and Müller, W. E. G., Differential effect of insulin and epidermal growth factor on mRNA translocation system and transport of specific poly(A+)mRNA and poly(A–)mRNA in isolated nuclei, *Biochemistry*, 29, 2368, 1990.

65. Moore, R. E., Goldsworthy, T. L., and Pitot, H. C., Turnover of 3'-polyadenylate-containing RNA in livers from aged, partially hepatectomized, neonatal, and Morris 5123C hepatoma-bearing rats, *Cancer Res.*, 40, 1449, 1980.

66. Müller, W. E. G., Bachmann, M., and Schröder, H. C., Molecular biological aspects of aging, in *Psychogeriatrics: An International Handbook*, Bergener, M., Ed., Springer, New York, 1987, 12.

67. Schröder, H. C. and Müller, W. E. G., Zellkern und Zellorganellen, in *Biologie des Alterns*, Platt, D., Ed., de Gruyter Verlag, Berlin, 1990, 25.

68. Schröder, H. C. and Müller, W. E. G., Age-correlated decrease in the nuclear restriction of mRNA, in *The Theoretical Basis of Aging Research, Proceedings of the 7th Wiener Symposium on Experimental Gerontology*, Robert, L. and Hofecker, G., Eds., Facultas, Wien, 1990, 123.

69. Yannarell, A., Schumm, D. E., and Webb, T. E., Age-dependence of nuclear RNA processing, *Mech. Ageing Dev.*, 6, 259, 1977.

70. Danner, D. B. and Schröder, H. C., Biologie des Alterns (Ontogenese und Evolution), in *Zukunft des Alterns und gesellschaftliche Entwicklung*, Baltes, P. B. and Mittelstraß, J., Eds., de Gruyter Verlag, Berlin, 1992, chap. 4.

71. Reff, M. E., RNA and protein metabolism, in *Handbook of the Biology of Aging*, Finch, C. E. and Schneider, E. L., Eds., Van Nostrand Reinhold, New York, 1985, 225.

72. Richardson, A. and Semsei, I., Effect of aging on translation and transcription, in *Review of Biological Research in Aging*, Vol. 3, Rothstein, M., Ed., Alan R. Liss, New York, 1987, 467.

73. Castle, T., Katz, A., and Richardson, A., Comparison of RNA synthesis by liver nuclei from rats of various ages, *Mech. Ageing Dev.*, 8, 383, 1978.

74. Semsei, I., Szeszak, F., and Nagy, I. Zs., In vivo studies on the age-dependent decreases of the rates of total and mRNA synthesis in the brain cortex of rats, *Arch. Gerontol. Geriatr.*, 1, 29, 1982.

75. Bolla, R. I. and Miller, J. K., Endogenous nucleotide pools and protein incorporation into liver nuclei from young and old rats, *Mech. Ageing Dev.*, 12, 107, 1980.

76. Müller, W. E. G., Rohde, H. J., Zahn, R. K., and Löhr, J., Alternsabhängige Avidin-Induktion. IV, *Akt. Gerontol.*, 6, 469, 1976.

77. Lindell, T. J., Duffy, J. J., and Byrnes, B., Transcription in aging: the response of rat liver nuclear RNA polymerases to cycloheximide in vivo, *Mech. Ageing Dev.*, 19, 63, 1982.

78. Britton, V. J., Sherman, F. G., and Florini, J. R., Effect of age on RNA synthesis by nuclei and soluble RNA polymerases from liver and muscle of C57BL/6J mice, *J. Gerontol.*, 27, 188, 1972.

79. Mainwaring, W. I. P., Changes in the ribonucleic acid metabolism of aging mouse tissues with particular reference to the prostate gland, *Biochem. J.*, 110, 79, 1968.

80. Bolla, R. and Denckla, W. D., Effect of hypophysectomy on liver nuclear ribonucleic acid synthesis in aging rats, *Biochem. J.*, 184, 669, 1979.

81. Bondy, S. C. and Roberts, S., Developmental and regional variations in ribonucleic acid synthesis on cerebral chromatin, *Biochem. J.*, 115, 341, 1969.

82. O'Meara, A. R. and Herrmann, R. L., A modified mouse liver chromatin preparation displaying age-related differences in salt dissociation and template activity, *Biochem. Biophys. Acta*, 269, 419, 1972.

83. Zeljabovskaja, S. M. and Berdysev, G. D., Composition, template activity and thermostability of the liver chromatin in rats of various age, *Exp. Gerontol.*, 7, 313, 1972.

84. Müller, W. E. G., Zahn, R. K., and Arendes, J., Age-dependent gene induction in quail oviduct. X. Alterations on the posttranscriptional level (enzymic aspect), *Mech. Ageing Dev.*, 14, 39, 1980.

85. Müller, W. E. G., Agutter, P. S., Bernd, A., Bachmann, M., and Schröder, H. C., Role of post-transcriptional events in ageing: consequences for gene expression in eukaryotic cells, in *The 1984 Sandoz Lectures in Gerontology*, Bergener, M., Ermini, M., and Staehelin, H. B., Eds., Academic Press, New York, 1984, 21.

86. Schröder, H. C., Biochemische Grundlagen des Alterns, *Chem. unserer Zeit*, 20, 128, 1986.

87. Lasky, L., Nozick, N. D., and Tobin, A. J., Few transcribed RNAs are translated in avian erythroid cells, *Dev. Biol.*, 67, 23, 1978.

88. Manley, J. L., Polyadenylation of mRNA precursors, *Biochim. Biophys. Acta*, 950, 1, 1988.

89. Proudfoot, N., Poly(A) signals, *Cell*, 64, 671, 1991.

90. Müller, W. E. G., Wenger, R., Bachmann, M., Ugarkovic, D., Courtis, N. C., and Schröder, H. C., Poly(A) metabolism and aging: a current view, *Arch. Gerontol. Geriatr.*, 9, 231, 1989.

91. Green, L. L. and Dove, W.F., Correlation between tubulin mRNA stability and poly(A) length over the cell cycle of *Physarum polycephalum*, *J. Mol. Biol.*, 200, 321, 1988.

92. Carlin, R. K., The poly(A) segment of mRNA: (1) Evolution and function and (2) the evolution of viruses, *J. Theor. Biol.*, 71, 323, 1978.

93. Tsiapalis, C. M., Dorson, J. W., and Bollum, F. J., Purification of terminal riboadenylate transferase from calf thymus gland, *J. Biol. Chem.*, 250, 4486, 1975.

94. Wahle, E., Purification and characterization of a mammalian polyadenylate polymerase involved in the 3′ end processing of messenger RNA precursors, *J. Biol. Chem.*, 266, 3131, 1991.

95. Müller, W. E. G., Endoribonuclease IV. A poly(A)-specific ribonuclease from chick oviduct. I. Purification of the enzyme, *Eur. J. Biochem.*, 70, 241, 1976.

96. Schröder, H. C., Zahn, R. K., Dose, K., and Müller, W. E. G., Purification and characterization of a poly(A)-specific exoribonuclease from a calf thymus, *J. Biol. Chem.*, 255, 4535, 1980.

97. Tsiapalis, C. M., Trangas, T., and Gounaris, A., Phosphorylation and activation of poly(A)-endoribonuclease from calf thymus gland, *FEBS Lett.*, 140, 213, 1982.

98. Schröder, H. C., Zahn, R. K., and Müller, W. E. G., Role of actin and tubulin in the regulation of poly(A) polymerase-endoribonuclease IV complex from calf thymus, *J. Biol. Chem.*, 257, 2305, 1982.

99. Müller, W. E. G., Zahn, R. K., Schröder, H. C., and Arendes, J., Age-dependent enzymatic poly(A) metabolism in quail oviduct, *Gerontology*, 25, 61, 1979.

100. Bernd, A., Schröder, H. C., Zahn, R. K., and Müller, W. E. G., Age-dependence of polyadenylate-stimulation of nuclear-envelope nucleoside triphosphatase, *Mech. Ageing Dev.*, 20, 331, 1982.

101. Schröder, H. C., Schenk, P., Baydoun, H., Wagner, K. G., and Müller, W. E. G., Occurrence of short-sized oligo(A) fragments during course of cell cycle and ageing, *Arch. Gerontol. Geriatr.*, 2, 349, 1983.

102. Pfeifer, K., Ushijima, H., Lorenz, B., Müller, W. E. G., and Schröder, H. C., Evidence for age-dependent impairment of antiviral 2′,5′-oligoadenylate synthetase/ribonuclease L-system in tissues of rat, *Mech. Ageing Dev.*, 67, 101, 1993.

103. Schröder, H. C., Messer, R., Breter, H.-J., and Müller, W. E. G., Evidence of ovalbumin heterogeneous nuclear RNA (hnRNA) processing in hen oviduct, *Mech. Ageing Dev.*, 30, 319, 1985.

104. Messer, R., Schröder, H. C., Breter, H.-J., and Müller, W. E. G., Differential polyadenylation pattern of ovalbumin precursor RNAs during development, *Mol. Biol. Rep.*, 11, 81, 1986.
105. Samarina, O. P. and Krichevskaya, A. A., Nuclear 30S RNP particles, in *The Cell Nucleus*, Busch, H., Ed., Academic Press, New York, 1981, 1.
106. Müller, W. E. G., Arendes, J., Zahn, R. K., and Schröder, H. C., Control of enzymic hydrolysis of polyadenylate segment of messenger RNA: role of polyadenylate-associated proteins, *Eur. J. Biochem.*, 86, 283, 1978.
107. Adams, D. S., Noonan, D., and Jeffery, W. R., The poly(adenylic acid) protein complex is restricted to the nonpolysomal messenger ribonucleoprotein of *Physarum polycephalum*, *Biochemistry*, 19, 1965, 1980.
108. Bernd, A., Batke, E., Zahn, R. K., and Müller, W. E. G., Age-dependent gene induction in quail oviduct. XV. Alterations of the poly(A)-associated protein pattern and of the poly(A) chain length of mRNA, *Mech. Ageing Dev.*, 19, 361, 1982.
109. Bernd, A., Zahn, R. K., Maidhof, A., and Müller, W. E. G., Analysis of poly-adenylate-protein complex of polysomal messenger RNA from mouse L cells, *Hoppe-Seyler's Z. Physiol. Chem.*, 363, 221, 1982.
110. Bernstein, P. and Ross, J., Poly(A), poly(A) binding protein and the regulation of mRNA stability, *TIBS*, 14, 373, 1989.
111. Blobel, G., A protein of molecular weight 78,000 bound to the polyadenylate region of eukaryotic messenger RNAs, *Proc. Natl. Acad. Sci. U.S.A.*, 70, 924, 1973.
112. Baer, B. W. and Kornberg, R. D., Repeating structure of cytoplasmic poly(A) ribonucleoprotein, *Proc. Natl. Acad. Sci. U.S.A.*, 77, 1890, 1980.
113. Tomcsanyi, T., Molnar, J., and Tigyi, A., Structural characterization of nuclear poly(A)-protein particles in rat liver, *Eur. J. Biochem.*, 131, 283, 1983.
114. Van Eekelen, C. A. G., Riemen, T., and van Venrooij, W. J., Specificity of the interaction of hnRNA and mRNA with proteins as revealed by in vivo cross-linking, *FEBS Lett.*, 130, 223, 1981.
115. Ono, T. and Cutler, R. G., Age-dependent relaxation of gene expression: increase of endogenous murine leukemia virus-related and globin-related RNA in brain and liver of mice, *Proc. Natl. Acad. Sci. U.S.A.*, 75, 4431, 1978.
116. Schröder, H.C., Superoxidradikale, Genexpression und Alterung: Reparable Schäden auf der Ebene der DNA und irreparable Schäden auf der Ebene der mRNA-Reifung, *Z. Gerontopsychologie & -psychiatrie*, 2, 259, 1989.
117. Schröder, H. C., Messer, R., Bachmann, M., Bernd, A., and Müller, W. E. G., Superoxide radical-induced loss of nuclear restriction of immature mRNA: a possible cause of ageing, *Mech. Ageing Dev.*, 41, 251, 1987.
118. Bernd, A., Schröder, H. C., Leyhausen, G., Zahn, R. K., and Müller, W. E. G., Alteration of activity of nuclear-envelope nucleoside triphosphatase in quail oviduct and liver in dependence on physiological factors, *Gerontology*, 29, 394, 1983.
119. Müller, W. E. G. and Schröder, H. C., Age-correlated alterations in the nucleocytoplasmic transport of mRNA, in *The Theoretical Basis of Aging Research, Proceedings of the 7th Wien Symposium on Experimental Gerontology*, Robert, F. and Hofecker, G., Eds., Facultas, Vienna, 1990, 117.
120. Schröder, H. C., Becker, R., Bachmann, M., Gramzow, M., Seve, A.-P., Monsigny, M., and Müller, W. E. G., Differential changes of nuclear-envelope-associated enzyme activities involved in nucleocytoplasmic mRNA transport in the devel-oping rat brain and liver, *Biochim. Biophys. Acta*, 868, 108, 1986.
121. Schröder, H. C., Bachmann, M., Bernd, A., Zahn, R. K., and Müller, W. E. G., Age-dependent changes of nuclear envelope protein phosphokinase and protein phosphatase activities. Significance for altered nucleo-cytoplasmic mRNA trans-location during development, *Mech. Ageing Dev.*, 27, 87, 1984.

122. Prochnow, D., Riedel, N., Agutter, P. S., and Fasold, H., Poly(A) binding proteins located at the inner surface of resealed nuclear envelope vesicles, *J. Biol. Chem.*, 265, 6536, 1990.

123. Schäfer, P., Aitken, S. J. M., Bachmann, M., Agutter, P. S., Müller, W. E. G., and Prochnow, D., Immunological evidence for the localization of a 110 kDa poly(A) binding protein from rat liver in nuclear envelopes and its phosphorylation by protein kinase C, *Cell. Molec. Biol.*, 39, 703, 1993.

124. Sippel, A. E., Hynes, N., Groner, B., and Schütz, G., Frequence distribution of messenger sequences within polysomal mRNA and nuclear RNA from rat liver, *Eur. J. Biochem.*, 77, 141, 1977.

125. Horbach, G. J. M. J., Princen, H. M. G., van der Kroef, M., van Bezooijen, C. F. A., and Yap, S. H., Changes in the sequence content of albumin mRNA and in its translational activity in the rat liver with age, *Biochim. Biophys. Acta*, 783, 60, 1984.

126. Dilella, A. G., Chiang, J. Y. L., and Steggles, A. W., The quantitation of liver cytochrome P 450-LM2 mRNA in rabbits of different ages and after phenobarbital treatment, *Mech. Ageing Dev.*, 19, 113, 1982.

127. Horbach, G. J., van der Boom, H., van Bezooijen, C. F., and Yap, S. H., Molecular aspects of age-related changes in albumin synthesis in female WAG/Rij rats, *Life Sci.*, 43, 1707, 1988.

128. Murty, C. V., Mancini, M. A., Chatterjee, B., and Roy, A. K., Changes in transcriptional activity and matrix association of alpha 2u-globulin gene family in the rat liver during maturation and aging, *Biochim. Biophys. Acta*, 949, 27, 1988.

129. Rath, P. C. and Kanungo, M. S., Age-related changes in the expression of cytochrome P-450 (b+e) gene in the rat after phenobarbitone administration, *Biochem. Biophys. Res. Commun.*, 157, 1403, 1988.

130. Chaudhari, N. and Hahn, W. E., Genetic expression in the developing brain, *Science*, 220, 924, 1983.

131. Chikaraishi, D. M., Complexity of cytoplasmic polyadenylated and nonpolyadenylated rat brain ribonucleic acids, *Biochemistry*, 18, 3249, 1979.

132. Lauc, G., Sève, A.-P., Hubert, J., Flögel-Mrsic, M., Müller, W. E. G., and Schröder, H. C., hnRNP CBP35·CBP67 interaction during stress response and ageing, *Mech. Ageing Dev.*, 70, 227, 1993.

133. Finch, C. E. and Landfield, P. W., Neuroendocrine and autonomic functions in aging mammals, in *Handbook of the Biology of Aging*, 2nd ed., Finch, C. E. and Schneider, E. L., Eds., Van Nostrand Reinhold, New York, 1985, 567.

134. de Kloet, E. R., Corticosteroids, stress, and aging, in *Aging and Cellular Defense Mechanisms*, Franceschi, C., Crepaldi, G., Cristofalo, V. J., and Vijg, J., Eds., *Ann. N.Y. Acad. Sci.*, 663, 357, 1992.

135. Heaphy, S., Finch, J. T., Gait, M. J., Karn, J., and Singh, M., Human immunodeficiency virus type 1 regulator of virion expression, rev, forms nucleoprotein filaments after binding to a purine-rich "bubble" located within the rev-responsive region of viral mRNAs, *Proc. Natl. Acad. Sci. U.S.A.*, 88, 7366, 1991.

Chapter **12**

TRANSLATION AND POST-TRANSLATIONAL MODIFICATIONS DURING AGING

Suresh I. S. Rattan

CONTENTS

0-8493-4786-6/95/$0.00+$.50
© 1995 by CRC Press, Inc.

I. INTRODUCTION

The genetic information encoded in DNA becomes functionally meaningful only when it is accurately transcribed and translated into RNA and
proteins, respectively. Whereas two types of RNA, transfer (t) RNA and
ribosomal (r) RNA, are themselves functional molecules, the genetic information transcribed into the third RNA, messenger (m) RNA, has to be
translated from a language of nucleic acids into a language of amino acids
in order to produce proteins, which are the functional products of the
genes. It has been estimated that in a human cell there are about 80,000
genes per haploid genome, of which about 22,000 are housekeeping genes
and the rest are tissue specific.[1] Furthermore, in order to become a functional protein, a newly synthesized polypeptide chain has to undergo a
wide variety of posttranslational modifications that determine its activity,
stability, specificity, and transportability.

Proteins are highly versatile macromolecules. They are necessary for
the organization of internal cellular structures, for the formation of the
energy-creating and metabolic-utilizing systems in the cell, for the transport of ions and larger molecules over the cell membranes, and for maintaining intra- and intercellular communication pathways. Proteins interact with all other macromolecules, including DNA, RNA, carbohydrates,
and lipids, and they are required for maintenance and repair at all levels
of biological organization. Protein synthesis is thus crucial for the survival
of a living system, and any disturbance at this level can cause large
imbalances and deficiencies. Inhibition of protein synthesis is followed
rapidly by cell death. If the processes of protein synthesis and posttranslational modification become less accurate, this can result in the loss of
activity and specificity of proteins and have far-reaching and damaging
consequences for the cell and the organism. Several theories of aging
imply directly or indirectly a role of alterations in protein synthesis and
posttranslational modifications as important determinants of the failure of
maintenance and the failure of homeostasis.[2-4]

A decline in the rate of total protein synthesis is one of the most
common age-associated biochemical changes observed in a wide variety
of cells, tissues, organs and organisms, including human beings. The

implications and consequences of slower rates of protein synthesis are manifold in the context of aging and age-related pathology. For example, slower protein synthesis can result in: (1) a decrease in the availability of enzymes for the maintenance, repair, and normal metabolic functioning of the cell; (2) the inefficient removal of inactive, abnormal, and damaged macromolecules in the cell; (3) inefficiency of the intracellular and intercellular signaling pathways including the receptors; and (4) lower level of production and secretion of hormones, antibodies, neurotransmitters, and the components of the extracellular matrix.

Although there is a considerable variability in the extent of decline among different tissues and cell types, the fact remains that the bulk protein synthesis slows down during aging. Furthermore, it has been shown that the conditions, such as calorie restriction, that increase the life span and retard the aging process in many organisms, also slow down the age-related decline in protein synthesis.[5] These observations reinforce the view that retardation of protein synthesis is an integral part of the aging process. For critical analyses of studies on age-related changes in protein synthesis, the limitations of various methods used to measure protein synthesis, and the differences in results obtained due to the cell-type and species-specific differences, the reader should refer to other reviews.[6-10]

Furthermore, it should be pointed out that the age-related slowing down of bulk protein synthesis does not mean that the synthesis of each and every protein uniformly becomes slower during aging. For example, a significant increase in the heterogeneity of protein synthesis during aging has been observed in *Drosophila*[11] and rat liver cells.[12] Therefore, age-related changes in protein synthesis are regulated both at the transcriptional and the pretranslational levels by changes in the availability of individual mRNA species for translation, and at the translational level by alterations in the components of the protein synthetic machinery of the cell. The aim of this article is to present a review of what is known about the changes in various components of the protein-synthetic machinery and the changes in posttranslational modifications of proteins during aging.

II. REGULATION OF PROTEIN SYNTHESIS DURING AGING

Eukaryotic protein synthesis is a highly complex process that requires about 200 small and large components to function effectively and accurately in order to translate one mRNA molecule while using large quantities of cellular energy. There are three major components of the translational apparatus: (1) the translational particle, the ribosome; (2) the charging system and the amino acid transfer system; and (3) the translational

TABLE 1.

Major Components of the Translational Machinery

Component	Subcomponents	Function
Translational particle		
Ribosome	40S and 60S subunits, 4 rRNAs and about 80 ribosomal proteins	Recognizing and translating the genetic codons in mRNA
Charging system		
Amino acids	At least 20	Building blocks for proteins
tRNAs	About 60	Matching codons with respective amino acids
Aminoacyl-tRNA-synthetases	At least 20	Adding correct amino acids to specific tRNAs
Translational factors		
Initiation factors	About 24 proteins	Making 80S initiation complex
Elongation factors	4 Proteins	Addition of amino acids to growing peptide chain
Release factor	1 Protein	Terminating protein synthesis

factors. The protein-synthesizing apparatus is highly organized and its macromolecular components are not freely diffusible within cells.[13] Table 1 gives an overview of the components and the subcomponents involved in eukaryotic protein synthesis, along with their major functional characteristics.

Protein synthesis can be envisaged as proceeding in three steps — initiation, elongation, and termination — followed by folding and, in many cases, by posttranslational modifications which give the protein a functional tertiary structure.

A. Initiation of Protein Synthesis

The translation of an mRNA molecule begins with the formation of a so-called initiation complex between the ribosome and the initiator codon. It is an intricate process which consumes energy and involves at least seven initiation factors (eIFs; e stands for eukaryotic) consisting of 24 different subunits, two subunits of ribosomes, and an initiating tRNA called methionyl (Met)-tRNA$_i$. Translational initiation begins by the dissociation of inactive 80S ribosomes to generate free 60S and 40S subunits. This dissociation is dependent on the activity of two initiation factors, eIF-3 and eIF-6, which keep subunits apart by binding to the 40S and the 60S subunits, respectively.[14,15] The next step is the formation of the 43S ternary complex of Met-tRNA$_i$, GTP, and eIF-2. Thereafter, through a process that is still largely a mystery, the 43S complex binds to mRNA recognizing its m[7]G cap at the 5' end. Three initiation factors, eIF-4A, 4B, and 4F, are required for optimal binding of mRNA. The binding of 43S complex to the capped 5'-end of mRNA is followed by scanning until the first AUG codon is encountered.[16] Once the correct positioning occurs, and the match is made between the anticodon of the Met-tRNA$_i$ and the start codon, the GTP molecule bound to eIF-2 is hydrolyzed in a reaction promoted by eIF-5. The hydrolysis of GTP causes the release of the initiation factors from the surface of the 40S ribosomal subunit, and it allows the attachment of the 60S subunit by triggering the release of eIF-6. The formation of the 80S initiation complex culminates in the formation of the first peptide bond at the ribosomal P-site, a step mediated by initiation factor eIF-4D. The whole process of the formation of the 80S initiation complex takes about 2 to 3 seconds in cell-free assays and is thought to occur much more rapidly *in vivo*.[16]

Each mRNA can participate in multiple rounds of initiation, thus giving rise to a string of ribosomes called polysomes, engaged at different stages of translation. It is estimated that an efficiently translated mRNA at 37°C initiates protein synthesis once every 5 to 6 seconds.[17] How many times an mRNA can be translated depends on several aspects of its structure, including the context surrounding the AUG codon and its lifetime.[18] What is important in a biological context is that the initiation step is considered to be the main target for the regulation of protein synthesis during the cell cycle, growth, development, hormonal response, and under stress conditions including heat shock, irradiation, and starvation.[16,17]

With respect to aging, however, the rate of initiation appears to remain unaltered. For example, the conversion of isolated 40S and 60S ribosomal subunits into the 80S initiation complex has been reported to decrease by less than 15% in old *Drosophila*,[19] rat liver and kidney,[20] and mouse liver and kidney.[21] On the other hand, since the polysomal fraction of the cellular ribosomes decreases during aging,[19] it suggests that the activity of an anti-ribosomal-association factor, eIF-3, may increase during aging. Similarly, the activity of eIF-2, which is required for the formation of the ternary complex of Met-tRNA$_i$, GTP, and eIF-2, has been reported to decrease in rat tissues during development and aging.[22-24] A decline in the amount (20 to 58%) and activity (30%) of GDP/GTP exchange factor eIF-2β has been reported in the brains and livers of 10-month-old Sprague-Dawley rats as compared with 1- and 4- month-old animals.[25] Similar studies on other eIFs and in other aging systems are yet to be performed. Recent developments in our understanding of the functioning and of posttranslational modifications of various eIFs during cell growth, proliferation, stress, and pathological conditions have revealed a need for further detailed studies on eIFs in the context of aging and for a reinvestigation of the regulation of protein synthesis at the level of initiation.

TABLE 2.

Changes in the Characteristics of Ribosomes During Aging

Characteristic	Change	Aging Systems[a]
Number of ribosomes	Decrease	Rat brain, liver; Drosophila; nematodes
Translational capacity	Decrease	Nematodes; rat liver
Binding to aminoacyl-tRNA	Decrease	Rat liver, kidney; nematodes; Drosophila
Thermal stability	Decrease	Nematodes; Drosophila
	No change	Mouse liver
Fidelity of poly(U) translation	No change	Rat liver, brain, kidney; mouse liver
Sensitivity to aminoglycosides	Increase	Human fibroblasts; rat liver
rRNA synthesis	Decreased	Mouse liver; rat heart
rRNA content	Increase	Human fibroblasts
Ribosomal protein pattern	No change	Mouse liver; Drosophila

[a]   For complete references to each system, see Reference 9.

1. Ribosomes

Ribosomes are cellular organelles that comprise at least 4 types of rRNA and about 80 proteins, and are the pivotal link where the language of nucleic acids is translated into a growing chain of amino acids. In the case of ribosomal proteins, the amino acid sequences of about 35 proteins out of a total of about 80 have been determined. However, the exact roles of the various rRNAs, the proteins, and their mutual interactions in determining the activity, efficiency, and accuracy of the ribosomes is not very well understood at present. Several studies have been performed on the age-related changes in the number of ribosomes, their thermal stability, their binding to aminoacyl-tRNA, the levels of ribosomal proteins and rRNAs, the sensitivity to aminoglycoside antibiotics, and the fidelity of ribosomes (Table 2).

Although there is a slight decrease in the number of ribosomes in old animals, this does not appear to be a rate-limiting factor for protein synthesis, because ribosomes remain abundant in the cell. Instead, several studies indicate that the biochemical and biophysical changes in ribosomal characteristics may be more important for translational regulation during aging. For example, the ability of aged ribosomes to translate synthetic poly(U) or natural globin mRNA decreases significantly.[26,27] A decrease in the translational capacity of ribosomes has also been observed in rodent tissues such as muscle, brain, liver, lens, testis, and parotid gland, and in various organs of Drosophila.[28,29]

The reasons for the functional changes observed in aging ribosomes are not known at present. Some attempts have been made to study the effect of aging on rRNAs and ribosomal proteins. For example, an extensive loss of rRNA gene activity in several tissues of aging beagles, mice and rats, and human lymphocytes and fibroblasts has been reported.[30] Although a threefold increase in the content of rRNA has been reported in late passage senescent human fibroblasts,[31] it is not clear if the quantity and quality of individual rRNA species undergo alterations during aging, or what effect such a change might have on the functioning of ribosomes. Similarly, although an increase in the levels of mRNA for ribosomal protein L7 has been reported in aged human fibroblasts[32] and rat preadipocytes,[33] there are no differences between the electrophoretic patterns of the ribosomal proteins from young and old *Drosophila* and mouse liver.[28,29]

a. Ribosomal Accuracy

Age-related changes in the functioning of ribosomes have also been studied by determining the accuracy of translation of synthetic templates or natural mRNAs. Earlier attempts to estimate the error frequencies during translation *in vitro* of the poly(U) template were inconclusive, because the error frequencies encountered in the assays were several times greater than the estimates of natural error frequencies (for a detailed discussion of this, see References 34 to 36).

Using natural mRNA of CcTMV coat protein for translation by cell extracts prepared from young and old human fibroblasts, a sevenfold increase in cysteine misincorporation during cellular aging has been observed.[37,38] Furthermore, an aminoglycoside antibiotic, paromomycin (Pm), which is known to reduce ribosomal accuracy during translation *in vivo* and *in vitro*, induces more errors in the translation of CcTMV coat protein mRNA by cell extracts prepared from senescent human fibroblasts than in translation by extracts from young cells.[37,38] Similarly, an increase in the Pm-induced error frequency of poly(U) translation by liver ribosomes from old rats as compared with those from young animals has been reported.[39] Further indirect evidence that indicates changes in the ribosome during cellular aging can be drawn from studies on the increase in the sensitivity of cells to the life-shortening and aging-inducing effects of Pm and another aminoglycoside antibiotic, G418.[40,41]

Other studies on ribosomal accuracy during aging have been performed on animal tissues such as chick brain, mouse liver, and rat brain, liver, and kidney. These failed to reveal any major age-related differences in the capacity and accuracy of ribosomes to translate poly(U) in cell-free extracts.[27,39,42-45] Similarly, the accuracy of mouse liver ribosomes did not change with age, as shown by cell-free assays that measured the incorporation of radioactive lysine during the translation of trout protamine mRNA, which does not have codons for lysine.[46] Therefore, even in the absence of any conclusive evidence for or against age-related changes in ribosomal accuracy, it is clear that certain significant and crucial changes do occur in ribosomes during aging, and that this needs further investigation.

B. Elongation of Protein Synthesis

The formation of the 80S initiation complex is followed by the repetitive cyclic event of peptide chain elongation, which is a series of reactions catalyzed by elongation factors (EFs; in eukaryotes also denoted as eEFs). The binding of an aminoacyl (aa)-tRNA carrying the appropriate amino acid is directed by EF-1α bound to GTP. The placement of the aa-tRNA in the A site is accompanied by the hydrolysis of GTP and the release of the EF-1α·GDP complex. The GDP on EF-1α is exchanged by GTP through a process that involves EF-1βγ, thereby regenerating an active EF-1α. The second step of elongation in protein synthesis is the peptidyltransferase reaction, in which a peptide bond is formed between the amino acid in the P-site and the amino acid coupled to aa-tRNA in the A-site. This reaction is catalyzed by the intrinsic activity of the ribosome. The movement, or translocation, of the dipeptide-tRNA from the A-site to the P-site is achieved by the action of EF-2 while another molecule of GTP is hydrolyzed. The deacylated tRNA is pushed away from the ribosome after a transient halt at the so-called exit (E) site. At this point, all the components involved in the elongation cycle become ready to undergo the next cycle. In terms of energy consumption, addition of each new amino acid to a growing polypeptide chain costs four high-energy phosphates coming from two molecules of ATP during aminoacylation and two molecules of GTP during elongation. Various estimates of the elongation rates in eukaryotic cells give a value in the range of 3 to 6 amino acids incorporated per ribosome per second, which is several times slower than the prokaryotic elongation rate of 15 to 18 amino acids incorporated per second.[15-17,47]

With regard to aging, a slowing down of the elongation phase of protein synthesis has been suggested as being crucial in bringing about the age-related decline in total protein synthesis. This is because a decline of up to 80% in the rate of protein elongation has been reported on the basis of estimates of the rate of binding of phenylalanyl-tRNA to ribosomes in poly(U)-translating cell-free extracts from old *Drosophila*, nematodes, and rodent organs.[28,29,48] *In vivo*, a twofold decrease in the rate of polypeptide chain elongation in old WAG albino rat liver and brain cortex has been observed by comparing the kinetics of radioactive leucine incorporation into nascent or still growing, and completed or released, polypeptides.[49] Similarly, a decline of 31% in the rate of protein elongation in the livers of male Sprague-Dawley rats has been reported by measuring the rate of polypeptide chain assembly, which was 5.7 amino acids per second in young animals and 4.5 amino acids per second in 2-year-old animals.[50]

However, these estimates of protein elongation rates have been made for proteins of "average" size. It will be important to see if there is differential regulation of protein elongation rates for different proteins during aging.

1. Elongation Factors

There are commonly two elongation factors in eukaryotes, EF-1 and EF-2 (a third factor, EF-3, is reported only in yeast). These mediate protein-chain elongation and are highly conserved during evolution.[51] EF-1 is comprised of three subunits and it is found in differently aggregated heavy or light forms, depending on the relative amounts of EF-1α and EF-1βγ. Sequences of EF-1α genes, cDNAs, and protein from more than 15 different species have been determined and found to be highly conserved during evolution.[51] Some other interesting features of EF-1α include its high abundance (between 3 and 10% of the cell's soluble protein), and multiple copies or isoforms of the gene that undergo cell-type- and/or developmental-stage-specific expression.[52,53] Furthermore, EF-1α appears to have several other functions in addition to its involvement in protein synthesis. For example, EF-1α has been reported to bind to cytoskeletal elements; it is associated with endoplasmic reticulum; it is part of the valyl-tRNA-synthetase complex; it is associated with the mitotic apparatus; it is involved in maintaining the accuracy of protein synthesis and protein degradation; and its overexpression increases the susceptibility of mammalian cells to transformation.[15,54,55]

With regard to aging, the activity of EF-1 declines with age in rat livers and *Drosophila*, and the drop parallels the decrease in protein synthesis.[28,29] This decline in the activity of EF-1 has been correlated only with EF-1α, as no changes were observed in the EF-1βγ-mediated activity. Using more specific cell-free stoichiometric and catalytic assays, a 35 to 45% decrease in the activity and amounts of active EF-1α has been reported for serially passaged senescent human fibroblasts, and for old mouse and rat livers and brains.[56-58] Another line of evidence that indicates an important role of EF-1α in aging and longevity is the experiments on the germ-line insertion of an extra copy of the EF-1α gene under the regulation of a heat shock promoter, resulting in a longer life span of transgenic *Drosophila* at high temperature.[59] However, this relative increase in the life span of transgenic insects at high temperature, but not at normal temperature, was not accompanied by any increase in the levels of mRNA, protein, or the activity of EF-1α.[60] Similarly, the increased longevity of EF-1α high-fidelity mutants of a fungus *Podospora anserina* suggests that the life-prolonging effects of EF-1α may be due to its role in maintaining the fidelity of protein synthesis.[61] Future studies on other aging systems, particularly human cells and rodents, will clarify the role of EF-1α in the regulation of both protein synthesis and longevity.

The reasons for decline in the activity and amounts of active EF-1α appear to lie at several levels. In *Drosophila*, for example, a decrease of more than 95% in the level of translatable mRNA for EF-1 has been reported.[62] In the case of aging human fibroblasts, rat livers, and *Drosophila*, only about 20 to 30% decline in the amount of EF-1α mRNA has been observed by hybridizing total cellular RNA with EF-1α-specific cDNA probes.[60,63] In contrast to this, a 50-fold increase in RNA transcripts hybridizing to EF-1α cDNA in quiescent and senescent human fibroblasts cells has been reported,[64] which may reflect an overestimation due to the sequence homology of EF-1α with another protein, statin, whose amounts increase in nondividing senescent cells.[65] Studies in which two-dimensional gel-electrophoretic methods were used to determine the total levels of EF-1α protein did not show any major differences during cellular aging of human fibroblasts in culture.[7] Thus, it is not clear at present whether the levels of EF-1α mRNA and protein decrease significantly during aging. Posttranslational modifications such as methylation and phosphorylation of EF-1α, regulating its activity, are discussed in Section III.

In the case of EF-2, which catalyzes the translocation of peptidyl-tRNA on the ribosome during the elongation cycle, conflicting data have been obtained regarding the changes during aging. For example, no difference in the rate of translocation was observed in the translation of poly(U) by cell-free extracts prepared from young and old *Drosophila* and from rodent organs.[28,29] Similarly, although the proportion of heat-labile EF-2 increases during aging, the specific activity of EF-2 purified from old rat and mouse liver remains unchanged.[66] In contrast, a decline of more than 60% in the amount of active EF-2 has been reported during aging of human fibroblasts in culture, measured indirectly by determining the content of diphtheria toxin-mediated ADP-ribosylatable EF-2 in cell lysates.[67] However, the same assay failed to detect any age-related change in the amount of ADP-ribosylatable EF-2 in the livers from calorie-restricted or freely fed rats.[68] Further studies are required to determine whether there are any qualitative or quantitative changes in EF-2 at the levels of transcription, translation, and posttranslational modification, and how such changes are related to the regulation of protein synthesis during aging.

2. tRNA and Aminoacyl-tRNA Synthetases

tRNAs are the molecules that physically bring the amino acids onto the template codons of mRNAs bound to ribosomes. There is at least one tRNA for each codon which is translatable into an amino acid, but there is no tRNA for the stop codons UAA, UAG, and UGA. For several amino acids, for example glycine, alanine, valine, leucine, serine, and arginine, there are four to six isoacceptor tRNA species, and their relative abundance is correlated with the codon usage in the mRNAs.[69] Sequences of a large number of tRNAs and their genes have been determined. All tRNAs are between 70 and 95 nucleotides long and can be folded into a cloverleaf secondary structure. A unique characteristic of tRNA is the presence of several modified nucleotides, which are found near and around the anticodon loop. More than 50 modified nucleotides have been discovered in eukaryotic tRNAs and these include dihydrouridine (D), inosine (I), N^6-isopentenyladenosine (i^6A), queusine (Q), and wyosine (Y). Although the exact mechanisms are not known, these modified nucleotides in tRNA are considered to be involved in the recognition of codons.

The function of a tRNA in transferring the amino acid to the ribosome-mRNA complex is dependent upon a specific enzyme that catalyzes the ligation of the appropriate amino acid to its acceptor arm at the 3' end. This process, aminoacylation of a tRNA, is also known as "charging", and the enzymes involved in this process are called aminoacyl-tRNA synthetases (aaRS) or, more accurately, aminoacyl-tRNA ligases. A group of isoaccepting tRNAs are charged only by the single aaRS specific for their amino acid.[69]

Levels of tRNAs and aaRS have been considered to be rate-limiting for protein synthesis. According to one of the molecular theories of aging, called the codon restriction theory,[70] a random loss of various isoaccepting tRNAs will progressively restrict the readability of codons, resulting in inefficiency and inaccuracy of protein synthesis. There is some evidence that a shift in the pattern of isoaccepting tRNAs occurs during development and aging in some plants, nematodes, insects, and rat liver and skeletal muscle,[71] but its significance in aging is not well understood. Similarly, a 30- to 60-fold increase in the amount of UAG suppressor tRNA has been reported in the brain, spleen, and liver of old mice, and has been related to increased expression of Moloney murine leukemia virus (MO-MuLV) in fibroblasts.[72]

Other characteristics of tRNAs that have been studied as a function of aging include the rate of synthesis, total levels, aminoacylation capacity, and nucleoside composition (Table 3). There is no generalized pattern that emerges from these studies, and the reported changes vary significantly among different species.

The aminoacylation capacity of different tRNAs varies to different extents during aging, and the reasons for this variability are not known.[73] However, the fidelity of aminoacylation did not differ significantly between cell-free extracts prepared from young and from old Sprague-Dawley[74] and Fischer 344 rat livers.[75] Therefore, more studies are required to establish the changes in the structural and functional aspects of individual tRNAs, including their stability, accuracy, and turnover, and in this way elucidate their role in the regulation of protein synthesis during aging.

TABLE 3.

Changes in the Characteristics of tRNA During Aging

Characteristic	Change	Aging systems[a]
Rate of synthesis	Decrease	Mouse liver, kidney heart, muscle
Total levels	Decrease	Mouse liver, kidney, heart, muscle
	Increase	Mouse brain
Capacity to accept amino acids	Variable	Rat liver
Methylation	Decrease	Nematodes; rat and mouse liver, kidney; human fibroblasts
Pattern of isoacceptors	Unstable	Soybean cotyledon; nematodes; *Drosophila*; rat liver
	Stable	Mouse liver, brain; *Drosophila*
Nucleoside composition	No change	Mosquitoes; mouse liver
Modified nucleoside queuine (Q) level	Decrease	Mosquitoes; mouse liver
	Increase	Rat liver
6-Isopentenyl adenosine level	Increase	Rat liver

a   For complete references to each system see Reference 9.

In the case of the aaRSs, an increase or decrease in the specific activities of almost all of them has been reported in various organs of aging mice without any apparent correlation with tissue, cell type, or protein-synthetic activity. A significant decline in the specific activities of 17 aminoacyl-tRNA synthetases has been reported in the liver, lung, heart, spleen, kidney, small intestine, and skeletal muscle of aging female mice[76] and during development and aging of *C. elegans*.[77] Similarly, an increase in the proportions of the heat-labile fraction of several of these enzymes has been reported in the liver, kidney, and brain of old rats.[73] However, no universal pattern can be seen for the changes in the activities of various synthetases in different organs or in different animals. Although an age-related decrease in the efficiency of aaRS can be crucial in determining the rate and accuracy of protein synthesis, direct evidence in this respect is lacking at present.

3. Amino Acids

Cell proliferation and survival can be severely affected by deprivation of a single amino acid.[78,79] However, direct studies on the changes in amino-acid pools during aging have been very few. The levels of various amino acids have been reported to change during aging in insects.[80,81] These changes are not large enough to become rate-limiting for total protein synthesis. Indirect evidence that the levels of normal amino acids may be crucial for survival and longevity comes from studies on the life-shortening effects of amino-acid analogues, such as p-fluorophenylalanine (pFPA), canavanine, and ethionine on *Drosophila* and human fibroblasts.[82,83] Similarly, adult mice fed with pFPA had a reduced life span.[84] What is clear from the limited amount of published data on amino acid levels during aging is that the availability of amino acids is not a rate-limiting factor in the regulation of protein synthesis during aging.

C. Termination of Protein Synthesis

The cycle of peptide-chain elongation continues until one of the three stop codons (UAA, UAG, UGA) is reached. There is no aa-tRNA complementary to these codons and, instead, a release factor (RF) binds to the ribosome and induces the hydrolysis of both the aminoacyl linkage and a GTP molecule, releasing the completed polypeptide chain from the ribosome. Studies on aging *Drosophila* and old rat livers and kidneys have shown that the release of ribosome-bound N-formylmethionine, a measure of the rate of termination, was not affected with age.[28,29] Direct estimates of the activity of RF during aging have not yet been made.

Thus it is clear that the regulation of protein synthesis during aging is not completely understood at present. The age-related decline in the rate of total protein synthesis that has been observed in a wide variety of aging systems appears to be regulated primarily at the elongation step. Although some changes in the elongation factors during aging have been reported, the exact molecular mechanisms of the interactions among ribosomes, aa-tRNAs, and initiation and elongation factors remain to be elucidated. Furthermore, the age-related structural and functional changes in the ribosome and their effects on the ribosomal efficiency and accuracy remain to be fully understood.

III. POSTTRANSLATIONAL MODIFICATIONS DURING AGING

Although faithful translation of the genetic information encoded in mRNA into a polypeptide chain is a prerequisite for accurate protein synthesis, it is not enough to guarantee efficient functioning of the protein. More than 200 types of posttranslational modification of proteins have been described that determine the activity, stability, specificity, transportability, and life span of a protein. Age-related changes in the functioning of proteins can be due to inefficient protein synthesis and/or to an altered pattern of posttranslational modification.[85] For example, although total protein synthesis slows down during aging, the translational processes are never shut off completely. Numerous studies on the biochemical basis of protein function and turnover during various biological processes indicate the crucial role of posttranslational modifications.

The term "posttranslational modification" covers: (1) covalent modifications that yield derivatives of individual amino acid residues, for example, phosphorylation, methylation, ADP-ribosylation, oxidation, and glycation; (2) proteolytic processing through reactions involving the polypeptide backbone; and (3) nonenzymic modifications, for example, deamidation, racemization, and spontaneous changes in protein conformation.

A. Phosphorylation

Phosphorylation of serine, threonine, and tyrosine residues is one of the most common types of posttranslational modification of proteins. At present, about 200 proteins have been reported to be phosphorylated in human cells and the identities of about 40 phosphorylated proteins is known, as seen by two-dimensional gel-electrophoresis.[86] The coordinated activities of protein kinases, which catalyze phosphorylation, and protein phosphatases, which catalyze dephosphorylation, are involved in the regulation of several biological processes, including protein synthesis, cell division, signal transduction, cell growth and development, and aging.[85,87,88] Table 4 gives a list of major proteins whose activities are regulated by phosphorylation.

1. Cell Proliferation

Inhibition of DNA synthesis and the loss of proliferative capacity is the ultimate characteristic of normal diploid cells undergoing aging *in vitro* and *in vivo*. Although several putative inhibitors of DNA synthesis have been identified in senescent cells, little is known about the mechanisms of action and the regulation of activity of these inhibitors.[89] It is possible that the activity of some of these inhibitors is regulated by phosphorylation. Furthermore, several studies have shown age-related alterations in the cell-cycle-regulated expression of various genes such as *c-fos*, *c-jun*, *JunB*, *c-myc*, *c*-Ha-*ras*, *p53*, *cdc2*, *cycA*, *cycB*, *cycD* and retinoblastoma gene *RB1*.[32,90-93] Although phosphorylation is involved in regulating the activities of the gene products of almost all these genes,[94] a decrease in phosphorylated cyclin E and Cdk2[93] and failure to phosphorylate *RB1* gene product p110[Rb] and *cdc2* product p34[cdc2] during cellular aging have been reported up to now.[95,96] It will be important to find out if there are age-related alterations in the phosphorylation state of other cell-cycle-related gene products, including various transcription factors.

TABLE 4.

Some Proteins Whose Activities are Modulated by Phosphorylation

Biological Process	Effect of phosphorylation	
	Increased activity	Decreased activity
DNA synthesis and cell proliferation	DNA polymerase α, histones	Products of *cdc*-series genes, retinoblastoma gene product
Protein synthesis	S6 ribosomal protein, initiation factors, eIF-3, 4B, 4F, aminoacyl-tRNA-synthetases	Initiation factor eIF-2, elongation factors EF-1α, β, EF-2
Structural organization and metabolism	Vimentin, lamin, neurofilament proteins, microtubules, glycogen phosphorylase, tyrosine hydroxylase	Synapsin
Signal transduction	Growth factor receptors, G protein subunits $\alpha_{i\text{-}2}$, α_z	Adrenergic and muscarinic receptors

Of the various components involved in the synthesis of DNA, a decline in the specific activity of DNA polymerase α has been reported for nondividing senescent human fibroblasts[97,98] and for old mice.[99] It is possible that this change is due to a decrease in the phosphorylation of DNA polymerase α, as observed during cell-cycle-related changes in the activity of this enzyme in normal and leukemic human cells.[100,101] Direct studies on the phosphorylation status of DNA polymerase α during aging are yet to be performed. Similarly, it is not known whether the age-related decline in the fidelity of DNA polymerase α during aging is related to altered levels of phosphorylation.[102]

Alterations of phosphorylation have also been observed for vimentin, lamin, histones, and nonhistone proteins during the mammalian cell cycle.[103] At present, there are no data available for the age-related changes in phosphorylation of these proteins. However, a decline of 50% in the phosphorylation of two acidic proteins and an increase of 300% in the phosphorylation of one basic protein in the microsomal and nuclear fraction of aging rat hepatocytes has been reported.[104]

2. The Translational Apparatus

Various components of the protein-synthetic apparatus undergo phosphorylation and dephosphorylation and thus regulate the rates of protein synthesis.[15,17] For example, the phosphorylation of eIF-2 correlates with inhibition of initiation reactions, and consequently with the inhibition of protein synthesis, by affecting the process of guanine nucleotide exchange.[105] Conditions such as starvation, heat shock, and viral infection, which inhibit the initiation of protein synthesis, induce the phosphorylation of eIF-2 in various cells. Similarly, stimuli such as insulin and phorbol esters modulate the phosphorylation of eIF-3, eIF-4B, and eIF-4F by activating various protein kinases. As regards aging, the activity of eIF-2 has been reported to decrease in old rat brain.[23] However, it is not known whether the phosphorylation status of eIF-2 also changes during aging. Similarly, no studies have been carried out on age-related changes in other initiation factors.

At the level of protein elongation, the phosphorylation of elongation factors EF-1α and EF-2 appears to be involved in the regulation of their activities.[47] Since it has been reported that the activity and amounts of active EF-1α and EF-2 decrease significantly during aging, it will be interesting to see whether this decline is accompanied by a parallel change in the extent of phosphorylation of these enzymes. Incidentally, it has been reported that there is an increase in the levels of phosphorylated EF-1 and EF-2 during mitosis, when minimal protein synthesis occurs.[106] There is indirect evidence that an increase in the level of phosphorylated EF-2 due to increased activity of EF-2-specific protein kinase III in old rat livers[107] may account for reduced protein synthesis during aging.

Phosphorylation also occurs in other proteins that participate in the translational process. For example, a regulatory role in protein synthesis has been suggested for the phosphorylation of aa-tRNA synthetase.[108] However, it is not known to what extent the decline in the activity and the accumulation of heat-labile aa-tRNA synthetases, reported in studies performed on various organs of aging mice and rats,[73,76] is related to their phosphorylation. Similarly, phosphorylation of the S6 ribosomal protein correlates with the activation of protein synthesis.[109] Since senescent human fibroblasts fail to phosphorylate S6 protein in response to serum,[110] this could be one of the reasons for the decline in the rate of protein synthesis observed during aging.

3. Signal Transduction

Pathways of intracellular signal transduction depend on sequential phosphorylation and dephosphorylation of a wide variety of proteins. All phosphorylation reactions result from the action of a single or multiple kinases, and the ratio between two interconvertible forms of kinases acts as a control mechanism for many cellular functions.[111] Typical examples of protein kinases regulating cellular mechanisms are the protein kinase C (PKC; signal transduction), growth factors receptors (cell growth), glucocorticoid receptors (hormonal action), and the glycogen phosphorylase (energy metabolism).

Studies performed on aging cells have not shown any deficiency in the amount, activity, or ability of PKC.[85] There is also evidence that senescent human fibroblasts retain their ability to phosphorylate proteins in the PKC signal-transduction pathway.[112] It appears that the PKCs are largely unaltered in fibroblasts, although the body of information about phosphorylation mechanisms is still very limited.

Growth-factor receptors for EGF, FGF, PDGF, insulin, glucocorticoids, and several other hormones also possess protein kinase activity. Therefore, deficiencies in the phosphorylation process of receptors would be a logical explanation for the age-related decline of responsiveness to hormonal action and growth stimulation. However, there is no age-related decline in the autophosphorylation activity of various growth-factor receptors.[113-116] Similarly, most of the PKC-mediated pathways of intracellular signal transduction, which are brought in action in response to various mitogens, appear to remain unaltered in senescent fibroblasts[115-117] However, in the case of T lymphocytes in aging mice, a decline in both serine/threonine- and tyrosine-specific protein kinase signals after activation has been observed.[118,119]

Another area in which protein phosphorylation plays a crucial role is neuronal communication. Since one of the major characteristics of aging includes defective neuronal systems, it has been suggested that either a loss of activity of the mediating kinases or decreased substrate availability may be involved in this. Studies on aged rodents have demonstrated reduced cAMP-dependent phosphorylation, area-selective modifications of PKC activity and translocation ability, and impairment of the adenylate cyclase system during aging.[85] Similarly, the phosphorylation of glycogen phosphorylase increases its affinity for glycogen by inducing a conformational change of the amino terminus, while the presence of glucagon and glucose-6-phosphate leads to its dephosphorylation and inactivation.[85] The ratio between the active and inactive forms of the enzyme regulates the energy metabolism. Therefore, it will be interesting to find out if the age-related decline in the activity of glycogen phosphorylase reported for rat heart muscle and human aorta is an example of allosteric control due to changes in the phosphorylation pattern of this enzyme.[85]

It can thus be concluded that the phosphorylation of a wide variety of proteins can have significant influence in various biological processes, and it will be extremely useful to undertake detailed studies on this posttranslational modification in relation to the process of aging.

B. ADP-Ribosylation

The structure and function of many proteins is modulated by posttranslational ADP-ribosylation, which is the enzymic addition of a ADP-ribose derived from NAD^+. These proteins include the nuclear proteins topoisomerase I, DNA ligase II, endonuclease, histones H1, H2B, and H4, DNA polymerases α and β, and the cytoplasmic proteins adenyl cyclase and elongation factor EF-2.[51,120-122] Generally, the cytoplasmic enzymes called mono-ADP-ribosyltransferases catalyze the formation of a mono-ADP-ribosyl protein, while the nuclear enzyme poly(ADP-ribose)polymerase (PARP) catalyzes the addition of several ADP-ribosyl residues to proteins.[120,121] ADP-ribosylation of proteins is involved in various cellular processes such as the maintenance of chromatin structure, DNA repair, protein synthesis, cell differentiation, and cell transformation.[121]

As yet, no studies have been carried out regarding the changes in the extent of poly-ADP-ribosylation of any specific proteins during aging. However, indirect evidence suggests that poly-ADP-ribosylation of proteins may decrease during aging because the activity of PARP decreases in aging human fibroblasts, both as a function of donor age and during serial passaging *in vitro*.[123] Similarly, the direct relationship observed between maximum life span of a species and the activity of PARP in mononuclear leukocytes of 13 mammalian species indicates its important role in aging and longevity.[124,125]

One cytoplasmic protein that can be specifically ribosylated by at least two bacterial toxins, namely diphtheria toxin and exotoxin A, is the protein elongation factor EF-2. ADP-ribosylation of the diphthamide (modified histidine 715) residue of EF-2 results in the complete abolition of its catalytic activity.[51] There is some evidence that increased ADP-ribosylation of EF-2 is correlated with cellular aging. For example, the amount of EF-2 that can be ADP-ribosylated in the presence of diphtheria toxin in cell-free extracts decreases significantly during aging of human fibroblasts in culture.[67] However, no decline in the amount of ADP-ribosylatable EF-2 was observed in liver extracts prepared from calorie-restricted and freely fed Fischer 344 rats of different ages.[68] Therefore, it is not clear to what extent the decline in the activity of EF-2 correlates with the decline in the rate of protein synthesis during aging.

C. Methylation

Methylation of nitrogens of arginine, lysine, and histidine, and carboxyls of glutamate and aspartate residues, is a widely observed post-translational modification that is involved in many cellular functions.[126] A number of specific enzymes, comprising three major groups of protein methyltransferases, have been identified on the basis of the amino acids that become methylated.[127] Although most of our present understanding regarding the significance of protein methylation has come from studies on bacterial chemotaxis, muscle contraction, electron transport, processing of pituitary hormones, and gene expression, its role in aging is beginning to emerge.

Proteins whose activities are increased by methylation include alcohol dehydrogenase, histones, ribosomal proteins, cytochrome C, elongation factor EF-1α, myosin, myelin, and rhodopsin.[85] Of these, decreased methylation of histones in livers and brains of aging rats has been reported.[85] On the other hand, there is no difference in the extent of methylation of newly synthesized histones during cellular aging of human fibroblasts in culture.[85] Studies on the levels of methylated histidine, arginine, and lysine of myosin isolated from the leg muscles of aging rats, mice, and hamsters showed unchanged levels of histidine, decreased levels of arginine and trimethyllysine, and increased levels of monomethyllysine.[85]

During the aging of erythrocytes, there is an increase in the number of methyl groups per molecule of band 2.1 (ankyrin) and band 3 protein, which correlates with increased membrane rigidity of erythrocytes during aging.[128] Similarly, there is a severalfold increase in the number of methyl acceptor proteins in the eye lenses of aged humans and persons suffering from cataracts.[129] The number of carboxylmethylatable sites of cerebral membrane-bound proteins also increases in rat brain during aging.[130]

An interesting case of the role of protein methylation in modulating enzyme activity is that of elongation factor EF-1α, which contains dimethyllysines at residues 55 and 165, and trimethyllysines at 36, 79, and 318.[51] The increased activity of EF-1α during morphogenesis of the fungus *Mucor racemosus* is associated with its enhanced methylation levels.[51] Similarly, the levels of methylated EF-1α were significantly higher in SV40-transformed mouse 3T3 fibroblasts as compared with immortal 3T3 cells without viral transformation, as determined by two-dimensional gel electrophoresis.[131] However, no major differences in the levels of methylated and unmethylated EF-1α could be observed during aging of human fibroblasts by the same method.[7]

Until now, age-related changes in the methylation of other proteins such as ribosomal proteins, calmodulin, cytochrome C, and myosin have not been studied. It is clear that protein methylation is involved in diverse functions, including protein synthesis and turnover, and that it should be studied thoroughly in relation to the process of aging.

D. Proteolytic Processing

Many newly synthesized proteins undergo posttranslational proteolytic processing, in which conformational restraint on the inactive precursor is released and a biologically active protein is generated. Several inactive precursors of enzymes called zymogens, precursors of growth factors, peptide and protein hormones such as insulin, precursors of extracellular matrix, and many other secretory proteins including various proteases such as collagenase undergo proteolytic processing.

No systematic studies on age-related changes in posttranslational proteolytic processing of any proteins have been described. However, there is some evidence that alterations in proteolytic processing may be among the reasons for the appearance or disappearance of certain proteins during aging. For example, the appearance of the so-called "senescent cell antigen" on the surface of a wide variety of aging cells is considered to be derived from the proteolysis of band 3 protein.[132] The exposure of senescent cell-specific epitopes on fibronectin[133,134] may also be due to altered proteolytic processing. Progressive proteolysis of a 90-kDa protein, Tp-90 terminin, into Tp-60 and Tp-30 terminin in senescent cells and in cells committed to apoptosis has been reported.[135,136] Increased proteolysis of a conformationally more labile single-chain form of the lysosomal protease cathepsin B has been suggested as a reason for the age-related decline in its activity during the aging of human fibroblasts.[137] Similarly, it has been suggested that alterations in the activity of collagenase during aging of human fibroblasts may be due to structural and catalytic changes.[138,139]

E. Oxidation

The accumulation of inactive and abnormal proteins during aging is a widely observed phenomenon. One of the reasons for the inactivation of enzymes can be their oxidative modification by oxygen free radicals and by mixed-function oxidation (MFO) systems or metal-catalyzed oxidation (MCO) systems.[140] Since some amino acid residues, particularly proline, arginine, and lysine, are oxidized to carbonyl derivatives, the amount of carbonyl content of proteins has been used as an estimate of protein oxidation during aging. Some of the proteins that have been shown to undergo oxidation are listed in Table 5.

Increased levels of oxidatively modified proteins have been reported in human erythrocytes of higher density (considered as old), and in cultured human fibroblasts from normal old donors and from individuals suffering from progeria and Werner's syndrome.[140,141] Similarly, there was a twofold increase in the protein carbonyl content of the brain proteins of retired breeder Mongolian gerbils, which was reversed by treatment with a spin-trapping compound N-tert-butyl-α-phenylnitrone (PBN).[142] An age-related increase in the carbonyl content has also been reported for houseflies,[143] mouse organs,[144] and Drosophila.[145]

It has also been suggested that the loss of 11 lysine residues, presumed due to oxidation, may be the cause of the inactivation of 6-phosphogluconate dehydrogenase in rat livers and human erythrocytes during aging. Similarly, the loss of activity of rat liver malic enzyme during aging is related to the loss of histidine residues by oxidation.[146] Furthermore, oxidation of a cysteine residue in glyceraldehyde-3-phosphate dehydrogenase may be responsible for its inactivation during aging in rat muscles.[147,148] It has also been reported that the concentration of the oxidation products of human lens proteins and skin collagen increases along with the accumulation of oxidative forms of α-crystallin in patients with age-related cataracts.[140] However, the content of ortho-tyrosine and dityrosine, formed by the

TABLE 5.

Proteins That Become Inactive or
Denatured After Oxidation During Aging

Glyceraldehyde-3-phosphate dehydrogenase
Glucose-6-phosphate dehydrogenase
6-Phosphogluconate dehydrogenase
Fructose-1,6-diphosphatase
Lactate dehydrogenase
Glutamine synthetase
Ornithine decarboxylase
Liver malic enzyme
Superoxide dismutase
Lens crystallin
Ceruloplasmin
Collagen

oxidation of phenylalanine and tyrosine, respectively, did not increase in the aging human lens.[149]

Structural alterations introduced into proteins by oxidation can lead to the aggregation, fragmentation, denaturation, and distortion of secondary and tertiary structure, thereby increasing the susceptibility of oxidized proteins to proteolysis.[140,147] Thus, the accumulation of abnormal proteins during aging may be due to an impairment of the protein degradation processes and/or to defective protection from oxidative damage. If better methods can be developed for the accurate estimation of the levels of oxidation products of proteins, they may become valuable as biomarkers of aging.

F. Glycation

Glycation is one of the most prevalent covalent modifications, in which the free amino groups of proteins react with glucose to form a ketoamine called Amadori product. This is followed by a sequence of further reactions and rearrangements leading to the production of the so-called advanced glycosylation end products (AGEs).[150,151] Most commonly, it is the long-lived structural proteins such as lens crystallins, collagen, and basement membrane proteins which show the greatest susceptibility to glycation. The glycated proteins are more prone to form cross-links with other proteins, leading to structural and functional alterations.[150,151]

An increase in the levels of glycated proteins during aging has been observed in a wide variety of systems. For example, there is an increase in the level of glycated lysine residues of rat sciatic nerve, aorta, and skin collagen during aging.[152] Similarly, there is an increase in the glycation of human collagen and osteocalcin during aging.[153] There is also an increase in the levels of glycation of collagen, hemoglobin, and human lens crystallin in patients with diabetes.[85] Calorie-restricted rodents, whose aging is generally slowed down, have reduced levels of glycated hemoglobin as compared with freely fed animals.[154]

The formation and the accumulation of the AGEs are implicated in the physiology and pathology of senescence.[155,156] It has been observed that amounts of pentosidine (cross-linked glycated lysine and arginine) and carboxylmethyllysine increase with age in humans.[155,157] Pyrroline, another AGE protein, has been shown to increase in diabetics.[155] Similarly, with the use of AGE-specific antibodies, an AGE-modified form of human hemoglobin has been identified whose levels increase during aging and in patients with diabetes-induced hyperglycemia.[158] More studies are required in order to understand differences in the rates of formation and removal of glycated proteins in different species with different life spans and rates of aging.

G. Deamidation, Racemization, and Isomerization

Age-related changes in the catalytic activity, heat stability, affinity for substrate, and other physical characteristics such as the conformation of proteins, may also be due to the change in electrostatic charge introduced by conversion of a neutral amide group to an acidic group by deamidation.[159] Spontaneous deamidation of asparaginyl and glutaminyl residues of several proteins has been related with the observed accumulation of their inactive and heat-labile isoforms during aging.[147] For example, the sequential deamidation of two asparagine residues of triosephosphate isomerase is responsible for the differences between the isozymes present in aging cells and tissues, such as bovine eye lens, and human skin fibroblasts from old donors and patients with progeria and Werner´s syndrome.[160] Similarly, deamidation of glucose-6-phosphate isomerase produces the variant of the enzyme that accumulates in aging bovine lenses.[161]

The interconversion of optical isoforms of amino acids, called racemization, has been reported to increase during aging. For example, the concentration of D-aspartate in protein hydrolysates from human teeth, erythrocytes and eye lens increases with age.[162,163] The spontaneous prolyl *cis-trans* isomerization in proteins that may cause some of the so-called spontaneous conformational changes has been implicated in the age-related decline in the activity of certain enzymes.[141] However, no definitive examples of enzymes undergoing this kind of post-translational modification during aging are known. Neither is it known to what extent the conformational changes associated with old rat muscle phosphoglycerate kinase,[164,165] enolase and other enzymes[141] are associated with racemization and isomerization.

H. Other Modifications

In addition to the types of posttranslational modification mentioned above, there are some other modifications that determine the structure and function of various proteins and may have a role to play during aging. For example, the incorporation of ethanolamine into protein elongation factor EF-1α may be involved in determining its stability and interaction with intracellular membranes.[51] Whether this modification has any role in the regulation of the activity of EF-1α is not known at present. Similarly, the protein initiation factor eIF-5A contains an unusual amino acid, hypusine, which is synthesized posttranslationally as a result of a series of enzymically catalyzed alterations of a lysine residue.[166] Since the absence of hypusine in eIF-5A blocks the initiation of protein synthesis,[166] it will be interesting to investigate changes in this modification during aging when total protein synthesis slows down.

Protein tyrosine sulfation is another posttranslational modification that may have significance in protein alteration during aging because it is involved in determining the biological activity of neuropeptides and the intracellular transport of a secretory protein.[167] Similarly, prenylation, the covalent attachment of isoprenoid lipids on cysteine-rich proteins, is involved in the regulation of the activity of some G proteins, protooncogenic ras proteins, and the nuclear lamins A and B.[168] These studies have indicated a critical role for prenylation in the regulation of oncogenesis, nuclear structure, signal transduction, and cell cycle progression, functions very much related to the causative aspects of aging.

Detyrosination of microtubules[169] affecting the cytoskeletal organization and many other cellular functions may also be important during aging. Furthermore, the roles of chaperones in protein folding and conformational organization[170] have yet to be studied in relation to the aging process. However, ubiquitin marking of proteins for degradation and ubiquitin-mediated proteolysis do not decline during aging, since no change was found in the levels of ubiquitin mRNA and ubiquitin pools in aging human fibroblasts in protein degradation.[171]

Finally, according to the cross-linking theory of aging, the progressive linking together of large vital molecules, especially the proteins, results in the loss of cellular functions.[172] There is some evidence that both the pentose-mediated protein cross-linking[157] and the transglutaminase-mediated cross-linking[173] of proteins is involved in aging and cell death. For example, there is a strong correlation between pentosidine protein cross-links and pigmentation in senescent and cataract-affected human lens.[174] Similarly, an increase in transglutaminase activity during apoptosis, differentiation, and aging of human keratinocytes[175,176] indicates an important role of this modification in the process of aging.

In conclusion, it is clear that an efficient and accurate translational machinery and the posttranslational modification of proteins constitute the fundamental biochemical processes for cellular functioning and survival. Alterations at the level of protein synthesis and their postsynthetic modifications can have widespread detrimental effects on the maintenance and survival of cells, tissues, organs and organisms, leading to aging and death.

REFERENCES

1. Antequera, F. and Bird, A., Number of CpG islands and genes in human and mouse., *Proc. Natl. Acad. Sci. U.S.A.*, 90, 11995, 1993.
2. Holliday, R., Towards a biological understanding of the aging process, *Persp. Biol. Med.*, 32, 109, 1988.
3. Rattan, S. I. S. and Clark, B. F. C., Ageing: a challenge for biotechnology, *Trends Biotech.*, 6, 58, 1988.
4. Medvedev, Z. A., An attempt at a rational classification of theories of ageing, *Biol. Rev.*, 65, 375, 1990.
5. Yu, B. P., Food restriction research: past and present status, *Rev. Biol. Res. Aging*, 4, 349, 1990.
6. Makrides, S. C., Protein synthesis and degradation during aging and senescence, *Biol. Rev.*, 58, 343, 1983.
7. Rattan, S. I. S., Protein synthesis and the components of protein synthetic machinery during cellular aging, *Mutat. Res.*, 256, 115, 1991.
8. Ward, W. and Richardson, A., Effect of age on liver protein synthesis and degradation, *Hepatology*, 14, 935, 1991.
9. Rattan, S. I. S., Regulation of protein synthesis during ageing, *Eur. J. Gerontol.*, 1, 128, 1992.
10. Van Remmen, H., Ward, W. F., Sabia, R. V., and Richardson, A., Gene expression and protein degradation, in *The Handbook of Physiology: Aging*, Masoro, E., Ed., Oxford University Press, 1995, 171.
11. Fleming, J. E., Quattrocki, E., Latter, G., Miquel, J., Marcuson, R., Zuckerkandi, E., and Bensch, K. G., Age-dependent changes in proteins of *Drosophila melanogaster*, *Science*, 231, 1157, 1986.
12. Butler, J. A., Heydari, A. R., and Richardson, A., Analysis of effect of age on synthesis of specific proteins by hepatocytes, *J. Cell. Physiol.*, 141, 400, 1989.
13. Negrutskii, B. S., Stapulionis, R., and Deutscher, M. P., Supramolecular organization of the mammalian translation system, *Proc. Natl. Acad. Sci. U.S.A.*, 91, 964, 1994.
14. Rhoads, R. E., Initiation: mRNA and 60S subunit binding., in *Translation in Eukaryotes*, Trachsel, H., Ed., CRC Press, Boca Raton, FL, 1991, 109.
15. Merrick, W. C., Mechanism and regulation of eukaryotic protein synthesis, *Microbiol. Rev.*, 56, 291, 1992.
16. Kozak, M., The scanning model for translation: an update, *J. Cell Biol.*, 108, 229, 1989.
17. Hershey, J. W. B., Translational control in mammalian cells, *Annu. Rev. Biochem.*, 60, 717, 1991.
18. Kozak, M., An analysis of vertebrate mRNA sequences: intimations of translational control, *J. Cell Biol.*, 115, 887, 1991.

19. Webster, G. C., Webster, S. L., and Landis, W. A., The effect of age on the initiation of protein synthesis in *Drosophila melanogaster, Mech. Ageing Dev.,* 16, 71, 1981.
20. Gabius, H. J., Engelhardt, R., Deerberg, F., and Cramer, F., Age-related changes in different steps of protein synthesis of liver and kidney of rats, *FEBS Lett.,* 160, 115, 1983.
21. Blazejowski, C. A. and Webster, G. C., Effect of age on peptide chain initiation and elongation in preparations from brain, liver, kidney and skeletal muscle of the C57B1/6J mouse, *Mech. Ageing Dev.,* 25, 323, 1984.
22. Calés, C., Fando, J. L., Azura, C., and Salinas, M., Developmental studies of the first step of the initiation of brain protein synthesis, role for initiation factor 2, *Mech. Ageing Dev.,* 33, 147, 1986.
23. Castañeda, M., Vargas, R., and Galván, S. C., Stagewise decline in the activity of brain protein synthesis factors and relationship between this decline and longevity in two rodent species, *Mech. Ageing Dev.,* 36, 197, 1986.
24. Vargas, R. and Castañeda, M., Heterogeneity of protein synthesis initiation factors in developing and aging rat brain, *Mech. Ageing Dev.,* 26, 371, 1984.
25. Kimball, S. R., Vary, T. C., and Jefferson, L. S., Age-dependent decrease in the amount of eukaryotic initiation factor 2 in various rat tissues, *Biochem. J.,* 286, 263, 1992.
26. Nokazawa, T., Mori, N., and Goto, S., Functional deterioration of mouse liver ribosomes during aging: translational activity and the activity for formation of the 47S initiation complex, *Mech. Ageing Dev.,* 26, 241, 1984.
27. Sojar, H. T. and Rothstein, M., Protein synthesis by liver ribosomes from aged rats, *Mech. Ageing Dev.,* 35, 47, 1986.
28. Webster, G. C., Protein synthesis in aging organisms, in *Molecular Biology of Aging: Gene Stability and Gene Expression,* Sohal, R. S., Birnbaum, L. S., and Cutler, R. G., Eds., Raven Press, New York, 1985, 263.
29. Webster, G. C., Effect of aging on the components of the protein synthesis system, in *Insect Aging,* Collatz, K. G. and Sohal, R. S., Eds., Springer-Verlag, Berlin, 1986, 207.
30. Medvedev, Z. A., Age-related changes of transcription and RNA processing, in *Drugs and Aging,* Platt, D., Eds., Springer-Verlag, Berlin, 1986, 1.
31. Adam, G., Simm, A., and Braun, F., Levels of ribosomal RNA required for stimulation from quiescence increase during cellular aging in vitro of mammalian fibroblasts, *Exp. Cell Res.,* 169, 345, 1987.
32. Seshadri, T. and Campisi, J., Repression of c-fos transcription and an altered genetic program in senescent human fibroblasts., *Science,* 247, 205, 1990.
33. Kirkland, J. L., Hollenberg, C. H., and Gillon, W. S., Effects of aging on ribosomal protein L7 messenger RNA levels in cultured rat preadipocytes, *Exp. Gerontol.,* 28, 557, 1993.
34. Holliday, R., *Genes, Proteins, and Cellular Aging,* Van Nostrand Reinhold, New York, 1986.
35. Holliday, R., Testing molecular theories of cellular aging, in *Thresholds on Ageing: The 1984 Sandoz Lectures in Gerontology,* Bergeber, M., Ermini, E., and Stahelin, H. B., Eds., Academic Press, London, 1985, 21.
36. Kirkwood, T. B. L., Holliday, R., and Rosenberger, R. F., Stability of the cellular translation process, *Int. Rev. Cytol.,* 92, 93, 1984.
37. Luce, M. C. and Bunn, C. L., Altered sensitivity of protein synthesis to paromomycin in extracts from aging human diploid fibroblasts, *Exp. Gerontol.,* 22, 165, 1987.

38. Luce, M. C. and Bunn, C. L., Decreased accuracy of protein synthesis in extracts from aging human diploid fibroblasts, *Exp. Gerontol.*, 24, 113, 1989.
39. Butzow, J. J., McCool, M. G., and Eichhorn, G. L., Does the capacity of ribosomes to control translational fidelity change with age?, *Mech. Ageing Dev.*, 15, 203, 1981.
40. Holliday, R. and Rattan, S. I. S., Evidence that paromomycin induces premature ageing in human fibroblasts, *Monogr. Devl. Biol.*, 17, 221, 1984.
41. Buchanan, J. H., Stevens, A., and Sidhu, J., Aminoglycoside antibiotic treatment of human fibroblasts: intracellular accumulation, molecular changes and the loss of ribosomal accuracy, *Eur. J. Cell Biol.*, 43, 141, 1987.
42. Hardwick, J., Hsieh, W. H., Liu, D. S. H., and Richardon, A., Cell-free protein synthesis by kidney from the aging female Fischer 344 rat, *Biochim. Biophys. Acta*, 652, 204, 1981.
43. Filion, A. M. and Laughrea, M., Translation fidelity in the aging mammal. Studies with an accurate in vitro system on aged rats, *Mech. Ageing Dev.*, 29, 125, 1985.
44. Laughrea, M. and Latulippe, J., The poly(U) translation capacity of Fischer 344 rat liver does not deteriorate with age and is not affected by dietary regime, *Mech. Ageing Dev.*, 45, 137, 1988.
45. Mori, N., Mizuno, D., and Gato, S., Conservation of ribosomal fidelity during ageing, *Mech. Ageing Dev.*, 10, 379, 1979.
46. Mori, N., Hiruta, K., Funatsu, Y., and Goto, S., Codon recognition fidelity of ribosomes at the first and second positions does not decrease during aging, *Mech. Ageing Dev.*, 22, 1, 1983.
47. Ryazanov, A. G., Rudkin, B. B., and Spirin, A. S., Regulation of protein synthesis at the elongation stage. New insights into the control of gene expression in eukaryotes, *FEBS Lett.*, 285, 170, 1991.
48. Richardson, A. and Semsei, I., Effect of aging on translation and transcription, *Rev. Biol. Res. Aging*, 3, 467, 1987.
49. Khasigov, P. Z. and Nikolaev, A. Y., Age-related changes in the rates of polypeptide chain elongation, *Biochem. Int.*, 15, 1171, 1987.
50. Merry, B. J. and Holehahn, A. M., Effect of age and restricted feeding on polypeptide chain assembly kinetics in liver protein synthesis *in vivo*, *Mech. Ageing Dev.*, 58, 139, 1991.
51. Riis, B., Rattan, S. I. S., Clark, B. F. C., and Merrick, W. C., Eukaryotic protein elongation factors, *Trends Biochem. Sci.*, 15, 420, 1990.
52. Lee, S., Francoeur, A.-M., Liu, S., and Wang, E., Tissue-specific expression in mammalian brain, heart, and muscle of S1, a member of the elongation factor-1α gene family, *J. Biol. Chem.*, 267, 24064, 1992.
53. Knudsen, S. M., Frydenberg, J., Clark, B. F. C., and Leffers, H., Tissue-dependent variation in the expression of elongation factor-1α isoforms: isolation and characterisation of a cDNA encoding a novel variant of human elongation factor 1α, *Eur. J. Biochem.*, 215, 549, 1993.
54. Song, J. M., Picologlou, S., Grant, C. M., Firoozan, M., Tuite, M. F., and Liebman, S., Elongation factor EF-1α gene dosage alters translational fidelity in *Saccharomyces cerevisiae*, *Mol. Cell. Biol.*, 9, 4571, 1989.
55. Tatsuka, M., Mitsui, H., Wada, M., Nagata, A., Nojima, H., and Okayama, H., Elongation factor-1α gene determines susceptibility to transformation, *Nature*, 359, 333, 1992.
56. Cavallius, J., Rattan, S. I. S., and Clark, B. F. C., Changes in activity and amount of active elongation factor-1α in aging and immortal human fibroblast cultures, *Exp. Gerontol.*, 21, 149, 1986.
57. Rattan, S. I. S., Cavallius, J., Hartvigsen, G., and Clark, B. F. C., Amounts of active elongation factor-1α and its activity in livers of mice during ageing, *Trends in Aging Research/ Colloque INSERM*, 147, 135, 1986.

58. Rattan, S. I. S., Cavallius, J., Bhatia, P., and Clark, B. F. C., Protein elongation factor-1α in aging rodent brain., in *Aging — A Multifactorial Discussion*, Subba Rao, K., and Prabhakar, V., Eds., Association of Gerontology Publishers, India, 1987, 125.

59. Shepherd, J. C. W., Walldorf, U., Hug, P., and Gehring, W. J., Fruitflies with additional expression of the elongation factor EF-1α live longer, *Proc. Natl. Acad. Sci. U.S.A.*, 86, 7520, 1989.

60. Shikama, N., Ackermann, R., and Brack, C., Protein synthesis elongation factor EF-1α expression and longevity in *Drosophila melanogaster*, *Proc. Natl. Acad. Sci. U.S.A.*, 91, 4199, 1994.

61. Silar, P. and Picard, M., Increased longevity of EF-1α high-fidelity mutants in *Podospora anserina*, *J. Mol. Biol.*, 235, 231, 1994.

62. Webster, G. C. and Webster, S. L., Specific disappearance of translatable messenger RNA for elongation factor one in aging *Drosophila melanogaster*, *Mech. Ageing Dev.*, 24, 335, 1984.

63. Cavallius, J., Rattan, S. I. S., and Clark, B. F. C., A decrease in levels of mRNA for elongation factor-1α accompanies the decline in its activity and the amounts of active enzyme in rat livers during ageing, *Topics Aging Res. Eur.*, 13, 125, 1989.

64. Giordano, T., Kleinsek, D., and Foster, D. N., Increase in abundance of a transcript hybridizing to elongation factor 1 α during cellular senescence and quiescence, *Exp. Gerontol.*, 24, 501, 1989.

65. Ann, D. K., Lin, H. H., Lee, S., Tu, Z. J., and Wang, E., Characterization of the statin-like S1 and rat elongation factor 1α as two distinctly expressed messages in rat, *J. Biol. Chem.*, 267, 699, 1992.

66. Takahashi, R., Mori, N., and Goto, S., Accumulation of heat-labile elongation factor 2 in the liver of mice and rats., *Exp. Gerontol.*, 20, 325, 1985.

67. Riis, B., Rattan, S. I. S., Derventzi, A., and Clark, B. F. C., Reduced levels of ADP-ribosylatable elongation factor-2 in aged and SV40-transformed human cells, *FEBS Lett.*, 266, 45, 1990.

68. Rattan, S. I. S., Ward, W. F., Glenting, M., Svendsen, L., Riis, B., and Clark, B. F. C., Dietary calorie restriction does not affect the levels of protein elongation factors in rat livers during ageing, *Mech. Ageing Dev.*, 58, 85, 1991.

69. Lapointe, J. and Giegé, R., Transfer RNAs and aminoacyl-tRNA synthetases, in *Translation in Eukaryotes*, Trachsel, H., Ed., CRC Press, Boca Raton, FL, 1991, 35.

70. Strehler, B. L., Hirsch, G., Gusseck, D., Johnson, R., and Bick, M., Codon restriction theory of ageing and development, *J. Theor. Biol.*, 33, 429, 1971.

71. Vinayak, M., A comparison of tRNA populations of rat liver and skeletal muscle during aging, *Biochem. Int.*, 15, 279, 1987.

72. Schröder, H. C., Ugarkovic, D., Müller, W. E. G., Mizushima, H., Nemoto, F., and Kuchino, Y., Increased expression of UAG suppressor tRNA in aged mice: consequences for retroviral gene expression, *Eur. J. Gerontol.*, 1, 452, 1992.

73. Takahashi, R., Mori, N., and Goto, S., Alteration of aminoacyl tRNA synthetases with age: accumulation of heat-labile moleculaes in rat liver, kidney and brain, *Mech. Ageing Dev.*, 33, 67, 1985.

74. Mays-Hoopes, L. L., Cleland, G., Bochantin, J., Kalunian, D., Miller, J., Wilson, W., Wong, M. K., Johnson, D., and Sharma, O. K., Function and fidelity of aging tRNA: *in vivo* acylation, analog discrimination, synthetase binding and *in vitro* translation, *Mech. Ageing Dev.*, 22, 135, 1983.

75. Takahashi, R. and Goto, S., Fidelity of aminoacylation by rat-liver tyrosyl-tRNA synthetase. Effect of age, *Eur. J. Biochem.*, 178, 381, 1988.

76. Gabius, H. J., Goldbach, S., Graupner, G., Rehm, S., and Cramer, F., Organ pattern of age-related changes in the aminoacylation synthetase activities of the mouse, *Mech. Ageing Dev.*, 20, 305, 1982.

77. Gabius, H. J., Graupner, G., and Cramer, F., Activity patterns of aminoacyl-tRNA synthetases, tRNA methylases, arginyltransferase and tubulin:tyrosine ligase during development and ageing of *Caenorhabditis elegans*, *Eur. J. Biochem.*, 131, 231, 1983.

78. Tanaka, H., Zaitsu, H., Onodera, K., and Kimura, G., Influence of the deprivation of a single amino acid on cellular proliferation and survival in rat 3Y1 fibroblasts and their derivatives transformed by a wide variety of agents, *J. Cell. Physiol.*, 136, 421, 1988.

79. Kilberg, M. S., Hutson, R. G., and Laine, R. O., Amino acid-regulated gene expression in eukaryotic cells, *FASEB J.*, 8, 13, 1994.

80. Sharma, S. P. and Rai, N., Amino acid variation during ageing of *Callosobruchus maculatus* Fabr. (Coleoptera), *Zool. Orient.*, 1, 26, 1984.

81. Levenbook, L., Protein synthesis in relation to insect aging: an overview, in *Insect Aging*, Collatz, K. G. and Sohal, R. S., Eds., Springer-Verlag, Berlin, 1986, 200.

82. Harrison, B. J. and Holliday, R., Senescence and the fidelity of protein synthesis in *Drosophila*, *Nature*, 213, 990, 1967.

83. Ryan, J. M., Duda, G., and Cristofalo, V. J., Error accumulation and aging in human diploid cells, *J. Gerontol.*, 29, 616, 1974.

84. Holliday, R. and Stevens, A., The effect of an amino acid analogue, *p*-fluorophenylalanine, on longevity of mice, *Gerontology*, 24, 417, 1978.

85. Rattan, S. I. S., Derventzi, A., and Clark, B. F. C., Protein synthesis, posttranslational modifications and aging, *Ann. N.Y. Acad. Sci.*, 663, 48, 1992.

86. Celis, J. E., et al., Comprehensive two-dimensional gel protein databases offer a global approach to the analysis of human cells: the transformed amnion cells (AMA) master database and its link to genome DNA sequence data, *Electrophoresis*, 11, 989, 1990.

87. Roach, P. J., Multisite and hierarchal protein phosphorylation, *J. Biol. Chem.*, 266, 14139, 1991.

88. Hubbard, M. J. and Cohen, P., On target with a new mechanism for the regulation of protein phosphorylation, *Trends Biochem. Sci.*, 18, 172, 1993.

89. Smith, J. R., Inhibitors of DNA synthesis derived from senescent human diploid fibroblasts, *Exp. Gerontol.*, 27, 409, 1992.

90. Shay, J. W., Pereira-Smith, O. M., and Wright, W. E., A role for both RB and p53 in the regulation of human cellular senescence, *Exp. Cell Res.*, 196, 33, 1991.

91. Stein, G. H., Drullinger, L. F., Robetorye, R. S., Pereira-Smith, O. M., and Smith, J. R., Senescent cells fail to express cdc2, cyc A, and cyc B in response to mitogen stimulation, *Proc. Natl. Acad. Sci. U.S.A.*, 88, 11012, 1991.

92. Won, K.-A., Xiong, Y., Beach, D., and Gilman, M. Z., Growth-regulated expression of D-type cyclin genes in human diploid fibroblasts, *Proc. Natl. Acad. Sci. U.S.A.*, 89, 9910, 1992.

93. Dulic´, V., Drullinger, L. F., Lees, E., Reed, S., and Stein, G. H., Altered regulation of G1 cyclins in senescent human diploid fibroblasts: accumulation of inactive cyclin E—Cdk2 and cyclin D1—Cdk2 complexes, *Proc. Natl. Acad. Sci. U.S.A.*, 90, 11034, 1993.

94. Murray, A. W., Turning on mitosis, *Curr. Biol.*, 3, 291, 1993.

95. Stein, G. H., Besson, M., and Gordon, L., Failure to phosphorylate the retinoblastoma gene product in senescent human fibroblasts, *Science*, 249, 666, 1990.

96. Richter, K. H., Afshari, C. A., Annab, L. A., Burkhart, B. A., Owen, R. D., Boyd, J., and Barrett, J. C., Down-regulation of cdc2 in senescent human and hamster cells, *Canc. Res.*, 51, 6010, 1991.

97. Krauss, S. W. and Linn, S., Studies of DNA polymerases α and β from cultured human cells in various replicative states, *J. Cell. Physiol.*, 126, 99, 1986.

98. Pendergrass, W. R., Angello, J. C., Saulewicz, A. C., and Norwood, T. H., DNA polymerase α and the regulation of entry into S phase in heterokaryons, *Exp. Cell Res.*, 192, 426, 1991.

99. Srivastava, V., Tilley, R., Miller, S., Hart, R., and Busbee, D., Effects of aging and dietary restriction on DNA polymerases: gene expression, enzyme fidelity, and DNA excision repair, *Exp. Gerontol.*, 27, 593, 1992.

100. Cripps-Wolfman, J., Henshaw, E. C., and Bambara, R. A., Alterations in the phosphorylation and activity of DNA polymerase α correlate with the change in replicative DNA synthesis as quiescent cells reenter the cell cycle, *J. Biol. Chem.*, 264, 19478, 1989.

101. Nasheuer, H. P., Moore, A., Wahl, A. F., and Wang, T. S. F., Cell cycle-dependent phosphorylation of human DNA polymerase α, *J. Biol. Chem.*, 266, 7893, 1991.

102. Srivastava, V. K., Millar, S., Schroeder, M. D., Hart, R. W., and Busbee, D., Age-related changes in expression and activity of DNA polymerase α: some effects of dietary restriction, *Mutat. Res.*, 295, 265, 1993.

103. Westwood, J. T., Church, R. B., and Wagenaar, E. B., Changes in protein phosphorylation during the cell cycle of Chinese hamster ovary cells, *J. Biol. Chem.*, 260, 10308, 1985.

104. Heydari, A. R., Butler, J. A., Waggoner, S. M., and Richardson, A., Age-related changes in protein phosphorylation by rat hepatocytes, *Mech. Ageing Dev.*, 50, 227, 1989.

105. Samuel, C. E., The eIF-2a protein kinases, regulators of translation in eukaryotes from yeast to humans, *J. Biol. Chem.*, 268, 7603, 1993.

106. Celis, J. E., Madsen, P., and Ryazanov, A. G., Increased phosphorylation of elongation factor 2 during mitosis in transformed human amnion cells correlates with a decreased rate of protein synthesis, *Proc. Natl. Acad. Sci. U.S.A.*, 87, 4231, 1990.

107. Riis, B., Rattan, S. I. S., Palmquist, K., Nilsson, A., Nygård, O., and Clark, B. F. C., Elongation factor 2-specific calcium and calmodulin dependent protein kinase III activity in rat livers varies with age and calorie restriction, *Biochem. Biophys. Res. Commun.*, 192, 1210, 1993.

108. Clemens, M. J., Does phosphorylation play a role in translational control by eukaryotic aminoacyl-tRNA synthetase?, *Trends Biochem. Sci.*, 15, 172, 1990.

109. Tas, P. W. L. and Martini, O. H. W., Regulation of ribosomal protein S6 phosphorylation in heat-shocked HeLa cells, *Eur. J. Biochem.*, 163, 553, 1987.

110. Kihara, F., Ninomyia-Tsuji, J., Ishibashi, S., and Ide, T., Failure in S6 protein phosphorylation by serum stimulation of senescent human diploid fibroblasts, TIG-1, *Mech. Ageing Dev.*, 20, 305, 1986.

111. Hunter, T., A thousand and one protein kinases, *Cell*, 50, 823, 1987.

112. Shigeoka, H. and Yang, H. C., Early kinase C dependent events in aging human diploid fibroblasts, *Mech. Ageing Dev.*, 55, 49, 1990.

113. Cristofalo, V. J., Phillips, P. D., Sorger, T., and Gerhard, G., Alterations in the responsiveness of senescent cells to growth factors, *J. Gerontol.*, 44, B55, 1989.

114. Cristofalo, V. J., Pignolo, R. J., and Rotenberg, M. O., Molecular changes with in vitro cellular senescence, *Ann. N.Y. Acad. Sci.*, 663, 187, 1992.

115. De Tata, V., Ptasznik, A., and Cristofalo, V. J., Effect of tumor promoter phorbol 12-myristate 13-acetate (PMA) on proliferation of young and senescent WI-38 human diploid fibroblasts, *Exp. Cell Res.*, 205, 261, 1993.

116. Farber, A., Chang, C., Sell, C., Ptasznik, A., Cristofalo, V.J., Hubbard, K., Ozer, H.L., Adamo, M., Roberts, C.T., LeRoith, D., Dumenil, G., and Baserga, R., Failure of senescent human fibroblasts to express the insulin-like growth factor-1 gene, *J. Biol. Chem.*, 268, 17883, 1993.

117. Derventzi, A., Rattan, S. I. S., and Clark, B. F. C., Phorbol ester PMA stimulates protein synthesis and increases the levels of active elongation factors EF-1α and EF-2 in ageing human fibroblasts, *Mech. Ageing Dev.*, 69, 193, 1993.

118. Patel, H. R. and Miller, R. A., Age-associated changes in mitogen-induced protein phosphorylation in murine T lymphocytes, *Eur. J. Immunol.*, 22, 253, 1992.

119. Miller, R. A., Aging and immune function: cellular and biochemical analyses, *Exp. Gerontol.*, 29, 21, 1994.

120. Simbulan, C. M. G., Suzuki, M., Izuta, S., Sakurai, T., Savoysky, E., Kojima, K., Miyahara, K., Shizutsa, Y., and Yoshida, S., Poly(ADP-ribose) polymerase stimulates DNA polymerase α by physical association, *J. Biol. Chem.*, 268, 93, 1993.

121. Shall, S., ADP-ribosylation of proteins: a ubiquitous cellular control mechanism, *Adv. Exp. Med. Biol.*, 231, 597, 1988.

122. Balestrieri, C., Giovane, A., Quagliuolo, L., and Servillo, L., Post-translational modifications of the elongation factor-2, *Adv. Exp. Med. Biol.*, 231, 627, 1988.

123. Dell'Orco, R. T. and Anderson, L. E., Decline of poly(ADP-ribosyl)ation during in vitro senescence in human diploid fibroblasts, *J. Cell. Physiol.*, 146, 216, 1991.

124. Grube, K. and Bürkle, A., Poly(ADP-ribose) polymerase activity in mononuclear leukocytes of 13 mammalian species correlates with species-specific life span, *Proc. Natl. Acad. Sci. U.S.A.*, 89, 11759, 1992.

125. Bürkle, A., Grube, K., and Küpper, J.-H., Poly(ADP-ribosyl)ation: its role in inducible DNA amplification, and its correlation with the longevity of mammalian species, *Exp. Clin. Immunogenet.*, 9, 230, 1992.

126. Paik, P. W. and Kim, S., *Protein Methylation*, John Wiley & Sons, New York, 1980, 258.

127. Clarke, S., Protein carboxyl methyltransferases: two distinct classes of enzymes, *Annu. Rev. Biochem.*, 54, 479, 1985.

128. Mays-Hoopes, L. L., Macromolecular methylation during aging, *Rev. Biol. Res. Aging*, 2, 361, 1985.

129. McFadden, P. N. and Clarke, S., Protein carboxyl methyltransferase and methyl acceptor proteins in aging and cataractus tissue of the human eye lens, *Mech. Ageing Dev.*, 34, 91, 1986.

130. Sellinger, O. Z., Kramer, C. M., Conger, A., and Duboff, G. S., The carboxylmethylation of cerebral membrane-bound proteins increases with age, *Mech. Ageing Dev.*, 43, 161, 1988.

131. Coppard, N. J., Clark, B. F. C., and Cramer, F., Methylation of elongation factor 1α in mouse 3T3B and 3T3B/SV40 cells, *FEBS Lett.*, 164, 330, 1983.

132. Kay, M. M. B., Molecular aging of membrane molecules and cellular removal, in *Biomedical Advances in Aging*, Goldstein, A. L., Ed., Plenum Press, New York, 1990, 147.

133. Porter, M. B., Pereira-Smith, O. M., and Smith, J. R., Novel monoclonal antibodies identify antigenic determinants unique to cellular senescence, *J. Cell. Physiol.*, 142, 425, 1990.

134. Porter, M. B., Pereira-Smith, O. M., and Smith, J. R., Common senescent cellspecific antibody epitopes on fibronectin in species and cells of varied origin, *J. Cell. Physiol.*, 150, 545, 1992.

135. Hébert, L., Pandey, S., and Wang, E., Commitment to cell death is signaled by the appearance of a terminin protein of 30 kDa, *Exp. Cell Res.*, 210, 10, 1994.

136. Wang, E., Are all nonproliferating cells similar?, *Exp. Gerontol.*, 27, 419, 1992.

137. Di Paolo, B. R., Pignolo, R. J., and Cristofalo, V. J., Overexpression of the twochain form of cathepsin B in senescent WI-38 cells, *Exp. Cell Res.*, 210, 500, 1992.

138. Baur, E. A., Kronberger, A., Stricklin, G. P., Smith, L. T., and Holbrook, K. A., Age-related changes in collagenase expression in cultured embryonic and fetal human skin fibroblasts., *Exp. Cell Res*, 161, 484, 1985.

139. Sottile, J., Mann, D. M., Diemer, V., and Millis, A. J. T., Regulation of collagenase and collagenase mRNA production in early- and late-passage human diploid fibroblasts, *J. Cell. Physiol.*, 138, 281, 1989.

140. Stadtman, E. R., Protein oxidation and aging, *Science*, 257, 1220, 1992.
141. Stadtman, E. R., Protein modification in aging, *J. Gerontol.*, 43, B112, 1988.
142. Carney, J. M., Starke-Reed, P. E., Oliver, C. N., Landum, R. W., Cheng, M. S., Wu, J. F., and Floyd, R. A., Reversal of age-related increase in brain protein oxidation, decrease in enzyme activity, and loss in temporal and spatial memory by chronic administration of the spin-trapping compound N-tert-butyl-α-phenylnitrone, *Proc. Natl. Acad. Sci. U.S.A.*, 88, 3633, 1991.
143. Sohal, R. S., Agarwal, S., Dubey, A., and Orr, W. C., Protein oxidative damage is associated with life expectancy of houseflies, *Proc. Natl. Acad. Sci. U.S.A.*, 90, 7255, 1993.
144. Sohal, R. S., Ku, H.-H., and Agarwal, S., Biochemical correlates of longevity in two closely related rodent species, *Biochem. Biophys. Res. Commun.*, 196, 7, 1993.
145. Orr, W. C. and Sohal, R. S., Extension of life-span by overexpression of superoxide dismutase and catalase in *Drosophila melanogaster*, *Science*, 263, 1128, 1994.
146. Gordillo, E., Ayala, A., Bautista, J., and Machado, A., Implication of lysine residues in the loss of enzymatic activity in rat liver 6-phosphogluconate dehydrogenase found in aging, *J. Biol. Chem.*, 264, 17024, 1989.
147. Gafni, A., Altered protein metabolism in aging, *Annu. Rev. Gerontol. Geriatr.*, 10, 117, 1990.
148. Gafni, A., Age-related effects in enzyme metabolism and catalysis, *Rev. Biol. Res. Aging*, 4, 315, 1990.
149. Wells-Knecht, M. C., Huggins, T. G., Dyer, D. G., Thorpe, S. R., and Baynes, J. W., Oxidized amino acids in lens protein with age. Measurement of o-tyrosine and dityrosine in the aging human lens, *J. Biol. Chem.*, 268, 12348, 1993.
150. Harding, J. J., Beswick, H. T., Ajiboye, R., Huby, R., Blakytny, R., and Rixon, K. C., Non-enzymic post-translational modification of proteins in aging: a review, *Mech. Ageing Dev.*, 50, 7, 1989.
151. Lis, H. and Sharon, N., Protein glycosylation: structural and functional aspects, *Eur. J. Biochem.*, 218, 1, 1993.
152. Oimomi, M., Maeda, Y., Hata, F., Kitamura, Y., Matsumoto, S., Hatanaka, H., and Baba, S., A study of the age-related acceleration of glycation of tissue proteins in rats, *J. Gerontol.*, 43, B98, 1988.
153. Miksík, I. and Deyl, Z., Changes in the amount of ε-hexosyllysine, UV absorbance, and fluorescence of collagen with age in different animal species, *J. Gerontol.*, 46, B111, 1991.
154. Masoro, E. J., Katz, M. S., and McMahan, C. A., Evidence for the glycation hypothesis of aging from the food-restricted rodent model, *J. Gerontol.*, 44, B20, 1989.
155. Lee, A. T. and Cerami, A., Role of glycation in aging, *Ann. N.Y. Acad. Sci.*, 663, 63, 1992.
156. Kristal, B. S. and Yu, B. P., An emerging hypothesis: synergistic induction of aging by free radicals and Maillard reactions, *J. Gerontol.*, 47, B107, 1992.
157. Sell, D. R. and Monnier, V. M., Structure elucidation of a senescence cross-link from human extracellular matrix. Implication of pentoses in the aging process, *J. Biol. Chem.*, 264, 21597, 1989.
158. Makita, Z., Vlassara, H., Rayfield, E., Cartwright, K., Friedman, E., Rodby, R., Cerami, A., and Bucala, R., Hemoglobin-AGE: a circulating marker of advanced glycosylation, *Science*, 258, 651, 1992.
159. Liu, D. T.-Y., Deamidation: a source of microheterogeneity in pharmaceutical proteins, *Trends Biotech.*, 10, 364, 1992.
160. Gracy, R. W., Yüksel, K. Ü., Chapman, M. L., Cini, J. K., Jahani, M., Lu, H. S., Oray, B., and Talent, J. M., Impaired protein degradation may account for the accumulation of "abnormal" proteins in aging cells, in *Modifications of Proteins During Aging*, Adelman, R. C. and Dekker, E. E., Eds., Alan R. Liss, New York, 1985, 1.

161. Cini, J. K. and Gracy, R. W., Molecular basis of the isozyme of bovine glucose-6-phosphate isomerase, *Arch. Biochem. Biophys.*, 249, 500, 1986.

162. Stadtman, E. R., Covalent modification reactions are marking steps in protein turnover, *Biochemistry*, 29, 6323, 1990.

163. Brunauer, L. S. and Clarke, S., Age-dependent accumulation of protein residues which can be hydrolyzed to D-aspartic acid in human erythrocytes, *J. Biol. Chem.*, 261, 12538, 1986.

164. Yuh, K.-C. and Gafni, A., Reversal of age-related effects in rat muscle phosphoglycerate kinase, *Proc. Natl. Acad. Sci. U.S.A.*, 84, 7458, 1987.

165. Zúniga, A. and Gafni, A., Age-related modifications in rat cardiac phosphoglycerate kinase. Rejuvenation of the old enzyme by unfolding-refolding, *Biochim. Biophys. Acta*, 955, 50, 1988.

166. Park, M. H., Wolff, E. C., and Folk, J. E., Hypusine: its post-translational formation in eukaryotic initiation factor 5A and its potential role in cellular regulation, *BioFactors*, 4, 95, 1993.

167. Huttner, W. B., Protein tyrosine sulfation, *Trends Biochem. Sci.*, 12, 361, 1987.

168. Marshall, C. J., Protein prenylation: a mediator of protein-protein interactions, *Science*, 259, 1865, 1993.

169. Tint, I. S., Bershadsky, A. D., Gelfand, I. M., and Vasiliev, J. M., Post-translational modification of microtubules is a component of synergic alterations of cytoskeleton leading to formation of cytoplasmic processes in fibroblasts, *Proc. Natl. Acad. Sci. U.S.A.*, 88, 6318, 1991.

170. Morimoto, R. I., Chaperoning the nascent polypeptide chain, *Curr. Biol.*, 3, 101, 1993.

171. Pan, J.-X., Short, S. R., Goff, S. A., and Dice, J. F., Ubiquitin pools, ubiquitin mRNA levels, and ubiquitin-mediated proteolysis in aging human fibroblasts, *Exp. Gerontol.*, 28, 39, 1993.

172. Bjorksten, J. and Tenhu, H., The cross-linking theory of aging — added evidence, *Exp. Gerontol.*, 25, 91, 1990.

173. Birckbichler, P. J., Anderson, L. E., and Dell'Orco, R. T., Transglutaminase, donor age, and in vitro cellular senescence, *Adv. Exp. Med. Biol.*, 231, 109, 1988.

174. Nagaraj, R. H., Sell, D. R., Prabhakaram, M., Ortwerth, B. J., and Monnier, V. M., High correlation between pentosidine protein cross-links and pigmentation implicates ascorbate oxidation in human lens senescence and cataractogenesis, *Proc. Natl. Acad. Sci. U.S.A.*, 88, 10257, 1991.

175. Fesus, L., Daview, P. J. A., and Piacentini, M., Apoptosis: molecular mechanisms in programmed cell death, *Eur. J. Cell Biol.*, 56, 170, 1991.

176. Saunders, N. A., Smith, R. J., and Jetten, A. M., Regulation of proliferation-specific and differentiation-specific genes during senescence of human epidermal keratinocyte and mammary epithelial cells, *Biochem. Biophys. Res. Commun.*, 197, 46, 1993.

Chapter 13

CARBONYL TOXIFICATION HYPOTHESIS OF BIOLOGICAL AGING

Dazhong Yin and Ulf T. Brunk

CONTENTS

0-8493-4786-6/95/$0.00+$.50
© 1995 by CRC Press, Inc.

Carbonyl modification (e.g., cross-linking and aldehyde-thiol reactions) of biomolecules, a common consequence of free radical/Maillard reactions, is an important process of biological aging. In spite of detoxification of carbonyls by a family of carbonyl dehydrogenases and other biomolecules (e.g., glutathione), even healthy organisms contain micromolar amounts of carbonyls, particularly carbonyls with di- and multifunctional groups (DMcarbonyls), e.g., malondialdehyde, hydroxylalkenals, methylglyoxal, and deoxyosones, which are all biologically toxic. DMcarbonyls react readily at physiological pH with almost all important biomolecules, e.g., proteins, lipids, carbohydrates, and nucleic acids, causing a variety of biological alterations, e.g., protein cross-linking, which affect most (if not all) aspects of body organization and function. DMcarbonyls, derived from both free radical and Maillard reactions, are biomarkers that are correlated with glutathione depletion, membrane destruction, enzyme inhibition, immune disturbances, mutations, inhibition of cell replication, etc. DMcarbonyls are also known precursors of advanced glycation end products, age pigments (lipofuscin) in postmitotic cells, lens cataracts, and collagen cross-linking. Considering that free radical-related oxidative stress, glycation reactions (which are mainly oxygen independent) and dietary carbonyls represent different sources of DMcarbonyls; each of these may be regarded as potential initiators, or promoters, of carbonyl toxification and, thus, of the aging process. DMcarbonyl modification of biomolecules, therefore, is hypothesized to be a central process related to organismic aging.

I.   INTRODUCTION

Gerontological studies performed at the organismic, cellular, and molecular levels have generated numerous theories that attempt to explain the events leading to biological senescence. In general, theories of aging have been either programmatic, postulating that aging is due to an inherent genetic program, or stochastic, suggesting that aging results from environmental damage.

Most theories of aging place emphasis on alterations of specific parts of cells and organisms. For example, the membrane theory of aging emphasizes the lipid bilayer of cellular membranes[1] while paying less attention to proteins which are the focus of the protein modification hypothesis of aging.[2] Other aspects are stressed by the cross-linking theory of aging,[3] the lysosomal theory of aging,[4] and the finite proliferation concept of aging.[5] It has long been known that the metabolic rate is a distinct factor related to life span.[6] Mammals induced to hibernate exhibit a significant increase in longevity as compared with controls,[7] and insects maintained under flightless conditions live up to 2.5 times longer than those permitted to fly.[8] Although the metabolic rate is found to be an important factor associated with the rate of aging, it fails to identify the cause of aging. Circumstantial evidence for causative factors of aging is provided by the free radical and glycation theories of aging, which suggest that oxidation, induced by oxygen-derived radicals and reactions between reducing sugars and proteins, are important in animal senescence.[9-12] Because both the free radical and glycation reactions are considered to be important, and because the two concepts are recently found interrelated and complementary in explaining aging phenomena, Kristal and Yu[13] proposed a free radical-glycation/Maillard reaction hypothesis of aging, attempting to construct a unified theory of aging. The combination of these two theories would provide an explanation for several unsolved problems of the aging process. However, the key mechanism (the essence) of biological aging is still unclear. It should be noted that a common aging-related biological process, carbonyl-cross-linking-related alterations of a variety of biomolecules, is pointed out as the result of both free radical and Maillard reactions.[14] This review focuses on biochemical reactions known to be associated with the aging process, stresses the differences and similarities between free radical and glycation reactions, and proposes that toxification by di- and multicarbonyls is a ubiquitous and inevitable process that underlies biological aging.

II. AGING AND SOME RELATED DEFENSE SYSTEMS

Several defense systems, such as antioxidative and repair mechanisms, are known to be consistently correlated with life expectancy and, possibly, even life span.[15] Since aerobic organisms are constantly exposed to oxygen-derived radicals and related oxidants, they have developed a variety of antioxidative compounds and enzymes, collectively referred to as the antioxidative defenses. However, this defense system is not perfect, and damage to cellular lipids, proteins, nucleic acids, and carbohydrates still happens. Consequently, a second line of defense exists, consisting of a number of enzymes (proteinases, lipases, and nucleases) that degrade most of the damaged elements while undamaged components are conserved for reutilization.[16,17] Together, these two defense systems are highly efficient and allow the biological machinery to survive a variety of physiological and pathological modifications. For example, the human body may sustain billions of free radical attacks per second.[18]

Nevertheless, biological changes beyond the capacity of the defense systems are evident in animal senescence. Accumulation of altered biological components is often observed in long-lived extracellular materials, such as collagen and elastic tissues.[3,19] In postmitotic cells, such as cardiac myocytes and neurones,[20,21] age pigments (lipofuscin) are characteristic manifestations of aging.[12,22,23]

III. THE FREE RADICAL THEORY OF AGING AND DMCARBONYLS

According to the free radical theory of aging, senescence and a variety of degenerative diseases associated with it are attributed primarily to the deleterious attack of oxygen free radicals on cellular constituents, including chromosomes, mitochondrial DNA, and connective tissues.[24,25] Univalent reduction of oxygen gives rise to damaging oxidative species:

$$O_2 \rightarrow O_2^{-\cdot} \rightarrow H_2O_2 \rightarrow HO^{\cdot} \rightarrow H_2O$$

The processes by which oxygen free radicals, e.g., superoxide and hydroxyl radicals, damage biomolecules have been extensively studied and well reviewed.[26,27] However, the stepwise oxidation of biomolecules has been less well considered. Ignoring various biological components, we may describe the gradual oxidation process of essential biological compounds as in Scheme I:

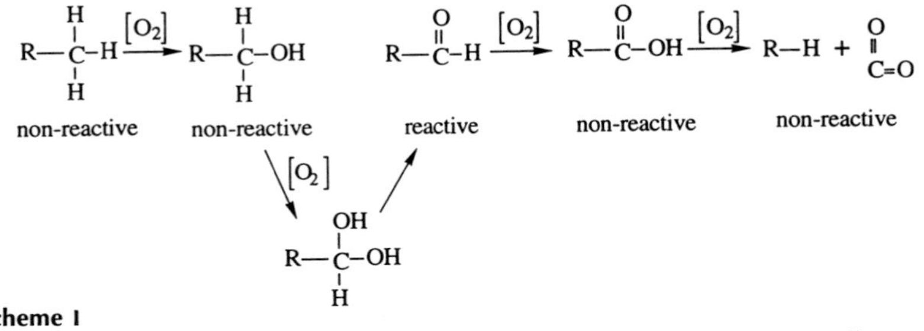

Scheme I
Principle of stepwise oxidation of biomolecules (R; saturated or unsaturated)

Among these, carbonyl compounds (biomolecules that contain a carbon-oxygen double bond, or carbonyl group, mainly aldehydes and ketones) are active intermediates, particularly when they are conjugated with a secondary functional group (e.g., α,β-unsaturated aldehydes). Carbonyl compounds have the potential to react with a variety of biomolecules such as proteins and nucleic acids.[28] Carbonyls conjugated with some additional functional groups in the vicinity of the primary aldehyde group are termed di-, multicarbonyl compounds (DMcarbonyls) in this review. Such DMcarbonyls include 2-ketoaldehydes, hydroxylenals, enals, dienals, trienals, osones, and various reductones that are all very reactive and toxic to almost all cellular and extracellular biomolecules.[29,30] Two of the most intensively studied DMcarbonyls are malondialdehyde[31] and 4-hydroxylnonenals.[30] A large body of knowledge about their biological occurrence, mechanism of formation, reactivity, and biotoxicity has been obtained mainly through studies of lipid peroxidation.

IV. LIPID PEROXIDATION AND BIOCHEMICAL REACTIVITY OF DMCARBONYLS

Based on early data obtained by food chemists, lipid peroxidation is the most intensively studied and best understood process in free radical biochemistry. Lipid peroxidation is initiated mainly by hydrogen abstraction from unsaturated fatty acids by oxygen-centered radicals or transition metal-related complexes, followed by the formation of hydroperoxides in the presence of oxygen. The ensuing degradation of the hydroperoxides results in a variety of derivatives including various carbonyl and DMcarbonyl products.[26,32] A comprehensive review of this field was compiled by Esterbauer and colleagues[30] and a list of DMaldehydes that have so far been identified as autoxidation products of unsaturated fatty acids is given in Table 1.

DMaldehydes react readily, even at neutral pH and room temperature, with many important biochemical groups such as amino, thiol, or hydroxyl.[30] Reversible reactions between carbonyls and amino groups form Schiff bases. A secondary functional group in aldehydes increases the reactivity potential and may induce further irreversible reaction products, or result in cross-linking reactions.[3] Napetschnig[33] has shown that 4-hydroxylalkenals can react with nearly all amino acids under appropriate conditions. Reactions between 4-hydroxylalkenals and amino groups in proteins[34] and nucleic acids has been demonstrated as well.[35] Reactions between carbonyls and thiol compounds have received particular attention since the addition of some DMcarbonyls (e.g., 4-hydroxylalkenals) to tissues, cells, or cell fractions causes a rapid loss of SH groups.[30] Glutathione and cysteine easily react in neutral solutions with 4-hydroxylalkenal[36,37] with the formation of a five-membered cyclic hemiacetal. Although the thiol-ether linkage that binds aldehydes to the protein-SH group is stable, it is reversible and, thus, may be removed from the protein

TABLE 1.

Di- and Multifunctional Carbonyls Discovered From Lipid Peroxidation

2-Butenal	2-Pentenal	2-Hexenal
2-Octenal	2-Nonenal	2-Decenal
2-Undecenal	2,4-Heptadienal	2,4-Octadienal
2,4-Nonadienal	2,4-Decadienal	2,4,7-Decatrienal
2-Ketohexanal	2-Ketoheptanal	2-Ketononanal
4-Hydroxy-2-hexenal	4-Hydroxy-2-octenal	4-Hydroxy-2-nonenal
But-2-en-1,4-dial	4-Hydroperoxy-2-nonenal	

by an excess of low molecular weight thiols, such as glutathione and cysteine.

Due to their reactivity, the carbonylic products, particularly DMcarbonyls of lipid peroxidation, are implicated in various types of cell damage including depletion of glutathione, protein modification, disturbance of calcium homeostasis, retardation of respiration and glycolysis, cell membrane destruction, tissue injuries, enzyme inhibition, and decreased DNA, RNA, and protein synthesis.[30] It should be noted that DMcarbonyl toxification during oxidative stress has mainly been studied on models using relatively high concentrations of DMcarbonyls.[30]

V. DMCARBONYLS AND MAILLARD REACTION-RELATED AGING PHENOMENA

DMcarbonyls may also arise from another type of biochemical reaction, namely Maillard or, more precisely, glycation reactions, which have also been studied early-on by food scientists.[38] A distinct feature of the glycation reaction is that it is based on reactions between reducing sugars and free amino groups, and is not dependent on either lipids or oxygen. The reversible formation of a Schiff base during glycation leads to a fairly stable ketoamine compound called an Amadori product. The degradation of the Amadori product then results in a variety of di- and multifunctional carbonyl compounds as is shown in Scheme II.[38,39] Because glucose is the most abundant sugar, and because it is elevated in diabetes, most glycation studies have focused on this sugar. Whereas fructose and pentose react more actively than glucose, almost all reducing sugars, whether of the aldose or ketose type, can initiate the Maillard reaction *in vivo*.[12]

Reactive DMcarbonyls (secondary products) produced during the Maillard reaction are less well studied and only a few have been identified, for example, deoxyosones,[39] furfural, and pyruvaldehyde.[38] Since the secondary products from Maillard reactions have been only recently emphasized, the effect of Maillard reaction products is often inappropriately referred to as the "effects of advanced glycation end products (AGE)".[40,41]

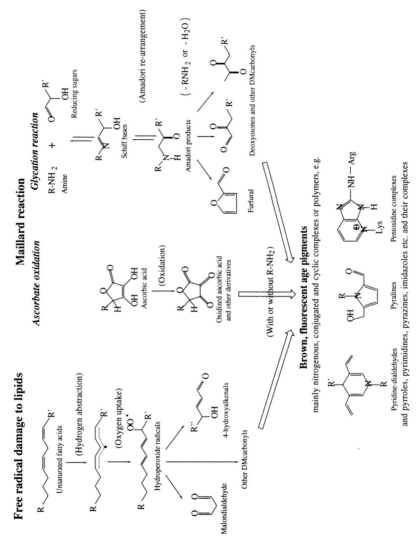

Scheme II

Formation mechanisms of di- and multifunctional carbonyls (DMcarbonyls) and further reactions.

Although some AGE may contain the conjugated DMcarbonyl structure shown in Scheme II, a majority of AGE (according to the definition of AGE) lack reactive groups and would be chemically stable in biological systems. However, the toxicity of the products (including both the secondary, and the end products) of the Maillard reaction has been extensively investigated.[12]

Most biochemical alterations, structural and functional, relating to Maillard reactions are considered to be due to ubiquitous cross-linking between various biomolecules and, in particular, different protein molecules.[39,42] Glycation studies have shown that the most dramatic age-related changes occur in nonrenewable tissues.[43,44] For example, during aging, the human lens crystalline becomes progressively less soluble, and acquires protein-bound yellow chromophores and fluorophores as brownish-yellow cataracts.[45] This browning is promoted by diabetes due to glucose-related Maillard reactions.[46] Diabetes-related glycation has also been reported to cause increased blood viscosity and adhesiveness, thickening of glomerular basement membranes in the kidney, poor wound healing, and decreased lung expansion volume.[41]

Collagen-rich tissues are found prone to damage related to Maillard reactions. With age, there is a loss of elasticity in skin, arteries, lungs, and joints.[47] The Maillard reaction has also been proposed to be responsible for the decreased ability of immune cells in old age to penetrate tissues and fight infections.[47] Maillard reaction products have also been found to cause many age-related changes in the genetic material and cause a decline in DNA replication, probably due to decrease of the proliferative response to mitogen stimulation.[41]

It is interesting to note that both lipid peroxidation and the Maillard reaction are found associated with an LDL alteration that results in its increased uptake by macrophages with formation of foam cells as an early event of atherosclerosis.[48-50]

VI. CARBONYL MODIFICATION, AN IMPORTANT PROCESS IN AGE PIGMENT FORMATION

DMcarbonyls are secondary products of lipid peroxidation and glycation reactions. Further reactions between carbonyls and various biomolecules are found to induce the formation of polymerized or cross-linked lipofuscin-like pigments, or fluorophores.[12,51-54] When comparing different studies in this area, it is interesting to note that the same fluorometric method to measure blue fluorescence has been utilized by both free radical and Maillard reaction scientists. The fluorophores, however, have been called lipofuscin-like age pigments by free radical scientists[51,53] and

AGE by the Maillard reaction scientists.[54,55] Although the fluorophores originate from different biomolecules, the formation mechanisms of the fluorophores are actually in the same category as shown in Scheme II, i.e., they are formed due to carbonyl-related cross-linking/polymerization reactions. Protein-associated nitrogen usually plays an important role in the cross-linking reaction. In addition to biomolecular cross-linkings, the reaction products are often conjugated and cyclic because such processes are thermodynamically favored. The nitrogenous, conjugated, and cyclic structure of the product contributes to coloration of the complex, which is found to be brownish, and sometimes fluorescent. Some components of this type are demonstrated in Scheme II, e.g., complexes of pyridines, pyrroles, pyralines, pyrimidines, imidazoles, pentosidines, etc. The coloration is a ubiquitous process in biological materials and may occur at temperatures as low as −10 °C and will be accelerated by increased temperature or exposure to air.[38,56] This coloration is known as Maillard reaction browning when food is kept in storage for a long period, and is correlated with the formation of age pigments (lipofuscin) in aged humans and animals.

Since experiments on glycation-related aging processes are usually performed during exposure to ambient oxygen, the formation mechanisms of age pigment in free radical and Maillard reactions are found interrelated and sometimes termed as "autoxidative glycation" or "glycoxidation".[57,58] The interplay between free radicals and glycation has been comprehensively reviewed by Kristal and Yu.[13] While elevated glucose levels may cause peroxidation of membrane lipids,[59] oxidative stress may, in turn, strongly accelerate the Maillard reaction.[57]

Striking discrepancies of fluorescence data in studies on age pigment exist with reports of both yellow-red fluorescence and blue fluorescence, depending on the technique used. These findings have strongly challenged the current understanding of the formation mechanisms of age pigments.[60] This discrepancy has recently been explained as being due to a universal red-shift of the fluorescence when highly concentrated fluorophores are studied, as is the case in microfluorometry.[61,62] Based on this finding, *in situ* lipofuscin may reasonably be considered as accumulates, or complexes, of both free radical-related age pigments and advanced glycation end products.

Convincing evidence has also been found that a substantial component of age pigment in the human retinal pigment epithelium is *N*-retinylidene-*N*-retinyl-ethanolamine which is derived from the reaction of retinaldehydes with the membrane lipid phosphatidylethanolamine.[63]

Furthermore, the accumulation of aberrant proteins is another event that characterizes the phenomenon of aging at the molecular level. Stadtman[2] and others have demonstrated that protein carbonyls are closely related to oxidatively modified, inactivated enzymes (e.g., glutamine synthetase) or aged proteins. Protein carbonyls are thus also regarded as one of the hallmarks of aging.

VII. DIFFERENCES BETWEEN THE FREE RADICAL AND GLYCATION THEORIES OF AGING

It is very important to point out that free radical damage to lipids and proteins, causing formation of DMcarbonyls, is oxygen-dependent, whereas the glycation reaction resulting in brown, fluorescent AGE is not. The Maillard reaction-related browning, according to Hodge,[38] in broad sense includes (1) glycation (reducing sugar-amino group) reactions, (2) caramelization, and (3) ascorbic acid-related oxidation. The former two reactions, unlike the third, do not depend on the presence of oxygen. Since caramelization takes place only at a high temperature, such as during cooking, it is not associated with the aging process and will not be discussed further. Glycation, representing the essential reaction of the broadly defined Maillard reaction (actually, glycation is the reaction that Maillard studied 80 years ago), is oxygen independent, although the process may be greatly interfered with and promoted by oxygen free radicals. The differences between the free radical and glycation reactions are shown in Scheme II. In the glycation reaction, neither the formation of Schiff bases nor the process of Amadori rearrangement are oxygen dependent. Although the further degradation of Amadori products may be strongly promoted by oxygen free radicals, or transition metals, the degradation may still occur due to deamidation, dehydration, or fission leading to the formation of DMcarbonyls.[38] Considering that the conversion of ascorbate to di- or polycarbonyl compounds is oxidation dependent,[38,64] these reactions should be distinguished from glycation and may better be considered as oxidative stress-related rather than glycation-related reactions. The dependence on oxygen is the second and crucial difference between the oxidative stress and the glycation mechanisms. This significant difference between the two aging mechanisms has not been stressed before, partly because of the similarity of the brownings caused by the ascorbate and glycation reactions, as observed in early studies, but mainly because the two aging theories have only recently been integrated.[13]

The occurrence of DMcarbonyl formation, which may be independent of oxidative damage, suggests that even if all free radical attacks could be prevented by an improved antioxidative defense system, DMcarbonyls would still form due to glycation reactions. As soon as DMcarbonyls are produced, further reactions between DMcarbonyls and various biomolecules are not dependent on either oxygen or reducing sugars.

Subsequent reactions are then governed by thermodynamic rules, i.e., the tendency of net entropy to increase, which favor cross-linking or polymerization of almost all biomolecules. Repair enzymes can only degrade (although at high efficiency) altered biomolecules but do not protect biomolecules from reacting with DMcarbonyls. The latter can often pass through membranes and travel long distances in cells and tissues.[30]

VIII. DETOXIFICATION OF CARBONYL COMPOUNDS IN BIOLOGICAL SYSTEMS

A further question is whether DMcarbonyl poisoning of organisms is prevented by some biological defense system. In general, carbonyls from whatever source, including the diet, may be dismutated or oxidized by carbonyl dehydrogenases.[30] A large family of these enzymes has indeed been discovered during the past decade.[65] In most animals, the liver contains the highest amount of carbonyl dehydrogenases,[30] probably mainly contributing to detoxification of dietary carbonyls. The concentration of DMcarbonyls in the human diet ranges from a few to several hundred times higher than that of the human body.[66] No studies have been carried out so far to quantify the degree to which DMcarbonyls of the body are produced as the result of oxidative stress vs. other causes. The prolongation of the life span of some rodents by caloric restriction may be related to the decreased intake of DMcarbonyls.

As described above, carbonyls and DMcarbonyls may also react with glutathione to form carbonyl-glutathione conjugates. However, the competition between glutathione and other thiol and amino groups of proteins and other biomolecules should be considered. Nevertheless, cellular glutathione has been repeatedly reported to decrease during aging.[67] Glutathione transferase can efficiently catalyze carbonyl-glutathione conjugation.[30] It has been reported, however, that mouse liver glutathione transferase shows only weak activity towards 4-hydroxylnonenals,[30] which may suggest critical genetic differences among animal species with respect to DMcarbonyl detoxification.

α,β-Unsaturated carbonyls have also been found in many other biological interactions, such as the base-propenals, which are oxidation products of sugars attached to DNA bases; acrolein and crotonaldehyde, which are air pollutants; and *trans,trans*-muconaldehyde, which is a microsomal metabolite of benzene.[68] Pyruvaldehyde, also named methylglyoxal (MG), is another example of a cytotoxic and genotoxic DMcarbonyl. MG exists widely in food and beverages[69] and may be produced during Maillard reactions.[38] In biological systems, however, MG may also be synthesized by several metabolic pathways. For example, MG is synthesized from dihydroxylacetone phosphate when catalyzed by MG synthetase; MG may also be made from aminoacetone during the catabolism of L-threonine.[70,71] On the other hand, MG may be eliminated by several biological pathways, including (1) conversion into D-lactate by the glutathione-requiring glyoxalase system, and (2) oxidation to pyruvate catalyzed by MG dehydrogenases.[70] Although the functions of MG and its conversion to lactic acid by glyoxalase in biological system are still unclear, the glyoxalase system was found to be clearly related to DNA synthesis and cell proliferation, which may provide insights into cellular senescence.[70]

Aminoguanidine is reported to be an effective drug in the prevention of diabetes-induced, glycation-related aging phenomena, for instance retinopathy or arterial wall protein cross-linking.[72,73] However, detoxification of DMcarbonyls by aminoguanidine, with a hydrazine as the reactive group in the molecule, is only competitive and also of only limited effectiveness.

IX. DMCARBONYL TOXIFICATION MAY BE A CENTRAL PROCESS IN BIOLOGICAL AGING

As mentioned previously, the formation of lens cataract, collagen cross-linking, and the accumulation of lipofuscin in postmitotic cells are remarkable phenomena of the aging process. All these are found associated with DMcarbonyl-induced cross-linking and polymerization of biomolecules.[3,12,19,30] Considering that oxidative stress, glycation reactions, and dietary carbonyls all are sources of DMcarbonyls, each of these may be considered to be an important initiator, or promoter, of carbonyl toxification as illustrated in Scheme III.

The physiological concentration of DMcarbonyls, measured as thiobarbituric acid reactive substance (TBARS), are in the range of 0.3 to 5.0 nmol/mL in normal human plasma,[30] whereas the concentration of protein carbonyls are about 3.0 nmol/mg protein in healthy humans.[2,30] Various types of free radical damage, e.g., ionizing radiation, metal-catalyzed oxidation, and oxidation by ozone or nitrogen oxides, may cause a direct and acute effect to biomolecules and increase cellular carbonyls, which may then reinforce carbonyl toxification *in vivo*. Lipid peroxidation was reported to increase progressively with advancing age, such that TBARS values of liver, brain, kidney, and testis from old rats are significantly higher than those of younger ones.[74] Likewise, Yagi and colleagues have demonstrated that the plasma TBARS values of diabetic patients are higher than those of controls, i.e., 5.5 vs. 3.5 nmol/ml.[75] The carbonyl toxification hypothesis of aging is also compatible with the finding that animals with a high metabolic rate have a shorter life span, probably because they also have an increased rate of carbonyl production.

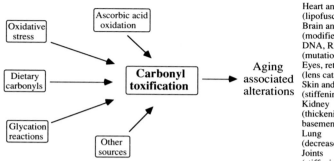

Heart and blood vessels
(lipofuscin, arteriosclerosis)
Brain and nerve cells
(modified neurons, age pigments)
DNA, RNA
(mutations, declined duplication)
Eyes, retinal pigment epithelium
(lens cataract, pigmentation)
Skin and elastic tissues
(stiffening, collagen crosslinking)
Kidney
(thickening of glomerulal
basement membrane)
Lung
(decreased expansion volume)
Joints
(stiffening)

Scheme III
Carbonyl toxification may represent a central process of biological aging.

Although animals possess well-developed defense systems against carbonyl toxification, still, their biomolecules are immersed in a carbonyl environment. The gradual physiological alterations induced by various carbonyls and DMcarbonyls, therefore, are ubiquitous and inevitable.

The recognition that the aging process involves an interplay among several networks of damaging agents and defense systems generates a complex picture of the aging process. The proposed hypothesis, the DMcarbonyl toxification theory of aging, based on several leading contemporary theories of organismic senescence, suggests a new approach towards the understanding of biological aging.

REFERENCES

1. Zs.-Nagy, I., A membrane hypothesis of aging, *J. Theor. Biol.*, 75, 189, 1978.
2. Stadtman, E. R., Protein oxidation and aging, *Science*, 257, 1220, 1992.
3. Bjorksten, J., The cross-linking theory of aging, *J. Am. Geriatr. Soc.*, 16, 408, 1968.
4. Hochschild, R., Lysosomes, membranes and aging, *Exp. Gerontol.*, 6, 153, 1971.
5. Hayflick, L., The cellular basis for biological aging, in *The Handbook of the Biology of Aging*, Hayflick, L. and Finch, C. E., Eds., Van Nostrand Reinhold, New York, 1977, 159.
6. Cutler, R. G., Antioxidants, aging and longevity, in *Free Radicals in Biology*, Vol. 6, Pryor, W. A., Ed., Academic Press, New York, 1984, 371.
7. Lyman, C. P., O'Brian, R. C., Green, G. C., and Papafrangos, E. G., Hibernation and longevity in the Turkish hamster *Mesocritus brandti*, *Science*, 212, 668, 1981.
8. Ragland, S. S. and Sohal, R. S., Mating behaviour, physical activity and aging in housefly, *Musca domestica*, *Exp. Gerontol.*, 8, 135, 1973.
9. Harman, D., Aging: a theory based on free radical and radiation chemistry, *J. Gerontol.*, 11, 289, 1956.
10. Emerit, I. and Chance, B., *Free Radicals and Aging*, Birkhäuser Verlag, Berlin, 1992.

11. Cerami, A., Hypothesis: glucose as a mediator of aging, *J. Am. Geriatr. Soc.*, 33, 626, 1985.

12. Baynes, J. W. and Monnier, V. M., *The Maillard Reaction in Aging, Diabetes, and Nutrition*, Alan R. Liss, New York, 1989.

13. Kristal, B. S. and Yu, B. P., An emerging hypothesis: synergistic induction of aging by free radicals and Maillard reaction, *J. Gerontol.*, 47, B107, 1992.

14. Yin, D., Lipofuscin-like fluorophores can result from reactions between oxidized ascorbic acid and glutamine, carbonyl-protein cross-linking may represent a common reaction in oxygen radical and glycation-related ageing processes, *Mech. Ageing Dev.*, 62, 35, 1992.

15. Pacifici, R. E. and Davies, K. J. A., Protein, lipid and DNA repair systems in oxidative stress: the free-radical theory of aging revisited, *Gerontology*, 37, 166, 1991.

16. Ames, B. N., Dietary carcinogens and anticarcinogens, *Science*, 221, 1256, 1983.

17. Davies, K. J. A., Intracellular proteolytic systems may function as secondary antioxidant defences: a hypothesis, *J. Free Rad. Biol. Med.*, 2, 155, 1986.

18. Esterbauer, H., Cytotoxicity and genotoxicity of lipid-oxidation products, *Am J. Clin. Nutr.*, Suppl. 57, 779S, 1993.

19. Fu, M. X., Knecht, K. J., Thorpe, S. R., and Baynes, J. W., Role of oxygen in cross-linking and modification of collagen by glucose, *Diabetes*, 41 (Suppl. 2), 42, 1992.

20. Brizzee, K. R. and Ordy, J. M., Cellular features, regional accumulation, and prospects of modification of age pigments in mammal, in *Age Pigments*, Sohal, R. S., Ed., Elsevier/North-Holland, Amsterdam, 1981, 101.

21. Strehler, B. L., *Time, Cells, and Aging*, Academic Press, New York, 1977.

22. Sohal, R. S., *Age Pigments*, Elsevier/North-Holland, Amsterdam, 1981.

23. Zs.-Nagy, I., *Lipofuscin-1987, State of the Art*, Excerpta Medica, Amsterdam, 1988.

24. Ames, B. N., Oxidants, antioxidants, and the degenerative diseases of aging, *Proc. Natl. Acad. Sci. U.S.A.*, 90, 7915, 1993.

25. Martin, G. R., Danner, D. B., and Holbrook, N. J., Aging — causes and defenses, *Annu. Rev. Med.*, 44, 419, 1993.

26. Halliwell, B. and Gutteridge, J. M. C., *Free Radicals in Biology and Medicine*, Clarendon Press, Oxford, 1989.

27. Cutler, R. G., Packer, L., Mori, A., and Bertram, J., *Oxidative Stress and Aging*, 1994, (in press).

28. Schauenstein, E., Esterbauer, H., Zollner, H., and Gore, T. P. H., *Aldehydes in Biological Systems*, Pion Limited, London, 1977.

29. Schauenstein, E. and Esterbauer, H., Formation and properties of reactive aldehydes, *Ciba Found. Symp.*, 67, 225, 1979.

30. Esterbauer, H., Schaur, R. J., and Zollner, H., Chemistry and biochemistry of 4-hydroxynonenal, malondialdehyde and related aldehydes, *Free Rad. Biol. Med.*, 11, 81, 1991.

31. Janero, D. R., Malondialdehyde and thiobarbituric acid-reactivity as diagnostic indices of lipid peroxidation and peroxidative tissue injury, *Free Rad. Biol. Med.*, 9, 515, 1990.

32. Comporti, M., Biology of disease, lipid peroxidation and cellular damage in toxic liver injury, *Lab. Invest.*, 53, 599, 1985.

33. Napetschnig, S., Reactions of Amino Acids With 4-Hydroxy-2,3-trans-pentenal and Therapy of Ehrlich Ascites Tumors With the Amino Acid Adducts, Thesis, University of Graz, Austria, 1981.

34. Jürgens, G., Lang, J., and Esterbauer, H., Modification of human low-density lipoprotein by the lipid peroxidation product 4-hydroxynonenal, *Biochim. Biophys. Acta*, 875, 103, 1986.

35. Winter, C. K., Segall, H. J., and Haddon, W. F., Formation of cyclic adducts of deoxyguanosine with the aldehydes trans-4-hydroxy-2-hexenal and trans-4-hydroxy-2-nonenal in vitro, *Cancer Res.*, 46, 5682, 1986.

36. Esterbauer, H., Zollner, H., and Scholz, H., Reaction of glutathione with conjugated carbonyls, *Z. Naturforsch*, 30, 466, 1975.

37. Esterbauer, H., Ertl, A., and Scholz, H., Reaction of cysteine with alpha, beta-unsaturated aldehydes, *Tetrahedron*, 32, 285, 1976.

38. Hodge, J. E., Dehydrated foods, chemistry of browning reactions in model systems, *J. Agric. Food Chem.*, 1, 928, 1953.

39. Monnier, V. M., Nonenzymatic glycosylation, the Maillard reaction and aging process, *J. Gerontol.*, 45, B105, 1990.

40. Cerami, A., Vlassara, H., and Brownlee, M., Role of advanced glycosylation products in complication of diabetes, *Diabetes Care*, 11 (Suppl. 1), 73, 1988.

41. Brownlee, M., Glycosylation products as toxic mediators of diabetic complications, *Annu. Rev. Med.*, 42, 159, 1991.

42. Brownlee, M. and Cerami, A., The biochemistry of the complication of diabetes mellitus, *Ann. Rev. Biochem.*, 50, 385, 1981.

43. Kohn, R. R. and Schnider, S. L., Glycosylation of human collagen, *Diabetes*, Suppl. 31, 47, 1982.

44. Monnier, V. M. and Cerami, A., Nonenzymatic browning in vivo: possible process for aging of long-lived proteins, *Science*, 211, 491, 1981.

45. Monnier, V. M. and Cerami, A., Nonenzymatic glycosylation and browning in diabetes and aging, studies on lens proteins, *Diabetes*, 31 (Suppl. 3), 57, 1982.

46. Stevens, V. J., Rouzer, C. A., Monnier, V. M., and Cerami, A., Diabetes cataract formation: potential role of glycosylation of lens crystallins, *Proc. Natl. Acad. Sci. U.S.A.*, 75, 2918, 1978.

47. Kohn, R. R. and Monnier, V. M., Normal aging and its parameters, in *Clinical Pharmacology in the Elderly*, Swift, C. G., Ed., Marcel Dekker, New York, 1987, 3.

48. Schonfeld, G., Diabetes, lipoproteins, and atherosclerosis, *Metabolism*, 34 (Suppl. 1), 45, 1985.

49. Witztum, J. L. and Koschinsky, T., Metabolic and immunological consequences of glycation of low density lipoproteins, in *The Maillard Reaction in Aging, Diabetes, and Nutrition*, Baynes, J. W. and Monnier, V. M., Eds., Alan R. Liss, New York, 1989, 219.

50. Esterbauer, H., Gebicki, J., Puhl, H., and Jürgens, G., The role of lipid peroxidation and antioxidants in oxidative modification of LDL, *Free Rad. Biol. Med.*, 13, 41, 1992.

51. Tappel, A. L., Lipid peroxidation and fluorescent molecular damage to membranes, in *Pathobiology of Cell Membranes*, Trump, B. F. and Arstila, A. U., Eds., Academic Press, New York, 1975, 145.

52. Wolman, M., Lipid pigments (chromolipids): their origin, nature, and significance, *Pathobiology Annual*, 10, 253, 1980.

53. Kikugawa, K., Fluorescent products derived from the reaction of primary amines and components in peroxidized lipids, *Adv. Free Rad. Biol. Med.*, 2, 389, 1986.

54. Brennan, M., Changes in solubility, non-enzymatic glycation, and fluorescence of collagen in tail tendons from diabetic rats, *J. Biol. Chem.*, 35, 20947, 1989.

55. Monnier, V. M., Kohn, R. P., and Cerami, A., Accelerated age-related browning of human collagen in diabetes mellitus, *Proc. Natl. Acad. Sci. U.S.A.*, 81, 583, 1984.

56. Davis, H. K. and Reece, P., Fluorescence of fish muscle: causes of change occurring during frozen storage, *J. Sci. Food Agric.*, 33, 1143, 1982.

57. Baynes, J. W., Role of oxidative stress in development of complications in diabetes, *Diabetes*, 40, 405, 1991.

58. Wolff, S., Jiang, Z. Y., and Hunt, J. V., Protein glycation and oxidative stress in diabetes mellitus and ageing, *Free Rad. Biol. Med.*, 10, 339, 1991.

59. Jain, S. K., Hyperglycemia can cause membrane lipid peroxidation and osmotic fragility in human blood cells, *J. Biol. Chem.*, 264, 21340, 1989.

60. Eldred, G. E. and Katz, M. L., The autofluorescent products of lipid peroxidation may not be lipofuscin-like, *Free Rad. Biol. Med.*, 7, 157, 1989.

61. Yin, D. and Brunk, U. T., Microfluorometric and fluorometric lipofuscin spectral discrepancies: a concentration-dependent metachromatic effect?, *Mech. Ageing Dev.*, 59, 95, 1991a.

62. Yin, D., Aging, age pigments, and concentration-dependent shift of autofluorescence, *Age*, 16, 80, 1994.

63. Eldred, G. E. and Lasky, M. R., Retinal age pigments generated by self-assembling lysosomotropic detergents, *Nature*, 361, 724, 1993.

64. Yin, D. and Brunk, U. T., Oxidized ascorbic acid and reaction products between ascorbic acid and amino acids might constitute part of age pigments, *Mech. Ageing Dev.*, 61, 99, 1991b.

65. Weiner, H., Crabb, D. W., and Flynn, T. G., *Enzymology and Molecular Biology of Carbonyl Metabolism*, Vol. 4, Plenum Press, New York, 1993.

66. Lang, J., Celotto, C., and Esterbauer, H., Quantitative determination of the lipid peroxidation product 4-hydroxynonenal by high-performance liquid chromatography, *Anal. Biochem.*, 150, 369, 1985.

67. Oberley, L. W. and Oberley, T. D., Free radicals, cancer, and aging, in *Free Radicals, Aging and Degenerative Diseases*, Johnson, J. E., Walford, R., Harman, D., and Miquel, J., Eds., Alan R. Liss, New York, 1986, 325.

68. Witz, G., Biological interactions of α,β-unsaturated aldehydes, *Free Rad. Biol. Med.*, 7, 333, 1989.

69. *Evaluation of Carcinogenic Risks to Humans*, IARC Monograph, 51, 443, 1991.

70. Thornalley, P. J., The glyoxalase system: new developments towards functional characterization of metabolic pathway fundamental to biological life, *Biochem. J.*, 269, 1, 1990.

71. Kalapos, M. P., Mechanisms leading to complications in diabetes mellitus: pathological role of α-oxoaldehydes, *Biochem. Educat.*, 20, 27, 1992.

72. Brownlee, M., Vlassara, H., Kooney, A., Ulrich, R., and Cerami, A., Aminoguanidine prevents diabetes-induced arterial wall protein cross-linking, *Science*, 232, 1629, 1986.

73. Hammes, H. P., Martin, S., Federlin, K., Geisen, K., and Brownlee, M., Aminoguanidine treatment inhibits the development of experimental diabetic retinopathy, *Proc. Natl. Acad. Sci. U.S.A.*, 88, 11555, 1991.

74. Uchiyama, M. and Mihara, M., Determination of malonaldehyde precursor in tissues by thiobarbituric acid test, *Anal. Biochem.*, 86, 271, 1978.

75. Sato, Y., Hotta, N., Sakamoto, N., Matsuoka, S., Ohishi, N., and Yagi, K., Lipid peroxide level in plasma of diabetic patients, *Biochem. Med.*, 21, 104, 1979.

Chapter 14

Amyloidosis and Aging

Per Westermark and Kenneth H. Johnson

CONTENTS

0-8493-4786-6/95/$0.00+$.50
© 1995 by CRC Press, Inc.

I. AMYLOID, AMYLOIDOSIS: BACKGROUND INFORMATION

The term *amyloidosis*, used for nearly 150 years to identify the deposition of amyloid fibrils in a variety of tissues, is sometimes misinterpreted to imply a single disease condition with a uniform pathogenesis. The *amyloidoses*, in fact, are represented by multiple individual disease conditions that often have quite different pathogenic mechanisms and clinical manifestations. The common denominator for all forms of localized or systemic amyloidosis is the deposition of nonbranching protein fibrils which have strong affinity for the dye Congo red and emit green birefringence when Congo red-stained specimens are viewed with polarized light. The Congophilia and marked insolubility of amyloid fibrils are attributed to the significant beta-pleated sheet conformation of the polymerized peptide subunits assembled within the amyloid fibrils.[1] Progressive deposition of insoluble amyloid fibrils is reflected by clinical signs or symptoms directly related to the specific sites of amyloid deposition.

The protein monomers that undergo abnormal self-aggregation to form the insoluble fibrils present in each form of amyloidosis are derived from one of several precursor proteins present in the blood or tissues. At present, at least 17 amyloid precursor proteins have been identified. Interestingly, many of the precursor proteins have a significant inherent amount of beta-pleated sheet structure. The repetitive protein subunits assembled within amyloid fibrils may represent the intact normal precursor protein, or they may represent enzymatically cleaved segments of the precursor protein. In some forms of amyloidosis (e.g., transthyretin (TTR)-derived familial amyloid polyneuropathies: FAPs), the protein subunits of the amyloid fibril are derived from mutant proteins which have amino acid substitutions at positions specific for the respective kindreds. An increased production and/or concentration of the precursor protein is also known to be associated with many forms of amyloidosis, and the increased concentration of precursor protein has been linked to the facilitation of precursor aggregation and fibrillogenesis.

II. GENERAL RELATIONSHIPS BETWEEN AMYLOIDOSIS AND AGING

In general, most forms of amyloidosis are seen with greater frequency in humans and animals as they age.[2,3] Amyloid deposits of one form or another, many of which were clinically inapparent, were reported in virtually all consecutive autopsies of individuals over 65 years of age in one study.[4] This association of amyloidosis with aging appears, at least partly, to be a reflection of an increasing cumulative risk for overt or occult diseases which either directly or indirectly favor factors that lead to fibrillogenesis of the respective amyloid precursor proteins. The specific mechanisms involved in the fibrillogenesis may be different and unique for each specific form of amyloidosis.

Reactive or AA-amyloidosis (i.e., so-called "secondary" amyloidosis), for example, is a systemic form of amyloidosis which occurs as a result of a variety of recurrent or chronic inflammatory and neoplastic diseases which can induce up to a thousandfold increase in the plasma levels of a specific precursor apolipoprotein (i.e., serum protein AA (apoSAA), reviewed in Reference 5). ApoSAA is an 11.5-kDa, 104-amino-acid acute-phase reactant that is produced primarily by the liver. When abnormal and incomplete enzymatic degradation of SAA occurs, an N-terminal 5- to 11-kDa protein (i.e., protein AA) is typically formed. The AA protein, composed of 44 to approximately 100 amino acid residues, can assemble to form the fibrils present in AA-amyloidosis. Elevated plasma apoSAA levels have been demonstrated consistently in a broad spectrum of recurrent or chronic inflammatory diseases and neoplastic diseases.[6] Leprosy, tuberculosis, osteomyelitis, pyelonephritis, bronchiectasis, ulcerative colitis, rheumatoid arthritis, ankylosing spondylitis, and neoplastic diseases (especially renal carcinoma) are historically documented examples of diseases predisposing to AA-amyloidosis. In addition to elevated apoSAA levels, the fibrillogenesis may also be importantly linked to abnormalities in the proteolysis of apoSAA which subsequently lead to formation of amyloidogenic AA molecules. In mink and mice, fibrillogenesis is also linked to certain isoforms of SAA. Thus, in the mouse only one of the two major plasma SAA isoforms is amyloidogenic. In humans, the situation is more complicated and SAA is encoded by at least three genes with allelic variations. At least five isoforms of apoSAA are known in humans.[7] Most of these isoforms have also been identified in amyloid deposits, although some more commonly than others. Existence of SAA isoforms that are more amyloidogenic than others may therefore contribute to the fact that only certain persons with longstanding high plasma levels of SAA develop AA-amyloidosis. Secondary structure predictions of human apoSAA$_1$ suggest that a region of beta-sheet configuration is represented by positions 34 to 45.[8] Nevertheless, experiments with synthetic peptides corresponding to different segments of the AA-protein indicate that the N-terminal region determines the fibrillogeneity.[9]

Systemic AL-amyloidosis (amyloidosis of Ig light-chain origin) is predominantly a disease of middle-aged and older individuals[10] who are predisposed to this form of amyloidosis by the presence of abnormal monoclonal Ig or Ig light chains in their serum (M-component) and/or urine (i.e., Bence Jones proteins). Two thirds of the patients with AL-amyloidosis are males with a mean age of 61 years;[10] up to 15% of humans with multiple myeloma have been reported to develop AL-amyloidosis.[1,11] The abnormal Ig components associated with these cases are derived from monoclonal populations of plasma cells associated with benign plasma cell dyscrasias or overt multiple myeloma. AL amyloidosis, which was earlier identified as so-called "primary" amyloidosis because of a lack of association with predisposing inflammatory or infectious diseases, is characterized by amyloid fibrils that are derived from either the intact monoclonal light chains or, much more commonly, N-terminal fragments of the variable region of these same Ig light chains. Approximately 15 to 20% of Bence Jones proteins appear to be amyloidogenic based on *in vitro* fibrillogenesis studies, but there is no evidence of a specific light-chain amino acid sequence which promotes amyloidogenesis in AL amyloidosis. However, lambda light chains are overrepresented in AL-amyloidosis and, especially, the lambda VI subgroup seems to be prone to form amyloid fibrils.[12] In addition to the organs symptomatically affected in AA-amyloidosis (especially kidneys) in one big group of AL-patients,[13] major AL-amyloid deposits in another group are seen in the heart, GI tract, skin, and joints. AL-amyloidosis thus involves mesenchymal tissues more frequently than AA-amyloidosis. Renal involvement with nephrotic syndrome is commonly a feature of both AA- and AL-amyloidosis, and is the most common clinical manifestation of AL-amyloidosis. Other clinical manifestations of AL-amyloidosis may include cardiomyopathy with ventricular arrhythmias, chronic diarrhea and/or malabsorption with weight loss, and carpal tunnel syndrome.[10]

III. FORMS OF AMYLOIDOSIS RECOGNIZED TO HAVE SPECIALLY IMPORTANT RELATIONSHIPS TO AGE-RELATED DISEASES

A number of forms of amyloidosis have an even more obvious and well-recognized association specifically with diseases of advanced age. Cerebral and cerebrovascular amyloidosis in Alzheimer's disease, islet amyloidosis in type II diabetes mellitus (DM), and cardiac amyloidosis in Senile Systemic Amyloidosis (SSA) are the most universally recognized examples of this more direct relationship between amyloidosis and aging. However, as will be apparent in our discussion of this group of age-linked forms of amyloidosis, it is often difficult to resolve in a completely satisfactory manner whether these forms of amyloidosis are primarily a cause, effect, or both cause and effect of the aging process.

A. Islet Amyloidosis and Type II Diabetes Mellitus (Noninsulin-Dependent Diabetes Mellitus: NIDDM)

Type II DM usually occurs in individuals during or after the fourth or fifth decade of life, and represents 85 to 90% of all cases of DM. This most common form of DM is known to have a strong hereditary influence which is demonstrated by the nearly 100% concordance found in identical twins. However, specific inherited gene defect(s) have not been delineated, and a variety of complex environmental factors are considered to contribute to the eventual expression of a possible genetic abnormality. Resistance to insulin-stimulated glucose uptake and disposal, together with an attenuated insulin response to glucose, are the clinical hallmarks of this form of DM, but the specific pathogenesis and primary defect involved in the evolution of this age-related form of DM remain unclear and is a source of considerable debate and controversy.

The frequent presence of amyloid deposits in the pancreatic islets of adult persons with type II DM was documented in the very early part of this century, and these deposits have been recognized for several decades to be a characteristic morphologic feature of more than 90% of humans with type II DM. However, the relationship between the pathogenesis of type II DM and these amyloid deposits restricted to the pancreatic islets has been regarded with considerable skepticism and controversy. This skepticism is at least partially related to the observation that islet amyloid is also known to occur in nondiabetic individuals. Studies in those species (e.g., humans, domestic cats, and nonhuman primates) that develop islet amyloidosis in association with age-related forms of DM have conclusively demonstrated, however, that there is both an increased frequency of islets that contain amyloid and a larger amount of amyloid per islet in diabetic patients than in age-matched controls.[14-16] The deposition of amyloid in pancreatic islets reduces the beta cell mass,[17,18] but this reduction is not sufficient per se to account for the diabetic state in these patients. The presence of a large amount of islet amyloid (Figure 1) should be regarded as a marker of attenuated islet function (i.e., glucose intolerance or overt DM) and delineation of its mechanisms of formation may be an important avenue of future research in type II DM.

A more intensive and serious interest in the relationship between islet amyloid and type II DM was elicited with the recent discovery that islet amyloid represents a concentrated and aggregated form of a previously unknown islet-derived hormone.[19-21] This previously unknown 37-amino-acid hormone, subsequently identified as islet amyloid polypeptide (IAPP)[20] or amylin,[22] belongs to a protein superfamily also including the neuropeptide calcitonin gene-related peptide (CGRP) and calcitonin (Figure 2). IAPP is nearly 50% identical to CGRP but with a short, unique, central segment important for the amyloid formation (see below). IAPP and its possible functions and relationship to type II DM have been the subject of several recent reviews.[23-25]

IAPP has been demonstrated to be synthesized and secreted predominantly by islet beta cells. IAPP is colocalized with insulin in the beta cell secretory vesicles[26,27] and is cosecreted in a biphasic pattern with insulin in

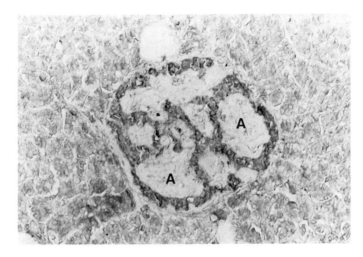

Figure 1
Islet of Langerhans from a patient with Type 2 diabetes mellitus. Most of the endocrine cells have been replaced by amyloid masses (A).

ACDTATCVTHRLAGLLSRSGGVVKNNFVPTNVGSKAF   CGRP1

KCNTATCATQRLANFLVHSSNNFGAILSSTNVGSNTY   IAPP

CGNLSTCMLGTYTQDF   NKFH   TFPQTAIGVGAP   Calcitonin

Figure 2
Amino acid sequences of three members of the calcitonin family: calcitonin gene-related peptide (CGRP), islet amyloid polypeptide (IAPP), and calcitonin, aligned for maximal identity. IAPP and calcitonin are both known as amyloid fibril proteins.

response to glucose and other secretagogues. On a molar basis the amount of IAPP secreted is about 1 to 10% of that of insulin, with basal blood levels of IAPP generally reported to be in the 2- to 15-pM range. Several potentially important biological functions for IAPP have been proposed and/or documented, but the most challenging putative role is as a glucoregulatory hormone which modulates or counterregulates the actions of insulin (e.g., reduces insulin-stimulated glucose uptake in skeletal muscle and impairs insulin suppression of hepatic glucose output).

The proposed role of IAPP as a counterregulatory hormone, thus modulating and balancing the effects of insulin, has potential ramifications related to better (i.e., more physiologic) glucose control in especially insulin-dependent diabetic patients.[28] Also of potential importance is the implication that exaggerated production and secretion of IAPP may play a key role in the development of the increased peripheral insulin resistance

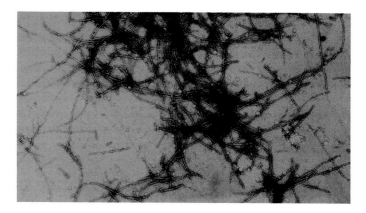

Figure 3
Fibrils formed from synthetic human IAPP. The fibrils are less than 10 nm in width and morphologically similar to native amyloid fibrils. They have the staining characteristics and X-ray diffraction properties of amyloid.

that is so characteristic of type II DM. The results of ongoing studies in many laboratories should help to further elucidate the proposed but questioned roles of IAPP regarding normal glucose regulation and its potential significance in the development of type II DM. It should be emphasized, however, that the reports of effects of IAPP on peripheral glucose regulation have usually been associated with IAPP plasma levels much above physiological concentrations.

1. Amyloidogenicity of IAPP

Like with many other amyloid fibril proteins, it has been shown that human IAPP has a strong intrinsic tendency to form insoluble fibrils with properties typical of amyloid fibrils[29] (Figure 3). This is in contrast to rat IAPP, which differs from human IAPP at only six amino acid positions[30,31] but which does not form fibrils *in vitro*. Interestingly, humans often develop islet amyloid while rats never do. In this way, a link between certain sequences in the fibril-forming protein and the occurrence of islet amyloid has been delineated. Although the islet amyloid deposits in humans, cats, and nonhuman primates are derived by self-aggregation of intact normal IAPP molecules, the fibrillogenic potential of the molecules appears to be importantly related to specific amino acid sequences inherently present in the central region (positions 24 to 28) of IAPP from these several species[29,32,33] (Figure 4).

Based on comparison of cDNA-predicted IAPP sequences of multiple species and *in vitro* fibrillogenesis studies utilizing synthetic IAPP decapeptides representing positions 20 through 29, the Gly-Ala-Ile-Leu-Ser sequence present at positions 24 to 28 appears most critically related

```
Human   IAPP20–29    SNNFGAILSS
Cat  IAPP20–29        – – – L – – – – – P
Mouse  IAPP20–29     – – – L–PV – PP
Hamster  IAPP20–29   N – – L– PV – – P
Human  CGRP20–29     CGVVKNNFVP
```

Figure 4
Amino acid sequence of IAPP, positions 20–29 of two species with occurrence of islet
amyloid (human and cat) and two species without (rat and hamster). The short
segment GAILS seems to determine whether or not IAPP forms amyloid fibrils. The
20–29 segment of human CGRP (not known as an amyloid protein) is completely
different from IAPP.

to fibrillogenesis of human and cat IAPP.[29,32] Overproduction of IAPP
(resulting in increased local concentration)[34] or aberrations in synthesis,
molecular processing, or release of IAPP[35] are additional potentially important factors involved in the facilitation of self-aggregation of IAPP to
form islet amyloid.

2. Future Studies

Ongoing and future studies concerning the relationships of IAPP and
IAPP-derived islet amyloid to the pathogenesis of type II DM will undoubtedly concentrate on the proposed role of IAPP as an inhibitor of
peripheral insulin action and its possible autocrine/paracrine actions.
However, future studies must also address the feasibility that states of
chronic insulin resistance, regardless of cause, induce hyperglycemia and
subsequent increased production of IAPP (and insulin), which (when
linked with concordant aberrations in processing of IAPP within the islets)
leads to amyloidogenesis, significant loss of beta cell mass, and the clinical
manifestations of type II diabetes. The possibility of defective IAPP synthesis, storage, or secretion should not be forgotten.

B. Amyloid and Alzheimer's Disease

Alzheimer's disease is a degenerative disease of the brain typically
characterized clinically by progressive loss of memory and cognitive ability (i.e., dementia) in elderly people. Severe debilitation and death usually
occur within 4 to 12 years following clinical onset. This most common
form of senile dementia, first described by Alzheimer in 1907, has been an
especially intense focus of investigation over the past 10 years. Major
emphasis has been placed on the significance and relationship of the
characteristic cerebral amyloid deposits to the complex pathogenesis of
Alzheimer's disease. In this relatively brief synopsis, we will primarily
provide an overview of current information and concepts regarding the

potential relationships of amyloid and amyloidogenesis to the pathogenesis of Alzheimer's disease. For a broader and more extensive perspective regarding this very complex disease, including the accumulating evidence of the etiologically heterogeneous nature of Alzheimer's disease, the reader is referred to several comprehensive and recent reviews in References 36 to 39.

Alzheimer's disease is characterized by three forms of cerebral lesions, all of which include the deposition of fibrils with characteristics of amyloid:

1. *Cerebral amyloid angiopathy* is manifested by amyloid deposition within and adjacent to cerebral and meningeal blood vessels;
2. *Neuritic plaques* are extracellular and multifocal aggregates, usually with compact cores of amyloid fibrils surrounded by a rim of silver-positive dystrophic neurites; and
3. So-called *neurofibrillary tangles* are Congophilic aggregates evident within neuronal cell bodies and neuronal processes.

Morphologically typical 8- to 10-nm amyloid fibrils are evident ultrastructurally in both of the extracellular amyloid forms (i.e., neuritic plaques and cerebrovascular amyloid deposits), whereas the intraneuronal aggregates with amyloid properties contain morphologically different and distinctive filamentous structures referred to as paired helical filaments (PHF).[40,41] Further biochemical distinction between the extracellular and intraneuronal amyloid fibrils has been provided by recent immunohistochemical and immunochemical studies as well as amino acid sequence analyses. Both neuritic plaque and cerebrovascular amyloid are formed from a 39- to 43-amino-acid protein[42-44] which has been variably identified as β, A4, or A4β protein (note: Aβ will be used to identify this protein in this chapter[45]).

1. The Aβ Protein

The 39- to 43-amino acid Aβ protein, which is the repetitive protein subunit present within the amyloid fibrils of cerebrovascular and neuritic plaque amyloid deposits, is derived from the proteolytic cleavage of a much larger transmembrane precursor protein, the Aβ precursor: βPP (often also referred to by the inexact name "amyloid protein precursor" (APP)). Alternative splicing of the primary transcript of the 18 exons in the single-copy βPP gene on the long arm of chromosome 21 gives rise to distinctive messengers coding for proteins which are 695, 714, 751, or 770 amino acids in length (reviewed in Reference 38). The βPPs are highly conserved in the animal kingdom, and they are expressed as a family of transmembrane proteins in a variety of mammalian cells (including both neural and nonneural cells).

The function(s) of the βPPs is still a question and focus of intense investigation. The overall structure resembles that of a receptor but no ligand has been identified. There are also indications that βPP can be cleaved close to the cell surface (within the amyloid domain) and secreted. These secreted forms may have important effects on cell growth. Furthermore, the largest of the βPPs (βPP$_{714}$, βPP$_{751}$, and βPP$_{770}$) are known to contain an amino acid sequence insert representing a serine protease inhibitor activity of the Kunitz type, while βPP$_{695}$ does not.

2. Mechanisms by Which Aβ Amyloid is Formed

There appears to be a growing consensus that an unraveling of the complex and elusive mechanisms involved in the normal and abnormal processing of βPPs will provide information fundamental to understanding the pathogenesis of Alzheimer's disease. Synthetic Aβ has a strong intrinsic tendency to form amyloid-like fibrils *in vitro*.[46,47] *In vitro* experiments have also shown that fibril formation rate from a Aβ solution is strongly enhanced by addition of trace amounts of preformed fibrils.[48] Therefore, formation of the first few fibrils may be of critical importance. Cleavage of βPP just outside the transmembrane region which is within the Aβ domain (at residue 16 of Aβ) results in the extracellular release of the major N-terminal part of βPP (see Reference 37). This cleavage abolishes the potential for amyloidogenesis by preventing the formation of intact Aβ. The proteolytic cleavage is assumed to be associated with an as yet unidentified membrane-associated secretase enzyme. However, there apparently are other alternative (intracellular) βPP processing routes associated with neurons, glial cells, and other cells within the brain that could leave the Aβ intact. The production of intact Aβ is likely crucial for amyloidogenesis, and the Aβ itself has a strong tendency to form amyloid-like fibrils *in vitro*. The assumption that Aβ (and thus amyloidogenesis) is only a product of abnormal processing of βPP is challenged, however, by the recent finding that Aβ is routinely produced as a soluble peptide *in vitro* by metabolically normal cells such as human neurons, glial cells, and endothelial cells.[49,50] Thus, there appears to be at least two different metabolic pathways for proteolytic cleavage of βPP. One of these pathways inhibits the formation of intact Aβ because of cleavage of the precursor molecule within the Aβ sequence. A second, perhaps intracellular pathway, cleaves the βPP molecule closer to the N-terminus, thus allowing the eventual production of intact Aβ following additional cleavage at the C-terminal end of the βPP molecule.[51]

It has been proposed that a balance between these different pathways exists in the normal aging process, but that this balance is disrupted or lost in Alzheimer's disease.[38] Like other amyloids, the local concentration of the fibrillogenic protein is probably important. It is also feasible that differences in the solubility of the variable-length normal or mutated Aβ produced are important determining factors as to whether fibrillogenesis does or does not occur, and thus whether or not the process does or does not become pathological.[39]

3. Familial Alzheimer's Disease

Further insights regarding the pathogenesis of Alzheimer's disease, especially as related to enzymatic processing of βPPs, will likely be provided by ongoing studies of familial cases of early onset disease which are linked to expression of mutant βPPs. Several βPP mutations involving either the Aβ region per se, or regions flanking the Aβ sequence, have been documented in cases of familial (autosomal dominant) Alzheimer's disease (reviewed in References 37 through 39). These cases not only provide additional support for the potential importance of βPPs in Alzheimer's disease, but they also provide an opportunity to study the effects of disordered metabolism and cleavage related to these precursor proteins. However, interestingly, one mutation within the Aβ domain, leading to an amino acid substitution (Gln for Glu at position 22 in Aβ), is not associated with Alzheimer's disease but with Dutch hereditary cerebral hemorrhage.[52] These individuals get Aβ amyloid in cerebral and meningeal vessels but do not develop typical Alzheimer brain pathology.[53]

Recently other hereditary factors linked to genes on chromosomes 14 and 19 (reviewed in Reference 38), have been implicated in the pathogenesis of Alzheimer's disease. The increased risk factor associated with chromosome 14 is associated with families of early onset Alzheimer's disease. The type 4 allele of the apolipoprotein E (apoE) gene, associated with chromosome 19, has been genetically associated with the common late onset familial and sporadic forms of Alzheimer's disease.[54] It was shown in the latter study[54] that the mean age of onset of Alzheimer's disease decreased from 84 to 68 years with an increasing number of the type 4 alleles, and homozygosity for the type 4 allele was associated with Alzheimer's disease in most individuals by age 80. The mechanism(s) by which apoE affects the Alzheimer's disease process is not known. ApoE (especially apoE4) binds to synthetic Aβ with great avidity *in vitro*[55] and, immunohistochemically, apoE is invariably present in plaque amyloid. However, apoE is also found in systemic amyloids of varying nature.[56] ApoE (like some other minor amyloid components) have been proposed to act as "pathological chaperones" by stabilizing the b-structure in amyloid fibril proteins.[56]

4. Neurofibrillary Tangle Proteins

The paired helical filaments (PHF) of the neurofibrillary tangles are commonly not regarded as typical amyloid fibrils. However, they exhibit amyloid-staining properties (used for practical recognition of amyloid) and show cross-b conformation in X-ray diffraction,[57] where they fulfill criteria for amyloid fibrils. PHF consist of abnormal accumulations of cytoskeletal proteins within which the microtubule-associated protein tau is a major component (reviewed in Reference 58). Tau exists normally as six different isoforms which all may be represented within PHFs. PHFs are supposed to develop from tau that is aberrantly and abnormally phospho-rylated,[58] which changes its binding to tubulin. The putative kinase(s) responsible for this phosphorylation has not been identified. Although tau is the major component of PHF, other components are also identified in PHF. Of putative importance is the fact that several investigators have identified Aβ not only in plaque amyloid but also in the tangles as well.[59-61]

5. Impact of Amyloid in the Pathogenesis of Dementia

Although amyloid deposition in several different morphologic forms are the morphological hallmarks of Alzheimer's disease, the importance of the amyloid deposits per se in the pathogenesis of dementia is a matter of debate, and the effects of both tangles and plaques on the cerebral function have not been clarified. In most studies there is no strong correlation between the degree of dementia and the quantities of plaques.[62] The number of tangles correlates slightly better with the degree of cognitive impairment.[63] The relationship between cerebral amyloid deposits and Alzheimer's disease is even further complicated by the knowledge that Aβ-derived amyloid deposits are not pathognomic of Alzheimer's disease in that they can also be demonstrated in the brains of elderly humans that have no clinical history of dementia.[63] Additionally, the sequential and pathogenetic relationships between the development of neurofibrillary tangles, amyloid-containing neuritic plaques, and cerebrovascular amy-loid deposits still is not clear. Regarding the latter question, it has been proposed that altered metabolism of βPPs contributes to a loss of neuronal calcium homeostasis which, in turn, is linked to neurofibrillary degenera-tion and neuritic plaque formation (see Reference 64). This scenario does not address the occurrence of cerebrovascular amyloidosis in Alzheimer's disease, however.

Regarding direct effects of amyloid fibrils on neurons, interesting and provocative results have been obtained *in vitro* with synthetic Aβ and Aβ-derived amyloid-like fibrils. These fibrils have been found to elicit direct toxic effects on neurons, both *in vitro* and when administered intracere-brally in experimental animals,[65] possibly by a tachykinin-like internal segment of Aβ.[66] Soluble Aβ may also form Ca^{2+} channels[67] and cause potassium channel dysfunction.[68] Some of these potentially very impor-tant findings, like much in Alzheimer pathogenesis, are a matter of debate, however.

Thus, the very complex and often-times incompletely understood relationships between amyloid deposits and the specific diseases they are associated with is well exemplified by Alzheimer's disease. Although there understandably is not universal acceptance of the primary importance of amyloid in the complex pathogenesis of Alzheimer's disease, there nevertheless is a significant amount of evidence which supports the possibility that abnormalities in the metabolism of the βPPs do play a central and causal role in the development of this disease.

C. Transthyretin [TTR]-Derived Senile Systemic Amyloidosis: SSA

The condition now identified as senile systemic amyloidosis (SSA), which is rarely seen in individuals under 70 years of age, was originally referred to as senile cardiac amyloidosis because when the disease is symptomatic the heart is usually affected more profoundly than other tissues or organs. However, this most common form of systemic amyloidosis associated with aging (affecting approximately 15% of persons 70 years of age or older) is now known to also involve many other organs.[69] In most organs or tissues the amyloid deposits are present mainly in vessel walls, but amyloid deposition in the heart is observed both within vessels and as a diffuse or multifocal infiltration between muscle cells in the ventricles and atria. In addition to the preponderant involvement of the heart, SSA is commonly observed in pulmonary vessels and alveolar walls.

There usually is a sparing of the specialized cardiac conduction tissue in SSA, which is in contradistinction to AL amyloidosis where deposits of amyloid often also affect the conduction system of the heart. Cardiac failure thus is a major cause of death in AL amyloidosis, whereas SSA is usually a more benign disease with mild cardiac symptoms. However, some individuals with SSA (mainly men) are more severely affected with heavy amyloid deposits in the myocardium which may give rise to cardiomegaly and congestive heart failure.[70]

The major constituent of the amyloid fibrils in SSA is transthyretin (TTR), which was originally called "prealbumin" because it migrates ahead of albumin on gel electrophoresis. TTR, which has no chemical relationship to albumin, is synthesized (mainly by the liver) as a 147-amino-acid proprotein chain.[71] After the signal sequence has been cleaved off, the 127-amino-acid TTR forms dimers and tetramers.[72] The circulating tetrameric form of TTR has binding sites for thyroxin and retinol-binding protein, and thus functions importantly in the transport of these substances.

TTR, which has substantial beta pleated-sheet structure,[72] also is the major protein precursor for several heredofamilial forms of predominantly late-onset amyloidosis (e.g., familial amyloid polyneuropathy (FAP), familial amyloid cardiomyopathy (FAC), and isolated vitreous amyloid (IVA) that affects individuals within certain Swedish, Portuguese, Japanese, Jewish, German, Swiss, Danish, Greek, or Italian kindreds. Investigations of these autosomal-dominant forms of amyloidosis have shown that specific point mutations in the TTR gene lead to single amino acid substitutions in TTR which are characteristic for each of the affected kindreds. To date more than 40 point mutations, distributed throughout the TTR-molecule, have been found in association with familial TTR-derived amyloidosis.[73] Although these mutations are generally considered to be importantly linked to the development of amyloidosis in affected individuals, there still is not a clear understanding of how these mutations are specifically related to fibrillogenesis. Furthermore, factors other than the presence of point mutations must also be of importance. For example, some individuals never develop amyloidosis although they synthesize a mutant TTR that is amyloidogenic in other individuals.[74]

A major question has been whether or not an amino acid substitution in the TTR precursor molecule is also a prerequisite for formation of the amyloid fibrils present in SSA.[75,76] The demonstration of a normal and complete TTR amino acid sequence representing the amyloid protein from a patient with SSA,[77] together with normal cDNA- and genomic DNA-predicted TTR sequences, respectively, in two additional SSA patients[78] (Gustavsson et al., unpublished data), show that TTR without amino acid substitutions is amyloidogenic in some individuals of advanced age. This fact also emphasizes the point that factors in addition to mutant TTR-variants are important for formation of TTR derived amyloid. In both SSA and the familial TTR-derived amyloidoses, the amyloid fibrils are generally found to contain intact TTR monomers, but TTR fragments of various length may also be incorporated into the amyloid fibrils associated with both of these conditions.[79] In fact, in both conditions (but especially SSA), TTR fragments may sometimes predominate over the presence of full-length TTR molecules. Interestingly, this fragmentation is not random since cleavage has been reported predominantly at positions 46, 49, and 52.[77,80] It still remains to be clarified as to whether proteolytic cleavage of TTR in SSA is a primary and significant event in fibrillogenesis in SSA, or whether cleavage only reflects a secondary event occurring within the already-formed amyloid fibril. It is quite possible, however, that cleavage leads to exposure of amyloidogenic protein segments that normally are hidden within the TTR molecule.[81]

D. Atrial Natriuretic Factor [ANF] and Isolated Atrial Amyloid [IAA]

Although early studies suggested that cardiac amyloidosis present in very aged patients (usually over 70 years of age) is a single disease entity, histochemical and immunohistochemical studies subsequently clearly showed that the hearts of aged individuals are the target of two entirely different but sometimes concurrent forms of amyloid.[82] IAA deposits, shown by amino acid sequence analysis to be derived from atrial natriuretic factor (ANF),[83,84] are restricted to the atria of the heart of aged patients. SSA deposits, derived from TTR, may be present both in the atrial and ventricular myocardium and also in other organs.[82] A study involving 72 persons over 70 years of age is illustrative of the comparative frequency of these two forms of cardiac amyloidosis which are linked to advanced age.[82] There were 47 of 72 patients (65%) who were shown to have amyloid deposits in the heart, and 39 of these 47 cardiac amyloid patients (83%) had deposits of only the IAA type; of the 8 remaining patients with cardiac amyloidosis, 3 had only the SSA type and 5 had both the IAA and SSA types of amyloidosis. The extremely common occurrence of IAA in persons of advanced age is further emphasized by a study showing that 78% of individuals 80 years of age or older had IAA deposits.[85]

In humans, ANF is a 28-amino-acid polypeptide hormone that is derived from the C-terminus of a 151-amino-acid preprohormone. ANF, which is stored in the endocrine granules present in atrial myocytes, has potent diuretic and natriuretic effects when released into the circulation (reviewed in Reference 86). The release of ANF is modulated by several factors, including the stretching of the atrial wall. Increased levels of ANF in the heart and plasma are seen in patients with heart disease, especially congestive heart failure.[87]

Immunohistochemical and immunoelectron microscopic studies in patients with IAA have shown that antisera to normal human ANF and to purified IAA protein label amyloid fibrils and ANF-containing granules in myocytes in a similar and specific fashion.[88,89] The ANF immunoreactive amyloid fibrils were distributed predominantly extracellulary in close association with the cell membranes of myocytes, although small amyloid deposits sometimes also appeared to be present intracellulary in muscle cells.[89] In the same study, it was shown that amyloid-like fibrils could be produced *in vitro* from normal human ANF. The specific mechanisms involved in the fibrillogenesis of ANF are not known, but the abnormally high atrial concentrations of ANF that have been shown to be present in patients with cardiac insufficiency are consistent with the high incidence of IAA in this state.[90] There is also an increased occurrence of IAA in other forms of heart disease.[91] However, there are only a few reports which document a correlation between IAA and clinical heart disease, and both the significance and pathogenesis of IAA are thus incompletely understood (for review, see Reference 92).

E. Miscellaneous Age-Related Amyloid Forms

There are several other amyloid forms that are commonly associated with aging. Among these are amyloid in the aorta,[93] seminal vesicles,[4] the pituitary gland,[5] and the intracellular, neurofibrillary tangle-like inclusions in the choroid plexus epithelial cells[96] and adrenal cortex.[97] All these forms are very common in old individuals and, in fact, the aorta and choroid plexus epithelial cells always contain some amyloid. However, the nature of the amyloid protein is not known for any of these forms of amyloidosis.

IV. FINAL REMARKS

It is clear from the discussions above that, although a significant amount of new information has been obtained over the past decade regarding amyloidosis, there are still many unknown factors that link the occurrence of several important forms of amyloidosis with aging. In all of the three more well-known age-related forms of amyloidosis (IAPP-derived islet amyloidosis, Aβ-derived cerebral amyloidosis, and TTR-derived senile systemic amyloidosis (SSA)), amyloid deposits are most commonly formed from a normal amyloid-protein precursor. Although specific mutations in βPP and TTR are not enough to cause disease (i.e., symptom-free carriers with amyloidogenic βPP and TTR variants have been identified), in both Aβ-derived and TTR-derived amyloidosis, mutations in the respective precursor proteins are associated with more pronounced formation of amyloid at a comparatively younger age. This suggests that the respective mutations primarily exaggerate a process that takes place in many (or most) individuals as they reach more advanced age, and that mechanisms normally exist which prevent formation of amyloid fibrils from those proteins which contain strongly amyloidogenic segments (e.g., IAPP, TTR, and βPP). Similar evidence for an association with mutations of the precursor protein has not been found in IAPP-derived islet amyloidosis, but we can not rule out the possibility that mutations in (pro)IAPP could be linked to early development of islet amyloidosis and diabetes. Further elucidation of the relationship between mutant amyloid fibril proteins and the process of amyloidogenesis on the one hand, and the relationship of amyloid deposits per se to the clinical disease on the other, will undoubtedly provide important new information and a better understanding of these different and common age-related diseases.

ACKNOWLEDGMENTS

The work from our own laboratories which has been included in this review was supported by the Swedish Medical Research Council (Project #5941), The Nordic Insulin Fund, the Swedish Diabetes Association, the National Institute of Diabetes and Digestive and Kidney Disease (grant #RO1 DK36734) and the Taylor Foundation.

REFERENCES

1. Glenner, G. G., Amyloid deposits and amyloidosis. The β-fibrilloses, *N. Engl. J. Med.*, 302, 1283 & 1333, 1980.
2. Cohen, A. S., Amyloidosis, *N. Engl. J. Med.*, 277, 522 & 628, 1967.
3. Schwartz, P., Amyloidosis, cause and manifestation of senile deterioration, Charles C. Thomas, Springfield, IL, 1970.
4. Wright, J. R., Calkins, E., Breen, W. J., Stolte, G., and Schultz, R. T., Relationship of amyloid to aging: review of the literature and systematic study of 83 patients derived from a general hospital population, *Medicine*, 48, 39, 1969.
5. Malle, E., Steinmetz, A., and Raynes, J. G., Serum amyloid A (SAA): an acute phase protein and apolipoprotein, *Atherosclerosis*, 102, 131, 1993.
6. Weinstein, P. S., Skinner, M., Sipe, J. D., Lokich, J. J., Zamcheck, N., and Cohen, A. S., Acute-phase proteins or tumour markers. The role of SAA, SAP, CRP and CEA as indicators of metastasis in a broad spectrum of neoplastic diseases, *Scand. J. Immunol.*, 19, 193, 1984.
7. Baba, S., Takahashi, T., Kasama, T., Fujie, M., and Shirasawa, H., A novel polymorphism of human serum amyloid A protein, SAA1γ, is characterized by alanines at both residues 52 and 57, *Arch. Biochem. Biophys.*, 303, 361, 1993.
8. Turnell, W., Sarra, R., Glover, I. D., Baum, J. O., Caspi, D., Baltz, M. L., and Pepys, M. B., Secondary structure prediction of human SAA₁. Presumptive identification of calcium and lipid binding sites, *Mol. Biol. Med.*, 3, 387, 1986.
9. Westermark, G. T., Engström, U., and Westermark, P., The N-terminal segment of protein AA determines its fibrillogenic property, *Biochem. Biophys. Res. Commun.*, 182, 27, 1992.
10. Kyle, R. A. and Bayrd, E. D., Amyloidosis: review of 236 cases, *Medicine*, 54, 271, 1975.
11. Cohen, A. S., Amyloidosis, in *Arthritis and Allied Conditions: A Textbook of Rheumatology*, 12th ed., McCarty, D. J. and Koopman, W. J., Eds., Lea & Febiger, Philadelphia, PA, 1993, 1427.
12. Solomon, A., Frangione, B., and Franklin, E. C., Bence Jones proteins and light chains of immunoglobulins. Preferential association of the V_{VI} subgroup of human light chains with amyloidosis AL(λ), *J. Clin. Invest.*, 70, 453, 1982.
13. Isobe, T. and Osserman, E. F., Patterns of amyloidosis and their association with plasma-cell dyscrasia, monoclonal immunoglobulins and Bence-Jones proteins, *N. Engl. J. Med.*, 290, 473, 1974.
14. Westermark, P., Quantitative studies of amyloid in the islets of Langerhans, *Upsala J. Med. Sci.*, 77, 91, 1972.
15. Johnson, K. H. and Stevens, J. B., Light and electron microscopic studies of islet amyloid in diabetic cats, *Diabetes*, 22, 81, 1973.
16. Westermark, P. and Wilander, E., The influence of amyloid deposits on the islet volume in maturity onset diabetes mellitus, *Diabetologia*, 15, 417, 1978.
17. Westermark, P. and Grimelius, L., The pancreatic islet cells in insular amyloidosis in human diabetic and non-diabetic adults, *Acta Pathol. Microbiol. Scand. A*, 81, 291, 1973.
18. Clark, A., Wells, C. A., Buley, I. D., Cruickshank, J. K., Vanhegan, R. I., Matthews, D. R., Cooper, G. J. S., Holman, R. R., and Turner, R. C., Islet amyloid, increased A-cells, reduced B-cells and exocrine fibrosis: quantitative changes in the pancreas in type 2 diabetes, *Diab. Res.*, 9, 151, 1988.
19. Westermark, P., Wernstedt, C., Wilander, E., and Sletten, K., A novel peptide in the calcitonin gene related peptide family as an amyloid fibril protein in the endocrine pancreas, *Biochem. Biophys. Res. Commun.*, 140, 827, 1986.

20. Westermark, P., Wernstedt, C., Wilander, E., Hayden, D. W., O'Brien, T. D., and Johnson, K. H., Amyloid fibrils in human insulinoma and islets of Langerhans of the diabetic cat are derived from a neuropeptide-like protein also present in normal islet cells, *Proc. Natl. Acad. Sci. U.S.A.*, 84, 3881, 1987.

21. Westermark, P., Wernstedt, C., O'Brien, T. D., Hayden, D. W., and Johnson, K. H., Islet amyloid in type 2 human diabetes mellitus and adult diabetic cats contains a novel putative polypeptide hormone, *Am. J. Pathol.*, 127, 414, 1987.

22. Cooper, G. J., Willis, A. C., Clark, A., Turner, A. C., Sim, R. B., and Reid, K. B. M., Purification and characterization of a peptide from amyloid-rich pancreases of type 2 diabetic patients, *Proc. Natl. Acad. Sci. U.S.A.*, 84, 8628, 1987.

23. Clark, A., Islet amyloid — an enigma of type-2 diabetes, *Diab. Metabol. Rev.*, 8, 117, 1992.

24. Johnson, K. H., O'Brien, T. D., Betsholtz, C., and Westermark, P., Islet amyloid polypeptide: mechanisms of amyloidogenesis in the pancreatic islets and potential roles in diabetes mellitus, *Lab. Invest.*, 66, 522, 1992.

25. Westermark, P., Johnson, K. H., O'Brien, T. D., and Betsholtz, C., Islet amyloid polypeptide — a novel controversy in diabetes research, *Diabetologia*, 35, 297, 1992.

26. Johnson, K. H., O'Brien, T. D., Hayden, D. W., Jordan, K., Ghobrial, H. K. G., Mahoney, W. C., and Westermark, P., Immunolocalization of islet amyloid polypeptide (IAPP) in pancreatic beta cells by means of peroxidase-antiperoxidase (PAP) and protein A-gold techniques, *Am. J. Pathol.*, 130, 1, 1988.

27. Lukinius, A., Wilander, E., Westermark, G. T., Engström, U., and Westermark, P., Colocalization of islet amyloid polypeptide and insulin in the B cell secretory granules of the human pancreatic islets, *Diabetologia*, 32, 240, 1989.

28. Young, A. A., Crocker, L. B., Wolfelopez, D., and Cooper, G. J. S., Daily amylin replacement reverses hepatic glycogen depletion in insulin-treated streptozotocin diabetic rats, *FEBS Lett.*, 287, 203, 1991.

29. Westermark, P., Engström, U., Johnson, K. H., Westermark, G. T., and Betsholtz, C., Islet amyloid polypeptide: pinpointing amino acid residues linked to amyloid fibril formation, *Proc. Natl. Acad. Sci. U.S.A.*, 87, 5036, 1990.

30. Betsholtz, C., Christmanson, L., Engström, U., Rorsman, F., Svensson, V., Johnson, K. H., and Westermark, P., Sequence divergence in a specific region of islet amyloid polypeptide (IAPP) explains differences in islet amyloid formation between species, *FEBS Lett.*, 251, 261, 1989.

31. Nishi, M., Chan, S. J., Nagamatsu, S., Bell, G. I., and Steiner, D. F., Conservation of the sequence of islet amyloid polypeptide in five mammals is consistent with its putative role as an islet hormone, *Proc. Natl. Acad. Sci. U.S.A.*, 86, 5738, 1989.

32. Betsholtz, C., Christmanson, L., Engström, U., Rorsman, F., Jordan, K., O'Brien, T. D., Murtaugh, M., Johnson, K. H., and Westermark, P., Structure of cat islet amyloid polypeptide and identification of amino acid residues of potential significance for islet amyloid formation, *Diabetes*, 39, 118, 1990.

33. Ashburn, T. T. and Lansbury, P. T., Interspecies sequence variations affect the kinetics and thermodynamics of amyloid formation: peptide models of pancreatic amyloid, *J. Am. Chem. Soc.*, 115, 11012, 1993.

34. Johnson, K. H., O'Brien, T. D., Jordan, K., and Westermark, P., Impaired glucose tolerance is associated with increased islet amyloid polypeptide (IAPP) immunoreactivity in pancreatic beta cells, *Am. J. Pathol.*, 135, 245, 1989.

35. Westermark, G. T., Christmanson, L., Terenghi, G., Permert, J., Betsholtz, C., Larsson, J., Polak, J. M., and Westermark, P., Islet amyloid polypeptide: demonstration of mRNA in human pancreatic islets by in situ hybridization in islets with and without amyloid deposits, *Diabetologia*, 36, 323, 1993.

36. Yankner, B. A. and Mesulam, M.-M., β-Amyloid and the pathogenesis of Alzheimer's disease, *N. Engl. J. Med.*, 325, 1849, 1991.
37. Anderton, B. H., Expression and processing of pathologic proteins in Alzheimer's disease, *Hippocampus*, 3, 227, 1991.
38. Mullan, M. and Crawford, F., Genetic and molecular advances in Alzheimer's disease, *Trends Neurosci.*, 16, 398, 1993.
39. Selkoe, D. J., Physiological production of the β-amyloid and the mechanism of Alzheimer's disease, *Trends Neurosci.*, 16, 403, 1993.
40. Wischik, C. M., Crowter, R. A., Stewart, M., and Roth, M., Subunit structure of paired helical filaments in Alzheimer's disease, *J. Cell Biol.*, 100, 1905, 1985.
41. Wisniewski, H. M., Merz, P. A., and Iqbal, K. I., Ultrastructure of paired helical filaments of Alzheimer's neurofibrillary tangle, *J. Neuropathol. Exp. Neurol.*, 43, 643, 1984.
42. Glenner, G. G. and Wong, C. W., Alzheimer's disease: initial report of the purification and characterization of a novel cerebrovascular amyloid protein, *Biochem. Biophys. Res. Commun.*, 120, 885, 1984.
43. Masters, C., Simms, G., Weinman, N. A., Multhaup, G., McDonald, B. L., and Beyreuther, K., Amyloid plaque core protein in Alzheimer disease and Down syndrome, *Proc. Natl. Acad. Sci. U.S.A.*, 82, 4245, 1985.
44. Wong, C. W., Quaranta, V., and Glenner, G. G., Neuritic plaques and cerebrovascular amyloid in Alzheimer disease are antigenically related, *Proc. Natl. Acad. Sci. U.S.A.*, 82, 8729, 1985.
45. Husby, G., Araki, S., Benditt, E. P., Benson, M. D., Cohen, A. S., Frangione, B., Glenner, G. G., Natvig, J. B., and Westermark, P., Nomenclature of amyloid and amyloidosis, *Bull. WHO*, 71, 105, 1993.
46. Fraser, P. E., Duffy, L. K., Omalley, M. B., Nguyen, J., Inouye, H., and Kirschner, D. A., Morphology and antibody recognition of synthetic beta-amyloid peptides, *J. Neurosci. Res.*, 28, 474, 1991.
47. Hilbich, C., Kisters-Woike, B., Reed, J., Masters, C. L., and Beyreuther, K., Aggregation and secondary structure of synthetic amyloid βA4 peptides of Alzheimer's disease, *J. Mol. Biol.*, 218, 149, 1991.
48. Jarrett, J. T., Berger, E. P., and Lansbury, P. T. J., The carboxy terminus of the β amyloid protein is critical for the seeding of amyloid formation: implications for the pathogenesis of Alzheimer's disease, *Biochemistry*, 32, 4693, 1993.
49. Haass, C., Schlossmacher, M. G., Hung, A. Y., Vigo-Pelfrey, C., Mellon, A., Ostaszewski, B. L., Lieberburg, I., Koo, E. H., Schenk, D., Teplow, D. and Selkoe, D. J., Amyloid beta-peptide is produced by cultured cells during normal metabolism, *Nature*, 359, 322, 1992.
50. Shoji, M., Golde, T. E., Ghiso, J., Cheung, T. T., Estus, S., Shaffer, L. M., Cai, X.-D., McKay, D. M., Tintner, R., Frangione, B., and Younkin, S. G., Production of the Alzheimer amyloid β protein by normal proteolytic processing, *Science*, 258, 126, 1992.
51. Golde, T. E., Estus, S., Younkin, L. H., Selkoe, D. J., and Younkin, S. G., Processing of the amyloid protein precursor to potentially amyloidogenic derivatives, *Science*, 255, 728, 1992.
52. Levy, E., Carman, M. D., Fernandez-Madrid, I. J., Power, M. D., Lieberburg, I., van Duinen, S. G., Bots, G. T. A. M., Luyendijk, W., and Frangione, B., Mutation of the Alzheimer's disease amyloid gene in hereditary cerebral hemorrhage, Dutch type, *Science*, 248, 1124, 1990.
53. Haan, J., Hardy, J. A., and Roos, R. A. C., Hereditary cerebral hemorrhage with amyloidosis — Dutch type: its importance for Alzheimer research, *Trends Neurosci.*, 14, 231, 1991.

54. Corder, E. H., Saunders, A. M., Strittmatter, W. J., Schmechel, D. E., Gaskell, P. C., Small, G. W., Roses, A. D., Haines, J. L., and Pericak-Vance, M. A., Gene dose of apolipoprotein E type 4 allele and the risk of Alzheimer's disease in late onset families, *Science*, 261, 921, 1993.

55. Strittmatter, W. J., Weisgraber, K. H., Huang, D. Y., Dong, L.-M., Salvesen, G. S., Pericak-Vance, M., Schmechel, D., Saunders, A. M., Goldgaber, D., and Roses, A. D., Binding of human apolipoprotein E to synthetic amyloid β peptide. Isoform-specific effects and implications for late-onset Alzheimer disease, *Proc. Natl. Acad. Sci. U.S.A.*, 90, 8098, 1993.

56. Wisniewski, T. and Frangione, B., Apolipoprotein E, a pathological chaperone protein in patients with cerebral and systemic amyloid, *Neurosci. Lett.*, 135, 235, 1992.

57. Kirschner, D. A., Abraham, C., and Selkoe, D. J., X-ray diffraction from intraneuronal paired helical filaments and extraneuronal amyloid fibers in Alzheimer disease indicates cross-β conformation, *Proc. Natl. Acad. Sci. U.S.A.*, 83, 503, 1986.

58. Trojanowski, J. Q. and Lee, V. M.-Y., Paired helical filament in Alzheimer's disease, *Am. J. Pathol.*, 144, 449, 1994.

59. Masters, C. L., Multhaup, G., Simms, G., Pottgiesser, J., Martins, R. N., and Beyreuther, K., Neuronal origin of a cerebral amyloid: neurofibrillary tangles of Alzheimer's disease contain the same protein as the amyloid of plaque cores and blood vessels, *EMBO J.*, 4, 2757, 1985.

60. Guiroy, D. C., Mellini, M., Miyazaki, M., Hilbich, C., Safar, J., Garruto, R. M., Yanagihara, R., Beyreuther, K., and Gajdusek, D. C., Neurofibrillary tangles of Guamanian amyotrophic lateral sclerosis, Parkinsonism-dementia and neurologically normal Guamanians contain a 4- to 4.5-kilodalton protein which is immunoreactive to anti-amyloid β/A4-protein antibodies, *Acta Neuropathol.*, 86, 265, 1993.

61. Perry, G., Cras, P., Siedlak, S. L., Tabaton, M., Kawai, M., β-protein immunoreactivity is found in the majority of neurofibrillary tangles of Alzheimer's disease, *Am. J. Pathol.*, 140, 283, 1992.

62. Terry, R. D., Mashliah, E., Salmon, D. P., Butters, N., DeTeresa, R., Hill, R., Hansen, L. A., and Katzman, R., Physical basis of cognitive alterations in Alzheimer's disease: synapse loss is the major correlate of cognitive impairment, *Ann. Neurol.*, 30, 572, 1991.

63. Crystal, H., Dickson, D., Fuld, P., Masur, D., Scott, R., Mehler, M., Masdeu, J., Kawas, C., Aronson, M., and Wolfson, L., Clinico-pathologic studies in dementia: nondemented subjects with pathologically confirmed Alzheimer's disease, *Neurology*, 38, 1682, 1988.

64. Crutcher, K. A., Anderton, B. H., Barger, S. W., Ohm, T. G., and Snow, A. D., Cellular and molecular pathology in Alzheimer's disease, *Hippocampus*, 3, 271, 1993.

65. Yankner, B. A., Dawes, L. R., Fisher, S., Villa-Komaroff, L., Oster-Granite, M. L., and Neve, R. L., Neurotoxicity of a fragment of the amyloid precursor associated with Alzheimer's disease, *Science*, 245, 417, 1989.

66. Yankner, B. A., Duffy, L. K., and Kirschner, D. A., Neurotrophic and neurotoxic effects of amyloid β protein: reversal by tachykinin neuropeptides, *Science*, 250, 279, 1990.

67. Arispe, N., Rojas, E., and Pollard, H. B., Alzheimer disease amyloid β protein forms calcium channels in bilayer membranes. Blockade by tromethamine and aluminum, *Proc. Natl. Acad. Sci. U.S.A.*, 90, 567, 1993.

68. Etcheberrigaray, R., Ito, E., Kim, C. S., and Alkon, D. L., Soluble β-amyloid induction of Alzheimer's phenotype for human fibroblast K+ channels, *Science*, 264, 276, 1994.

69. Pitkänen, P., Westermark, P., and Cornwell, G. G., III, Senile systemic amyloidosis, *Am. J. Pathol.*, 117, 391, 1984.

70. Johansson, B. and Westermark, P., Senile systemic amyloidosis: a clinicopathological study of twelve patients with massive amyloid infiltration, *Int. J. Cardiol.*, 32, 83, 1991.

71. Sasaki, H., Yoshioka, N., Takagi, Y., and Sakaki, Y., Structure of the chromosomal gene for human serum prealbumin, *Gene*, 37, 191, 1985.

72. Blake, C. C. F., Geisow, M. J., Oatley, S. J., Rérat, B., and Rérat, C., Structure of prealbumin: secondary, tertiary and quaternary interactions determined by Fourier refinement at 1.8 Å, *J. Mol. Biol.*, 121, 339, 1978.

73. Hesse, A., Altland, K., Linke, R. P., Almeida, M. R., Saraiva, M. J. M., Steinmetz, A., and Maisch, B., Cardiac amyloidosis: a review and report of a new transthyretin (prealbumin) variant, *Br. Heart J.*, 70, 111, 1993.

74. Alves, I. L., Almeida, M. R., Skare, J., Skinner, M., Kurose, K., Sakaki, Y., Costa, P. P., and Saraiva, M. J. M., Amyloidogenic and nonamyloidogenic transthyretin Asn 90 variants, *Clin. Genet.*, 42, 27, 1992.

75. Jacobson, D. R., Gorevic, P., and Buxbaum, J. N., A homozygous transthyretin variant associated with senile systemic amyloidosis: evidence for a late-onset disease of genetic etiology, *Am. J. Hum. Genet.*, 47, 127, 1990.

76. Nichols, W. C., Liepnieks, J. J., Snyder, E. L., and Benson, M. D., Senile cardiac amyloidosis associated with homozygosity for a transthyretin variant (Ile-122), *J. Lab. Clin. Med.*, 117, 175, 1991.

77. Westermark, P., Sletten, K., Johansson, B., and Cornwell, G. G., III, Fibril in senile systemic amyloidosis is derived from normal transthyretin, *Proc. Natl. Acad. Sci. U.S.A.*, 87, 2843, 1990.

78. Christmanson, L., Betsholtz, C., Gustavsson, Å., Johansson, B., Sletten, K., and Westermark, P., The transthyretin cDNA sequence is normal in transthyretin-derived senile systemic amyloidosis, *FEBS Lett.*, 281, 177, 1991.

79. Felding, P., Fex, G., Westermark, P., Olofsson, B.-O., Pitkänen, P., and Benson, L., Prealbumin in Swedish patients with senile systemic amyloidosis and familial amyloidotic polyneuropathy, *Scand. J. Immunol.*, 21, 133, 1985.

80. Nordlie, M., Sletten, K., Husby, G., and Ranløv, P. J., A new prealbumin variant in familial amyloid cardiomyopathy of Danish origin, *Scand. J. Immunol.*, 27, 119, 1988.

81. Gustavsson, Å., Engström, U., and Westermark, P., Normal transthyretin and synthetic transthyretin fragments form amyloid-like fibrils in vitro, *Biochem. Biophys. Res. Commun.*, 175, 1159, 1991.

82. Westermark, P., Johansson, B., and Natvig, J. B., Senile cardiac amyloidosis: evidence of two different amyloid substances in the aging heart, *Scand. J. Immunol.*, 10, 303, 1979.

83. Johansson, B., Wernstedt, C., and Westermark, P., Atrial natriuretic peptide deposited as atrial amyloid fibrils, *Biochem. Biophys. Res. Commun.*, 148, 1087, 1987.

84. Linke, R. P., Voigt, C., Störkel, F. S., and Eulitz, M., N-terminal amino acid sequence analysis indicates that isolated atrial amyloid is derived from atrial natriuretic peptide, *Virchows Arch. B*, 55, 125, 1988.

85. Cornwell, G. G. I., Murdoch, W. L., Kyle, R. A., Westermark, P., and Pitkänen, P., Frequency and distribution of senile cardiovascular amyloid, *Am. J. Med.*, 75, 618, 1983.

86. Rosenzweig, A. and Seidman, C. E., Atrial natriuretic factor and related peptide hormones, *Ann. Rev. Biochem.*, 60, 229, 1991.

87. Cody, R. J., Atlas, S. A., Laragh, J. H., Kubo, S. H., Covit, A. B., Ryman, K. S., Shaknovich, A., Pondolfino, K., Clark, M., Camargo, M. J. F., Scarborough, R. M., and Lewicki, J. A., Atrial natriuretic factor in normal subjects and heart failure patients. Plasma levels and renal, hormonal, and hemodynamic responses to peptide infusion, *J. Clin. Invest.*, 78, 1362, 1986.

88. Kaye, G. C., Butler, M. G., D'Ardenne, A. J., Edmondson, S. J., Camm, A. J., and Slavin, G., Isolated atrial amyloid contains atrial natriuretic peptide: a report of six cases, *Br. Heart J.*, 56, 317, 1986.

89. Johansson, B. and Westermark, P., The relation of atrial natriuretic factor to isolated atrial amyloid, *Exp. Mol. Pathol.*, 52, 266, 1990.

90. Johansson, B. and Westermark, P., in *Amyloid and Amyloidosis 1990*, Natvig, J. B., Førre, Ø., Husby, G., Husebekk, A., Skogen, B., Sletten, K., and Westermark, P., Eds., Kluwer, Dordrecht, 1991, 474.

91. Looi, L.-M., Isolated atrial amyloidosis. A clinicopathologic study indicating increased prevalence in chronic heart disease, *Hum. Pathol.*, 24, 602, 1993.

92. Westermark, P., Amyloid and polypeptide hormones: what is their interrelationship?, *Amyloid*, 1, 47, 1994.

93. Mucchiano, G., Cornwell, G. G. I., and Westermark, P., Senile aortic amyloid. Evidence of two distinct forms of localized deposits, *Am. J. Pathol.*, 140, 871, 1992.

94. Pitkänen, P., Westermark, P., Cornwell, G. G., III., and Murdoch, W., Amyloid of the seminal vesicles. A distinctive and common localized form of senile amyloidosis, *Am. J. Pathol.*, 110, 64, 1983.

95. Tashima, T., Kitamoto, T., Tateishi, J., Ogomori, K., and Nakagaki, H., Incidence and characterization of age-related amyloid deposits in the human anterior pituitary gland, *Virchows Arch. A*, 412, 323, 1988.

96. Eriksson, L. and Westermark, P., Intracellular neurofibrillary tangle-like aggregations. A constantly present amyloid alteration in the aging choroid plexus, *Am. J. Pathol.*, 125, 124, 1986.

97. Eriksson, L. and Westermark, P., Age-related accumulation of amyloid inclusions in adrenal cortical cells, *Am. J. Pathol.*, 136, 461, 1990.

Chapter **15**

EXTRACELLULAR MATRIX

L. Robert and J. Labat-Robert

CONTENTS

0-8493-4786-6/95/$0.00+$.50
© 1995 by CRC Press, Inc.

I. INTRODUCTION

Mammalian tissues are composed of cells and a more or less abundant extracellular matrix (ECM). Tissues particularly rich in ECM are designated as connective tissues (CT). There is, however, only a quantitative difference between CTs and other tissues. It was classically assumed that the only physiological role which can be ascribed to CTs is a mechanical one — to confer resistance, resilience, or elasticity to tissues exposed to a variety of mechanical stresses during life. This is particularly the case for the osteoarticular system, which is exposed during a lifetime to repeated and often violent mechanical stresses. It is no wonder that such repeated stresses progressively damage the tissues, resulting in pain, functional lesions, and finally in clinically recognizable and, most importantly, age-related diseases. In Table 1 we have listed some of the most important age-related diseases which directly or indirectly concern CTs.

This mechanistic view on CT-aging was largely refined during the last decades as a result of the explosive increase of our knowledge of ECMs.[1] The number of macromolecular constituents which were recognized increased rapidly, as shown in Table 2. From just three types of constituents recognized in the middle of this century — collagen, elastin, and acid mucopolysaccharides — we now have actually close to a hundred different macromolecules composing the ECM of vertebrate organisms. If we add the phylogenetically "older" forms of ECM macromolecules, for instance those of invertebrates, we end up with approximately several hundred different components. Since the early 1960s a fourth type of component was added to the above-mentioned three major components: structural glycoproteins (SGP). This nomenclature was proposed in order to distinguish tissue glycoproteins, apparently playing a "structural role", from circulating blood-borne glycoproteins.[2] Although fibronectin, the best-characterized component of this family, is present both in tissues and in blood, the above distinction between "structural" and circulating blood-borne glycoproteins still seems justified.

Meanwhile, "acid mucopolysaccharides" became proteoglycans (PG)[3,4] and the collagen family exploded into many subtypes as shown in Table 2.[5]

A final complication came recently with the recognition that alternative splicing of the primary transcripts of the genes of several ECM

TABLE 1.

Some of the Age-Related Diseases Concerning Connective Tissues

Disease	Relationship to Alteration of the Extracellular Matrix
Arteriosclerosis	Hardening of elastic arteries due to increase of collagen/elastin ratio, deposition of calcium and lipids in ECM components, essentially in elastin.
Osteoarthritis	Alteration of articular cartilage, degradation of proteoglycans, increase of fibronectin replacement by fibrous tissue and bone erosion.
Osteoporosis	Progressive loss of the mineralizable bone-matrix, composed of collagen type I and associated glycoconjugates.
Diabetes type II	Micro-angiopathy due to altered rates of synthesis (and degradation) of basement membrane components (increase in collagen IV, laminin, fibronectin, decrease in heparan sulfate-proteoglycan) Accelerated arteriosclerosis.

macromolecules produces a variety of isoforms, as was first shown for fibronectin and recently for some collagens and elastin.

It will appear evident from this introduction that it is beyond the scope of a chapter on CT-aging to propose an exhaustive description of all the varieties of ECM macromolecules. This short chapter, however, is devoted to a succinct description of some of the major characteristics of these four families of matrix components, essentially as related to their age-dependent modifications.

CTs are composed of cells and ECM macromolecules. In order to understand aging of the ECM one has to take into consideration the following three aspects of the problem:

1. Age-related modifications of the *biosynthesis* of ECM components.
2. *Postsynthetic* modifications of ECM macromolecules.
3. Modifications with age of *cell-matrix interactions*.

The first topic also concerns cell aging, which is adequately covered in other chapters of this book and will not be considered here in detail. The second topic is an important one since it was the first discovered by Verzar[53] in the middle of this century and has turned out to be of great importance for the aging process. Finally, the third topic, the most recent one, has to be considered in detail because it might well turn out to be one of the main components of the integrative mechanisms of cellular and molecular aging processes in the whole organism, and directly involved in information transfer between ECM and cells. This third topic was only recently recognized to be of general importance as a result of two main lines of research. The first was the recognition of the importance of cell-matrix interactions mediated by special classes of cell-membrane recep-

TABLE 2.

Macromolecular Components of Extracellular Matrix and Some of
Their Characteristics[a]

I. Collagens	There are at least 18 different types known in vertebrates, several more in invertebrates. The fibrous collagens, type I, II, and III confer mechanical resistance to tissues, type IV is the major component of basement membranes.
II. Elastin	Great micro heterogeneity due to alternative splicing of the primary transcript of a single gene at 8 exons. Its hydrophobicity is important for elasticity but predisposes elastin to interaction with lipids and Ca^{2+}. Degradation products present in circulating blood. Lends elasticity to vascular, pulmonary tissues, and skin, progressively lost with age.
III. Proteoglycans	Variable number of glycosaminoglycan chains linked covalenty to a variety of proteins (from one GAG chain in decorin to several hundred in syndecan). Hyaluronan is a very high mol wt GAG with no protein. They control fibrillogenesis, molecular traffic, ion balance, and hydration. Associated with cell membranes, fibers, and filling interstitial spaces.
IV. Structural glycoproteins	Mostly cell membrane-associated components, with recognition sites for cell membrane receptors. Key role in cell-matrix interactions. Modular structure, enabling them to interact with a variety of matrix components — fibronectin, laminins, nidogen, thrombospondin and several others were characterized in a variety of tissues.

[a] For more details see References.

tors. The second is the very recent recognition of the age-dependent modifications of these coupling mechanisms, directly affecting information transfer between cells and ECM. These three topics will therefore be considered in some detail.

II. MACROMOLECULAR COMPOSITION OF EXTRACELLULAR MATRIX

As shown on Table 2, the great variety of macromolecules identified in ECMs can be subdivided into four major classes or families: collagens and elastins forming the fibrous elements and proteoglycans and structural glycoproteins filling the gaps and mediating cell-matrix interactions. We should add a fifth family of components: the cell-membrane receptors, which will be mentioned shortly in the section devoted to cell-matrix interactions. The boundary between these four families is not as sharp as it will appear from this brief description.

A. Collagens

Known since antiquity, collagens have been the source of the first industries of mankind — leather, glue, and bone objects — and detailed knowledge on the molecular level dates from the mid-1960s. One major breakthrough was the recognition of the existence of a second isoform of collagen in cartilage — collagen type II.

Type I collagen, making up close to 30% of the proteins of vertebrates and type III, intermingled with type I in mixed fibers and type II in cartilage, form the bulk of the so-called fibrous, interstitial collagens. Known age-dependent changes essentially concern these subtypes and to a lesser extent type IV collagen, the major component of basement membranes. For the other types of collagens, please refer to the literature cited in the references. Although they are sometimes referred to as "minor" collagens, they are ubiquitous components of all ECMs and probably fulfill important functions still largely unexplored. A great deal is known about their structure and molecular properties. Their genes have been mostly sequenced but as far as their age-dependent modifications are concerned they remain largely unexplored.

B. Elastin

It would be more correct to speak plurally about elastins because of the recently recognized demonstration concerning the alternative splicing of eight exons of the human elastin gene.[6] This could result in a large number of variants, several of which can be easily separated by PAGE-immunoblots. The physiological significance of this potentially important microheterogeneity is not yet explored. The amino acid composition of elastin revealed a preponderance of aliphatic amino acids with about one third of glycine. Its secondary and tertiary structures together with this peculiar amino acid composition explain most of its physicochemical properties: strong hydrophobic interactions, entropic type of elasticity, exceptional resistance to physical, chemical, and enzymatic aggressions, but strong affinity for lipids and calcium. Elastin withstands boiling in 0.1 N NaOH, a procedure currently used for its purification.[7,8] It can however be rapidly "solubilized" by alkaline hydrolysis in aqueous-organic solvents.[9] The conformation of the β turns and β-pleated sheets with its molecular dimensions confers a strong affinity for calcium ions.[10] On its turn, the presence of calcium strongly increases the affinity of elastin for lipids as shown by its uptake of ^{14}C-cholesterol.[11] This potentiation of the affinity of elastin for lipids and calcium is retained by large peptides obtained by organo-alkaline hydrolysis (K-elastin). Several other physiologically important properties of elastin will be mentioned in later sections. For an extensive coverage of the literature see Reference 8.

C. Proteoglycans

These macromolecules were first characterized by the composition of their polysaccharide chains, named glycosaminoglycans (GAG).[3,4] Several types of GAGs were described since the early work of K. Meyer and A. Dorfman and many others in the 1950s and 1960s.[3] A major change in the conceptions concerning PGs occurred when Haskal and Sajdera at the Rockefeller Institute isolated by mild procedures PG aggregates and monomers from cartilage, revealing the complex nature of these large macromolecules recently designated as *syndecan*. During the last decade or so, it became clear that several distinct proteins can form the backbone of PGs. Ruoslahti's main contribution was to identify the amino acid sequence of these backbone proteins which command the fixation of many of the GAG-chains: Ser-Gly-X or threo for at least some of the PGs.[12] Several of the genes coding for these proteins were cloned and sequenced (for a review see Reference 1).

It became clear also that the large PG of cartilage, syndecan, represents an extreme case, with several hundred GAG-chains on a single protein. Other PGs, for instance *decorin*, were shown to bear only one single GAG-chain.[13,14] All intermediary situations were described. The designation of PGs shifted from the emphasis on GAG-chains (chondroitin 4- and 6-sulfate, heparan sulfate, dermatan sulfate, keratan sulfate)[14,15] to specific and sometimes fanciful names given according to the protein portions of PGs.[4] Two of the macromolecules of this class deserve a special mention. One is hyaluronan,[16] the other is heparin. Hyaluronan has no known protein component and is much larger than all other known GAGs. It is a polymer of $\geq 10^6$ mol. wt. of a disaccharide "monomer" of N-acetylglucosamine and glucuronic acid and is devoid of sulfate. It is synthesized by a special enzyme: hyaluronan synthetase, localized at the cell membrane.[16] It can retain a very large amount of water, occurs in several conformations,[17] and largely controls the pericellular molecular traffic. It also appears to be involved in the control of cell movements and cell proliferation, as will be discussed later.

Heparin has a similar structure to heparan sulfate chains of a special class of PGs (HSPGs) present on cell membranes and also in the ECM. This is probably the most heterogeneous GAG component, consisting of alternative disaccharide "subunits" composed of N-acetyl- and N-sulfated glucosamine and D-glucuronic and L-iduronic acids, this last one can also be sulfated. The membrane-bound forms of heparan sulfate PGs were shown to be involved in the retention of growth factors and in the regulation of their action on cell proliferation as involved in atherogenesis.[18,19]

More details on their structure and biological functions can be found in the cited references. Their age-dependent modifications will be described later.

D. Structural Glycoproteins

These compounds, also called matrix glycoproteins, belong to a class of high-molecular-weight proteins made of modules, blocks of amino acids structurally, and functionally autonomous mosaic proteins. They are elaborated by mesenchymal cells in tissues, although isoforms of some of them can be found in the circulating blood also. Some of these isoforms are synthesized in the liver. They fulfill an essential role by mediating cell-matrix interactions.This mediation is the result of their multimodular structure, consisting of distinct domains as shown on Figure 1 for fibronectin (FN). Some of these domains recognize cell membrane receptors, many of them being integrins, by some specific sequences as shown by Ruoslahti's work on the importance of the R-G-D sequence (arginine-glycine-aspartic acid) for some of them.[12] Several other sequences have since been described, for instance the V-G-V-A-P-G sequence (valine-glycine-valine-proline-glycine) for the elastin-laminin receptor.[23,24] Other domains recognize ECM macromolecules present on collagens, proteoglycans, or on elastin. They also play important "structural" roles in specialized ECM constructions as for instance basement membranes. Some of these glycoproteins exhibit age-dependent modifications which will be described in a later section. More details about this important class of ECM macromolecules can be found in the cited references.

III. AGE-DEPENDENT MODIFICATIONS OF EXTRACELLULAR MATRIX

For the purposes of this chapter, it is important to distinguish modifications of the matrix which result from (1) changes with age of gene regulation and posttranscriptional changes in the biosynthetic mechanisms of matrix components, and (2) those modifications which concern postsynthetic macromolecules and do not directly concern the regulations of their biosynthesis. These two types of age-dependent changes were sometimes confused, as shown by the evolution of the concept of "molecular aging" which started with the discovery by Gershon of modified, inactive enzymes in aging organisms, and continued with Orgel's error catastrophe theory, and ended with the convincing demonstration of postsynthetic modifications in all well-investigated cases.[25,26] They are presumably the result of the slowdown with age of the turnover of many

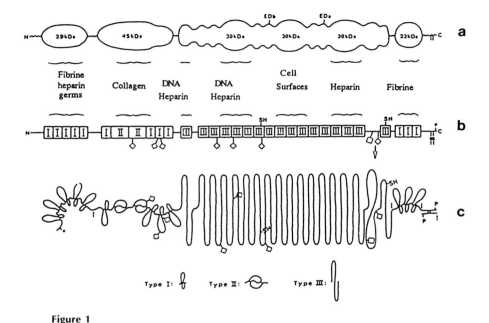

Figure 1
Homology domain structure of fibronectin shown in three different schematic models (a, b, c). Each of the three types of homologies is indicated by Roman numeral (I, II, and III) or by symbols (shown in the lower line). There are a total of 12 type I homology units, 2 type II units, and 17 type III homology units in the longest variant of fibronectin. Fragments, which can be obtained by enzymatic proteolysis, are indicated by their size and binding abilities. EDa and EDb are the "extra" type III domains present in some cellular fibronectins. V is the third alternatively spliced region. Arrows indicate plasmin split sites. (SH) Free sulfhydryl group (cysteine); (*) transglutaminase site; ($\diamond$) glucosamine-based oligosaccharide; ($\diamond$) galactosamine-based oligosaccharide; (P) phosphate group. The suggested antiparallel interchain disulfide bridge pattern in the C-terminus is indicated in the lower model; the other half of the dimer would go off the figure toward the right. (From Hynes, R. O., *Fibronectins,* Springer-Verlag, New York, 1990. With permission.)

cell and tissue constituents due to a decreased rate of biosynthesis and/or degradation.

A. Modifications of the Relative Rates of Synthesis of ECM Macromolecules During Aging

Several experimental models are used to explore the modifications of the biosynthetic processes during chronological aging — in animal experiments or on humans by the use of biopsies and explant culture techniques or, alternatively, and much more frequently, the Hayflick model[27,28] by determining in sequential cultures the modifications of biosynthesis of selected macromolecules. In several cases such experiments did address the transcriptional and translational levels. As many of the ECM macro-molecules on the genomic level are known (genes sequenced) and specific antibodies are also available, their biosynthesis could be studied at both these levels of regulation. We shall cite here some examples of studies conducted with this methodology in our laboratory over the last decades. The most convincing experiments concern both the cellular level (with the Hayflick model) and the *in vivo* or *ex vivo* situation. Results obtained using only the *in vitro* system have still to be confirmed *in vivo* because of the very different environmental situation and the absence of most intercellu-lar and intertissular regulatory influences in the *in vitro* system. Such combined experiments, using serial cell cultures as well as *in vivo* and *ex vivo* experiments, were carried out in our laboratory on the age-dependent modifications of the biosynthesis of collagens type I and III and fibronectin. We also shall mention similar experiments carried out on some catabolic enzymes as elastase-type endopeptidases.

1. Age-Dependent Modifications of the Rate of Biosynthesis of Interstitial Collagens and Fibronectin

These experiments were performed on serial cultures of human skin fibroblasts, on Werner-fibroblasts in collaboration with the team of Sam Goldstein, and on mice and rats of increasing age. Human skin and conjunctival biopsies were also used.[28,29,29a] As shown on Figure 2a the rate of total collagen synthesis decreases with age, but the relative rate of biosynthesis of collagen type III increases with age (Figure 2b). These results, obtained *ex vivo*, could be confirmed also in cell culture experi-ments and on human biopsy material concerning collagen type III in-crease.[30] Estimation of total collagen on human skin biopsy samples also showed a steady decrease of the hydroxyproline content per square mil-limeter of skin.[31] Total skin volume (expressed as skin thickness measured on histological sections of biopsies) also decreased with age.[32] Although the individual variations are very important, the average decrease was of the order of 6% per decade.

Fibronectin biosynthesis, however, was shown to increase with chro-nological age in blood plasma and skin[22] and also in serial cell cultures[29] (Figure 3a,b). The increased rate of synthesis of collagen III and fibronectin could be confirmed both at the transcriptional and translational levels. The comparison of Werner skin fibroblasts and *in vitro* aged (phase III) fibro-blasts, however, revealed a different mechanism for the regulation of gene expression in these two situations. The increased expression of the fibronectin gene in Werner fibroblasts was serum dependent, as it was in normal phase III fibroblasts, but much less.[29] It appears, therefore, that more than one mechanism may be involved at the level of gene regulation in the increased biosynthesis of fibronectin.

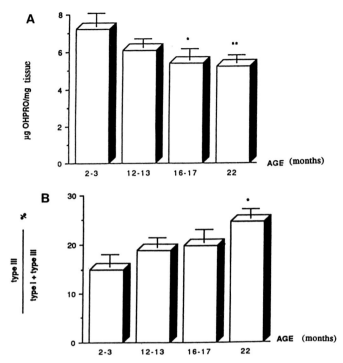

Figure 2
Modification of collagen content and of the ratio of collagen type III/I + III ratio as a function of age in mouse and human skin. (A) Decrease of total collagen content in mouse skin as a function of age (months) on a fresh weight basis; abscissa: age in months; ordinates: collagen content expressed as µg hydroxyproline per mg of fresh wt. (B) Increase in the proportion of collagen type III in mouse skin with age (months); abscissa as in (a); ordinates: type III to I + III ratio; significance:* $p < 0.05$;** $p < 0.01$. (From Boyer, B., Kern, P., Fourtanier, A. and Labat-Robert, J., *Exp. Gerontol.*, 26, 375, 1991. With permission.)

Using skin biopsies from normal and diabetic patients the increase of fibronectin could be confirmed at the tissue level (Figure 4a,b). This could also be shown in a Werner skin biopsy (Figure 4c). As diabetes and Werner syndrome are diseases considered to imitate some aspects of accelerated or premature aging, the above results can be considered as *in vivo* confirmations of the *in vitro* results.

Another condition related to accelerated aging is "photoaging". Mice skin samples from animals exposed to chronic UV radiation (both UVA and UVB) also exhibited an increased fibronectin biosynthesis (Figure 5). Interestingly, *in vivo* and *in vitro* treatment with heparin fragments (preparation designated CY 222 of Choay Laboratories[33]) effectively down-regulated both increased biosynthesis and message levels for fibronectin, and collagen type III. It appears, therefore, that this short-chain glycosami-

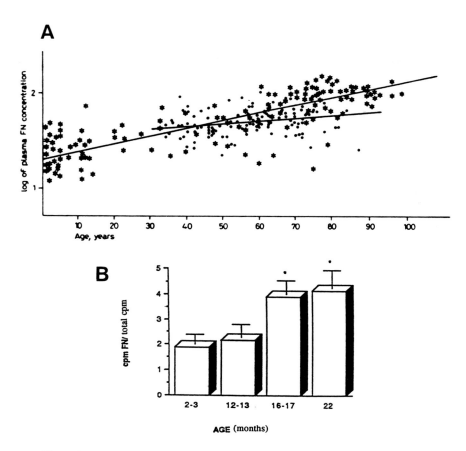

Figure 3
(A) Increase of plasma fibronectin in human plasma as a function of age. Abscissa: age in years; ordinates: log fibronectin concentration; (*) clinically healthy females; (●) breast cancer patients. (From Potarman, J. P., Le Dounal, V., Pouillard, J., Jollies, L., Labat-Robert, J., *Clin. Physiol. Biochem.*, 6, 12, 1988. With permission.) (B) Increase with age of fibronectin in mouse skin. Abscissa: age in months; ordinates: incorporation of ^{35}S-methionine in immunoprecipitable fibronectin by skin fibroblasts in explant cultures as a percentage of total incorporation. (*) Significance $p < 0.05$ to youngest value. (From Boyer, B., Kern, P., Fourtanier, A., and Labat-Robert, J., *Exp. Gerontol.*, 26, 375, 1991. With permission.)

noglycan of the heparin-type can interact with the gene regulatory steps and decrease the rate of transcription of genes coding for fibronectin and collagen type III.

Independently, Chandrasekhar and Millis[34] could show that fibronectin synthesized by phase III fibroblasts *in vitro* was deficient in its adhesive properties. It is not clear, however, if this is due to a modification of the structure of the molecule or to posttranslational modifications, for instance

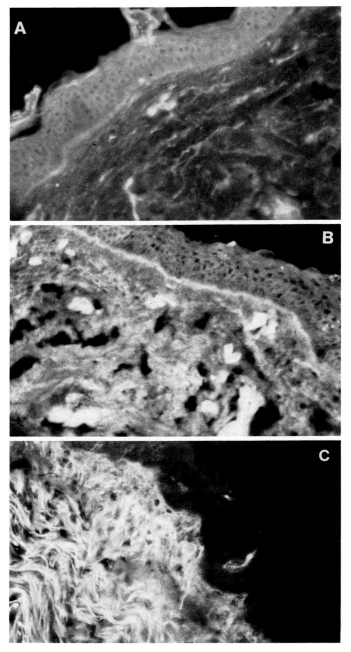

Figure 4
Increase of fibronectin immunofluorescence in human skin of diabetic patients (A) and a Werner patient (B) as compared to an age-matched clinically normal control (C). (From Labat-Robert, J. and Robert, L., *Exp. Gerontol.*, 23, 5, 1988. With permission.)

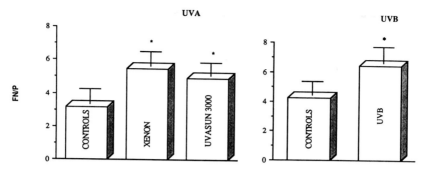

Figure 5
Increase of fibronectin in the skin of UV-irradiated mice as compared to controls. Both UVA and UVB radiations were administered for over 52 weeks, 5460 J/cm² total dose for UVA, and 12 weeks with a total dose of 4 J/cm² for UVB, using different UV lamps, xenon lamp, and UV sun, and fibronectin biosynthesis was examined in skin explant cultures by ³⁵S-methionine incorporation and expressed as % of incorporation in total proteins; *: $p < 0.05$ as compared to controls. (From Boyer, B., Fourtanier, A., Kern, P., and Labat-Robert, J., *J. Photochem. Photobiol.*, 14, 247, 1992. With permission.)

proteolytic cleavage. The studies of Pagani et al.[35] also confirmed the age-dependent modifications of the alternative splicing of the fibronectin gene. These modifications can concern two exons which can be included or omitted (forms A and B) and a third exon which can be subdivided (V region).[20,35]

The above results clearly show that age-dependent modifications of the expression of genes coding for ECM macromolecules occur both *in vivo* and *in vitro*. However, the detailed mechanisms of these changing regulations still remain to be elucidated. The effect of heparin fragments on these phenomena also suggests the possibility of therapeutical interventions at the level of gene regulation.

2. Basement Membrane Constituents — Collagen Type IV, Laminin, and Proteoheparan Sulfate

Among the earliest observations concerning age-dependent modifications of connective tissues, we have to mention those concerning the progressive increase of capillary basement membranes. Their thickness increases with age in normal individuals and more intensively in diabetics.[36] Results from several laboratories showed that this was also the case in kidney glomerular capillary basement membranes (Figure 6). The induction of diabetes in rats and mice by streptozotocin or the presence of a genetic diabetes (KK-mice) also produced an increase of capillary basement membrane thickness.[36]

Using both immunohistochemical and biochemical techniques, it could be shown that this increase concerns collagen type IV, laminin, and also fibronectin, although this last macromolecule is not considered as an

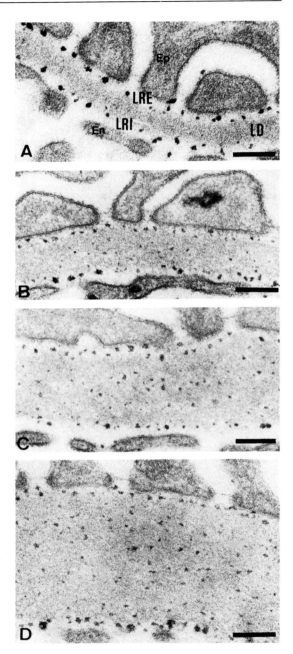

Figure 6
Increase of basement membrane thickness in renal glomerular capillaries with age of Wistar rats (WAG/RI strain, germ free). The anionic sites (heparan sulfate proteoglycans) are visualized by a cationic polyethylene label (dark spots). (A) At 3 months; (B) 10 months; (C) 20 months; (D) 30 months. (En) Endothelial cells; (Ep) epithelial cells; (LD) lamina densa; (LRE) lamina rara externa; (LRI) lamina rara interna. (Transmission electron microscopy by J. and M. Schaeverbeke, magnification × 130,000; bar: 0.1 nm.) (From Robert, L., *Le Vieillissement*, CNRS-Belin, Paris, 1994. With permission.)

integral component of basement membranes. It appeared, however, that antifibronectin antibodies clearly localize capillary contours in tissue sections and show their enlargment in diabetic biopsies (Figure 4).

Heparan sulfate proteoglycan decreases, however (see Figure 6), probably explaining the increased permeability of the thickened basement membranes.

Using streptozotocin to induce diabetes in mice also inoculated with the basement membrane producing EHS tumor, it could be shown that these tissues overproduce laminin as well as type IV collagen in explant cultures.[37] This was shown by the incorporation of ^{3}H-proline and ^{35}S-methionine followed by separation of collagen chains on PAGE and immunoprecipitation of laminin.

These phenomena reveal concordant modifications of the expression of several matrix coding genes: some amplified as collagen III, IV, laminin and fibronectin, some apparently downregulated as heparan sulfate proteoglycan. Some experiments suggested, however, that distinct mechanisms might be involved because the increase of collagen type III and of fibronectin could be dissociated. Indirect evidence was also obtained concerning the possibility of a qualitative "error" in gene expression in aging and diabetic basement membranes: electron microscopy of conjunctival capillary basement membranes performed by Kern et al. revealed in about half of diabetic patients the presence of striated collagen fibrils in the width of the enlarged basement membranes.[36]

An onion-sheet-like superposition of successive layers of basement membrane material was suggested by Vracko[38] for the explanation of these thickened basement membranes. The cellular origin of these constituents is therefore less certain than for those in close contact with the capillary endothelial cells considered to be the site of synthesis of most if not all basement membrane constituents.

The available experiments do not permit extensive speculation on the mechanisms underlying the above-described modifications of gene expression for interstitial collagen types, basement membrane constituents, and fibronectin. The described models, and especially the serial culture of cells for fibronectin and collagen gene expression, however, are suitable models for further research.

3. Proteoglycans (PGs) and Hyaluronan

The most investigated age-dependent changes concerning PGs concern articular cartilage. Osteoarthritis is strongly age-dependent and advances at different rates in a variety of cartilagenous tissues. The main feature is the progressive loss of the large PGs from cartilage. This results in the progressive increase of mechanical stress, abrasion of the articular surfaces, and inflammation (Figure 7). As the large PGs of cartilage (syndecan) are associated with hyaluronan, the degradation of hyaluronan by free radical mechanisms[39] or by endoglycosidases can alone strongly modify cartilage structure. It appears, however, that decreased biosynthe-

A

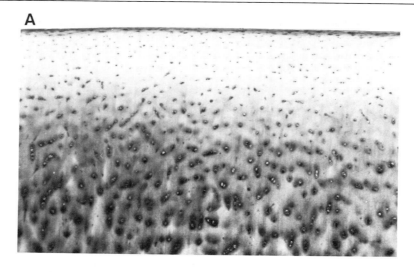

B

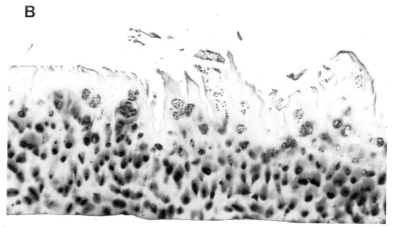

Figure 7
Degradation of articular cartilage during the development of osteoarthritis: (A) normal cartilage, (B) osteoarthritic cartilage. (From Mitrovic, D., *L'Année Gérontologique*, Serdi, Paris, 1991. With permission.)

sis and increased proteolytic degradation of cartilage PGs are also involved.[39,40]

Loss of hyaluronan may have some other effects also. It could be shown that degradation of pericellular hyaluronan triggers its increased resynthesis[42] and also cell proliferation.[43] If these mechanisms apply to the chondrocytes *in situ*, their proliferation could lead to loss of differentiation, resulting in a fibroblast-like phenotype, aggravating the fibrotic process of the cartilage. The capacity of cells to react to hyaluronan degradation by the above-mentioned mechanisms is decreased in phase III, senescent fibroblasts.[43] The biosynthesis of hyaluronan, however, appears to increase with age according to the studies of Lindqvist and Laurent.[44] Its concentration was shown to increase in human intervertebral discs with age by Scott et al.[45]

4. Elastin

Using a PCR amplification method and *in situ* hybridization for the determination of the elastin message, it could be shown recently that the rate of transcription of the elastin gene is high in several tissues and especially in the vascular wall in the embryo, but decreases during maturation.[46,47] It also could be shown on human skin fibroblasts obtained from donors of increasing age that the transcription of the elastin gene increases again during aging.[46] Confirmation of the age-dependent increase of elastogenesis was also obtained by morphometric procedures on human skin biopsies.[48,49] Figure 8a shows the increase with age of elastic fiber length and width in the reticular dermis taken at sun-protected sites and determined by morphometry.[48] However, this increase of elastin content is not accompanied by an increase of skin elasticity, which as a matter of fact decreases with age[50] (Figure 8b). This finding, confirmed on a large number of female and male volunteers, may be the result of postsynthetic modifications of elastin (see later).

B. Postsynthetic Modifications

As mentioned earlier, these modifications are the only ones firmly established in aging organisms at the level of postsynthetic macromolecules. Although the original findings of Gershon concerning the presence of inactive enzymes in aging nematodes were attributed to faulty biosynthetic mechanisms, this hypothesis had to be abandoned.[25,26] The error rate during the translational process is quite low, about 10^{-3} to 10^{-4} (one erroneous "choice" of aminoacyl tRNA in a thousand or ten thousand). It is not negligible, but it does not seem to increase with age. The most important limitation in correcting these errors appears to be the cost of "corrections" in terms of energy (ATP) converted to these purposes.[51] Those reactions which are considered as the most disturbing for the aging organism, however, are independent from these considerations because they are apparently noncatalyzed by enzymes. The reaction between glucose and other low-molecular-weight carbohydrates possessing a reducing group and free amino groups of proteins (ε-lysines especially) are the most important. These so-called nonenzymatic glycosylation (glycation) reactions first described by Maillard in 1912[52] were shown to concern many proteins. Although relatively slow, the speed of these reactions is not negligible with glucose even at its physiological concentration of about 1

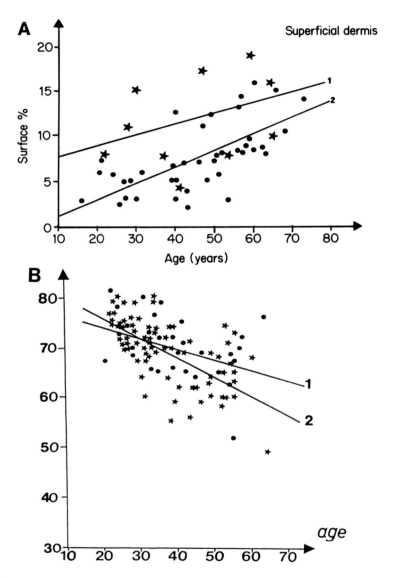

Figure 8
(A) Increase of elastin fiber content of the human skin with age; abscissa: age in
years; ordinates: relative surface area of elastic fibers in the papillary dermis of skin
biopsy sections evaluated by morphometry. (From Robert, C., Lesty, C., and Robert,
A. M., *Gerontology*, 34, 91, 1988. With permission.) (B) Decrease of skin elasticity with
age as measured by indentometry in a healthy population (employees of a pharmaceutical firm); abscissa: age in years; ordinates: % elastic rebound of skin after the
application of an "indentation" with a force of 10 g/cm²; (●) males, (∗) females.
(From Robert, C., Blanc, M., Lesty, C., Dikstein, S., and Robert, L., *Gerontology*, 34,
84, 1988. With permission.)

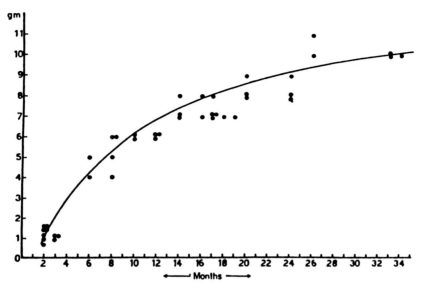

Figure 9
Increased "cross-linking" of collagen fibers with age as demonstrated by Verzar.[20]
Increase of the weight to be used with the age of the rats when the tendon was taken
in order to oppose thermal contraction. (From Verzar, F., in *Int. Rev. Connect. Tissue
Res.*, 2, 257, 1964. With permission.)

g/l in blood. In the clinical routine this reaction is quantified by the
determination of "glycosylated hemoglobin". The normal range of glycated
hemoglobin A1C is about $5 \pm 1.5\%$ of total hemoglobin. In hyperglycemic
states this reaction is speeded up proportionally to the blood-glucose
level. Although it concerns most proteins, the most harmful effects appear
to concern the more long-lived molecular species, for instance fibrous
collagens. The important discovery of Verzar concerning the progressive
cross-linking of collagen fibers with age[53] (Figure 9) is now attributed to
this reaction.[54] The result is the resistance to digestion of such cross-linked
fibers by collagenases and the lack of their turnover. This is one of the
reasons explaining the progressive hardening of the vascular wall with
age-arteriosclerosis.[55] Rapidly turning over matrix proteins are also concerned by the Maillard reaction, for instance fibronectin. Glycated
fibronectin was demonstrated in diabetic blood plasma and tissues.[56] The
adhesive properties of FN appear to be severely altered by glycation. This
may be one of the reasons for the structural alteration of diabetic connective tissues in general, and of the micro- and macrovascular wall in particular in diabetes. It also should be mentioned that lower molecular
weight aldehydes such as acetaldehyde derived from the metabolism of
ethanol, and even pentoses, react much faster than glucose with amino
groups.[57] Their role in the postsynthetic modifications deserves further

attention. Another important aspect of the Maillard reaction is the demonstration by Esposito et al.[58] of the presence of receptors on some cells, such as macrophages, that recognize Maillard products. In some model reactions such products were shown to be mutagenic. This observation also certainly deserves further attention. Other posttranslational modifications of matrix proteins are interactions with lipids and calcium, which are especially important for elastin and proteolytic degradation.

1. Collagens

Fibrous type I and III collagens are especially concerned by the abovementioned cross-linking process. The regular age-dependent increase of the resistance to thermal shrinkage of collagen fibers, shown to concern all vertebrates species investigated[53] is certainly one of the most important aspects of the post-synthetic aging process of matrix macromolecules.

2. Proteoglycans and Hyaluronan

As mentioned above their rates of biosynthesis were not systematically studied as a function of *in vitro* or *in vivo* aging. The older literature was reviewed previously.[41] The most conspicuous postsynthetic modifications concern the proteolytic degradation of proteoglycans in osteoarthritic cartilage, as is also shown in the model experiments initiated by Halpern et al.[59] by repeated injects proteolytic enzymes into the circulation. The progressive decrease of PGs in articular cartilage and in some intervertebral discs[40,45] with age is probably the result of decreased synthesis and increased degradation. Hyaluronan, although quite sensitive to free radical degradation as shown by Pigman,[39] was shown to increase in several tissues[44,45] suggesting that biosynthesis may well exceed degradation. This is especially the case in intervertebral discs, as shown recently by Scott et al.[45] As GAGs are considered mainly responsible for controlling tissue hydration and molecular traffic in interstitial spaces, the change in their concentration certainly affects these phenomena.

3. Structural Glycoproteins

The rapid glycation of fibronectin in diabetic hyperglycemic tissues and body fluids has already been mentioned. Fewer studies are available on other glycoproteins, such as laminin, for instance. As its biosynthesis increases in diabetic tissues and basement membranes, its glycation may contribute to the functional disturbances of capillary basement membranes in aging organisms in general and in diabetics in particular.

Another newly discovered aspect of postsynthetic modifications of matrix glycoproteins is the demonstration that some of the proteolytic fragments of fibronectin may have distinct and deleterious effects as potentiators of viral transformation[60] or the appearance of proteolytic activity associated with some of the larger fragments.[61] The importance of these findings for aging organisms deserves further studies.

4. *Elastin*

Elastic fibers are considered as long-lived tissue constituents.[8] Although mature elastic fibers are resistant to chemical and physical aggressions as well as to most proteases, they undergo posttranslational modifications leading to the loss of elasticity and increased susceptibility to elastase-type endopeptidases. The highly hydrophobic character of elastin as well as its secondary and tertiary structure explain its strong affinity to lipidic components and to calcium. In the presence of calcium salts elastin can retain much higher amounts of ^{14}C-cholesterol than in the presence of sodium salts.[11] Several cell types were shown to produce elastase-type endopeptidases which belong to nearly all classes of proteolytic enzymes.[8] The arterial wall was shown to accumulate lipids and calcium within its elastic fibers with age and much more so during atherogenesis.[62] Its elastase content also increases with age and becomes faster during the development of arteriosclerosis.[63] These age-dependent modifications of vascular elastic tissue play an important role in the age-dependent hardening of the arterial wall — arteriosclerosis. As the breakdown products of elastic fibers, elastin peptides were shown to be present in the circulating blood and to increase in several vascular diseases.[64] Their interactions with elastin receptors appear to be involved in cell-aging and in the progressive increase of the calcium content of the vascular wall.[65]

C. Modifications of Cell-Matrix Interactions

The discovery of cell membane receptors mediating cell-matrix interactions opened up a new important field for the investigation of reciprocal interactions between cells and extracellular matrix components. Several types of receptors were described; the most intensively studied matrix-receptor family are the integrins.[20-22]

Figure 10 shows their structure schematically, composed of two distinct, interacting peptide chains, α and β, both present as several isoforms. Their assortment entails them some specificity for their interaction with the matrix components, as shown on Table 3.

Other matrix-receptors are apparently involved in collagen-cell interaction, as was proposed for the anchorins.[66] A third type of cell receptor was shown to be involved in the mediation of cell interactions with elastin and laminin.[67-69] The 67-kDa subunit of this receptor appears to be a splice-isoform of β-galactosidase,[70] is located on the cell membrane, and can be

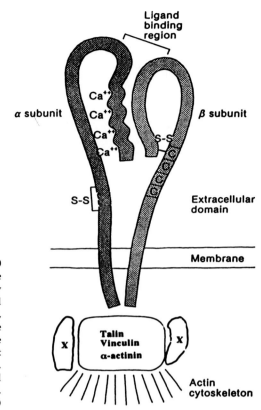

Figure 10
Schematic representation of the structure of integrins, formed by two separate peptide chains, α and β (both exist in several isoforms), with their ligand recognition site towards the matrix and the intracellular portion in contact with the cytoskeletal elements. X = Fibulin? (Albeda, S. M. and Buck, C. A., *Faseb J.*, 4, 2868, 1990. With permission.)

extracted and purified through its affinity for lactose and elastin peptides. This lectin-type subunit is apparently involved in the recognition of both laminin and elastin peptides[67] (Figure 11a).

Another cell-membrane-located glycoprotein, elastonectin, was shown to be involved in the mediation of the adhesion of cells to elastic fibers.[68,71] Its biosynthesis and membrane localization are induced by the activation of the elastin laminin receptor. This phenomenon may be important for the adhesive interaction of vascular smooth muscle cells with matrix components during the changes of wall tension induced by variations in blood pressure or the sympathetic nervous system modifying the tension of smooth muscle cells. Their adhesion to elastic fibers may transmit the variation of tension to the vascular wall (Figure 11b,c). Recently, we showed that the elastin receptor mediated an endothelium-dependent vasorelaxation.[72,72a] This effect is presumably the result of the coupling of the elastin-laminin receptor to the NO-synthetase, the EDRF*-releasing mechanism of the endothelial cells. Several other important cell reactions were shown to be mediated by the elastin-laminin receptor, for instance

* Endothelium-derived relaxing factor.

TABLE 3.

The Integrin Family

Name	Synonym	Ligand	Role of RGD
β1 integrins (VLAs):			
α1β1	VLA-1	LM, Coll I ct IV	No
α2β1	VLA-2	Coll I et IV	No (DGEA for coll I)
α3β1	VLA-3	FN, LM, Coll I	No
α4β1	VLA-4	CS1, CS5 du FN IIICS	No
α5β1	VLA-5	FN	Yes
α6β1	VLA-6	LM	No
α7β1	VLA-7	LM	
H36α7β1		LM	
αvβ1		VN, FN	Yes
β2 integrins (adhesion molecule of leukocytes: LEU-CAMs = CD18)			
αLβ2	LFA-1	I-CAM1 et 2	No
αMβ2	Mac-1	C3Bi, FX, Fb	Yes
αXβ2	p150,95	Fb, C3B(i?)	No GPRP
β3 integrins (cytoadhesins)			
αVβ3		Coll I, VN, Fb, vWF	Yes
		OP, BSP1	Yes
αIIBβ3	GpIIb-IIIa	Fb, FN, vWFVN, Tsp	Yes
β4 integrin (hemidesmosomes of certain epithelia, endothelia, and large vessels)			
α6β4	BM	LM	Yes
β5 integrin (vitronectin receptor)			
αVβ5		VN	Yes
β6 integrin			
αVβ6		FN	Yes
β7 integrin (adhesion molecule of B and T lymphocytes, immunoregulatory molecule)			
β7			
α4β7		FN	
β8 integrin			
αvβ8			

release of lytic enzymes and oxygen free radicals from leukocytes and control of ion fluxes, an increase in cellular Na^+ and Ca^{2+}, and a decrease in K^+.[68,69] One of the important consequences of the presence of matrix receptors on cells is the possibility to influence and redirect cell behavior during changing matrix conditions as observed with aging and in age-dependent diseases. Several authors demonstrated a profound modification of cell behavior by matrix components. This aspect of cell-matrix interaction appears to be of great importance for the aging process, the information transfer from the ECM to cells will change with age. As mentioned previously, most matrix components undergo postsynthetic modifications. Most of these modifications are on the epigenetic level. By their action on cells through the matrix receptors they can influence the gene expression of cells. This apparently pseudo-Lamarckian mechanism of modulation of gene expression by environmentally influenceable

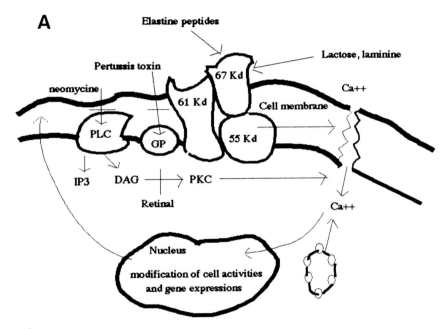

Figure 11
Interaction between cells and elastic fibers. (A) Schematic representation of the elastin receptor with its three subunits, the 67 kDa subunit reacting with elastin peptides, laminin, and lactose, and its transmission pathway, a G-protein that is inhibitable with pertussis toxin, phospholipase C, (inhib: neomycin) liberating inositol-3-phosphate (IP_3) and diacyl glycerol (DAG) activating phosphokinase C (PKC) (inhib: retinal), opening calcium channels and modifying cell function. (B) Demonstration of immunofluorescence of the cell membrane localized fibrous network which develops during the contact of the cell and the elastin fiber (elastonectin); fibroblasts in culture in presence of elastic fibers, as in (A). (C) Transmission electron microscopy of a fibroblast in culture in close contact with an elastic fiber (elast.). The arrows point to spots of increased thickness of the cell membrane in close contact with the fiber. (From Robert, L., *Le Vieillissement*, CNRS-Belin, Paris, 1994. With permission.)

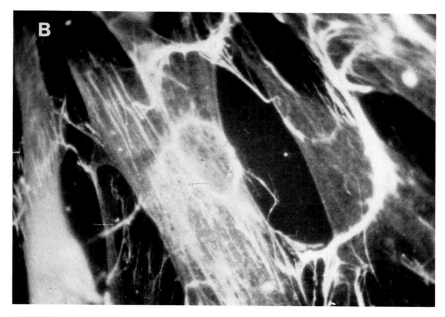

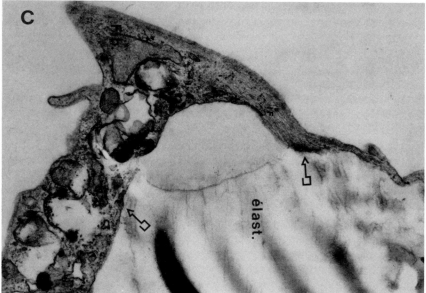

Figure 11 (continued)

modifications (nutrition, for instance) of tissue composition appears to be an important aspect of the age-dependent modifications of cell behavior.

IV. ROLE OF ECM IN ORGANISMIC AGING AND AGE-RELATED DISEASES

One of the major problems in aging research is the integration of results obtained on reductionistic model systems in the realm of the whole organism. Comparative studies on the Hayflick model and *in vivo* on the regulation of matrix biosynthesis sometimes revealed agreements and sometimes discrepancies between the results obtained *in vitro* and *in vivo*. Several of the matrix components are upregulated in the *in vitro* system and some only are increasing during chronological aging.[74] One of the reasons of possible discrepancies concerns the role of hormones, cytokines, and other regulatory factors in the *in vivo* situation that are not present during the *in vitro* serial passages of cells. It appears, therefore, logical to search for coordinating systems in order to pass from model experiments to the *in vivo* situation. Several such coordinating systems exist in the organism, for instance the nervous system, hormones, cytokines, and the extracellular matrix itself. The essential role of the ECM is to integrate cells in tissues, tissues in organs, and organs in the whole organism. This integrating role of ECM can be demonstrated, for instance, by the organization of the musculoskeletal system. Each muscle fiber is surrounded by a connective tissue sheet, the endomysium, the muscle itself by the perimysium, which is continuous with the tendon which, in its turn, fuses in the periosteum. There is a continuum between each muscle fiber and the bones moved by a given muscle system. The nature of the ECM at these sites is specifically adapted to the physiological role they have to perform. Therefore the qualitative and quantitative modifications of ECM components described previously will influence the whole physiological system that the matrix has to protect and integrate into functional units. Progressive cross-linking of collagen fibers will impair their function. The decrease of biosynthesis of the calcifiable matrix components of bones, collagen type I, and associated glycoproteins is the major factor of osteoporosis. Hormonal factors and vitamin D receptors appear to be involved in these regulations.

We already mentioned osteoarthritis and its main biochemical symptom, the progressive loss of the proteoglycans of the articular cartilage (Figure 7). Arteriosclerosis, the progressive hardening of elastic vessels, is attributed to cross-linking of collagen by the Verzar-Maillard reaction, the saturation of elastin with lipids and calcium and its proteolytic fragmentation.

Skin aging is very much dependent on the loss of cells and ECM. In most of these situations both decreased biosynthesis and increased degradation appear to be involved.

Another important factor is the progressive uncoupling of some cell membrane receptors involved in the mediation of cell-matrix interactions. This was shown to be the case for the elastin-laminin and fMLP receptors.[75] As shown on Figure 12a,b, with increasing age the calcium transients show a progressive slow-down of the capacity of the cells to recover their basic free intracellular calcium level. Approximately one third of all the elderly patients investigated in these studies were unable to downregulate the increased intracellular calcium after triggering PMN-leukocytes with the chemotactic peptide fMLP.[75] It could be shown that the mobilization of the inositol phosphate pathway by the elastin receptor also decreases very strongly in leukocytes from older (>65 years) individuals. Similar results were reported for other, unrelated receptors.[76] These results indicate that loss of receptors and/or their uncoupling may be a key factor in the loss of integrated cell function during the aging of the organism.

V. CONCLUSIONS

The succinct enumeration of some of the factors involved in connective tissue aging clearly indicates the importance of the changing matrix composition and function for the aging organism. The reported modifications can be traced to altered cell function and also to a large extent to postsynthetic modifications of matrix components. At a time when major emphasis and hope is placed on gene-controlled modifications it is important to realize the existence of such epigenetic factors playing a major role in organismic aging. As clearly shown by the ever-increasing details of cell-matrix interactions being discovered and the possibility to redirect cell behavior through modified matrix components, it does not appear farfetched to propose an important role for matrix-directed feedback mechanisms in cellular aging. It also appears from this brief description of ECM and its age-related modifications that cell-matrix interactions are intimately involved in information transfer from cells to the matrix during morphogenesis and back from the matrix to the cells during maturation and aging. The "nonprogrammed" epigenetic modification of ECM will strongly influence this information transfer (Figure 13). Its progressive deterioration during aging appears to be the result of postsynthetic modifications of matrix components (glycation, degradation, etc.), the action of their degradation products on cell receptors, and the apparent uncoupling of receptors from their transmission pathway as was exemplified by the aging of the elastin-laminin and fMLP receptors. These considerations

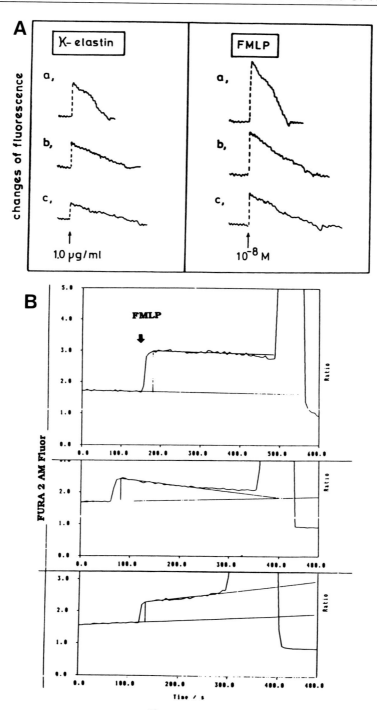

Figure 12

Figure 12

(A) Modifications with age of the calcium transients (free intracellular calcium) triggered by the addition of elastin peptides (k-elastin) or a chemotactic peptide (fMLP) to human polymorphonuclear leukocytes: (a) young individuals, <45 years; (b) old individuals, >65 years; (c) atherosclerotic old individuals. Quin-2 fluorescence recordings. Notice the slow-down of the return to base values of the increased intracellular calcium with age and pathology. (From Varga, Z., Kovacs, E. M., Paragh, G., Jacob, M. P., Robert, L., and Fülöp, T., *Clin. Biochem.*, 21, 127, 1988. With permission.) (B) Similar recording of free intracellular calcium in the PMN leukocytes of old inpatients of a retirement home (70 to 90 years), some demented, with fura-2 as indicator and fMLP as a trigger. Some patients could still reestablish the basal calcium values (middle curve) although slowly, for others (about 1/3 of the total examined) calcium homeostasis was lost, intracellular calcium continued to increase (bottom curve) or could not be decreased (upper curve). (From Ghuysen-Itard, A. F., Robert, L., Gourlet, V., Berr, C., and Jacob, M. P., *Gerontology*, 39, 163, 1993. With permission of S. Karger AG, Basel.)

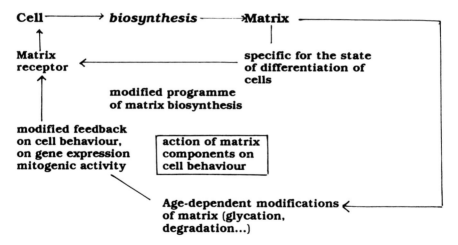

Figure 13

Informational feedback loops between cells and extracellular matrix components. The upper part of the scheme shows the feedback loops between cells which synthesize the matrix components and the postsynthetic matrix which regulates cell behavior by contacting the cell membrane receptors (integrins, elastin-laminin receptor). The lower part of the scheme shows the modifications of the above (normal) feedback loop as a result of the degradation of matrix components and by the action of degradation products, elastin peptides and fibronectin fragments, on cell receptors. This second feedback loop can result in deterioration of cell functions, as mentioned in the text.

should motivate the use of a variety of models for the better understanding of the aging mechanisms from the cellular to the organismic levels and the role of this reverse information transfer in aging and age-related diseases.

REFERENCES

1. Labat-Robert, J., Bihari-Varga, M., and Robert, L., Extracellular matrix, *FEBS Lett.*, 268, 386, 1990.
2. Labat-Robert, J., Timpl, T., and Robert, L., Structural glycoproteins in cell-matrix interactions, in *Frontiers of Matrix Biology*, Karger, Basel, 1986.
3. Balazs, E. A., *Chemistry and Molecular Biology of the Intercellular Matrix*, I, II, III, Academic Press, New York, 1970.
4. Scott, J. E., The nomenclature of glycosaminoglycans and proteoglycans, *Glycoconjugate J.*, 10, 419, 1993.
5. Fleischmajer, R., Olsen, B. R., and Kühn, K., Structure, molecular biology, and pathology of collagen, *Ann. N.Y. Acad. Sci.*, 580, 1990.
6. Indik, Z., Yeh, H., Ornstein-Golstein, N., Sheppard, P., Anderson, N., Rosenbloom, J. C., Peltonen, L., and Rosenbloom, J., Alternative splicing of human elastin mRNA indicated by sequence analysis of cloned genomic and complementary DNA, *Proc. Natl. Acad. Sci. U.S.A.*, 84, 5680, 1987.
7. Jacob, M. P. and Hornebeck, W., Isolation and characterization of insoluble and kappa-elastins, in *Frontiers of Matrix Biology*, Robert, L., Moczar, M., and Moczar, E., Eds., Karger, Basel, 1985.
8. Robert, L. and Hornebeck, W., *Elastin and Elastases*, CRC Press, Boca Raton, FL, 1989.
9. Kornfeld-Poullain, N. and Robert, L., Effets de différents solvants organiques sur la dégradation alcaline de l'élastine, *Bull. Soc. Chim. Biol.*, 50, 759, 1968.
10. Urry, D. W., Sequential polypeptides of elastin: structural properties and molecular pathologies, in *Frontiers of Matrix Biology*, Robert, A. M. and Robert, L., Eds., Karger, Basel, 1980.
11. Jacob, M. P., Hornebeck, H., and Robert, L., Studies on the interaction of cholesterol with soluble and insoluble elastins, *Int. J. Biol. Macromol.*, 5, 275, 1983.
12. Ruoslahti, E., Extracellular matrix in the regulation of cellular functions, in *Cell to Cell Interaction*, Burger, M. M., Sordat, B., and Zinkernagel, R. M., Eds., Karger, Basel, 1990, 88.
13. Sandell, L. J., Molecular biology of proteoglycans and link proteins, in *Biology of Proteoglycans*, Wight, T. N. and Mecham, R. P., Eds., Academic Press, New York, 1987, 27.
14. Scott, J., E., *Dermatan Sulphate Proteoglycans*, Portland Press, London, 1993.
15. Greiling, H. and Scott, J. E., *Keratan Sulphate*, Portland Press, London, 1989.
16. Balazs, E. A. and Laurent, T., The biology of hyaluronan, *Ciba Foundation Symposium 143*, John Wiley & Sons, New York, 1989.
17. Scott, J. E., Supramolecular organization of extracellular matrix glycosaminoglycans, in vitro and in the tissues, *FASEB J.*, 6, 2639, 1992.
18. Völker, W., Schmidt, A., and Buddecke, E., Cytochemical changes in a human arterial proteoglycan related to atherosclerosis, *Atherosclerosis*, 77, 117, 1989.

19. Hauss, W. H., Über die Rolle des Mesenchyms in der Genese der Arteriosklerose, *Virchows Arch. Abt. A Pathol. Anat.*, 359, 135, 1973.
20. Hynes, R. O., *Fibronectins*, Springer-Verlag, New York, 1990.
21. Albelda, S. M. and Buck, C. A., Integrins and other cell adhesion molelcules, *FASEB J.*, 4, 2868, 1990.
22. Labat-Robert, J., Glycoprotéines de structure et intégrines, *C.R. Soc. Biol.*, 187, 181, 1993.
23. Mecham, R. P., Hinek, A., Entwistle, R., Wrenn, D. S., Griffin, G. L., and Senior, R. M., Elastin binds to a multifunctional 67-kDa peripheral membrane protein, *Biochemistry*, 28, 3716, 1989.
24. Groult, V., Hornebeck, W., Ferrari, P., Tixier, J. M., and Robert, L., Mechanisms of interaction between human skin fibroblasts and elastin: differences between elastin fibres and derived peptides, *Cell Biochem. Funct.*, 9, 171, 1991.
25. Adelman, R. C. and Roth, G. S., Eds., *Altered Proteins and Aging*, CRC Press, Boca Raton, FL, 1983.
26. Robert, L., *Mécanismes Cellulaires et Moléculaires du Vieillissement*, Masson, Paris, 1983.
27. Hayflick, L., The limited in vitro lifetime of human diploid cell strains, *Exp. Cell. Res.*, 37, 614, 1965.
28. Macieira-Coelho, A., *Biology of Normal Proliferating Cells* In Vitro *Relevance for In Vivo Aging*, Karger, Basel, 1988.
29. Rasoamanantena, P., Labat-Robert, J., and Goldstein, S., Variations de la biosynthèse et quantification de l'ARNm de la fibronectine humaine au cours du vieillissement en culture, *C. R. Soc. Biol.*, 187, 238, 1993.
29a. Rasoamanantena, P., Thweatt, R., Labat-Robert, J., and Goldstein, S., Exper. Cell Res., 213, 121, 1994.
30. Kern, P., Sebert, B., and Robert, L., Increased type III/Type I collagen ratios in diabetic human conjunctival biopsies, *Clin. Physiol. Biochem.*, 4, 113, 1986.
31. Branchet, M. C., Boisnic, S., Frances, C., Lesty, C., and Robert, L., Morphometric analysis of dermal collagen fibers in normal human skin as a function of age, *Arch. Gerontol., Geriatr.*, 13, 1, 1991.
32. Branchet, M. C., Boisnic, S., Frances, C., and Robert, A. M., Skin thickness changes in normal aging skin, *Gerontology*, 36, 28, 1990.
33. Asselot-Chapel, C., Kern, P., and Labat-Robert, J., Biosyntheses of interstitial collagens and fibronectin by porcine aorta smooth muscle cells. Modulation by low molecular weight heparin fragments, *Biochim. Biophys. Acta*, 993, 240, 1989.
34. Chandrasekhar, S. and Millis, A. J. T., Fibronectin from aged fibroblasts is defective in promoting cellular adhesion, *J. Cell. Physiol.*, 103, 47, 1980.
35. Pagani, F., Zagato, L., Vergani, C., Casari, G., Sidoli, A., and Baralle, F. E., Tissue-specific splicing pattern of fibronectin messenger RNA precursor during development and aging in rat, *J. Cell. Biol.*, 113, 1223, 1991.
36. Robert, L., Kern, P., Regnault, F., Bouissou, H., Lagrue, G., Miskulin, M., and Robert, A.M., Correlation between basement membrane anomalies and the incorporation of ^{14}C-proline and ^{3}H-glucosamine in diabetic connective tissues, in *Biology and Chemistry of Basement Membranes*, Kefalides, N., A., Ed., Academic Press, New York, 1978, 503.
37. Asselot-Chapel, C., Biosynthèse des macromolécules de la matrice extracellulaire par les cellules mésenchymateuses. Régulation transcriptionnelle, modifications dans le diabète et modulation pharmacologique par des fragments d'héparine, Thèse de Doctorat, Université Paris XII, 1991.
38. Vracko, R., Basal lamina scaffold, in *Frontiers of Matrix Biology*, Robert, A. M., Boniface, R., and Robert, L., Eds., Karger, Basel, 1979, 78.

39. Pigman, W. and Rizwi, S., Hyaluronic acid and the ORD reaction, *Biochem. Biophys. Res. Commun.*, 1, 39, 1959.
40. Stuhlsatz, H. W. and Greiling, H., Proteoglycans and glycosaminoglycans of human joint cartilage in health, senescence and disease, in *Glycosaminoglycans and Proteoglycans in Physiological and Pathological Processes of Body Systems*, Varma, R. S. and Varma, R., Eds., Karger, Basel, 1982, 276.
41. Robert, L. and Moczar, M., Age-related proteoglycans and glycosaminoglycans, in *Glycosaminoglycans and Proteoglycans in Physiological and Pathological Processes of Body Systems*, Varma R.S. and Varma R., Eds., Karger, Basel, 1982, 440.
42. Larnier, C., Kerneur, C., Robert, L., and Moczar, M., Effect of testicular hyaluronidase on hyaluronate synthesis by human skin fibroblasts, *Biochim. Biophys. Acta*, 1014, 145, 1989.
43. Moczar, M. and Robert, L., Stimulation of cell proliferation by hyaluronidase during in vitro aging of human skin fibroblasts, *Exp. Gerontol.*, 28, 59, 1993.
44. Lindqvist, U. and Laurent, T. C., Serum hyaluronan and aminoterminal propeptide of type III procollagen: variation with age, *Scand. J. Clin. Lab. Invest.*, 52, 613, 1992.
45. Scott, J. E., Bosworth, T. R., Cribb, A. M., and Taylor, J. R., The chemical morphology of age-related changes in human intervertebral disc glycosaminoglycans from cervical, thoracic and lumbar nucleus pulposus and annulus fibrosus, *J. Anat.*, 184, 73, 1994.
46. Holzenberger, M., Leviinzi, S. A., Herzog, C. P., Deak, S. B., Robert, L., and Boyd, C., Quantitation of tropoelastin messenger RNA and assessment of alternative splicing in human skin fibroblasts by reverse transcriptase polymerase chain reaction, *PCR — Methods and Applications*, 3, 107, 1993.
47. Holzenberger, M., Ayer-LeoLievre, C., and Robert, L., Tropoelastin gene expression in the developing vascular system of the chicken: an in situ hybridization study, *Anat. Embryol.*, 188, 481, 1993.
48. Robert, C., Lesty, C., and Robert, A.M., Ageing of the skin: study of elastic fiber network. Modification by computerized image analysis, *Gerontology*, 34, 91, 1988.
49. Frances, C., Branchet, M. C., Boisnic, S., Lesty, C. L., and Robert, L., Elastic fibers in normal human skin. Variations with age: a morphometric analysis, *Arch. Gerontol. Geriatr.*, 10, 57, 1990.
50. Robert, C., Blanc, M., Lesty, C., Dikstein, S., and Robert, L., Study of skin ageing as a function of social and professional conditions: modification of the rheological parameters. Measured with a noninvasive method — indentometry, *Gerontology*, 34, 84, 1988.
51. Kirkwood, T. B. L., Rosenberger, R. F., and Galas, D. J., *Accuracy in Molecular Processes*, Chapman and Hall, London, 1986.
52. Maillard, L. C., Action des acides aminés sur les sucres; formation des mélanoïdes par voie méthodique, *C. R. Ac. Sci.*, 154, 66, 1912.
53. Verzar, F., Aging of the collagen fibers, in *International Review of Connective Tissue Research*, Hall, D. A., Ed., Academic Press, New York, 1964.
54. Cerami, A., Vlassara, H., and Brownlee, M., *Pour la Science*, Juillet 1987, 72.
55. Robert, L., Pathogénie de l'athérosclérose, in *Athérosclérose*, Jacotot, B., Ed., Sandoz, Rueil-Malmaison, 1993, 47.
56. Tarsio, J., Reger, L., and Furcht, L., Decreased interaction of fibronectin, type IV collagen, and heparin due to nonenzymatic glycation. Implication for diabetes mellitus, *Biochemistry*, 26, 1014, 1988.
57. Bajic, V., Robert, L., and Polonowski, J., Sur l'interaction entre aldéhydes et réductones et acides aminés et protéines. IV. Dosage des groupements basiques des protéines traitées à l'acétaldéhyde ou au glucose, *Experientia*, 12, 59, 1956.

58. Esposito, C., Gerlaich, H., Brett, J., Stern, D., and Vlassara, H., Endothelial receptor-mediated binding of glucose-modified albumin is associated with increased monolayer permeability and modulation of cell surface coagulant properties, *J. Exp. Med.*, 170, 1387, 1989.

59. Halpern, B. N., Morard, J. C., Juster, M., Robert, L., Abadie, A., and Coudert, A., Experimental collagen-like disease induced by repeated injections of papain, with evidence of auto-immune antibodies, *Ann. N. Y. Acad. Sci.*, 124, 395, 1965.

60. Barlatti, S., Adamoli, A., and De Petro, G., Presence and role of fibronectin fragments in transformed cells, in *Frontiers of Matrix Biology*, Labat-Robert, J., Timpl, R., and Robert, L., Eds., Karger, Basel, 1986, 174.

61. Xie, D. L. and Homandberg, B. A., Fibronectin fragments bind to and penetrate cartilage tissue resulting in proteinase expression and cartilage damage, *Biochem. Biophys. Acta*, 1182, 189, 1993.

62. Claire, M., Jacotot, B., and Robert, L., Characterization of lipids associated with macromolecules of the intercellular matrix of human aorta, *Conn. Tiss. Res.*, 4, 61, 1976.

63. Robert, L., Labat-Robert, J., and Hornebeck, W., Aging and atherosclerosis, in *Atherosclerosis Reviews*, Gotto, A. M. and Paoletti, R., Eds., Raven Press, New York, 1986, 143.

64. Fülöp, T., Wei, S. M., Robert, L., and Jacob, M. P., Determination of elastin peptides in normal and arteriosclerotic human sera by ELISA, *Clin. Physiol. Biochem.*, 8, 273, 1990.

65. Robert, L. and Labat-Robert, J., Cell-matrix interactions, their importance in ageing at the tissue level, *Eur. J. Gerontol.*, 2, 82, 1992.

66. Mollenhauer, J. and Von Der Mark, K., Anchorins, in *Frontiers of Matrix Biology*, Labat-Robert, J., Timpl, R., and Robert, L., Eds., Karger, Basel, 1986, 11, 110.

67. Mecham, R. P., Laminin receptors, *Annu. Rev. Cell. Biol.*, 7, 71, 1991.

68. Robert, L., Jacob, M. P., Fülöp, T., Timar, J., and Hornebeck,W., Elastonectin and the elastin receptor, *Pathol. Biol.*, 37, 736, 1989.

69. Varga, Z., Jacob, M. P., Robert, L., and Fülöp, T., Identification and signal transduction mechanism of elastin peptide receptor in human leukocytes, *FEBS Lett.*, 258, 5, 1989.

70. Hinek, A., Rabinovitch, M., Keeley, F., Okamura-Oho, Y., and Callahan, J., The 67-kDa elastin/laminin-binding protein is related to an enzymatically inactive, alternatively spliced form of β-galactosidase, *J. Clin. Invest.*, 91, 1198, 1993.

71. Hornebeck, W., Tixier, J. M., and Robert, L., Inducible adhesion of mesenchymal cells to elastic fibers: elastonectin, *Proc. Natl. Acad. Sci. U.S.A.*, 83, 5517, 1986.

72. Faury, G., Ristori, M. T., Verdetti, J., Jacob, M. P., and Robert, L., Effect of elastin peptides on vascular tonus, *J. Vascular Res.*, 5, in press.

72a. Role du Recepteur de l'Elastine Laminine dans la Vasoregulation, *C.R.Ac. Sci.*, 317, 807, 1994.

73. Labat-Robert, J., Kern, P., and Robert, L., Biomarkers of connective tissue aging; biosynthesis of fibronectin, collagen Type III and elastase, *Ann. N.Y. Acad. Sci.*, 673, 16, 1992.

74. Robert, L., Jacob, M. P., and Labat-Robert, J., Cell-matrix interactions in the genesis of arteriosclerosis and atheroma: effect of aging, *Ann. N.Y. Acad. Sci.*, 673, 331, 1992.

75. Ghuysen-Itard, A. F., Robert, L., Gourlet, V., Berr, C., and Jacob, M. P., Loss of calcium-homeostatic mechanisms in polymorphonuclear leukocytes of demented and nondemented elderly subjects, *Gerontology*, 39, 163, 1993.

76. Miyamoto, A., Villalobos-Molina, R., Kowatch, M. A., and Roth, G. S., Altered coupling of α_1-adrenergic receptor-G protein in rat parotid during aging, *Am. J. Physiol.*, 262, C1181, 1992.

77. Boyer, B., Kern, P., Fourtanier A., and Labat-Robert, J., Age-dependent variations of the biosynthesis of fibronectin and fibrous collagens in mouse skin, *Exp. Gerontol.*, 26, 375, 1991.

78. Labat-Robert, J. and Robert, L., Modifications of fibronectin in age-related diseases: diabetes and cancer, *Arch. Gerontol. Geriatr.*, 3, 1, 1984.

79. Labat-Robert, J. and Robert, L., Aging of the extracellular matrix and its pathology, *Exp. Gerontol.*, 23, 5, 1988.

80. Asselot, C., Labat-Robert, J., and Kern, P., Heparin fragments regulate collagen phenotype and fibronectin synthesis in the skin of genetically diabetic mice, *Biochem. Pharmacol.*, 38, 895, 1989.

81. Mitrovic, D., Vieillissement et arthrose, in *Année Gérontologique*, Albarède, J. L. and Vellas, P., Eds., Serdi, Paris, 1992.

82. Labat-Robert, J., Les intégrines, *Pathol. Biol.*, 40, 883, 1992.

83. Perdomo, J. J., Gounon, P., Schaeverbeke, M., Schaeverbeke, J., Groult, V., Jacob, M. P., and Robert, L., Interaction between cells and elastin fibers: an ultrastructural and immunocytochemical study, *J. Cell. Physiol.*, 158, 451, 1994.

84. Krstic, R. V., *Die gewebe des menschen und der Säugetiere*, Springer-Verlag, New York, 1982.

85. Varga, Z., Kovacs, E. M., Paragh, G., Jacob, M. P., Robert, L., and Fülöp, T., Effect of elastin peptides and N-formyl-methionyl-leucyl-phenylalanine on cytosolic free calcium in polymorphonuclear leukocytes of healthy middle-aged and elderly subjects, *Clin. Biochem.*, 21, 127, 1988.

Chapter 16

BRAIN METABOLISM DURING AGING

Siegfried Hoyer

CONTENTS

I. INTRODUCTION

Longevity is one of the oldest desires of mankind. During recent decades medical and social progress have increased the life expectancy of the population, at least in the highly developed countries. However, it is one of the paradoxes of modern and highly specialized medicine that the increase in life expectancy is not accompanied by maintained physical and/or mental health in every case. With age, mental health problems are manifested mainly as dementia and brain infarction. Therefore, it is of general importance to take age-related changes into account when considering the etiopathogenesis of such disorders. Brain morphology and oxidative metabolism undergo inherent variations during aging that may influence neuronal functions and may, thus, contribute to the degree of cellular damage in pathological conditions.

The oxidative metabolism of mature, healthy, nonstarved mammalian brain uses glucose exclusively to form energy as ATP to meet its functional and structural requirements.[1-4] Thus, glucose metabolism is centered in the brain and plays a pivotal role in maintaining cellular homeostasis. In this chapter, oxidative and energy metabolism of the brain will be discussed with respect to normal aging and its possible impacts on pathological conditions.

II. THE NORMALLY AGING BRAIN

A. Morphological Variations

It has been well documented in several studies that neuronal loss and changes in the dendritic arborization occur during normal aging. They are, however, regionally specific, and corresponding brain regions do not change similarly in rodents, non-human primates, and human beings in any case.

Studies in human cerebral cortex revealed that the total number of isocortical neurons is only moderately reduced with aging. A decreased density of large neurons[5,6] has been described, as well as its numerical constancy.[7,8] However, the extent and severity of morphological changes of pyramidal neurons obviously depend on their location within the various layers of the cerebral cortex.[7,9] There are also conflicting findings with respect to the density reduction of small neurons.[5,6,10] The ratio of pyramidal neurons vs. nonpyramidal neurons varied from about 85:15 in the 6th decade of life to about 92:8 in the 9th decade.[7,8] This loss is responsible for decreased cortical volume with age.

In spite of the preservation of the soma of pyramidal neurons, many of them show a destruction in dendritic arborization. The decrease of basal dendrites was more prominent in layer V pyramidal cells than in those of layer III.[11] On the other hand, pyramidal cells not undergoing any destruction develop proliferation of dendrites to compensate for neuronal loss. However, this capacity becomes lost in very old age.[12] In human hippocampus, the number of pyramidal cells decreased for both CA1 and CA4 subfields by 19% beyond the age of 68 years, and the number of granule cells diminished by 15%.[13] Total dendritic length of dentate gyrus granule cells increased between middle age and old age to compensate for neuronal loss, but showed regression in very old age.[14] This property was not found in CA2/3 pyramidal neurons, which showed no age-related dendritic changes.[15]

In rodents, the most frequently studied species in aging research, different results have also been reported with respect to cortical neuronal loss, which obviously depends on whether or not animals are old enough to have reached an age that produces neuronal loss. No changes in neuronal number and in laminar volumes were detected in layer II of the piriform cortex of Sprague-Dawley rats between 3 to 33 months of age.[16] In Sprague-Dawley rats, the thickness of area 17 and the number of nucleus-containing neuronal profiles of layer II through VIb, as well as the diameters of neuronal nuclei, were also found to be largely constant between 3 to 33 months of age.[17] However, in 47-month-old Sprague-Dawley rats, the cortical thickness of area 17 decreased by about 24%. The number of neuronal profiles of layer IV through VIa decreased by 17 to 22%, indicating neuronal loss; whereas, the diameters of neuronal nuclei did not show any age-related decline.[18] In a strain of Wistar-Kyoto rats, a rather uniform reduction of 20 to 30% in number and volume densities of cortical neurons was found and was most pronounced (43%) in the deepest lamina in 22- to 27-month-old rats when compared to 3-month-old ones. Granule neurons of lamina II exhibited no age-related changes in nuclear diameter, but large pyramidal cells of lamina V did.[19] In Sprague-Dawley rats of 24 months of age, a reduction of neuronal density was found.[20] In Fischer 344 rats, a diminution in neuron packing density of 18% was reported from 11 months through 29 months of age.[21] Dendritic length and number of segments remained unchanged in brain cortex of C57 BL/6N mice from 4 through 45 months of age.[22]

In hippocampus, a 14% neuronal loss could be shown in the strata pyramidale and oriens of the CA1 subfield from 11 months through 29 months of age in Fischer 344 rats.[21] This also held true for Wistar-Kyoto rats in which the number of hippocampal CA1 pyramidal neurons decreased from 3 through 22 to 27 months of age.[19] In Fischer 344 rats, a reduction in neuronal density by 25% of CA3 pyramidal cells could be demonstrated in 25- to 28-month-old animals as compared to 4- to 7-month-old ones.[23] Neurons with (^{3}H) corticosterone receptors were also lost in CA2 and CA3 subfields, but were not lost in the CA4 area in 24- to 26-month-old Fischer 344 rats as compared to 3- to 5-month-old animals.[24] In dentate gyrus, no age-related change in the number of granule cells could be found between 3 and 25 months of age in Fischer 344 rats,[25] nor in Sprague-Dawley rats from 4.5 to 6 through 29 to 30 months of age.[26] In the same study, neither synaptic density nor mean spine volume showed any age-related variation. On the other hand, a loss of synapses involving dendritic spines and shafts and axon terminals in dentate gyrus was reported in Fischer 344 rats from 3 through 25 months of age.[25] Studies on synaptic ultrastructure evaluated in cerebellar glomeruli and dentate gyrus supragranular layers clearly showed a decrease of volume density and surface density and of numerical density, and an increase in the size of contact areas during aging from 3 through 28 months in rats, and in human beings.[27,28]

More generally, and with respect to synapse/receptor function, the receptor is supposed to exist in two interconvertible forms: the l form, labile and diffusible; and the s form, stable and resistant to degradation, and immobilized. The s state derives from the l state and is irreversible.[29] If the l state is increasingly converted into the s state with advancing age, this conversion along with the age-related loss of synapses will contribute to decreased neuronal function and thus to diminished neuronal plasticity during aging. From these findings in human and rodent cerebral cortex and hippocampus, it may be assumed that the aging process causes structural changes of a different kind in cortical neurons in the layers III through VI, including pyramidal and nonpyramidal cells. In hippocampus, structural changes became most obvious in the subfields CA1 and CA4, but cell losses were also found in CA2 and CA3 subfields. However, the functionally most important age-related changes may occur at the site of synapses, and these structural changes may point to a particular vulnerability due to variations in energy metabolism (see below).

The synapse was found to be the site of the highest energy utilization as compared to other cellular compartments.[30] Aged mitochondria are less able to fulfil their energy requirement.[31] Synaptic mitochondria of cerebellar glomeruli showed variations (decrease) in numerical density and (increases) in average volume and average skeleton length during aging as compared to the adult life period of female Wistar rats.[32] In heart mitochondria, an age-dependent drastic diminution of the activity of adenine nucleotide translocase was demonstrated.[33,34] Furthermore, in cerebral cortex of primates, the activities of enzymes which catalyze oxidative phosphorylation in complex I and complex IV were age-dependently diminished.[35] The latter findings point to a damage to mitochondrial DNA which encodes the above complexes. Taken together, these above data may indicate distinct age-related abnormalities in both mitochondrial structure and function with impact on mitochondrial work such as energy production (see below).

III. GLUCOSE AND RELATED METABOLISM

A. The Normal Adult Brain

In nonnervous tissue, glucose metabolism is largely controlled by insulin and its signal transduction via the insulin receptor. The regulation of the signal transduction pathway is mediated by amplification and desensitization of responses to the receptor ligand insulin. Amplification of the insulin signal is forwarded by activation of tyrosine kinase, desensitization by activation of serine kinase.[36] Serine phosphorylation by cAMP-dependent kinases counteracts the effect of tyrosine phosphorylation[37] mediated by catecholamines, which have been shown to reduce the tyrosine kinase activity.[38]

There is increasing evidence that insulin in the brain acts similarly as in nonnervous tissue[39] although the origin of cerebral insulin is still an issue of controversial debate. Insulin receptors are widely distributed in the brain with highest densities in olfactory and limbic structures.[40,41]

The control of cerebral glucose metabolism includes various mechanisms. The uptake of glucose from arterial blood into the brain across the blood-brain barrier by means of a carrier-mediated transport mechanism is obviously insulin-dependent.[42-44] The glycolytic breakdown of glucose is controlled by the enzymes hexokinase and pyruvate kinase working in a concerted way under the predominance of phosphofructokinase.[45] The oxidation of the glycolytically formed pyruvate starts by means of the multienzyme complex pyruvate dehydrogenase.[46] Finally, the energy state of brain tissue influences cellular glucose metabolism via feedback mechanisms.

The mitochondrial multienzyme complex pyruvate dehydrogenase (PDH) occupies a preeminent place in glucose metabolism. It provides acetyl groups for subsequent oxidation and energy production on the one hand, and for acetylcholine synthesis on the other. The activity of the enzyme choline acetyltransferase, which catalyzes acetylcholine formation, is closely linked functionally to the PDH complex[47] and is stimulated by means of insulin.[48] The activation state of the PDH complex depends on its state of phosphorylation. Phosphorylation inhibits and dephosphorylation activates this multienzyme complex.[49,50] The activity of the dephosphorylated (active) form of PDH after membrane depolarization is increased by cytosolic Ca^{2+} in brain mitochondria more extensively than in synaptosomes. Calcium accumulation by mitochondria was found to be closely linked to PDH activity when fueled by pyruvate. Phosphorylation of the PDH alpha-subunit may interfere with the calcium-buffering capacity of mitochondria, as PDH activity was markedly reduced when Ca^{2+} uptake by mitochondria was inhibited. Thus, the activation state of the PDH-complex contributes to cellular Ca^{2+} homeostasis.[51,52] On the other hand, activation of PDH decreased in correlation with a reduction of pyruvate-supported calcium transport into mitochondria in the hippocampus after entorhinal cortex lesions.[53] Independently of the intramitochondrial Ca^{2+} concentration, the active dephosphorylated form of PDH increased by stimulation of insulin[54,55] and changed inversely with the concentration of adenine nucleotides.[54] PDH activity is reduced by its product acetyl CoA, e.g., when fatty acids or ketone bodies are used for oxidation.[56]

Under normal conditions, glucose carbon is rapidly transferred into amino acids via the tricarboxylic acid cycle (TCAC) and the gamma-aminobutyric acid (GABA) shunt.[57,58] Glutamate, glutamine, aspartate, and GABA are formed most abundantly.[59-61] At least two compartments of these acidic amino acids are assumed in the brain, one of which is a storage compartment. These glucoplastic amino acids may serve in part as a fuel reserve under emergency conditions when glucose is lacking. Additionally, glutamate and aspartate function as excitatory neurotransmitters active in nearly the whole brain but particularly in the entorhinal afferents and the Schaffer collaterals, both ending in the CA1 subfield of the hippocampus and also in its mossy fibers.[62] Cholinergic neurons receive glutamatergic afferents.[63-65] Upon K^+-evoked depolarization, aspartate, glutamate, and GABA were preferentially released from neocortical tissue, the efflux of glutamate being calcium dependent.[66] After its release from nerve endings, glutamate binds with high affinity to postsynaptic dendritic membranes.[67] Furthermore, glutamate induced release of GABA from cerebral cortex interneurons[68] and enhanced GABA-activated conductances in hippocampal pyramidal neurons at concentrations below that required for excitation.[69]

It thus becomes obvious that brain glucose metabolism, as well as metabolism of related compounds, may play a central and pivotal role in maintaining normal neuronal function. Disturbances in glucose metabolism may therefore give rise to neuronal damage, causing abnormal mental states.

B. The Aging Brain

It has been well documented in several studies that mental capacity is closely associated with the functioning of brain perfusion necessary for both substrate supply and waste product transportation, as well as with the functioning of oxidative and energy metabolism. There has been a protracted controversy as to whether or not cerebral blood flow and metabolism decrease with advancing age. From data reviewed in the literature, it may be deduced that there is a minor reduction of cerebral blood flow and utilization rates of oxygen and glucose between the 3rd to 4th and the 7th to 8th decades of life, with a more severe decrease in later life.[70] Thus, a threshold phenomenon with regard to brain perfusion and nutrition may be assumed with advancing age. The same holds true for the activities of phosphofructokinase,[71] choline acetyltransferse,[72] and acetylcholine esterase along with acetylcholine synthesis[73] in normally aging human brain. Furthermore, cAMP-dependent protein kinase and glutamate decarboxylase were markedly diminished beyond the age of 70 years. However, no age-related variations became obvious in Na^+-K^+-ATPase and Mg^{2+}-ATPase that break down ATP.[73] Reductions in the above brain parameters before this threshold of 70 years in human life may therefore be disease related rather than age related.

From animal studies, it may be deduced that in brain cortex and in some subcortical nuclei glucose consumption diminishes from development to adulthood, but not further with advanced age.[74-76] At the cellular level, a moderate but steady decline in the concentration of glycolytic compounds was found from development to senescence. However, the diminution was not evenly distributed with respect to the different periods of life. Glucose and fructose-1,6-diphosphate, and ATP, too, decreased the most from development to adulthood, whereas pyruvate and creatine phosphate fell most from adulthood to senescence.[77] The changes in glycolytic compounds are associated with age-related reductions in the activities of the enzymes hexokinase and phosphofructokinase, controlling glycolytic flux.[78,79] On the other hand, only slight variations are found in the oxidation processes of the tricarboxylic acid cycle and the respiratory chain with aging. The decrease in malate concentration found in senescent rats may be consistent with the reduced activity of malate dehydrogenase,[77,80] indicating diminished tricarboxylic acid cycle activity. Otherwise, no age-related changes were reported in the enzyme activities of pyruvate dehydrogenase complex (active and total), citrate synthase, NAD^+-isocitrate dehydrogenase, fumarase, and NAD^+ malate dehydrogenase,[81,82] although the finding about NAD^+-isocitrate dehydrogenase was inconsistent.[83] Studies on cytochrome a, a_3 as the final member of substrate oxidation that reacts directly with molecular oxygen revealed no aged-related changes.[84] However, in cerebral cortex of rats, oxygen consumption was found to decrease gradually with age[85] and $^{14}CO_2$ production diminished by around 30% in senescence. The neurotransmitters that derive from the breakdown of glucose in the brain also show reduced concentrations with aging. Acetylcholine synthesis declined to 65% in senescence as compared to young adulthood; acetylcholine release dropped to around 25% in the same study,[86] and to around 50% in another.[87] The number of muscarinic receptors in the dorsal hippocampus was reduced by 22% in aged rats.[88] In total, these findings are indicative of the reduced capacity of the acetylcholinergic system with age.

When glucose/energy metabolism and its control of the aging brain is considered, in particular, ante mortem, it has to be noted that in physically and mentally healthy senescent subjects a 23% reduction was found in the cerebral metabolic rate of glucose without any change in cerebral oxygen utilization.[89,90] When ATP formation is calculated on the basis of these data, a slight fall (by around 5%) becomes obvious. This also holds true for experimental animals: the availability of energy was reduced by 5% in parietotemporal cerebral cortex of 104-week-old rats compared with 52-

week-old rats under resting conditions[135] but dropped by 15% in very old (130 weeks of age) rats.[77]

As discussed above, diverse variations are found in cerebral glucose metabolism during aging. This fact may point to a dysregulation of the neuronal insulin signal transduction pathway. Thus, ^{125}I-insulin binding was found to be decreased in the olfactory bulb, but not in the frontal cortex, hippocampus, and hypothalamus in aged rats.[91] In human B cells, and not proven for the brain as yet, aging altered the activation and expression of phosphotyrosine kinases of endogenous proteins.[92] Whether or not the tyrosine kinase of the insulin receptor is also involved remains to be established.

Both the pre- and postsynaptic efficiency in the noradrenergic system was reduced, with only slight changes in the noradrenergic concentration in the aging brain, but no changes were noted in noradrenaline turnover.[93-97] At first view, these findings along with the reduced activity of cAMP-dependent protein kinase[73] renders it less likely that the noradrenergic system is increased in its capacity during aging to inhibit the activity of tyrosine kinase of the insulin receptor. However, it was recently demonstrated that aging prolonged the stress-induced release of noradrenaline in rat hypothalamus.[98] Otherwise, recent studies have provided evidence that glucocorticoids counteract the effect of insulin in the brain (Plaschke and Hoyer, in preparation). After stress, the circulating glucocorticoid concentrations remained elevated longer in aged animals, whereas there was a decline to basal levels in young animals.[99,100] It is tempting to assume that this effect leads to a glucocorticoid-mediated decrease in tyrosine phosphorylation of the neuronal insulin receptor, as was demonstrated for skeletal muscle.[101]

The glucose-derived amino acids glutamate and aspartate diminished in aged brain. However, it is controversial as to whether or not the synthesis of glutamate from glucose remained unchanged[102] or reduced, since the conversion of glucose carbon into glutamate, glutamine, GABA, aspartate, and alanine was diminished in the cerebrum with aging.[103] As mentioned above, the basal release of glutamate in striatum and hippocampus increased with aging, thus raising its extracellular concentration; whereas, the level after K^+ stimulation remained unaffected.[104] Glutamate binding to hippocampal membranes increased progressively, due to the growing number of binding sites rather than an increase in their affinity for glutamate.[105]

One additional aspect related to cerebral glucose metabolism needs to be considered: the activity of free radicals which are potent in cellular destruction via proteolysis and lipid peroxidation.[106] The formation of free radicals was shown to increase with advancing age.[107-109] Tissue lactacidosis dramatically enhanced the formation of free radicals in brain tissue, obviously by its mediation of an increased dissociation of catalytic iron from proteins of the transferrin type.[110]

A discussion of the age-related changes in glucose and related metabolism does not provide an answer to why some biological parameters, which are considered to be important in maintaining normal neuronal function, start to become abnormal past the 7th to 8th decade of human life and late in the life of rodents, while other parameters remain unchanged. The majority of biological abnormalities in the nondiseased aging process of the brain may point to a first slight incipient perturbation of neuronal homeostasis.[111] This includes reductions in neuronal glucose utilization due to a decreased glycolytic flux, slight aberrations in glucose oxidation, diminished synthesis and release of acetylcholine, and increases in the concentrations of cytosolic Ca^{2+}, extracellular glutamate and glutamate binding, as well as an enhancement of free radical formation and its augmentation under lactacidosis. In all probability, these metabolic variations in the "milieu interieur" may give rise to the morphological destruction of highly vulnerable neurons during aging. Under resting conditions, these variations may be sufficiently compensated for even in old age. However, in stress situations such a compensation may fail or be retarded, and functional normalization may be jeopardized.

It has been demonstrated that the changes in cerebral glucose metabolism were more severe in aged animals when compared to adult ones.[112] Recovery of the energy pool in the cerebral cortex after arterial hypoglycemia was found to be more markedly compromised in aged than in adult animals, as was the restoration of the cerebral amino acid pool. On the other hand, the concentration of ammonia more than doubled in aged brains when compared to adult ones.[113] Cerebral ischemia caused a more pronounced fall in the adenosine nucleotide level in aged than in adult animals, and the delayed decrease in energy-rich phosphates in the postischemic recirculation period was more severe in aged than in young adult animals.[114,115]

Intensive mental activation increased the cerebral cortex energy pool (sum of adenine nucleotides, and sum of ATP + creatine phosphate) by 25 and 13% in adult, and by 21 and 9% in aged animals, indicating that an age-dependent decline in the size of the energy pool could not be prevented by short-term mental activation. The diminution of the energy pool with aging was even more marked after mental activation than after mental rest. Mental activation induced an increase in ATP turnover up to 24 months of age in male Wistar rats (aged animals).[135] However, at the age of 30 months (very old animals), ATP turnover fell drastically although ATP formation was found to be unchanged. These changes are thought to be due to an age-related reduction in mitochondrial function, as was mentioned above.[32-35]

From the data discussed above, it becomes evident that aging leads to inherent changes in fundamental metabolic principles at the cellular and molecular levels. These changes are accentuated under stress. Anabolic capacities, and the capacities of cellular repair and cellular defense on the one side, and the degree of vulnerability on the other, may be assumed to diverge with aging.[116,118]

As discussed above in more detail, the stress-induced demand for energy cannot be sufficiently met in the aged brain so that energy-dependent processes are compromised. Among numerous such processes, one was found to be of central importance during the aging process: mixed function oxidation (MFO), also termed metal-catalyzed oxidation (MCO).[119] Continuous intracellular protein turnover includes oxidative inactivation by various enzymatic and nonenzymatic MFO processes that precede proteolysis.[120-124] The oxidation of amino acids to carbonyl derivatives, mediated by the formation of oxygen free radicals, is synergistically affected by nucleoside diphosphates and triphosphates and by bicarbonate,[123] and the degradation of proteins is ATP-dependent.[125-127] An age-related increase in superoxide radical formation at plasma membranes appears earlier in the brain than in the heart and liver.[128] Consistent with these observations, the amount of oxidized proteins increases in the brain cortex during normal aging.[129-131] Thus, the aged brain may be characterized by an imbalance between enhanced formation of oxidized, damaged proteins and the cellular capacity to degrade them, because protease activities are reduced.[129] Thus, this metabolic imbalance as a whole may contribute considerably to neuronal vulnerability and may render the aged brain prone to functional and structural abnormalities.

IV. THE PRINCIPLE OF CRITICALITY

In the physical sciences, the term criticality is used to describe a self-organized metalabile steady state. Criticality can progress to supercriticality, which is able to induce a catastrophic reaction, subsequently approaching another metalabile steady state. Snowslides, for example, can be explained in this manner.[132,133] Although the principle of criticality has not yet been proven for biological systems, in all probability it is applicable here, too. The model of coupled synchronization has been demonstrated to exist in biological systems, and this model may be assumed to be very closely related to criticality,[134] i.e., the uncoupling of synchronization may induce supercriticality.

To give a simplified example: take, for example, an area of distinct size containing a small number of groups of dominoes at some distance from each other, which represents the degree of vulnerability. If one of the dominoes in one of the groups falls (increased vulnerability due to a damaging event), only the near neighbors of this domino fall as well (subcriticality: compensation of damage in young adulthood). Criticality is the state when the number of dominoes increases so that the groups approach one another. Now, if one domino falls, the dominoes of several, but not all groups, also fall (adulthood). When the given area is nearly completely filled with dominoes (increase of uncoupled synchronization, high degree of vulnerability in old age), should only one domino fall then the whole system collapses (supercriticality: vulnerability shifts to damage).

As has been discussed above, numerous smaller but permanent aberrations in glucose/energy metabolism and in related metabolism occur in the brain from adulthood to senescence. This pattern may reflect a distinct metalabile steady state in aged neurons. Any small additional abnormality, even one that is ineffective in itself, may change the former steady state and may cause a catastrophic reaction representing another new but detrimental steady state. In this context, age may be considered as a risk factor for neuronal damage and, thus, for age-related brain disorders such as sporadic dementia of the Alzheimer type and Parkinson's disease.

V. CONCLUSIONS

Aging is a fateful process which leads to inherent changes of fundamental biological principles at the structural, cellular, and molecular levels. As far as oxidative glucose/energy metabolism and related metabolism is concerned, reduced energy availability, diminished formation of glucose-derived neurotransmitters, enhanced formation of free radical formation, and decreases in clearing and repair capacities are involved, obviously due to an imbalance between amplification and desensitization of the neuronal insulin receptor. Such a pivotal variation at the control level of neuronal glucose metabolism may be assumed to induce cascade-like changes altering the metalabile steady state of the cell, i.e., changing the state of criticality. The multiplicity of slight variations may indicate that not only one metabolic change governs the process of aging. The divergence between anabolic and catabolic metabolic processes may be assumed to increase with aging, becoming particularly evident after stress situations. In these terms, the aging brain may be considered to be at risk for (permanent) neuronal damage and, thus, age-related mental disabilities.

REFERENCES

1. Gibbs, E. L., Lennox, W. G., Nims, L. F., and Gibbs, F. A., Arterial and cerebral venous blood. Arterial-venous differences in man, *J. Biol. Chem.*, 144, 325, 1942.
2. Gottstein, U., Bernsmeier, A., and Sedlmeyer, I., Der Kohlenhydratstoffwechsel des menschlichen Gehirns. I. Untersuchungen mit substratspezifischen enzymatischen Methoden bei normaler Hirndurchblutung, *Klin. Wschr.*, 41, 943, 1963.

3. Hoyer, S., Der Aminosäurenstoffwechsel des normalen menschlichen Gehirns, *Klin. Wschr.*, 48, 1239, 1970.

4. Siesjö, B. K., *Brain Energy Metabolism*, John Wiley & Sons, Chichester, 1978, chap. 1 and 6.

5. Brody, H., Organization of the cerebral cortex. III. A study of aging in the human cerebral cortex, *J. Comp. Neurol.*, 102, 511, 1955.

6. Henderson, G., Tomlinson, B. E., and Gibson, P. H., Cell counts in human cerebral cortex in normal adults throughout life using an image analysing computer, *J. Neurol. Sci.*, 46, 113, 1980.

7. Braak, H. and Braak, E., Ratio of pyramidal cells versus non-pyramidal cells in the human frontal isocortex and changes in ratio with aging and Alzheimer's disease, *Prog. Brain Res.*, 70, 185, 1986.

8. Braak, H. and Braak, E., Morphology of the human isocortex in young and aged individuals: Qualitative and quantitative findings, *Interdiscipl. Topics Gerontol.*, 25, 1, 1988.

9. Haug, H., Kuhl, S., Mecke, E., Sass, N. L., and Wasner, K., The significance of morphometric procedures in the investigation of age changes in cytoarchitectonic structures of human brain, *J. Hirnforsch.*, 25, 353, 1984.

10. Terry, R. D., De Teresa, R., and Hansen, L. A., Neocortical cell counts in normal human adult aging, Ann. Neurol., 21, 530, 1987.

11. Nakamura, S., Akiguchi, I., Kameyama, M., and Mizuno, N., Age-related changes of pyramidal cell basal dendrites in layers III and V of human motor cortex. A quantitative Golgy-study, *Acta Neuropathol.*, 65, 281, 1985.

12. Coleman, P. D. and Flood, D. G., Dendritic proliferation in the aging brain as a compensatory repair mechanism, *Prog. Brain Res.*, 70, 227, 1986.

13. Mouritzen Dam, A., The density of neurons in the human hippocampus, *Neuropathol. Appl. Neurobiol.*, 5, 249, 1979.

14. Flood, D.G., Buell, S.J., Horwitz, G.J., and Coleman, P.D., Dendritic extent in human dentate gyrus granule cells in normal aging and senile dementia, *Brain Res.*, 402, 205, 1987.

15. Flood, D. G., Guarnaccia, M., and Coleman, P. D., Dendritic extent in human CA2/3 hippocampal pyramidal neurons in normal aging and senile dementia, *Brain Res.*, 409, 88, 1987.

16. Curcio, C. A., McNelly, N. A., and Hinds, J. W., Aging in the rat olfactory system. Relative stability of piriform cortex contrasts with changes in olfactory bulb and olfactory epithelium, *J. Comp. Neurol.*, 235, 519, 1985.

17. Peters, A., Feldman, M. L., and Vaugham, D. W., The effect of aging on the neuronal population within area 17 of adult rat cerebral cortex, *Neurobiol. Aging*, 4, 273, 1983.

18. Peters, A., Harriman, K. M., and West, C. D., The effect of increased longevity, produced by dietary restriction, on the neuronal population of area 17 in rat cerebral cortex, *Neurobiol. Aging*, 8, 7, 1987.

19. Knox, C. A., Effects of aging and chronic arterial hypertension on the cell population in the neocortex and archicortex of the rat, *Acta Neuropathol.*, 56, 139, 1982.

20. Mufson, E. J. and Stein, D. G., Behavioral and morphological aspects of aging. An analysis of rat frontal cortex, in *The Psychobiology of Aging: Problems and Perspectives*, Stein, D. G., Ed., Elsevier/North Holland, Amsterdam, 1980, 99.

21. Brizzee, K. R. and Ordy, J. M., Age pigments, cell loss and hippocampal function, *Mech. Ageing Dev.*, 9, 143, 1979.

22. Coleman, P. D., Buell, S. J., Magagna, L., Flood, D. G., and Curcio, C. A., Stability of dendrites in cortical barrels of C 57 BL/GN mice between 4 and 45 months, *Neurobiol. Aging*, 7, 101, 1986.

23. Landfield, P. W., Braun, L. D., Pitler, T. A., Lindsey, J. D., and Lynch, G., Hippocampal aging in rats: a morphometric study of multiple variables in semithin sections, *Neurobiol. Aging,* 2, 265, 1981.

24. Sapolsky, R. M., Krey, L. C., McEwen, B. S., and Rainbow, T. C., Do vasopressin-related peptides induce hippocampal corticosterone receptors? Implications for aging?, *J. Neurosci.,* 4, 1479, 1984.

25. Bondareff, W., Synaptic atrophy in the senescent hippocampus, *Mech. Ageing Dev.,* 9, 163, 1979.

26. Curcio, C. A. and Hinds, J. W., Stability of synaptic density and spine volume in dentate gyrus of aged rats, *Neurobiol. Aging,* 4, 77, 1983.

27. Bertoni-Freddari, C., Fattoretti, P., Casoli, T., Meier-Ruge, W., and Ulrich, J., Morphological adaptive response of the synaptic junctional zones in the human dentate gyrus during aging and Alzheimer's disease, *Brain Res.,* 517, 69, 1990.

28. Bertoni-Freddari, C., Fattoretti, P., Casoli, T., Pieroni, M., Meier-Ruge, W., and Ulrich, J., Neurobiology of the aging brain: morphological alterations at synaptic regions, *Arch. Gerontol. Geriatr.,* 12, 253, 1991.

29. Changeux, J. P. and Danchin, A., Selective stabilization of developing synapses as a mechanism for the specification of neuronal network, *Nature,* 264, 705, 1976.

30. Kadokaro, M., Crane, A. M., and Sokoloff, L., Differential effects of electric stimulation of sciatic nerve on metabolic activity in spinal cord and dorsal root ganglion in the rat, *Proc. Natl. Acad. Sci. U.S.A.,* 82, 6010, 1985.

31. Corbisier, P. and Remacle, J., Influence of the energetic pattern of mitochondria in cell aging, *Mech. Ageing Dev.,* 71, 47, 1993.

32. Bertoni-Freddari, C., Fattoretti, P., Casoli, T., Spagna, C., Meier-Ruge, W., and Ulrich, J., Morphological plasticity of synaptic mitochondria during aging, *Brain Res.,* 628, 193, 1993.

33. Nohl, H. and Krämer, R., Molecular basis of age-dependent changes in the activity of adenine nucleotide translocase, *Mech. Ageing Dev.,* 14, 137, 1980.

34. Kim, J. H., Shrago, E., and Elson, C. E., Age-related changes in respiration coupled to phosphorylation. II. Cardiac mitochondria, *Mech. Ageing Dev.,* 46, 279, 1988.

35. Bowling, A. C., Mutisya, E. M., Walker, L. C., Price, D. L., Cork, L. C., and Beal, M. F., Age-dependent impairment of mitochondrial function in primate brain, *J. Neurochem.,* 60, 1964, 1993.

36. Häring, H. U., The insulin receptor: signalling mechanism and contribution to the pathogenesis of insulin resistance, *Diabetilogia,* 34, 848, 1991.

37. Roth, R. A. and Beaudoin, J., Phosphorylation of purified insulin receptor by cAMP kinase, *Diabetes,* 36, 123, 1987.

38. Häring, H. U., Kirsch, D., Obermaier, B., Ermel, B., and Machicao, F., Decreased tyrosine kinase activity of insulin receptor isolated from rat adipocytes rendered insulin- resistant by catecholamine treatment in vitro, *Biochem. J.,* 234, 59, 1986.

39. Hoyer, S., Prem, L., Sorbi, S., and Amaducci, L., Stimulation of glycolytic key enzymes in cerebral cortex by insulin, *NeuroReport,* 4, 991, 1993.

40. Hill, J. M., Lesniak, M. A., Pert, C. B., and Roth, J., Autoradiographic localization of insulin receptors in rat brain: prominence in olfactory and limbic areas, *Neuroscience,* 17, 1127, 1986.

41. Unger, J. W., Livingston, J. N., and Moss, A. M., Insulin receptors in the central nervous system: localization, signaling mechanisms and functional aspects, *Progr. Neurobiol.,* 36, 343, 1991.

42. Bachelard, H. S., Specific and kinetic properties of monosaccharide uptake into guinea pig cerebral cortex in vitro, *J. Neurochem.,* 13, 213, 1971.

43. Hertz, M. M., Paulson, O. B., Barry, D. L., Christansen, J. S., and Swendsen, P. A., Insulin increases glucose transfer across the blood-brain barrier, *J. Clin. Invest.*, 67, 597, 1981.

44. Kahn, C. R., The molecular mechanism of insulin action, *Ann. Rev. Med.*, 36, 429, 1985.

45. Newsholme, E. A. and Start, C., Regulation in metabolism, John Wiley & Sons, Chichester, 1973, chap. 3.

46. Garland, P. B. and Randle, P. J., Control of pyruvate dehydrogenase in the perfused rat heart by the intracellular concentration of acetyl-coenzyme A, *Biochem. J.*, 91, 6C, 1964.

47. Perry, E. K., Perry, R. H., Tomlinson, B. E., Blessed, G., and Gibson, P. H., Coenzyme A acetylating enzymes in Alzheimer's disease: possible cholinergic "compartment" of pyruvate dehydrogenase, *Neurosci. Lett.*, 18, 105, 1980.

48. Kyriakis, J. M., Hausman, R. E., and Peterson, S. W., Insulin stimulates choline acetyltransferase activity in cultured embryonic chicken retina neurons, *Proc. Natl. Acad. Sci. U.S.A.*, 84, 7463, 1987.

49. Linn, T. C., Pettit, F. H., and Reed, L. J., Alpha-keto acid dehydrogenase complexes. X. Regulation of the activity of the pyruvate dehydrogenase complex from beef kidney mitochondria by phosphorylation and dephosphorylation, *Proc. Natl. Acad. Sci. U.S.A.*, 62, 234, 1969.

50. Linn, T. C., Pettit, F. H., Hucho, F., and Reed, L. J., Alpha-keto acid dehydrogenase complexes. XI. Comparative studies of regulatory properties of the pyruvate dehydrogenase complex from kidney, heart, and liver mitochondria, *Proc. Natl. Acad. Sci. U.S.A.*, 64, 227, 1969.

51. Browning, M., Baudry, M., Bennett, W. F., and Lynch, G., Phosphorylation-mediated changes in pyruvate dehydrogenase activity influence pyruvate-supported calcium accumulation by brain mitochondria, *J. Neurochem.*, 36, 1932, 1981.

52. Hansford, R. G. and Castro, F., Role of CA^{2+} in pyruvate dehydrogenase interconversion in brain mitochondria and synaptosomes, *Biochem. J.*, 227, 129, 1985.

53. Baudry, M., Fuchs, J., Kessler, M., Arst, D., and Lynch, G., Entorhinal cortex lesions induce a decreased calcium transport in hippocampal mitochondria, *Science*, 216, 411, 1982.

54. Jope, R. and Blass, P. J., The regulation of pyruvate dehydrogenase in brain in vivo, *J. Neurochem.*, 26, 709, 1976.

55. Denton, R. M., McCormack, J. G., and Thomas, A. P., Hormonal regulation of intramitochondrial metabolism, *Biol. Chem. Hoppe-Seyler*, Suppl. 367, 64, 1986.

56. Garland, P. B., Newsholme, E. A., and Randle, P. J., Regulation of glucose uptake by muscle. IX. Effects of fatty acids and ketone bodies, and of alloxan-diabetes and starvation, on pyruvate metabolism and on lactate/pyruvate and L-glycerol 3-phosphate/dihydroacetone phosphate concentration ratios in the rat heart and rat diaphragm muscles, *Biochem. J.*, 93, 665, 1964.

57. Sacks, W., Cerebral metabolism of isotopic glucose in normal human subjects, *J. Appl. Physiol.*, 10, 37, 1957.

58. Sacks, W., Cerebral metabolism of doubly labeled glucose in human in vivo, *J. Appl. Physiol.*, 20, 117, 1965.

59. Barkulis, S. S., Geiger, A., Kawikata, Y., and Aquilar, V., A study of the incorporation of ^{14}C derived from glucose into free amino acids of the brain cortex, *J. Neurochem.*, 5, 339, 1960.

60. Geiger, A., Kawikata, Y., and Barkulis, S. S., Major pathways of glucose utilization in the brain in brain perfusion experiments in vivo and in situ, *J. Neurochem.*, 5, 323, 1960.

61. Wong, K. L. and Tyce, G. M., Glucose and amino acid metabolism in rat brain during sustained hypoglycemia, *Neurochem. Res.*, 8, 401, 1983.

62. Strange, P. G., The structure and mechanism of neurotransmitter receptors. Implications for the structure and function of the central nervous system, *Biochem. J.*, 249, 309, 1988.

63. Malthe-Sorensen, D., Skrede, K., and Fonnum, F., Calcium dependent release of D-³H-aspartate from the dorsal septum after electrical stimulation of the fimbria in vitro, *Neuroscience*, 5, 127, 1980.

64. Walaas, I. and Fonnum, F., Biochemical evidence for glutamate as a transmitter in hippocampal efferents to the basal forebrain and hypothalamus in the rat brain, *Neuroscience*, 5, 1691, 1980.

65. Davies, S. W., McBean, G. J., and Roberts, P. J., A glutamatergic innervation of the nucleus basalis/substantia innominata, *Neurosci. Lett.*, 45, 105, 1984.

66. Smith, C. C. T., Bowen, D. M., and Davison, A. N., The evoked release of endogenous amino acids from tissue prisms of human neocortex, *Brain Res.*, 269, 103, 1983.

67. Rothman, S. M. and Olney, J. W., Glutamate and the pathophysiology of hypoxic-ischemic brain damage, *Ann. Neurol.*, 19, 105, 1986.

68. Drejer, J., Honore, T., and Schousboe, A., Excitatory amino acid-induced release of ³H-GABA from cultured mouse cerebral cortex interneurons, *J. Neurosci.*, 7, 2910, 1987.

69. Stelzer, A. and Wong, R. K. S., GABA response in hippocampal neurons are potentiated by glutamate, *Nature*, 337, 170, 1989.

70. Hoyer, S., Senile dementia and Alzheimer's disease. Brain blood flow and metabolism, *Prog. Neuropsychopharmacol. Biol. Psychiatr.*, 10, 447, 1986.

71. Meier-Ruge, W., Hunziker, O., Iwangoff, P., Reichlmeier, K., and Schultz, U., Effect of age on morphological and biochemical parameters of the human brain, in *The Psychobiology of Aging: Problems and Perspectives*, Stein, D. C., Ed., Elsevier/North Holland, Amsterdam, 1980, 297.

72. Davies, P., Neurotransmitter-related enzymes in senile dementia of the Alzheimer type, *Brain Res.*, 171, 319, 1979.

73. Bowen, D. M., Smith, C. B., White, P., Flack, R. H. A., Carrasco, L. H., Gedye, J. L., and Davison, A. N., Chemical pathology of the organic dementias. II. Quantitative estimation of cellular changes in post-mortem brain, *Brain*, 100, 427, 1977.

74. London, E. D., Nespor, S. M., Ohata, M., and Rapoport, S. I., Local cerebral glucose utilization during development and aging in the Fischer-344 rat, *J. Neurochem.*, 37, 317, 1981.

75. Smith, C. B., Goochee, C., Rapoport, I., and Sokoloff, L., Effects of aging on local rates of cerebral glucose utilization in the rat, *Brain*, 103, 351, 1980.

76. Takei, H., Fredericks, W. R., London, E. D., and Rapoport, S. I., Cerebral blood flow and oxidative metabolism in conscious Fischer-344 rats of different ages, *J. Neurochem.*, 40, 801, 1983.

77. Hoyer, S., The effect of age on glucose and energy metabolism in brain cortex of rats, *Arch. Gerontol. Geriatr.*, 4, 193, 1985.

78. Iwangoff, P., Armbruster, R., Enz, A., Meier-Ruge, W., and Sandoz, P., Glycolytic enzymes from human autoptic brain cortex: normally aged and demented cases, in *Biochemistry of Dementia*, Roberts, P. J., Ed., John Wiley & Sons, Chichester, 1980, 258.

79. Leong, S. W. and Clark, J. B., Regional enzyme development in rat brain. Enzymes associated with glucose utilization, *Biochem. J.*, 218, 131, 1984.

80. Benzi, G., Arrigoni, E., Dagani, F., Marzatico, F., Curti, D., Polgatti, M., and Villa, R. F., Aging and brain enzymes, in *The Aging Brain, Neurological and Mental Disturbances*, Barbagello-Sangiorgi, G. and Exton-Smith, A. N., Eds., Plenum Press, New York, 1980, 1.

81. Leong, S. F., Lim, J. C. K., and Clark, J. B., Energy-metabolizing enzymes in brain regions of adult and aging rats, *J. Neurochem.*, 37, 1548, 1981.

82. Deshmukh, D. R., Owen, O. E., and Patel, M. S., Effect of aging on the metabolism of pyruvate and 3-hydroxybutyrate in nonsynaptic and synaptic mitochondria from rat brain, *J. Neurochem.*, 34, 1219, 1980.

83. Patel, M. S., Age-dependent changes in the oxidative metabolism in rat brain, *J. Gerontol.*, 32, 643, 1977.

84. Sylvia, A. L. and Rosenthal, M., The effect of age and lung pathology on cytochrome a, a_3 redox levels in rat cerebral cortex, *Brain Res.*, 146, 109, 1978.

85. Peng, M.-T., Peng, Y.-L., and Chen, F.-N., Age-dependent changes in the oxygen consumption of the cerebral cortex, hypothalamus, hippocampus and amygdaloid in rats, *J. Gerontol.*, 32, 517, 1977.

86. Gibson, G. E. and Peterson, C., Aging decreases oxidative metabolism and the release and synthesis of acetylcholine, *J. Neurochem.*, 37, 978, 1981.

87. Pedata, F., Slavikova, J., Kotas, A., and Pepeu, G., Acetylcholine release from rat cortical slices during postnatal development and aging, *Neurobiol. Aging*, 4, 31, 1983.

88. Lippa, A. S., Critchett, D. J., Ehlert, F., Yamamura, H. I., Enna, S. J., and Bartus, R. T., Age-related alterations in neurotransmitter receptors: an electrophysiological and biochemical analysis, *Neurobiol. Aging*, 2, 3, 1981.

89. Dastur, D. K., Lane, M. H., Hansen, D. B., Kety, S. S., Butler, R. N., Perlin, S., and Sokoloff, L., Effects of aging on cerebral circulation and metabolism in man, in *Human Aging — A Biological and Behavioural Study*, Birren, J. E., Butler, R. N., Greenhouse, S. W., Sokoloff, L., and Yarrow, M. R., Eds., U.S. Department of Health, Education and Welfare, National Institute of Mental Health, DHEW Publ. No 986, Washington, D.C., 1963, 59.

90. Dastur, D. K., Cerebral blood flow and metabolism in normal human aging, pathological aging, and senile dementia, *J. Cereb. Blood Flow Metab.*, 5, 1, 1985.

91. Tchilian, E. Z., Zhelezarov, I. E., Petkov, V. V., and Hadjiivanova, C. I., ^{125}I-insulin binding is decreased in olfactory bulbs of aged rats, *Neuropeptides*, 17, 193, 1990.

92. Whisler, R. L. and Grants, I. S., Age-related alterations in the activation and expression of phosphotyrosine kinases and protein kinase C (PKC) among human B cells, *Mech. Ageing Dev.*, 71, 31, 1993.

93. Walker, C. and Walker, J. P., Properties of adenylate cyclase from senescent rat brain, *Brain Res.*, 54, 391, 1973.

94. Schmidt, M. J. and Thornberry, J. F., Cyclic AMP and cyclic CMP accumulation in vitro in brain regions of young, old and aged rats, *Brain Res.*, 139, 169, 1978.

95. Jones, R. S. G. and Olpe, H. R., Altered sensitivity of forebrain neurones to iontophoretically applied noradrenaline in aging rats, *Neurobiol. Aging*, 4, 97, 1983.

96. McIntosh, H. H. and Westfall, T. C., Influence of aging on catecholamine levels, accumulation, and release in F-344 rats, *Neurobiol. Aging*, 8, 233, 1987.

97. Venero, J. L., de la Roza, C., Machado, A., and Cano, J., Age-related changes on monoamine turnover in hippocampus of rats, *Brain Res.*, 631, 89, 1993.

98. Perego, C., Vetrugno, C. C., De Simoni, M. G., and Algeri, S., Aging prolongs the stress-induced release of noradrenaline in rat hypothalamus, *Neurosci. Lett.*, 157, 127, 1993.

99. Sapolsky, R. M., Krey, L. C., and McEwen, B. S., Glucocorticoid-sensitive hippocampal neurons are involved in terminating the adrenocortical stress response, *Proc. Natl. Acad. Sci. U.S.A.*, 81, 6174, 1984.

100. Sapolsky, R. M., Krey, L. C., and McEwen, B. S., The neuroendocrinology of stress and aging: the glucocorticoid cascade hypothesis, *Endocrine Rev.*, 7, 284, 1986.

101. Giorgino, F., Almahfouz, A., Goodyear, L. J., and Smith, R. J., Glucocorticoid regulation of insulin receptor and substrate IRS-1 tyrosine phosphorylation in rat skeletal muscle in vivo, *J. Clin. Invest.*, 91, 2020, 1993.

102. Dekoning-Verest, I. F., Glutamate metabolism in aging rat brain, *Mech. Ageing Develop.*, 13, 83, 1980.

103. Tyce, G. M. and Wong, K.-L., Conversion of glucose to neurotransmitter amino acids in the brains of young and aging rats, *Exp. Gerontol.*, 15, 527, 1980.

104. Freeman, G. B. and Gibson, G. E., Selective alteration of mouse brain neurotransmitter release with age, *Neurobiol. Aging*, 8, 147, 1987.

105. Baudry, M., Arst, D. S., and Lynch, G., Increased (^{3}H) glutamate receptor binding in aged rats, *Brain Res.*, 223, 195, 1981.

106. Davies, K. J. A. and Goldberg, A. L., Oxygen radicals stimulate intracellular proteolysis and lipid peroxidation by independent mechanisms in erythrocytes, *J. Biol. Chem.*, 262, 8220, 1987.

107. Harman, D., The aging process, *Proc. Natl. Acad. Sci. U.S.A.*, 78, 7124, 1981.

108. Leibovitz, B. E. and Siegel, B. V., Aspects of free radical reactions in biological systems: aging, *J. Gerontol.*, 35, 45, 1980.

109. Scarpa, M., Rigo, A., Viglino, P., Stevanato, R., Bracco, F., and Battistin, L., Age dependence of the level of the enzymes involved in the protection against active oxygen species in the rat brain, *Proc. Soc. Exp. Biol. Med.*, 185, 129, 1987.

110. Rehncrona, S., Hauge, H. N., and Siesjö, B. K., Enhancement of iron-catalyzed free radical formation by acidosis in brain homogenates: difference in effect by lactic acid and CO_2, *J. Cereb. Blood Flow Metab.*, 9, 65, 1989.

111. Khachaturian, Z. S., Towards theories of brain aging, in *Handbook of Studies on Psychiatry and Old Age*, Kay, D. W. K. and Burrows, G. D., Eds., Elsevier, Amsterdam, 1984, 7.

112. Degrell, I., Krier, C., and Hoyer S., Carbohydrate and energy metabolism of the aging rat brain in severe arterial hypoxemia, in *Neuropathology and Neuropharmacology*, (Aging Vol. 21), Cervos-Navarro, J. and Sarkander, H. I., Eds., Raven Press, New York, 1983, 289.

113. Benzi, G., Pastoris, O., Villa, R. F., and Giuffrida-Stella, A. M., Effect of aging on cerebral cortex energy metabolism in hypoglycemia and posthypoglycemic recovery, *Neurobiol. Aging*, 5, 205, 1984.

114. Hoyer, S. and Krier, C., Ischemia and the aging brain. Studies on glucose and energy metabolism in rat cerebral cortex, *Neurobiol. Aging*, 7, 23, 1986.

115. Hoyer, S. and Betz, K., Abnormalities in glucose and energy metabolism are more severe in the hippocampus than in the cerebral cortex in postischemic recovery in aged rats, *Neurosci. Lett.*, 94, 167, 1988.

116. Hefti, F., Nerve growth factor (NGF) promotes survival of septal cholinergic neurons after fimbrial transections, *J. Neurosci.*, 6, 2155, 1986.

117. Koh, S. and Loy, R., Age-related loss of nerve growth factor sensitivity in rat basal forebrain neurones, *Brain Res.*, 440, 396, 1988.

118. Vijayan, V. K. and Cotman, C. W., Lysosomal enzyme changes in young and aged control and entorhinal-lesioned rats, *Neurobiol. Aging*, 4, 13, 1983.

119. Fucci, L., Oliver, C. N., Coon, M. J., and Stadtman, E. R., Inactivation of key metabolic enzymes by mixed-function oxidation reactions: possible implication in protein turnover and ageing, *Proc. Natl. Acad. Sci. U.S.A.*, 80, 1521, 1983.

120. Levine, R. L., Oliver, C. N., Fulks, R. M., and Stadtman, E. R., Turnover of bacterial glutamine synthetase: oxidative inactivation precedes proteolysis, *Proc. Natl. Acad. Sci. U.S.A.*, 78, 2120, 1981.

121. Fisher, M. T. and Stadtman, E. R., Oxidative modification of Escherichia coli glutamine synthetase. Decrease in the thermodynamic stability of protein structure and specific changes in the active conformation, *J. Biol. Chem.*, 267, 1872, 1992.

122. Stadtman, E. R., Protein oxidation and aging, *Science,* 257, 1220, 1992.

123. Stadtman, E. R. and Berlett, B. S., Fenton chemistry. Amino acid oxidation, *J. Biol. Chem.,* 266, 17201, 1991.

124. Stadtman, E. R. and Oliver, C. N., Metalcatalyzed oxidation of proteins. Physiological consequences, *J. Biol. Chem.,* 266, 2005, 1991.

125. Hershko, A., Ciechanover, A., and Rox, I. A., Resolution of the ATP-dependent proteolytic system from reticulocytes: A component that interacts with ATP, *Proc. Natl. Acad. Sci. U.S.A,* 76, 3107, 1979.

126. Goldberg, A. L. and Boches, F. S., Oxidized proteins in erythrocytes are rapidly degraded by the adenosine triphosphate-dependent proteolytic system, *Science,* 215, 1107, 1982.

127. Okada, M., Ishikawa, M., and Mizushima, Y., Identification of a ubiquitin- and ATP-dependent protein degradation pathway in rat cerebral cortex, *Biochim. Biophys. Acta,* 1073, 514, 1991.

128. Sawada, M., Sester, U., and Carlson, J. S., Superoxide radical formation and associated biochemical alterations in the plasma membrane of brain, heart, and liver during the lifetime of the rat, *J. Cell. Biochem.,* 48, 296, 1992.

129. Carney, J. M., Starke-Reed, P. E., Oliver, C. N., Landum, R. W., Cheng, M. S., Wu, J. F., and Floyd, R. A., Reversal of age-related increase in brain protein oxidation, decrease in enzyme activity, and loss in temporal and spatial memory by chronic administration of the spin-trapping compound N-tert-butyl-alpha-phenylnitrone, *Proc. Natl. Acad. Sci. U.S.A.,* 88, 3633, 1991.

130. Smith, C. D., Carney, J. M., Starke-Reed, P. E., Oliver, C. N., Stadtman, E. R., Floyd, R. A., and Markesbery, W. R., Excess brain protein oxidation and enzyme dysfunction in normal aging and in Alzheimer's disease, *Proc. Natl. Acad. Sci. U.S.A.,* 88, 10540, 1991.

131. Mecocci, P., MacGarvey, U., Kaufman, A. E., Koontz, D., Shoffner, J. M., Wallace, D. C., and Beal, M. F., Oxidative damage to mitochondrial DNA shows marked age-dependent increases in human brain, *Ann. Neurol.,* 34, 609, 1993.

132. Bak, P., Tang, C., and Wiesenfeld, K., Self-organized criticality, *Physic. Rev. A,* 38, 364, 1988.

133. Held, G. A., Solina, D. H., Keane, D. T., Haag, W. J., Horn, P. M., and Grinstein, G., Experimental study of critical-mass fluctuations in an evolving sandpile, *Physic. Rev. Lett.,* 65, 1120, 1990.

134. Mirollo, R. E. and Strogatz, S. H., Synchronization of pulse-coupled biological oscillators, *SIAM J. Appl. Math.,* 50, 1645, 1990.

135. Deutschke, K., Nitsch, R. M., and Hoyer, S., Short-term mental activation accelerates the age-related decline if high-energy phosphates in rat cerebral cortex, *Arch. Gerontol. Geriatr.,* 19, 43, 1994.

Chapter **17**

CENTRAL NEUROTRANSMISSION IN THE ELDERLY

Hervé Allain and Danièle Bentué-Ferrer

CONTENTS

0-8493-4786-6/95/$0.00+$.50
511

I. INTRODUCTION

Aging of the brain is accompanied, in all species, by modifications of its main components, and more particularly of the neurotransmission networks.[1] The abundant data obtained in animals is in sharp contrast to the scarcity and fragmentariness of those obtained in man. This is due to the heterogeneity of brain aging in man, the increasing incidence of brain pathology as a function of age and, above all, to the difficulties of *in vivo* accessibility to the healthy aged brain (Table 1). Beyond the mere description of abnormalities of neurotransmitters and synaptic functions, it is now important to consider the theoretical and practical consequences. It is also possible that the data acquired by modern functional neuroimaging techniques such as magnetic resonance imaging (MRI) or positron emission tomography (PET-Scan) modify the current description.[2]

II. NEUROTRANSMISSION NETWORKS

A. The Dopaminergic System

Age–related impairment of the dopaminergic systems has been known for 15 years. It mainly involves the nigrostriatal pathway, without totally sparing the mesocorticolimbic one. With regard to enzymatic activities, tyrosine hydroxylase (TH) decreases sharply and early in man.[3] In the putamen, its seems that in the later years of life the level of TH activity is very reduced, close to that of patients with Parkinson's disease where the nigrostriatal dopaminergic system is almost totally impaired.

The dihydroxyphenylalanine (DOPA)–decarboxylase activity also decreases with age, although in smaller proportions than TH. Meanwhile, the activities of monoamine oxidase inhibitor enzymes, of catechol-*O*-methyl transferase (COMT) typically increase, suggesting increased degradation of catecholamines — dopamine in particular. According to Rinne

TABLE 1.

Neurotransmission and Aging: Methodological Difficulties

1. Neurochemical data are difficult to obtain in healthy elderly subjects
2. Limitations of *in vivo* paraclinical investigations in man
3. Classic confusion between normal senescence and age–related pathologies
4. Inadequacy between animal and human data
5. Scarcity of data on receptor response and postsynaptic events according to age
6. Lack of systematic studies on psychotropic drugs in healthy and ill subjects
7. Multiplicity of cellular impacts of psychotropic drugs
8. Increasing number of neurotransmitter or modulator substances (adenosine, peptides, amino acids,...)
9. Neuronal density and brain shrinkage are not taken into account

TABLE 2.

Neurobiology of Aging

Dopaminergic System		Cholinergic System	
Receptor D_1 and D_2	↓	ACh cerebral receptor binding	±↓
TH activity	↓	Cerebral CAT activity ↓	
DA striatal concentrations	↓		
Noradrenergic system (NA)		**GABAergic System**	
Cerebral NA concentration	↓	Thalamus GABA concentration ↓	
CSF NA concentration	↓	Benzodiazepine receptor binding?	
Na^+–dependent neuroendocrine responses:			
Cortisol	↑±		
GH	↓		
Serotoninergic System		**Amino-Excitatory System**[59]	
Cerebral 5-HT concentration	=		
Cerebral 5-HT2 binding	↓	Glutamate concentration ↑ or =	
Neuropeptidic System			
β-Endorphine, enkephalin	↓		
Vasopressin	↑		
Substance P	↓		
CRF	↑		
Galanin	↑		

et al.[4] the number of D1 receptors (binding of ^{3}H-SCH 23390, a selective antagonist of D1 receptors) decreases with age, both in the caudate nucleus and in the putamen. The average rate of decrease per decade is 3.8%. The dissociation constant is not modified by age in these two structures. The same applies to the D2 receptors (binding of ^{3}H-spiroperidol), with higher decrease rates of 4.8%, without any modification of the dissociation constant. The D1/D2 ratio is unrelated to age. These modifications are not sex–related. These binding studies have confirmed earlier findings and are consistent with results obtained *in vivo* by CT-scan, by positron emission tomography (PET) using ^{76}Br-bromospiperone for the study of D2 receptors. The discordance of some results obtained elsewhere for D1 receptors[5] probably relates only to the ligand specificity, SCH 23390 being the most specific one currently available. In man, the exact topographic localization (pre- or post-synaptic) of this receptor decline in the striatum has not been determined, due to the lack of autoradiographic studies like those performed in rats.[6] In that animal species, it has been shown that the striatal subregions were not affected equally by the aging process,[6,7] the loss of D2 binding sites occurring predominantly in the postero-lateral part of the striatum.

These topographic differences are not found, within the same species, when studying the presynaptic markers of dopaminergic function, such as the striatal tissular concentrations of dopamine, homovanillic acid (HVA) or dihydroxyphenyl- acetic acid (DOPAC); these markers are evenly decreased in the striatum.[6] This shows that the effect of aging on dopaminergic receptors can be dissociated from its influence on the dopaminergic innervation of the striatum, which suggests an independent control of the pre- and post-synaptic sides of the synapse.

Regarding the spontaneous release of endogenous dopamine, some authors think that this would be reduced, even if the DOPA accumulation in the striatum, the nucleus accumbens and olfactive tubercules, induced by haloperidol treatment, remains unchanged. This decrease in spontaneous release is still controversial. In contrast, it seems that the increased release which follows nerve end depolarization is reduced, reflecting impaired coupling between neuronal electric activation and neuromediator release. An increase in the influence of acetylcholine towards dopamine release in the striatum of aged rats could also reflect a lower effectiveness of the self-regulating mechanisms normally involved to limit dopamine release. At the molecular level, the effectiveness of D1 receptor stimulation to activate cAMP-dependent cellular phosphorylation appears to be sharply reduced, while the inhibitor effect of D2 receptors on cAMP production would be unaffected by age.

Lastly, from the pharmacological standpoint, differences in behavioral reactivity to the various dopaminergic agonists have been shown to occur with age.[8] In addition, the response to D2 agonists is not altered with age, whereas that of D1 agonists is disrupted, possibly leading to a loss of the physiological regulation of D1- D2 functions.[9,10] Chronic treatment by pergolide could play a protective role in aged rats against the nigrostriatal anatomic lesions of senescence. Prolactin, after a 7-day course in aged rats, restores the same number of dopaminergic receptors as found in young animals, thereby illustrating the role of peripheral hormones on central synaptic functions.

B. The Noradrenergic System

The issue of a possible age-linked decrease in noradrenergic activity is still controversial. However, it seems that age is associated with neuronal loss in the locus coeruleus, the starting point of the main ascending noradrenergic system, essentially distributed between the neocortex and the hippocampal cortex. The results concerning tissue concentrations of noradrenaline are variable and conflicting, according to the species studied, and there are also nonnegligible interindividual variations within the same species. The capacities for noradrenaline release in the cerebral cortex are not influenced by age; the same is true for the modulation of this release by autoreceptors.[11]

Several studies have shown the age-independent reduction of the beta–adrenoceptor function, whereas conflicting reports have been made on the modifications of α-adrenoceptors.[12] However, chronic fluphenazine treatment induces a greater hypersensitivity of these receptors in aged animals than in young ones. This suggests that there is a compensating response of alpha receptors to pharmacological stimulation during aging, which could make up for their reduction in number.

Regarding the pharmacology of β receptors during aging, it has been shown that chronic administration of desipramine induced a significant decrease in the density of ^{3}H-dihydroalprenolol binding sites in aged rats, even if baseline values were already lower than in young animals. This shows that the adaptive mechanisms that lead to a downregulation of β adrenoceptors in the cerebral cortex after prolonged antidepressant treatment, for instance, are still functional with age. However, it has also been shown that the β-adrenergic receptors of aged brains did not develop the hypersensitivity normally induced by reserpine treatment. Lastly, the effect of noradrenaline on the electrophysiological responses of Purkinje cells or cortical cells is reduced in old animals. The activity of locus coeruleus neurones (firing) also decreases with age.

C. The Serotoninergic System

Investigations on the effect of aging on the serotoninergic systems are still very incomplete and have often given conflicting results. Some studies have shown a significant decrease in serotonin (5HT) concentrations and its synthesis enzyme, tryptophan hydroxylase, in the nuclei that contain the 5HT cellular body, and in the terminal ends of these neurons in the septum and the hippocampus. Conversely, unchanged concentrations have been found in the brain as a whole, or even increased in some regions.[13] The serotoninergic activity, as assessed by the 5HIAA/5HT ratio (5HIAA = 5-hydroxyindolacetic acid), measured in the cerebral cortex, is increased in old rats. This increased ratio is in fact due to a decrease in the baseline level of 5HT and a concomitant increase in its metabolite. These alterations are due to several mechanisms, such as the increased activity of monoamine oxidase, linked to age, decreased clearance of the metabolite, or age-dependent modifications of serum tryptophan levels.[13]

Human studies are not very conclusive, and postmortem 5HT and 5HIAA assays do not show constant modifications according to age, in the various regions of the brain.[14] Assessment of serotoninergic receptor activity in man, using PET with C^{11}-labelled ^{3}N-methyl-spiredone as a ligand, reveals a linear decrease in the 5HT-2 receptors, in the caudate nucleus, the putamen, the frontal cortex, between the age of 19 and 73 years.[15] These results have been confirmed by postmortem binding studies in the frontal cortex. This apparent decrease in 5HT receptors could reflect a loss of serotoninergic cellular bodies and constitute an adaptive response to the availability of 5HT and its receptors.

Receptor binding studies have also been conducted in animals. The reduced number of 5HT-2 receptors was also observed. High affinity 5HT recapture sites are reduced with age, and the density of ^{3}H-imipramine binding, which follows an allosteric relation with these recapture sites, is significantly increased; this was also observed in elderly humans.[16] In total, these biochemical and receptor binding studies are still too fragmented to provide an answer to the question of whether these modifications of the serotoninergic system are merely an epiphenomenon, or if they constitute a true causal relationship with aging.

D. The Cholinergic System

The development of specific antibodies directed against choline acetyl transferase (CAT), an enzyme synthesizing acetylcholine (ACh), a marker of presynaptic cholinergic neuron integrity, and the use of cellular enzyme labeling have made it possible to refine histological techniques. This was at the origin of several studies which morphologically explored the central cholinergic systems. Using Butcher's pharmacohistological technique, which marks the cells with acetylcholinesterase activity, a 26% decrease in the size of marked central nuclei has been demonstrated in rats. The neuronal density of these regions is also lower in old rats; thus, marked neurons would be lost and the remaining ones would exhibit signs of morphologic alterations.[17]

Nevertheless, the acetylcholinesterase activity is not entirely specific for cholinergic neurons, and the absence of marking may simply reflect an alteration of acetylcholinesterase synthesis rather than an impairment of neuron viability. In fact, CAT remains the most specific marker of cholinergic neurons. Its concentration in man decreases linearly with age, especially in the frontotemporal cortex and the hippocampus. Immunohistological studies also seem to show a neuronal loss in the ACh system produced by Meynert's basal nucleus, tempered by physiological aging and enhanced in Alzheimer's disease.

The age-dependent decline in cholinergic activity in central brain structures is also supported by an analysis of cholinergic receptors. In that respect, it has been shown that there was a reduction of muscarinic receptors in the frontal cortex, the hippocampus, the caudate nucleus, and the putamen of elderly subjects.[18] Besides, the decrease in M2 receptors, which occurs in parallel to CAT activity, suggests the presynaptic localization of these receptors on the ACh neuron.

Electrophysiological responses to ACh of hippocampal pyramidal cells are compromised in elderly rats. Cingular cortex neurons are also less sensitive to ACh. Spontaneous release of septo-hippocampal cholinergic neurons are altered with age. The conductivity of fibers from Meynert's basal nucleus is reduced in the cerebral cortex.

Few pharmacological studies assessing the age-dependent variations in receptor response to ACh have been conducted in normal subjects. Old rats given scopolamine (blocking ACh receptors) develop amnesia; conversely, various cholinomimetic drugs are capable of improving responses to memory and learning tests in aged animals. All these facts support the important role of cholinergic systems in the cognitive disorders of senescence, with the reservation that it is not easy to elaborate on a single mediator knowing the modifications already described in other systems.

E. The GABAergic System

As early as 1976, a reduction in glutamate decarboxylase (GAD) activity was observed in certain regions of the brain, the thalamic nuclei being those most affected, while the striatum was spared. Likewise, gamma-aminobutyric acid (GABA) concentrations were reduced in elderly subjects, again in the thalamic region.

Studies on ^{3}H-GABA and ^{3}H-muscimol binding revealed an age-related decrease in the number of GABA receptors, but only in the hippocampus and in the cerebral cortex in rats. Functional studies using specific pharmacologic agents are contradictory and do not permit clear conclusions as to the role of these receptors in aging. Also conflicting are the results involving receptors to benzodiazepines, which are functionally and anatomically linked to the GABA receptors in the brain, and which are either increased or reduced in number.[19] Further investigations are necessary, especially since this inhibitory neurotransmitter is implicated in a number of networks, functions, or pathological conditions.

F. The Amino-Excitatory System

Few studies have so far explored the effect of aging on amino-excitatory neurotransmission. The main two biochemical techniques used as the presynaptic functional index of this neurotransmission are the sodium-dependent high-affinity capture of D-^{3}H-aspartate or L-^{3}H-glutamate, and Ca^{2+}-dependent and K^+-stimulated glutamate release, as assessed on fine sections of nervous tissue or synaptosomes. Many cortical and subcortical regions have been explored in animals according to age. The hippocampus and the cerebellum are not sites of significant modifications of D-^{3}H-aspartate capture, which suggests that no amino-excitatory terminal ends are lost at that level, unless compensatory mechanisms are involved. In contrast, this parameter decreases in other explored regions (neocortex, striatum, Meynert's basal nucleus, amygdala, thalamus).[20] This decrease is not gradual, but appears to stabilize at midlife and even to correct itself with age, which may perhaps be explained by a concomitant but slower increase in the transporter affinity. This arrest in the capture decrease at midlife could also reflect a compensation of the loss process by neuronal connections. Glutamate release has also been studied in rats; it is not altered with age at the Meynert's nucleus basalis level, an observation which contradicts the excitotoxic origin of cholinergic cell loss in that nucleus which is markedly observed in cases of pathological aging (Alzheimer's disease).

Analyzing concentrations reveals an increase in glutamate and/or aspartate in the striatum, the pallidus, and the locus niger, which is consistent with cellular destruction as a result of the aging process. More specifically, in the striatum, the increased glutamate concentration is not consistently homogeneous with the known heterogeneity of that structure. The increase preferentially involves the lateral part of the striatum;[21] this also corresponds to the mediolateral gradient of the density of D2 receptor in the striatum of adult rats. Taking into account the fact that, in rodents, striatal D2 receptors are lost during normal aging, and that D2 receptor activation inhibits glutamatergic release in the striatum, it is conceivable that the observed increase in glutamic acid levels is due to a disinhibition of its release by the loss of D2 receptors. These amino-excitatory systems illustrate the fact that all structures containing the same neurotransmitter are not equally subjected to the aging process, and moreover, even within the same structure senescence can have heterogeneous consequences.

G. The Neuropeptidic System

Data on the possible peptide modifications linked to normal aging is extremely fragmented, although well supported in pathological situations (Table 3). β-endorphin and enkephalin are decreased, and vasopressin is increased in elderly mice. Increased hypothalamic release of somastostatin was observed *in vitro* in elderly rats. Substance P (essentially in the hippocampus) and neurotensin levels are decreased.[22]

In man, β-endorphin and β-lipotropin levels are reversely correlated to age; this decrease is markedly enhanced in cases of dementia of the Alzheimer type (DAT).[23] The galanine and corticotrophin releasing factor (CRF) level is positively correlated to age. The feedback which, under stress, reduces the activity of the hypothalamo-pituitary-adrenal axis, and which appears to be mediated by cortisol receptors in the hippocampus, would be less active in the elderly. Lastly, the adrenocorticotropic hormone (ACTH) level was found reduced in the cerebrospinal fluid, without any currently possible interpretation of these abnormalities. To a number of authors, however, the peptide content of the cortex or the cerebrospinal fluid appears to be little altered with age;[24] for a review, see Leake and

TABLE 3

Neuropeptides in Pathological Situations

Neuropeptide	Disease		
	Alzheimer	Lewy Body Type Dementia	Depression
Arginine Vasopressin	↓ or ↑	→ ←	↓ or ↑
CCK	↓		→ ←
Corticotrophin	↓		→ ←
CRF	↑	↓	→ ← ↑
Neuropeptide Y	↓		
β-Endorphin	↓		↑
Substance P	↓		↑
Somatostatin	↓		↓

Note: ↓ Decrease; ↑ increase; → ← unchanged.

Ferrier[24]: corticotrophin, cholecystokinin, β-endorphin, somatostatin, neurotensin, substance P, alpha-melanine stimulating hormone (α-MSH), CRF, and vasoactive intestinal peptide (VIP).

III. PRACTICAL AND THEORETICAL CONSEQUENCES

A. Therapeutics

1. Neuroleptics

Elderly subjects are more exposed than the young[25] to the adverse effects of neuroleptics, which all have, schematically speaking, antidopaminergic, anticholinergic, and adrenolytic properties: extrapyramidal syndrome and dyskinesia resulting from the nigrostriatal dopaminergic deficiency;[26,27] orthostatic hypotension by baroreflex impairment;[28] and cognitive and amnestic disorders by cholinergic neuron loss. New atypical neuroleptics (clozapine, amisulpride, and risperidone) appear less prone to induce such side effects.

2. Benzodiazepines

The increased sensitivity of elderly subjects to the sedative and amnestic effects of anxiolytics and hypnotics has been recognized.[29,30-32] Indeed, the age-related pharmacokinetic modifications of these molecules could in part explain these phenomena; in contrast, their impact on the GABAergic system, itself connected to other systems (adrenergic and cholinergic), could account for this sensitivity.

3. Antidepressants

Tricyclic substances are nowadays hardly recommended in elderly subjects, even if their effectiveness appears to be the same as in younger adults;[33] the least anticholinergic and the least adrenolytic are to be chosen by priority.[9] New-generation antidepressants and serotoninergic drugs seem a more logical choice, equals to the new monoamine oxidase inhibitors (MAOIs) such as moclobemide or brofaromine, which are free of the classic side effects of former MAOIs (tyramine effect, blood pressure changes, etc.).[33,34] CRF antagonists could constitute choice antidepressants for the elderly, bearing in mind that fluoxetine has such a property.[35]

4. Other Drugs

Pharmacovigilance has taught us that a number of nonpsychotropic drugs can induce neurological or psychiatric adverse effects, especially in the elderly (antihypertension, antibiotics, etc.). Here again, the explanation may come from the preexistent synaptic dysfunction . This reflection was at the basis of our review on the nonpsychotropic drugs responsible for sleep disorders in the elderly.[36]

B. Pathology

Since the discovery of the close correlation between the drop in dopamine levels in the nigrostriatal system and the motor signs of Parkinson's disease, similar reasonings have been applied, although with less success, to other pathologies. Lesions of the cholinergic neurons in Meynert's nucleus basalis are a constant in Alzheimer's disease; this disorder is thought to be at the origin of the amnestic disorders initially occurring in the disease. Likewise, certain behavioral disorders in demented subjects are to be related to the central serotoninergic deficiency. On the other hand, from the pathophysiological standpoint, there is a new interrogation as to why such a neurotransmission system will be impaired in a more or less selective manner. This opens up constructive lines of research: the role of MAOI in the genesis of free radicals, the role of excitatory amino acids and calcium influx in cell death and in cell metabolic content disturbances, the role of peptides on the trophicity and function of synaptic cells, etc.[37] In any case, interrogations still remain as to the quality and validity of a therapeutical response to a given drug, depending on whether one, two, or several main neurotransmission circuits are altered.

C. Pharmacology

The pharmacology of the aging brain is in full expansion. Among the main avenues being explored, restoration of synaptic functions remains a

TABLE 4.

Nonsynaptic Diffusion Neurotransmission (NDN)

1. Neuromodulation
     Nitric oxide
     Carbon oxide
2. Receptor Plasticity
     Up/Down Regulation
     Glycine, Polyamines, Glutamate Receptors
3. Glial Cells
     Receptors
     Calcium
     Phospholipase A_2; Phosphokinase C
4. Dendritic Information Processing

priority. This has been made possible, in particular, by agonists specific for the various receptors and subtypes. This is particularly true in the dopaminergic domain, in serotoninergy, and in cholinergy. Symptomatic treatments are already being evaluated clinically in major pathological areas such as Alzheimer's disease, dementia, accelerated cognitive decline, and specific behavioral and psychiatric disorders of the elderly.

Another line already well explored consists of antagonizing the so-called degenerative processes, using widely varied pathways: modification of glutamatergic transmission, modification of intracellular calcium pools, A and B MAOIs, and modification of ionic channels. In clinical pharmacology, the interest of studies in healthy[38] or ill elderly subjects now appears to be evident.

IV. CRITICAL READING

The theories of the 1980s gave the synaptic, hence the neurotransmitter functions, a preferential and exaggerated role in brain physiology.[39] However, it is striking that there are no strict correlations between neuropathological changes and cerebral performance — cognitive and mental in particular.[40] Interneuronal transmission of information has now to consider not only the purely synaptic aspects of communication (the "wiring transmission"), but also the often indirect, nonsynaptic channels (the "volume transmission").[41] Besides the mechanisms of neuronal plasticity,[42] few data are currently available on the role of age on the main actors of this nonsynaptic diffusion neurotransmission (NDN) (Table 4), whether these are the nitric oxide[43] of glial cells or astrocytes[44] or even substances with hormonal activity, such as melatonin.[45] This crucial deficiency has to be underlined, not only because it authorizes more pertinent pathophysiological hypothesis, but mainly because it opens new prospects and perspectives for pharmacology. Very schematically, the drugs destined to improve amnestic performance, or to correct the deficiencies that accompany Alzheimer's disease, can be developed without the need to apply theoretical synaptology.[46-48] This approach also permits a better understanding of the circadian rhythms characteristic of aging (sleep, vigilance, mood, memory, and nutritional behavior), as well as the chronopharmacology of the main psychotropic drugs.[49]

Recent data on the processing of information in brain, and in particular the process of spatial integration at the dendritic level,[50] for instance, indicate that any drug having an effect at these elementary level by globally altering the output of the system. Conversely, fragilization of these networks with age and pathology now provides keys to explain the classic symptoms observed in the elderly.

V. CONCLUSION

Qualitative and functional impairment at the synaptic level constitutes one of the most fundamental characteristics of the aging brain. Aminergic systems appear to be altered earlier and more severely, even in the absence of pathology. The description of such abnormalities deserves to be known, for a better use of the drugs in the elderly, and also to base research hypothesis on brain aging; the ultimate aim is indeed to treat diseases that have long been incurable, but it is also to ensure comfort and a good quality of mental and cognitive functioning to the end of life. The importance of this issue is very well illustrated by the increasing number of recent papers reporting either the use of psychotropic drugs by the elderly[51] (in particular, anxiolytics[52-54] and antidepressants[55,56]) or the interest in drugs prescribed in senile dementia[57] or neuronal death conditions.[58,59]

REFERENCES

1. Allain, H., Bentué-Ferrer, D., and Reymann, J. M., Neurotransmission et vieillissement cérébral, *Neuropsychobiology*, 4, 557, 1989.
2. Perani, D., Bressi, S., Cappa, S. F., Vallar, G., Alberoni, M., Grassi, F., et al., Evidence of multiple memory systems in the human brain, a ^{18}F FDG PET metabolic study, *Brain*, 116, 903, 1993.
3. Hornykiewicz, O., Dopamine changes in the aging human brain: functional consideration, in *Aging*, Vol. 23, A. Agnoli, Ed., Raven Press, New York, 1983.
4. Rinne, J. O., Lonnberg, P., and Marjamaki, P., Age-dependent decline in human brain dopamine D1 and D2 receptors, *Brain Res.*, 508, 349, 1990.
5. Morgan, D. G., Marcusson, J. O., Nyberg, P., Wester, P., Winblad, B., Gordon, M. N., and Finch, C. E., Divergent changes in D1 and D2 dopamine binding sites in human brain during aging, *Neurobiol. Aging*, 8, 195, 1987.

6. Marshall, J. F. and Rosenstein, A. J., Age-related decline in rat striatal dopamine metabolism is regionally homogeneous, *Neurobiol. Aging*, 11, 131, 1990.
7. Strong, R., Regionally selective manifestations of neostriatal aging, *Ann. N.Y. Acad. Sci.*, 515, 161, 1988.
8. Allain, H., Van den Driessche, J., Reymann, J. M., Pape, D., and Bentué-Ferrer, D., Influence de l'âge sur les réactions comportementales du rat à certains agonistes et antagonistes dopaminergiques, *J. Pharmacol.*, 11, 289, 1980.
9. Allain, H., Bentué-Ferrer, D., and Decombe, R., Pharmacologie des antidépresseurs et démences séniles, in *Démences et Dépressions*, Fondation Nationale de Gérontologie, Maloine, Paris, 1990, 111.
10. Allain, H., Bentué-Ferrer, D., Reymann, J. M., and Martinet, J. P., Systèmes dopaminergiques et fonctions cognitives, *Neuropsychobiology*, 4, 17, 1990.
11. Schlicker, E., Betz, R., and Gothert, M., Investigation into the age-dependence of release of serotonin and noradrenaline in the rat brain cortex and of autoreceptor-mediated modulation of release, *Neuropharmacology*, 28, 811, 1989.
12. Bickford-Wimer, P. C., Parfitt, K., and Hoffer, B. J., Desipramine and noradrenergic neurotransmission in aging: failure to respond in aged laboratory animals, *Neuropsychopharmacology*, 26, 597, 1987.
13. Timiras, P. S. and Cole, G., Changes in brain 5-HT with aging and modification through precursor availability, in *Aging Brain and Ergot Alkaloids*, Vol. 23, Agnoli, Crepaldi, Spano and Trabucchi, Eds., Raven Press, New York, 1983, 23.
14. Bucht, G., Adolfsson, R., Grottfries, C. G., Roos, B. E., and Winblad, B., Distribution of 5-hydroxytryptamine and 5-hydroxyindolacetic acid in human brain in relation to age, drug influence, agonal status, circadian variation, *J. Neural. Transm.*, 51, 186, 1981.
15. Wong, D. F., Wagner, Jr., Dannals, R. F., Links, J. M., Frost, J. J., Ravert, H. T., Wilson, A. A., Rosenbaum, A. E., Gjedde, A., Douglass, K. H., Pentronis, J. D., Folstein, M. F., Toung, J. K. T., Burns, H. D., and Kuhar, M. J., Effects of age on dopamine and serotonin receptors measured by positron tomography in the living human brain, *Science*, 226, 1393, 1984.
16. Severson, J. A., Marcusson, T. O., Osterburg, H. H., Fich, C. E., and Winblad, B., Elevated density of 3-H-imipramine binding in aged human brain, *J. Neurochem.*, 45, 1382, 1985.
17. Altavista, M. C., Rossi, P., Bentivoglio, A. R., Grociani, P., and Albanese, A., Aging is associated with a diffuse impairment of forebrain cholinergic neurons, *Brain Res.*, 508, 51, 1990.
18. Rinne, J. O., Muscarinic and dopaminergic receptors in the aging human brain, *Brain Res.*, 404, 162, 1987.
19. Kochman, R. L. and Sepulveda, C. K., Aging does not alter the sensitivity of benzodiazepine receptors to GABA modulation, *Neurobiol. Aging*, 7, 363, 1986.
20. Najlerahim, A., Francis, P. T., and Bowen, D. M., Age-related alterations in excitatory amino acid neurotransmission in rat brain, *Neurobiol. Aging*, 11, 155, 1990.
21. Donzanti, B. A. and Unga, A. K., Alterations in neurotransmitter amino acid content in the aging rat striatum are sub-region dependent, *Neurobiol. Aging*, 11, 159, 1990.
22. Ferrier, I. N., Cross, A. J., Johnson, J. A., Roberts, G. W., Crow, T. J., et al., Neuropeptides in Alzheimer type dementia, *J. Neurol. Sci.*, 62, 159, 1983.
23. Facchinetti, F., Petraglia, F., Nappi, G., Martignoni, E., Antoni, G., Parrini, D., and Genazzani, A. R., Different patterns of central and peripheral beta-endorphin, beta-lipotropin and ACTH throughout life, *Peptides*, 4, 744, 1983.

24. Leake, A. and Ferrier, I. N., Alterations in neuropeptides in aging and disease: pathophysiology and potential for clinical intervention, *Drugs & Aging*, 3, 408, 1993.

25. Gilleard, C. J., Morgan, K., and Wade, B. E., Patterns of neuroleptic use among institutionalized elderly, *Acta Psychiatr. Scand.*, 68, 419, 1983.

26. Lohr, J. B. and Brach, S. H., Association of psychosis and movement disorders in the elderly, *Psychiatr. Clin. North Am.*, 11, 61, 1988.

27. Smith, J. M. and Baldessarini, R. J., Changes in prevalence, severity and recovery in tardive dyskinesia with age, *Arch. Gen. Psychiatry*, 37, 1368, 1980.

28. Gribbin, B., Pickering, T. G., and Sleight, P., Effect of age and high blood pressure on baroflex sensitivity in man, *Cir. Res.*, 29, 424, 1971.

29. Bourin, M., *Les Benzodiazépines*, Ellipses, Paris, 1989.

30. Pomora, N., Stanley, B., and Block, R., Adverse effects of single therapeutic doses of diazepam on performance in normal geriatric subjects: relationship to plasma concentrations, *Psychopharmacology*, 342, 1984.

31. Pomora, N., Stanley, B., and Block, R., Increased sensitivity of the elderly to the central depressant effect of diazepam, *J. Clin. Psychiatry*, 46, 185, 1985.

32. Rickels, K., Schweizer, E., and Lucki, I., Benzodiazepine side-effects, in *American Psychiatric Association, Annual Review*, Vol. 6, American Psychiatry Association Press, Washington D.C., 1987.

33. Georgotas, A., McCue, R. E., and Hapwoth, W., Comparative efficacy and safety of MAOIs versus TCAs in treating depression in the elderly, *Biol. Psychiatry*, 21, 1155, 1986.

34. Allain, H., Lieury, A., Brunet-Bourgin, F., Mirabaud, C., Trebon, P., Le Coz, F., and Gandon, J. M., Antidepressants and cognition: comparative effects of moclobemide, viloxazine and maprotiline, *Psychopharmacology*, 106, 556, 1992.

35. De Bellis, M. D., Gold, P. W., Geracioti, T. D., Listwak, S. J., and Kling, M. A., Association of fluoxetine treatment with reductions in CSF concentrations of corticotropin–releasing hormone and arginine vasopressin in patients with major depression, *Am. J. Psychiatr.*, 150, 655, 1993.

36. Menard, G., Allain, H., Beneton, C., and Delamaire, D., Médicaments non psychotropes et sommeil chez la personne âgée, *Psychol. Med.*, 24, 829, 1992.

37. Mizuno, Y., Mori, H., and Kondo, T., Potential of neuroprotective therapy in Parkinson's disease, *CNS Drugs*, 1, 45, 1994.

38. Allain, H., Le Coz, F., and Bureau, M., Le volontaire sain âgé: une nécessité, *Thérapie*, 48, 239, 1993.

39. Allain, H. and Reymann, J. M., Dix ans passés en psychopharmacologie, *Synapse*, 103, 71, 1994.

40. Jellinger, K. A., Histopathologic validation of dementia disorders of the aged, *Neurol. Neurobiol.*, 54, 79, 1990.

41. Bach-y-Rita, P., Non synaptic diffusion neurotransmission (NDN) in the brain, *Neurochem. Int.*, 93, 297, 1993.

42. Mori, N., Toward understanding of the molecular basis of loss of neuronal plasticity in aging, *Age & Aging*, 22, S5, 1993.

43. Bruhwyler, J., Chleide, E., Liegeois, J. F., and Carreer, F., Nitric oxide: a new messenger in the brain, *Neurosci. Biobehav. Rev.*, 17, 373, 1993.

44. Finkbeiner, S. M., Glial calcium, *Glia*, 9, 83, 1993.

45. Hardeland, R., Reiter, R. J., Poeggeler, B., and Tan, D. X., The significance of the metabolism of the neurohormone melatonin: antioxidative protection and formation of bioactive substances, *Neurosci. Biobehav. Rev.*, 17, 347, 1993.

46. Allain, H., Belliard, S., de Certaines, J., Bentué-Ferrer, D., Bureau, M., and Lacroix, P., Potential biological targets for anti-Alzheimer drugs, *Dementia*, 4, 347, 1993.

47. Allain, H., Raoul, P., Lieury, A., Le Coz, F., and Gandon, J. M., Effect of two doses of Gingko biloba extract (EGb 761) on the dual-coding test in elderly subjects, *Clin. Ther.*, 15, 549, 1993.
48. Allain, H., Lieury, A., and Gandon, J. M., Psychopharmacology of memory components, in *Human Psychopharmacology*, Vol. 44, Hindmarch, I. and Stonier, P. D., Eds., John Wiley & Sons, London, 1993, 143.
49. Nagayama, H., Chronopharmacology of psychotropic drugs: circadian rhythms in drug effects and its implications to rhythms in the brain, *Pharmacol. Ther.*, 59, 31, 1993.
50. Midtgaard, J., Processing of information from different sources: spatial synaptic integration in the dendrites of vertebrate CNS neurons, *Trends Neurosci.*, 17, 166, 1994.
51. Ghose, K., CNS drugs for elderly patients, *Drugs & Aging*, 4, 275, 1994.
52. Stoudemire, A. and Moran, M. G., Psychopharmacologic treatment of anxiety in the medically ill elderly patient: special considerations, *J. Clin. Psychiatry*, 54 (Suppl. 5), 27, 1993.
53. Markowitz, P. J., Treatment of anxiety in the elderly, *J. Clin. Psychiatry*, 54 (Suppl. 5), 64, 1993.
54. Shorr, R. I. and Robin, D. W., Rational use of benzodiazepines in the elderly, *Drugs & Aging*, 4, 9, 1994.
55. Preskorn, S. H., Recent pharmacologic advances in antidepressant therapy for the elderly, *Am. J. Med.*, 94 (Suppl. 5A), 2, 1993.
56. Nyth, A. L., Gottfries, C. G., Lyby, K., et al., A controlled multicenter clinical study of citalopram and placebo in elderly depressed patients with and without concomitant dementia, *Acta Psychiatr. Scand.*, 86, 138, 1992.
57. Benešuová, O., Neuropathology of senile dementia and mechanism of action of nootropic drugs, *Drugs & Aging*, 4, 285, 1994.
58. Lees, G. J., Contributory mechanisms in the causation of neurodegenerative disorders, *Neuroscience*, 54, 287, 1993.
59. Sanchez-Prieto, J., Herrero, I., Miras-Portugal, M. T., and Mora, F., Unchanged exocytotic release of glutamic acid in cortex and neostriatum of the rat during aging, *Brain Res. Bull.*, 33, 357, 1994.

Chapter **18**

AGE-RELATED CHANGES IN NEUROPEPTIDERGIC NEURONS IN THE HUMAN HYPOTHALAMUS

Jiang-Ning Zhou and Dick F. Swaab

CONTENTS

0-8493-4786-6/95/$0.00+$.50
© 1995 by CRC Press, Inc.

I. INTRODUCTION

Since 72-year-old Brown-Sèquard, more than one century ago, injected himself with testicular extracts and claimed remarkable physical and mental signs of rejuvenation,[1] a close relationship between endocrine changes and aging has been supposed.[2] Because of its central role in endocrine regulation, the hypothalamus has received the constant attention of gerontologists.[3-5] Over the past decades there has been remarkable progress in the knowledge of hypothalamic neuropeptidergic systems in relation to aging, to which several technical developments have contributed. In the first place, the isolation and characterization of hypothalamic peptides[6-8] have made subsequent immunocytochemical localization of neuropeptides possible in the human hypothalamus.[9] It is now generally accepted that neuropeptides may either be released into the circulation as hormones, or act as neurotransmitters or neuromodulators when released from synapses, and may then influence central processes.[10] In addition, many, if not all, hypothalamic peptides are colocalized with classical transmitters, e.g., acetylcholine, gamma-aminobutyric acid (GABA), or amines such as dopamine.[11] Since the classical neurotransmitters show clear changes with aging,[12-14] changes in the colocalizing neuropeptides may also be expected. Another reason to stress the importance of the hypothalamus for the aging process is that some hypothalamic systems themselves have been causally implicated in aging of the brain[15,16] and in the life span.[17] The present chapter tries to relate functional changes in aging with alterations in neuropeptidergic neurons of the human hypothalamus.

The hypothalamus is a complex, heterogeneous structure containing a number of nuclei which are often characterized by specific neuropeptides.[9] Basically, there are two types of hypothalamic peptidergic neurons. The first one is the neuroendocrine type, which releases its peptide as a hormone into the general circulation in the neurohypophysis, e.g., vasopressin (AVP) and oxytocin (OXT), or into the portal circulation of the pituitary, e.g., AVP, luteinizing hormone-releasing hormone (LHRH), thyrotropin-releasing hormone (TRH), and corticotropin-releasing hormone (CRH). The second type of hypothalamic peptidergic neuron is the one that sends its axon into the brain[18] where it terminates synaptically on other neurons, acting as a neurotransmitter or neuromodulator.[10] The same peptide may be present in both types of neurons, e.g., AVP is present in the hypothalamo-neurohypophysial-system (HNS) as a neurohormone and also in the suprachiasmatic nucleus as a neurotransmitter or neuromodulator.

II. SUPRACHIASMATIC NUCLEUS

The suprachiasmatic nucleus (SCN) is the major circadian pacemaker of the mammalian brain and coordinates hormonal and behavioral circadian rhythms.[19] A relatively large number of neuropeptides have been identified in the human SCN. Neurons that are immunoreactive for vasopressin (AVP), vasoactive intestinal polypeptide (VIP), neuropeptide-Y (NPY), neurotensin (NT), and somatostatin (SOM) are present in the SCN in a characteristic anatomical orientation (Figure 1).[20-23] Typical for the human SCN, as compared to monkeys and other animals, are the very large populations of NT and NPY neurons.[23] Colocalization of different neuropeptides in the SCN has been found mainly in rat but also in human.[24,25] For example, VIP-producing neurons in the SCN were shown to colocalize galanin, AVP,[25] gastrin releasing peptide (GRP),[26] or GABA.[27]

Recent observations have revealed marked changes in the volume of AVP subpopulation and AVP cell number of the human SCN in relation to the season.[28,29] In addition, a day-night fluctuation in the number of AVP expressing neurons in the SCN was found to be present, but only in young subjects,[30] which suggests a diminution of circadian fluctuations of the SCN in human aging. Age-related changes in circadian rhythms have indeed been reported in man as well as in other species.[31-33] Furthermore, a decrease in the number of AVP cells and total cell number was found in subjects aged 80 to 100, while these changes were even more pronounced in Alzheimer's disease patients than in controls (Figure 2).[21]

A different pattern from that of the AVP neurons was found recently in the number of VIP expressing neurons of the human SCN during aging (Figure 3).[34,35] The VIP cell number in the female SCN remained very stable during the life span. In males, however, the number of VIP neurons in the SCN reached its peak value in young males (10 to 40 years of age). Subsequently, a dramatic decrease in the number of VIP neurons in SCN was found in the middle-aged subjects (41 to 65 years of age). A significant reduction in the number of VIP expressing neurons was found in the old-age group (65 to 92 years of age). An age-dependent sex difference was observed in the SCN: males of 10 to 40 years of age had twice as many VIP neurons in the SCN as females. Due to the age-related fluctuations in VIP cell number in males, this sex difference was reversed in the middle-aged

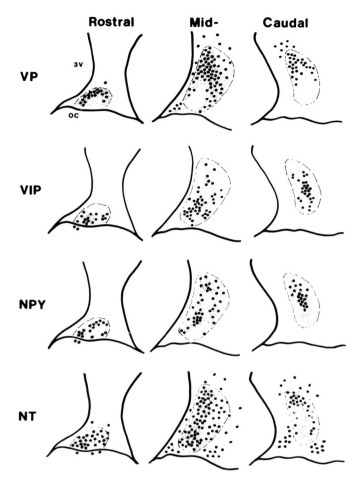

Figure 1
Diagram showing the organization of the human suprachiasmatic nucleus (SCN).
The distribution of vasopressin (VP), vasoactive intestinal polypeptide (VIP),
neurotensin (NT), and neuropeptide-Y (NPY) neurons and fibers is shown at three
levels, from rostral to caudal. (From Moore, R. Y., *Progress in Brain Research*, Swaab,
D. F., Hofman, M. A., Mirmiran, M., Ravid, R., and Van Leeuwen, F. W., Eds.,
Elsevier, Amsterdam, 1992. With permission.)

group, the females having twice as many VIP neurons in the SCN. After
65 years, sex differences were no longer found (Figure 3).[34,35] Since the
SCN is the clock of the brain, the morphological sex differences may be
related to sex differences that have been found in circadian control mechanisms of hamsters[36] and humans.[37] In addition, it has been found in rat that
VIP expressing neurons from the SCN directly innervate LHRH neurons
that are involved in reproductive functions.[38] Although such a connection

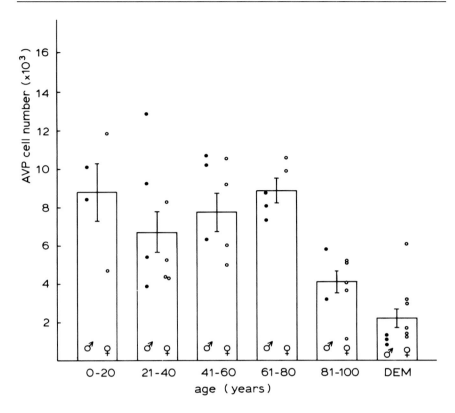

Figure 2
The number of vasopressin (AVP) immunoreactive neurons in the human SCN. The
number of AVP neurons in the 81- to 100-year-old group decreased as compared to
the 61- to 80-year-old subjects ($p < 0.02$). Data are represented as mean ± SEM. (From
Swaab, P. F., Roozendaal, B., Ravid, R., Velis, D. N., Gooren, L., and Williams, R. S.,
Progress in Brain Research, Vol. 72, De Kloet, R. et al., Eds., Elsevier, Amsterdam,
1987. With permission.)

should be confirmed in the human hypothalamus, the sex difference in the
number of VIP neurons in the SCN and the difference in the AVP subnucleus
of the SCN according to sexual orientation also suggests a possible role of
the biological clock in reproduction or sexual behavior.[39,40] Females showed
a very stable number of VIP neurons in the SCN with aging, whereas a
decrease in the number of VIP neurons in the SCN was found in middle-
aged males (Figure 3).[35] It is tempting to relate the changes in the peptidergic
neurons of the SCN to functional changes, e.g., in circadian rhythmicity.

Although the number of AVP neurons in the SCN in 60- to 80-year-old
subjects did not differ from the number found in young subjects,[41] the
circadian fluctuation in the number of AVP neurons in the human SCN
diminished in subjects older than 50 years.[30] The number of AVP neurons

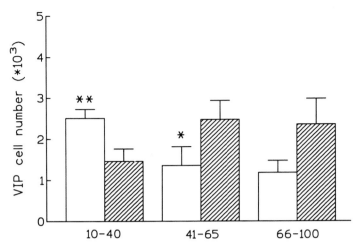

Figure 3
Lifespan changes in the number of vasoactive intestinal polypeptide (VIP) immunoreactive neurons in the human SCN. The blank bar indicates the males, the
hatched bar indicates the females. The SCN of young males (10 to 40 years) contains
twice as many neurons as that of young females ($p < 0.02$). This sex difference
reverses in middle-aged subjects ($p < 0.02$). Since the number of VIP neurons decreased after 40 years, the cell number is significantly lower in elderly males than
in young males ($p < 0.05$). (From Zhou, J. N., Hofman, M. A., and Swaab, D. F.,
Neurobiol. Aging, in press. With permission.)

did not decrease until after 80 years of age,[21] suggesting that the circadian
fluctuations in AVP neurons disappear earlier in the process of aging than
the number of neurons expressing AVP.

The relation between VIP and changed circadian fluctuations is less
clear. Circadian changes were found in plasma VIP levels in elderly males
(74 to 85 years) and in subjects that were 10 years younger (65 to 75
years).[42,43] However, these blood levels of VIP probably do not come from
SCN neurons. The stability of VIP neurons, especially in the female SCN,
might be related to some stable rhythms in normal human aging, such as
the rhythmicity of temperature, prolactin, or cortisol.[44-47] On the other
hand, it has been proposed that the decreased AVP cell number might be
the basis for circadian disturbances in aging and Alzheimer's disease.[21]
Some observations suggest that a certain degree of plasticity remains
present in the SCN neurons in aging.[32] SCN neurons in old rats seem to
continue to respond to increased input, since increased amounts of light
improved and restored circadian rhythms in these animals.[48] Such a
nonpharmacological treatment of disturbances of the sleep-wake pattern
may be of clinical importance, not only in aging but also in Alzheimer's
disease, where it may reduce nightly restlessness.[32]

Other changes in peptidergic SCN neurons may also be present in aging. A dense plexus of substance P (SP) immunoreactive axons that overlaps the distribution of VIP expressing perikarya has recently been reported in the human SCN (Moore et al., personal communication, 1994). Interestingly, the number of SP neurons in the SCN of aged hamsters was increased three to four times compared with adult animals, day and night.[49] However, observations on this peptidergic neuron population during the process of aging have not yet been performed in humans.

III. SEXUALLY DIMORPHIC NUCLEUS (INTERMEDIATE NUCLEUS, INAH-1)

The sexually dimorphic nucleus of the preoptic area (SDN) is identical to the intermediate nucleus as mentioned by Braak and Braak,[50] and to the INAH-1 described by Allen et al.[51] In girls, the SDN shows a decreasing cell number during prepubertal development, leading to sexual dimorphism.[52] The SDN in the young adult human brain is twice as large in males as in females and contains twice as many cells.[53] During aging, a decrease in cell number is found in both sexes. In males the cell number decreases strongly after 50 years of age, in females a second phase of cell loss appears after the age of 70 (Figure 4).[52,54] The sharp decline in cell numbers in the SDN later in life might be related to the hormonal changes which accompany both male and female senescence[54] and to the decrease in male sexual activity,[55] although the causality of such a relationship has not yet been established. A good marker for the neuronal content of the majority of SDN neurons is not available at present. Only a few TRH neurons have so far been identified in this nucleus.[56] Such TRH-positive neurons have also been identified in the rat.[57]

IV. PARAVENTRICULAR AND SUPRAOPTIC NUCLEUS

The paraventricular (PVN) and supraoptic (SON) nucleus and their axons form the hypothalamo-neurohypophyseal-system (HNS). Immuno-cytochemical studies have established that in addition to oxytocin (OXT) and vasopressin (AVP), a large number of other neuropeptides are synthesized by neurons of the PVN and SON.

A. Vasopressin and Oxytocin

AVP and OXT are produced by the magnocellular neurosecretory system of the hypothalamic SON and PVN projecting to the neurohypo-

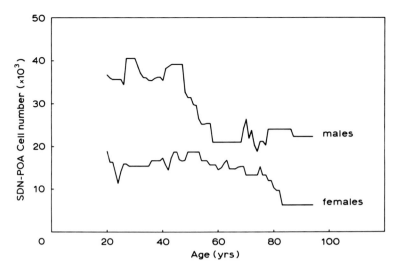

Figure 4

Age-related changes in the total cell number of the sexually dimorphic nucleus of the human hypothalamus. The general trend in the data is enhanced by using smoothed growth curves. Note that in males the SDN cell number steeply declines between the ages of 50 and 60 years, whereas in females a more gradual cell loss is observed around the age of 80 years. These curves demonstrate that the reduction in cell number in the human SDN in senescence is a nonlinear, sex-dependent process. (From Hofman, M. A. and Swaab, D. F., *J. Anat.,* 164, 55, 1989. With permission.)

physis where they are released into the circulation. AVP acts as an antidiuretic hormone on the kidney[58] and as a vasopressor on the blood vessels.[59] OXT is involved in labor and lactation[60] and in other reproductive processes.[9] In addition to these functions, magnocellular OXT- and AVP-containing cells in the SON and PVN coexpress tyrosine hydroxylase, suggesting the possibility of dopamine production.[61,62] AVP neurons of the PVN project into the brain,[18] and animal experiments suggest that they may influence central processes such as certain aspects of memory.[63,64] Peptides have been given as substitution therapy in disorders where a deficiency in these systems was presumed. However, clinical trials in which AVP or its analogs were administered to patients with Alzheimer's disease (AD) yielded inconsistent results.[65] OXT also has central effects, e.g., on the inhibition of food intake and on maternal and reproductive behavior.[66,67] In males, OXT might be involved in sexual arousal and ejaculation.[68] In rodents, depending on the strain, either activation or deterioration of the HNS during aging has been reported.[69] In contrast to the rodent data, nearly all human data point to an activation of the HNS with aging, especially of the vasopressinergic neurons. The mean profile area of AVP cells increased after the age of 80 years, suggesting an increased peptide production from this age onwards.[70] The OXT cells in these nuclei showed no such change.[70] Neuronal hypertrophy has also been described in unidentified human SON and PVN neurons in aging.[71] Although the correlation between cell size and peptide production is well established in adulthood, one might wonder whether this relationship would also persist in senescence. Since, for example, lipofuscin is known to accumulate in many types of aging nerve cells, this may theoretically cause an enlargement of cytoplasmic volume. Therefore, nucleolar size, which is a reliable parameter for neurosecretory activity, was also determined in the AVP and OXT cells in the same human material. A significantly increased nucleolar diameter was again found in AVP neurons of the SON and PVN in senescent subjects and not in the OXT cells.[72]

These findings confirmed the idea that the previously observed increase in cell size was indeed due to enhanced neurosecretory activity. However, it could not be excluded from those data that the observed activation of neurosecretory AVP cells was a compensation for cell loss from the PVN or SON. Total cell number, and OXT and AVP cell numbers, have therefore also been determined in the PVN and SON. The results revealed that no significant differences in volume or total cell number were present in either the PVN or SON between young and old control subjects.[73-75] Furthermore, a gradual increase in the number of AVP expressing neurons was even observed in the human PVN and SON with aging (Figure 5).[76] These findings are in line with the increased cellular[70] and nucleolar size[72] that indicated increased AVP synthesis in this nucleus during aging. To further substantiate the hyperactivity of HNS neurons in aging, the size of the Golgi apparatus (GA) was determined in the human SON and PVN in a recent study. The GA, indeed, showed a clear increase in size and intensity with age in controls and Alzheimer patients (Figure 6).[77] All these indications for activation of AVP are supported by the presence of a gradual increase in human plasma AVP levels during aging.[4,78,79] In addition, an increase in AVP secretion upon osmotic stimulation was found in elderly subjects.[80-84] Since the activation of AVP neurons in aging is probably due to loss of AVP receptors in the kidney,[85,86] the observed activation of the HNS in senescence might be considered as a compensatory activation. This mechanism, however, must still be confirmed in humans.

The number of OXT expressing neurons in the PVN was found to remain constant during aging (Figure 7),[87] which is in line with the absence of morphological signs of activation in these cells in senescence.[70,72] The remarkable stability of the activated SON and PVN neurons in aging, and also in Alzheimer's disease, supports our concept that activated neurons may be able to withstand the processes of aging or neurodegeneration better — a hypothesis that is paraphrased as "use it or lose it".[88]

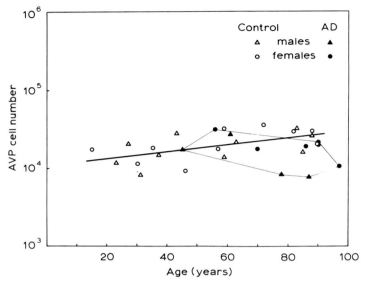

Figure 5
Linear regression between AVP cell number in PVN and age. A significant correlation between age and cell number was found in control subjects (r = 0.583, n = 20; *p* <0.01). Old control subjects had a significantly higher cell number as compared with young controls. This increase in AVP expressing neuron number with age does not occur in Alzheimer's disease (AD), as indicated by the minimum convex polygon. (From Van der Woude, P. F., Goudsmit, E., Wierda, M., Purba, J. S., Hofman, M. A., Bogte, H., and Swaab, D. F., *Neurobiol. Aging*, in press. With permission.)

B. Corticotropin-Releasing Hormone

Corticotropin-releasing hormone (CRH) immunoreactive neurons are restricted to the PVN in the human hypothalamus.[89,90] As in rat, the CRH neurons of the human PVN are parvicellular.[90] However, in the rat the CRH neurons are localized in a strictly defined subnucleus of the PVN,[91-93] while they are spread throughout the entire PVN in humans, except for the most rostral part where they are absent.[90] CRH plays a key role in the stress response of the hypothalamic-pituitary-adrenal (HPA) axis. CRH neurons appeared to be activated in aging as was shown by a number of parameters. In the first place, the number of CRH immunoreactive neurons in the human increases in the PVN (Figure 8).[94] Another sign of activation of CRH neurons is an increase in the coexpression of AVP as appeared from animal experiments.[93] Interestingly, an age-dependent increase in the colocalization of AVP was also found in the parvicellular CRH neurons in the human PVN with aging.[90] Colocalization was especially noted in older control subjects (aged 43 to 91 years), whereas no colocalization was present in younger subjects (aged 23 to 37 years). In addition, an increase in cortisol with age was found in post-mortem cerebrospinal fluid.[95]

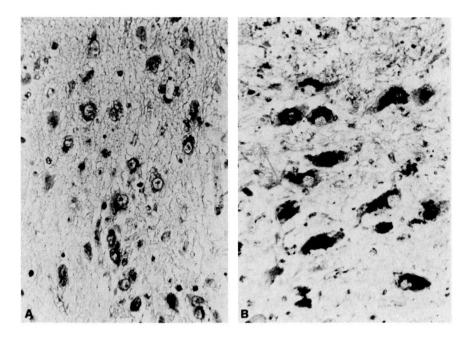

Figure 6
Activation of the Golgi apparatus in supraoptic and paraventricular nucleus (SON) and (PVN) neurons of the human hypothalamus as indicated by an increase in size and staining intensity of MG-160, a structural sialoglycoprotein of the medial cisternae. (A) Supraoptic neuron from a 29-year-old control, and (B) from a 73-year-old control. From Lucassen, P. J., Ravid, R., Gonatas, N. K., and Swaab, D. F., *Brain Res.*, 632, 105, 1993. With permission.)

All these findings are in agreement with hormone measurements in the periphery, indicating an activation of the HPA-axis during aging.[91,96] Moreover, resistance of cortisol secretion to dexamethasone suppression increases with age in controls.[97,98] Hyperactivity of the HPA-axis is proposed to have severe long-term consequences, since increased levels of corticosteroids have been hypothesized to lead to irreversible hippocampal damage.[16] The hippocampus normally inhibits CRH neurons[99] and hippocampal lesions may, therefore, subsequently lead to more hyperactivity of CRH neurons. A positive feedback loop would then develop, leading to more CRH activation and more brain damage. Whether such a mechanism is indeed operative in the human brain in aging and AD remains, however, to be proven. There are also observations which do not agree with an activation of the HPA-axis in aging. Measurements of plasma adrenocorticotropin (ACTH) in 25 young and 28 elderly humans revealed no significant differences.[100] Older people did not show significant change in ACTH response after having undergone major surgery. In addition, rhythms of ACTH and cortisol secretion showed no significant

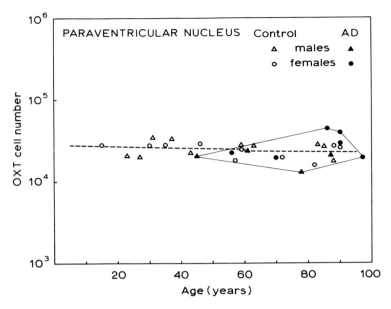

Figure 7

Linear regression between oxytocin (OXT) cell number in the PVN and age. Data of male and female control patients did not differ and were pooled. No statistically significant correlations were observed in either young or old control subjects. Values of male and female Alzheimer's disease (AD) patients are delineated by the minimum convex polygon and were within the range of the controls. (From Wierda, M., Goudsmit, E., Van der Woude, P. F., Purba, J. S., Hofman, M. A., Bogte, H., and Swaab, D. F., *Neurobiol. Aging*, 12, 511, 1991. With permission.)

change with age in healthy elderly subjects. Using frequent plasma sampling techniques,[47] older subjects also had a normal circadian cortisol rhythm, although the cycle peaked at an earlier hour. These data indicate that the regulatory capacity of the HPA-axis function, though this function is only slightly elevated under basal conditions in elderly subjects, may be diminished. However, on the basis of the activation of CRH neurons we observed in the PVN,[90,94] central effects of increased CRH activity should also be considered. Increased activity of CRH neurons that project into the brain may lead to symptoms of depression, since CRH when administered centrally in laboratory animals leads to signs and symptoms that are very similar to the symptoms of major depression.[101] In addition, extremely activated CRH neurons were indeed observed in depressed patients.[94]

C. Thyrotropin-Releasing Hormone (TRH)

The distribution of TRH neurons in the human hypothalamus has been studied only recently.[56] The majority of TRH-containing neurons was

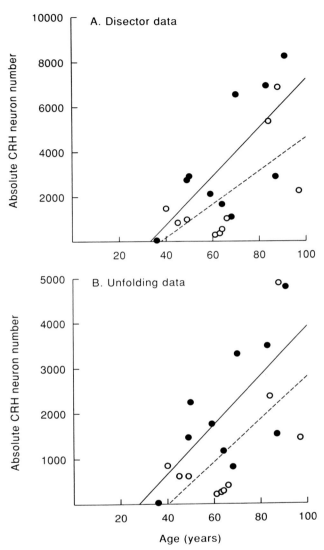

Figure 8
Linear regression between age and absolute CRH cell number in the PVN estimated by the disector method (A) and the unfolding method (B). Filled circles and solid lines indicate control subjects; open circles and dashed lines indicate Alzheimer's disease patients. A significant correlation was found between age and absolute CRH cell number for control subjects with both the disector and unfolding methods (respectively, rho = 0.66, p = 0.02; rho = 0.62, p = 0.03). (From Raadsheer, F. C., Oorschot, D. F., Verwer, R. W. H., Tilders, F. J. H., and Swaab, D. F., *J. Comp. Neurol.*, 339, 447, 1994. With permission.)

present in the PVN, especially in the dorsocaudal part of this nucleus. It is thought that these neurons project to the median eminence and regulate thyroid stimulating hormone (TSH) release. The TRH neurons in the PVN were mostly parvicellular, but a few magnocellular TRH-positive neurons were observed as well. The SON did not show any TRH immunoreactivity. High densities of TRH-positive fibers were seen, not only in the median eminence but also in other hypothalamic areas, e.g., in the PVN, ventromedial nucleus (VM), and in the perifornical area. The large number of TRH-containing fibers apparently terminating on neurons suggests important physiological functions of this neuropeptide as a neurotransmitter or neuromodulator in the human brain. Hypothalamic TRH levels and TRH secretion are reduced in old (24 to 28 months) rats.[102,103] Up to now, no data are available concerning age-related TRH changes in the human hypothalamus. Increased basal TSH concentrations were reported in eldery people[104] as well as in aged rats.[105] These changes point to the possibility that hypothalamic TRH may be compensatorily increased in elderly subjects. It seems worthwhile, therefore, to study age-related changes of TRH in the human hypothalamus.

D. Other Peptides

The human PVN and SON contain a number of other peptidergic neurons such as prosomatostatin[106] and LHRH.[107] Recently, positive VIP neurons were found to be present in the PVN and SON.[34,35] In humans, the VIP neurons are spread all over the PVN and are not localized in a particular subnucleus as was found in the rat.[108] In addition, colocalization of galanin has been found in the human SON and PVN, mainly with AVP and less with OXT.[25] This means that changes of galanin in the HNS can also be expected in aging.

V. INFUNDIBULAR (ARCUATE) NUCLEUS

The horseshoe-shaped infundibular (or arcuate) nucleus[50] contains a large number of neurotransmitters and neuropeptides, e.g., catecholamine-containing neurons,[61] somatostatin, neuropeptide Y, and neurotensin. Various neuroendocrine cell types that are involved in the hypothalamo-pituitary-gonadal (HPG) axis are located in this nucleus.

A. Luteinizing Hormone-Releasing Hormone (LHRH)

LHRH is less widely distributed in the brain than many other neuropeptides. LHRH-containing cell bodies are located predominantly in the

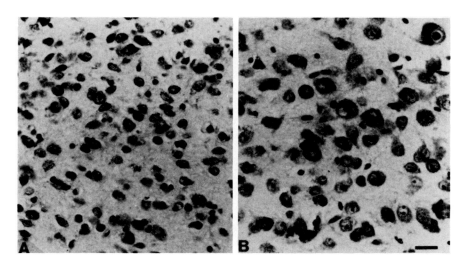

Figure 9
Representative photomicrographs of cresyl violet-stained sections of the infundibular nucleus of premenopausal (A) and postmenopausal (B) women. The hypertrophied neurons are distinguished not only by increased soma size, but also by large nuclei, nucleoli, and increased Nissl substance. Bar is 20 μm for both photomicrographs. (From Rance, N. E., *Progress in Brain Research,* Swaab, D. F., Hofman, M. A., Mirmiran, M., Ravid, R., and Van Leeuwen, F. W., Eds., Elsevier, Amsterdam, 1992. With permission.)

infundibular nucleus and preoptic area.[109,107,110] LHRH-immunoreactive fibers project to the median eminence, septum, stria terminalis, ventral pallidum, dorsomedial thalamus, olfactory stria, and the anterior olfactory area of the human brain.[111] Recently, a much wider distribution and greater number of LHRH neurons was found in the human hypothalamus using *in situ* hybridization.[112] In this study, three subtypes of LHRH neurons were found as well as two types of small-sized neurons located primarily in the hypothalamus, suggesting that different functional subgroups of LHRH neurons exist in the human brain.[112] The colocalization of delta sleep-inducing peptide (DSIP) and LHRH, as found in the arcuate nucleus of aged human subjects, suggests that DSIP may also play a physiological role in LHRH neurons.[113]

The menopause represents a dramatic alteration in the function of the HPG axis in women. As a consequence of decreased levels of sex hormones, neuronal hypertrophy has been reported in the human infundibular nucleus in old men and postmenopausal women.[114,115] The mean profile area of infundibular neurons from old men and postmenopausal women was significantly larger than that of young subjects (Figure 9). The density of hypertrophied neurons was also increased. Furthermore, the hypertrophied neurons contained increased amounts of neurokinin B, substance P, and estrogen receptor mRNA, which indicated an increased neuronal activity as well.[116,117] LHRH neurons are also found in this nucleus, but the hypertrophied neurons themselves do not contain this peptide. The neurokinin B-containing neurons are probably involved in the regulation of the HPG-axis and have been related to menopausal flushes.[114] The sensitivity of LH to LHRH did not decrease in elderly males.[118-120] On the other hand, a decreased sensitivity to sex steroid feedback was found in elderly (80 years) postmenopausal women as compared to younger post-menopausal women (55 years).[121] No data on changes in the exact number of LHRH expressing neurons in relation to aging in the human hypothalamus are available at present.

B. Growth Hormone-Releasing Hormone (GHRH) and Somatostatin

In the rat the majority of GHRH-immunoreactive neurons are located in the arcuate nucleus.[122,123] Together with the inhibiting somatostatin neurons that are situated in the periventricular nucleus,[124] they regulate the secretion of growth hormone (GH), which is not only necessary for normal infant and childhood growth but also for the regulation of normal body composition and metabolism in adulthood.[125] A current hypothesis states that a defective GH secretion may be one of the pacemakers of aging.[126,127] In addition, Morimoto[128] showed that the intensity of GHRH immunoreactivity in the median eminence of 20-month-old rats is markedly reduced in comparison with that of young rats. Interestingly, however, the number of immunoreactive neurons in the GHRH and somatostatin-containing neuronal perikarya in the hypothalamus in old colchicine-treated rats did not differ.[128] These observations indicate that in old animals GHRH and somatostatin-containing neurons remain present and have the capacity to synthesize the respective peptides. However, either the production, transport rate, or release of GHRH should be changed in aging. Indeed, De Gennaro Colonna et al.[129] reported a reduction in GHRH peptide and mRNA levels in the hypothalamus of (20-month) old male Sprague-Dawley rats. Both decreased somatostatin gene expression[130,131] and increased somatostatin secretion have been reported in the rat.[132] Endocrine studies indicate the presence of changes in GH regulation in human aging. In elderly people the response of GH to GHRH was shown to be significantly reduced.[133,134] It has even been reported that GH responses to GHRH decline after 30 to 40 years in men and after menopause in women.[135-137] Furthermore, the feedback effects of circulating GH on GHRH that are present in adult rats were not detectable in aged rats.[129] Although it has been suggested that a decreased GHRH or increased somatostatinergic activity are the main events underlying the age-related decline of GH secretion,[138] no direct evidence is available about the changes of GHRH or somatostatin neurons in the human hypothalamus with aging.

VI. LATERAL TUBERAL NUCLEUS

The lateral tuberal nucleus (nucleus tuberalis lateralis, NTL) can only be recognized in man and higher primates. The only neuropeptide found so far that is characteristic for NTL neurons is somatostatin.[9,124] In addition, some galanin and LHRH immunoreactive fibers have been found in the NTL.[25,107] A dense innervation of prosomatostatin fibers, most probably derived from the NTL interneurons, were recently found in the NTL.[124] Receptors for CRH, somatostatin, muscarinic cholinergic receptors, benzodiazepin receptors, and N-methyl-D-aspartate (NMDA) receptors have been localized in the NTL.[139] In adulthood the NTL contains about 60,000 neurons. It has been shown that the number of NTL neurons may gradually decline with age. Although no significant correlation between NTL cell number and age was found, this may, however, be due to the small sample, especially in the oldest age group.[139] No clear changes in the somatostatin immunoreactive neurons were observed in human NTL with aging.[124]

VII. CONCLUSION

The main conclusion of the present review is that the aging process causes differential changes in the hypothalamus. Aging may start around middle-age in some peptidergic systems (e.g., the decreased number of VIP neurons in middle-aged males and the sharp decline of SDN neurons after 50 years). On the other hand, many more systems remain perfectly intact and are even activated (e.g., the unchanged number of VIP neurons in the female SCN and the increased number of CRH and AVP neurons of the PVN in the course of aging). The latter pattern argues against the idea that normal aging leads to a general decline in cellular functions, i.e., by "wear and tear".

Activation of some groups of nerve cells within the physiological range seems to lead to maintenance of neurons during aging. This "use it or lose it" hypothesis might explain why certain neurons degenerate in aging while others do not, and why recovery of various neuronal systems during aging can be obtained by restoration of the missing stimulus.[88] The finding that some peptidergic neurons are activated during aging may have important functional consequences, e.g., the involvement of activated CRH neurons in the development of depression. In addition, the presence of activated peptidergic neurons may have consequences for the treatment of elderly people with such peptides. When neuropeptides are given to elderly people, it should be taken into account that the release of many of them is already significantly increased.

Treatment of old and demented people with AVP and analogues was based upon the presumption that AVP levels in the brain were decreased,[65] whereas it was shown later that the endogenous activity of AVP cells in the HNS was increased in old people. It can be concluded that the multitude of changes in the various hypothalamic nuclei may be the basis for many functional changes in aging, i.e., both endocrine and central alterations. We suspect, however, that only a small proportion of such changes has, at present, been revealed.

ACKNOWLEDGMENTS

Brain material was obtained from the Netherlands Brain Bank, Amsterdam (coordinator Dr. R. Ravid). The authors are indebted to NUFFIC for financial support to Jiang-Ning Zhou, to Drs. M.A. Hofman, P. Lucassen, E. Van Someren, and A. Salehi for their excellent remarks, to Ms. W.T.P. Verweij for her secretarial help and for helping to revise the English, and to Mr. G. Van der Meulen for his photographic work.

REFERENCES

1. Brown-Sèquard, C. R., Des effects produits chez l'homme par des injections souscutanees d'un liquid retire des testicles de cobaye et de chien, *C.R. Soc. Biol.*, 41, 415, 1889.
2. Beach, F. A., Historical origins of modern research on hormones and behavior, *Horm. Behav.*, 15, 325, 1981.
3. Dilman, V. M., Age-associated elevation of hypothalamic threshold to feedback control, and its role in development, ageing and disease, *Lancet*, i, 1211, 1971.
4. Frolkis, V. V., Bezrukov, V. V., Duplenko, Y. K., and Genis, E. D., The hypothalamus in aging, *Exp. Gerontol.*, 7, 169, 1972.
5. Groen, J. J., General physiology of aging, *Geriatrics*, 14, 318, 1959.
6. Guillemin, R., Sakiz, E., and Ward, D. N., Further purification of TSH releasing from sheep hypothalamic tissues, with observations on the amino acid composition, *Proc. Soc. Exp. Biol. Med.*, 118, 1132, 1965.
7. Schally, A., Bowers, C., Redding, T., and Barrett, J., Isolation of thyrotropin releasing factor (TRF) from porcine hypothalamus, *Biochem. Biophys. Res. Commun.*, 25, 165, 1966.
8. Burgus, R. and Guillemin, R., Hypothalamic releasing factors, *Ann. Rev. Biochem.*, 39, 499, 1970.

9. Swaab, D. F., Hofman, M. A., Lucassen, P. J., Purba, J. S., Raadsheer, F. C., and Van de Nes, J. A. P., Functional neuroanatomy and neuropathology of the human hypothalamus, *Anat. Embryol.* (Berl.), 187, 317, 1993.

10. Buijs, R. M., Chemical transmission in the brain. The role of amines, amino acid and peptides, in *Progress in Brain Research,* Buijs, R. M., Pévet, P. and Swaab, D. F., Eds., Elsevier, Amsterdam, 1983, 167.

11. Hökfelt, T., Johansson, O., Holets, V., Meister, T., and Melander, T., Distribution of neuropeptides with special reference to their coexistence with classical neurotransmitter, in *Psychopharmacology: The Third Generations of Progress,* Meltzer, H. Y., Ed., Raven Press, New York, 1987, 401.

12. Meites, J., Importance of the endocrine system in aging processes, *Adv. Biochem. Psychopharmacol.,* 43, 283, 1987.

13. Meites, J., Aging: hypothalamic catecholamines, neuroendocrine immune interactions and dietary restriction, *Proc. Soc. Exp. Biol. Med.,* 195, 304, 1990.

14. Horniekiewicz, O., Neurotransmitter changes in human brain during aging, in *Modification of Cell to Cell Signals During Normal and Pathological Aging,* Govani, S. and Battaini, F., Eds., Springer-Verlag, Berlin, 1987, 169.

15. Landfield, P., Baskin, R., and Pitler, T., Brain aging correlates: retardation by hormonal-pharmacological treatments, *Science,* 214, 581, 1981.

16. Sapolsky, R., Krey, L., and McEwen, B., Prolonged glucocorticoid exposure reduces hippocampal neuron number: implications for aging, *J. Neurosci.,* 5, 1222, 1985.

17. Bodansky, M. and Engel, S. L., Oxytocin and the life-span of male rats, *Nature,* 210, 751, 1966.

18. Fliers, E. and Swaab, D. F., Neuropeptide changes in aging and Alzheimer's disease, *Prog. Brain Res.,* 70, 141, 1986.

19. Rusak, B. and Zucker, I., Neural regulation of circadian rhythms, *Physiol. Rev.,* 59, 449, 1979.

20. Stopa, E. G., King, J. C., Lydic, R., and Schoene, W. C., Human brain contains vasopressin and vasoactive intestinal polypeptide neuronal subpopulations in the suprachiasmatic region, *Brain Res.,* 297, 159, 1984.

21. Swaab, D. F., Fliers, E., and Partiman, T. S., The suprachiasmatic nucleus of the human brain in relation to sex, age and senile dementia, *Brain Res.,* 342, 37, 1985.

22. Mai, J. K., Kedziora, O., Teckhaus, L., and Sofroniew, M. V., Evidence for subdivisions in the human suprachiasmatic nucleus, *J. Comp. Neurol.,* 305, 508, 1991.

23. Moore, R. Y., The organization of the human circadian rhythm, the human hypothalamus in health and disease, in *Progress in Brain Research,* Vol. 93, Swaab, D. F., Hofman, M. A., Mirmiran, M., Ravid, R., and Van Leeuwen, F. W., Eds., Elsevier, Amsterdam, 1992, 101.

24. Albers, E., Liou, S., Stopa, E., and Zoeller, T., Interaction of colocalized neuropeptides: functional significance in the circadian timing system, *J. Neurosci.,* 11, 846, 1991.

25. Gai, W. P., Geffen, L. B., and Blessing, W. W., Galanin immunoreactive neurons in the human hypothalamus: colocalization with vasopressin-containing neurons, *J. Comp. Neurol.,* 298, 265, 1990.

26. Okamura, H., Murakami, S., Uda, K., Sugano, T., Takahashi, Y., Yanaihara, C., Yanahara, N., and Ibata, Y., Coexistence of vasoactive intestinal peptide (VIP), peptide histidine isoleucine amide (PHI), and gastrin releasing peptide (GRP)-like immunoreactivity in neurons of the rat suprachiasmatic nucleus, *Biomed. Res.,* 7, 295, 1986.

27. Francois-Bellan, A. M., Machidian, P., Dusticier, G., Tonon, M. C., Vaudry, H., and Bosler, O., GABA neurons in the rat suprachiasmatic nucleus: involvement in chemospecific circuitry and evidence for GAD-peptide colocalization, *J. Neurocytol.*, 19, 939, 1990.

28. Hofman, M. A. and Swaab, D. F., Seasonal changes in the suprachiasmatic nucleus of man, *Neurosci. Lett.*, 139, 257, 1992.

29. Hofman, M. A., Purba, J. S., and Swaab, D. F., Annual variations in the vasopressin neuron population of the human suprachiasmatic nucleus, *Neuroscience*, 53, 1103, 1993.

30. Hofman, M. A. and Swaab, D. F., Alterations in circadian rhythmicity of the vasopressin-producing neurons of the human suprachiasmatic nucleus (SCN) with aging, *Brain Res.*, 657, 281, 1994.

31. Van Gool, W. A. and Mirmiran, M., Aging and circadian rhythms, aging of the brain and Alzheimer's disease, *Progress in Brain Research*, Vol 70, Swaab, D. F., Fliers, E., Mirmiran, M., Van Gool, W. A., and Van Haaren, F., Eds., Elsevier, Amsterdam, 1986, 255.

32. Van Someren, E. J. W., Mirmiran, M., and Swaab, D. F., Non-pharmacological treatment of sleep and wake disturbances in aging and Alzheimer's disease: chronobiological perspectives, *Behavioral Brain Res.*, 57, 235, 1993.

33. Witting, W., Kwa, I. H., Eikelenboom, P., Mirmiran, M., and Swaab, D. F., Alterations in the circadian rest-activity rhythm in aging and Alzheimer's disease, *Biol. Psychiat.*, 27, 563, 1990.

34. Swaab, D. F., Zhou, J. N., Ehlhart, T., and Hofman, M. A., Development of vasoactive intestinal polypeptide neurons in the human suprachiasmatic nucleus in relation to birth and sex, *Dev. Brain Res.*, 79, 249, 1994b.

35. Zhou, J. N., Hofman, M. A., and Swaab, D. F., Vasoactive intestinal polypeptide neurons in the human suprachiasmatic nucleus in relation to sex, age and Alzheimer's disease, *Neurobiol. Aging,* (in press, 1995).

36. Davis, F. C., Darrow, J. M., and Menaker, M., Sex difference in the circadian control of hamster wheel-running activity, *Am. J. Physiol.*, 244, R93, 1983.

37. Wever, R. A., Characteristics of circadian rhythms in human function, *J. Neural. Transm.*, Suppl. 21, 323, 1986.

38. Van Der Beek, E. M., Wiegant, V. M., Van Der Donk, H. A., Van Den Hurk, R., and Buijs, R. M., Lesions of the suprachiasmatic nucleus indicate the presence of a direct vasoactive intestinal polypeptide-containing projection to gonadotrophin-releasing hormone neurons in the female rat, *J. Neuroendocrinol.*, 5, 137, 1993.

39. Swaab, D. F. and Hofman, M. A., An enlarged suprachiasmatic nucleus in homosexual men, *Brain Res.* 537, 141, 1990.

40. Swaab, D. F., Gooren, L. J. G., and Hofman, M. A., The human hypothalamus in relation to gender and sexual orientation, the human hypothalamus in health and disease, *Progress in Brain Research*, Vol. 93, Swaab, D. F., Hofman, M. A., Mirmiran, M., Ravid, R., and Van Leeuwen, F.W., Eds., Elsevier, Amsterdam, 1992, 205.

41. Hofman, M. A. and Swaab, D. F., Diurnal and seasonal rhythms of neuronal activity in the suprachiasmatic nucleus of humans, *J. Biol. Rhythms*, 8, 283, 1993a.

42. Rolandi, E., Franceshini, R., Cataldi, A., and Barreca, T., Twenty-four-hour secretory pattern of vasoactive intestinal polypeptide in the elderly, *Gerontology*, 36, 356, 1990.

43. Cugini, P., Lucia, P., Di Palma, L., Re, M., Leone, G., Battisti, P., Canova, R., Gasbarrone, L., and Cianetti, A., Vasoactive intestinal peptide fluctuates in human blood with a circadian rhythm, *Regul. Pept.*, 34, 141, 1991.

44. Prinz, P. N., Christie, C., Smallwood, R., Vitaliano, P., Bokan, J., Vitiello, M., and Martin, D., Circadian temperature variation in healthy aged and in Alzheimer's disease, *J. Gerontol.*, 39, 30, 1984.

45. Touitou, Y., Fèver, M., Lagoguey, M., Carayon, A., Bogdan, A., Reinberg, A., Beck, H., Cesselin, F., and Touitou, C., Age- and mental health-related circadian rhythms of plasma levels of melatonin, prolactin, luteinizing hormone and follicle-stimulating hormone in man, *J. Endocrinol.*, 91, 467, 1981.

46. Touitou, Y., Sulon, J., Bogdan, A., Touitou, C., Reinberg, A., Beck, H., Sodoyez, J., Demey-Ponsart, E., and Van Cauwenberghe, H., Adrenal circadian system in young and elderly human subjects: a comparative study, *J. Endocrinol.*, 93, 201, 1982.

47. Sherman, B., Wysham, C., and Pfohl, B., Age-related changes in the circadian rhythm of plasma cortisol in man, *J. Clin. Endocrinol. Metab.*, 61, 439, 1985.

48. Witting, W., Mirmiran, M., Bos, N. P. A., and Swaab, D. F., Effect of light intensity on diurnal sleep-wake distribution in young and old rats, *Brain Res. Bull.*, 30, 157, 1993.

49. Reuss, S. and Burger, K., Substance P-like immunoreactivity in the hypothalamic suprachiasmatic nucleus of Phodopus sungorus relation to daytime, photoperiod, sex and age, *Brain Res.*, 638, 189, 1994.

50. Braak, H. and Braak, E., The hypothalamus of the human adult: chiasmatic region, *Anat. Embryol.*, 176, 315, 1991.

51. Allen, L., Hines, M., Shryne, J., and Gorski, R., Two sexually dimorphic cell groups in the human brain, *J. Neurosci.*, 9, 497, 1989.

52. Swaab, D. F. and Hofman, M. A., Sexual differentiation of the human hypothalamus ontogeny of the sexually dimorphic nucleus of the preoptic area, *Dev. Brain Res.*, 44, 314, 1988.

53. Swaab, D. F. and Fliers, E., A sexually dimorphic nucleus in the human brain, *Science*, 228, 1112, 1985.

54. Hofman, M. A. and Swaab, D. F., The sexually dimorphic nucleus of the preoptic area in the human brain: a comparative morphometric study, *J. Anat.*, 164, 55, 1989.

55. Vermeulen, A., Androgens and male senescence, in *Testosterone: Action, Deficiency, Substitution*, Nieschlag, E. and Behre, H. M., Eds., Springer-Verlag, New York, 1990, 629.

56. Fliers, E., Noppen, N. W. A. M., Wiersinga, W. M., Visser, T., and Swaab, D. F., Distribution of thyrotropin-releasing hormone (TRH)-containing cells and fibers in the human hypothalamus, 350, 311, 1994.

57. Simerly, R. B., Gorski, R. A., and Swanson, L. W., Neurotransmitter specificity of cells and fibers in the medial preoptic nucleus: an immunohistochemical study in the rat, *J. Comp. Neurol.*, 246, 343, 1986.

58. Handler, J. S. and Orlof, J., Antidiuretic hormone, *Ann. Rev. Physiol.*, 43, 611, 1981.

59. Cowley, A. W. and Barber, B. J., Vasopressin vascular and reflex effects — a theoretical analysis, the neurohypophysis: structure, function and control, *Progress in Brain Research*, Cross, B. A. and Leng, G., Eds., Elsevier, Amsterdam, 1983, 415.

60. Swaab, D. F. and Boer, K., Function of pituitary hormones in human parturition — a comparison with data in the rat, in *Human Parturition*, Keirse, M. J. N. C., Anderson, A. B. M., and Gravenhorst, B. J., Eds., Martinius Nijhoff, The Hague, 1979, 49.

61. Spencer, S., Saper, C. B., Joh, T., Reis, D. J., Goldstein, M., and Raese, J. D., Distribution of catecholamine-containing neurons in the normal human hypothalamus, *Brain Res.*, 328, 730, 1985.

62. Panayotacopoulou, M. and Swaab, D. F., Development of tyrosine hydroxylase-immunoreactive neurons in the human paraventricular and supraoptic nucleus, *Dev. Brain Res.,* 72, 145, 1993.

63. De Wied, D., Central actions of neurohypophysial hormones, the neurohypophysis: structure, function and control, in *Progress in Brain Research,* Cross, B. A. and Leng, G., Eds., Elsevier, Amsterdam, 1985, 155.

64. De Wied, D. and Van Ree, J. M., Neuropeptides: animal behaviour and human psychopathology, *Eur. Arch. Psychiatry Neurol. Sci.,* 238, 323, 1989.

65. Jolles, J., Neuropeptides and the treatment of cognitive deficits in aging and dementia, aging of the brain and Alzheimer's disease, in *Progress in Brain Research,* Swaab, D. F., Fliers, E., Mirmiran, M., Van Gool, W. A., and Van Haaren, F., Eds., Elsevier, Amsterdam, 1986, 429.

66. Carter, L. S., Oxytocin and sexual behavior, *Neurosci. Biobehav. Rev.,* 16, 131, 1992.

67. Insel, T. R., Oxytocin — a neuropeptide for affiliation: evidence from behavioral, receptor autoradiographic, and comparative studies, *Psychoneuroendocrinology,* 17, 3, 1992.

68. Murphy, M. R., Seckl, J. R., Burton, S., Checkley, S. A., and Lightman, S. L., Changes in oxytocin and vasopressin secretion during sexual activity in men, *J. Clin. Endocrinol. Metab.,* 65, 738, 1987.

69. Goudsmit, E., Neijmeijer-Leloux, A., and Swaab, D. F., The human hypothalamo-neurohypophyseal system in relation to development, aging and Alzheimer's disease, *Prog. Brain Res.,* 93, 237, 1992.

70. Fliers, E., Swaab, D. F., Pool, C. W., and Verwer, R. W., The vasopressin and oxytocin neurons in the human supraoptic and paraventricular nucleus: changes with aging and in senile dementia, *Brain Res.,* 342, 45, 1985.

71. Vogels, O. J., Broere, C. A., and Nieuwenhuys, R., Neuronal hypertrophy in the human supraoptic and paraventricular nucleus in aging and Alzheimer's disease, *Neurosci. Lett.,* 109, 62, 1990.

72. Hoogendijk, J. E., Fliers, E., Swaab, D. F., and Verwer, R. W., Activation of vasopressin neurons in the human supraoptic and paraventricular nucleus in senescence and senile dementia, *J. Neurol. Sci.,* 69, 291, 1985.

73. Hofman, M. A., Fliers, E., Goudsmit, E., and Swaab, D. F., Morphometric analysis of the suprachiasmatic and paraventricular nuclei in the human brain: sex differences and age-dependent changes, *J. Anat.,* 160, 55, 1988.

74. Hofman, M. A., Goudsmit, E., Purba, J. S., and Swaab, D. F., Morphometric analysis of the supraoptic nucleus in the human brain, *J. Anat.,* 172, 259, 1990.

75. Goudsmit, E., Hofman, M. A., Fliers, E., and Swaab, D. F., The supraoptic and paraventricular nuclei of the human hypothalamus in relation to sex, age and Alzheimer's disease, *Neurobiol. Aging,* 11, 529, 1990.

76. Van der Woude, P. F., Goudsmit, E., Wierda, M., Purba, J. S., Hofman, M. A., Bogte, H., and Swaab, D. F., No vasopressin cell loss in the human hypothalamus in aging and Alzheimer's disease, *Neurobiol. Aging,* (in press, 1995).

77. Lucassen, P. J., Ravid, R., Gonatas, N. K., and Swaab, D. F., Activation of the human supraoptic and paraventricular nucleus neurons with aging and in Alzheimer's as judged from increasing size of Golgi apparatus, *Brain Res.,* 632, 105, 1993.

78. Phillips, P. A., Johnston, C. I., and Gray, L., Disturbed fluid and electrolyte homeostasis following dehydration in elderly people, *Age & Ageing,* 22, S26, 1993.

79. Kirkland, J., Lye, M., Goddard, C., Vargas, E., and Davies, I., Plasma arginine vasopressin in dehydrated elderly patients, *Clin. Endocrinol.,* 20, 451, 1984.

80. Helderman, J. H., Vestal, R. E., Rowe, J. W., Tobin, J. D., Andres, R., and Robertson, G. L., The response of arginine vasopressin to intravenous ethanol and hypertonic saline in man, the impact of aging, *J. Gerontol.,* 33, 39, 1978.

81. Rowe, J. W., Minaker, K. L., Sparrow, D., and Robertson, G. L., Age-related failure of volume-pressure-mediated vasopressin release, *J. Clin. Endocrinol. Metab.*, 54, 661, 1982.

82. Crawford, G. A., Johnson, A. G., Gyory, A. Z., and Kelly, D., Change in arginine vasopressin concentrations with age [letter], *Clin. Chem.*, 39, 2023, 1993.

83. Faull, C. M., Holmes, C., and Baylis, P. H., Water balance in elderly people: is there a deficiency of vasopressin?, *Age & Ageing*, 22, 114, 1993.

84. Bursztyn, M., Bresnahan, M., Gavras, I., and Gavras, H., Effect of aging on vasopressin, catecholamines, and alpha 2-adrenergic receptors, *J. Am. Geriatr. Soc.*, 38, 628, 1990.

85. Ravid, R., Fliers, E., Swaab, D.F., and Zurcher, C., Changes in vasopressin and testosterone in the senescent Brown-Norway (BN/BiRij) rat, *Gerontology*, 33, 87, 1987.

86. Herzberg, N.H., Goudsmit, E., Kruisbrink, J., and Boer, G. J., Testosterone treatment restores reduced vasopressin binding sites in the kidney of the aging rat, *J. Endocrinol.*, 123, 59, 1989.

87. Wierda, M., Goudsmit, E., Van der Woude, P. F., Purba, J. S., Hofman, M. A., Bogte, H., and Swaab, D. F., Oxytocin cell number in the human paraventricular nucleus remains constant with aging and in Alzheimer's disease, *Neurobiol. Aging*, 12, 511, 1991.

88. Swaab, D.F., Brain aging and Alzheimer's disease,"wear and tear" versus "use it or lose it", *Neurobiol. Aging*, 12, 317, 1991.

89. Pelletier, G., Desy, L., Cote, J., and Vaudry, H., Immunocytochemical localization of corticotropin-releasing factor-like immunoreactivity in the human hypothalamus, *Neurosci. Lett.*, 41, 259, 1983.

90. Raadsheer, F. C., Sluiter, A. A., Ravid, R., Tilders, F. J., and Swaab, D. F., Localization of corticotropin-releasing hormone (CRH) neurons in the paraventricular nucleus of the human hypothalamus; age-dependent colocalization with vasopressin, *Brain Res.*, 615, 50, 1993.

91. Merchenthaler, I., Vigh, S., Petrusz, P., and Schally, A. V., Immunocytochemical localization of corticotropin-releasing factor (CRF) in the rat brain, *Am. J. Anat.*, 165, 385, 1982.

92. Swanson, L., Sawchenko, P. E., and Lind, R. W., Regulation of multiple peptides in CRF parvicellular neurosecretory neurons: implications for the stress response, *Prog. Brain Res.*, 68, 169, 1986.

93. Sawchenko, P. F. and Swanson, L. W., Organization of CRF immunoreactive cells and fibers in the rat brain; immunohistochemical studies, in *Corticotropin Releasing Factor: Basic and Clinical Studies of a Neuropeptide*, De Souza, E. B. and Nemeroff, C. B., Eds., CRC Press, Boca Raton, FL, 1990, 29.

94. Raadsheer, F. C., Oorschot, D. F., Verwer, R. W. H., Tilders, F. J. H., and Swaab, D. F., Age-related increase in the total number of corticotropin-releasing hormone neurons in the human paraventricular nucleus in controls and Alzheimer's disease: comparison of the disector with an unfolding method, *J. Comp. Neurol.*, 339, 447, 1994.

95. Swaab, D. F., Raadsheer, F. C., Endert, E., Hofman, M. A., Kamphorst, W., and Ravid, R., Increased cortisol levels in aging and Alzheimer's disease in postmortem cerebrospinal fluid, *J. Neuroendocrinol.*, 6, 681, 1994.

96. Dodt, C., Dittman, J., Hruby, J., Späth-Schwalbe, E., Born, J., Schüttler, R., and Fehm, H. L., Different regulation of adrenocorticotropin and cortisol secretion in young, mentally healthy elderly, and patients with senile dementia of Alzheimer's type, *J. Clin. Endocrinol. Metab.*, 72, 272, 1991.

97. Oxenkrug, G. F., Pomara, N., McIntyre, I. M., Brancinnier, R. J., Stanly, M., and Gershon, S., Aging and cortisol resistance to suppression by dexamethasone: a positive correlation, *Psychiatry Res.*, 10, 125, 1983.

98. Rosenbaum, A. H., Schatzberg, A. F., MacLaughlin, R. A., Snyder, K., Jiang, N. S., Ilstrup, D., Rothschild, A.J., and Kliman, B., The dexamethasone suppression test in normal control subjects: comparison of two assays and effect of age, *Am. J. Psychiatry*, 141, 1550, 1984.

99. Herman, J.P., Schafer, M.K.H., Young, E.A., Thompson, R., Douglass, J., Akil, H., and Watson, S. J., Evidence for hippocampal regulation of neuroendocrine neurons of the hypothalamo-pituitary-adrenocortical axis, *J. Neurosci.*, 9, 3072, 1989.

100. Blichert-Toft, M., Secretion of corticotrophin and somatotrophin by the senescent adenohypophysis in the man, *Acta Endocrinol.*, 78 (Suppl. 195), 15, 1975.

101. Holsboer, F., Psychiatric implications of altered limbic-hypothalamic-pituitary-adrenocortical activity, review, *Eur. Arch. Psychiatry Neurol. Sci.*, 238, 302, 1989.

102. Pekary, A. E., Carlson, H. E., Tadataka, Y., Sharp, B., Walfish, P. G., and Hershman, J. M., Thyrotropin-releasing hormone levels decrease in hypothalamus of aging rats. *Neurobiol. Aging*, 5, 221, 1984.

103. Pekary, A. E., Mirell, C. J., Turner, L. F., Walfish, P. G., and Hershman, J. M., Hypothalamic secretion of thyrotropin releasing hormone decline in aging rats, *J. Gerontol.*, 42, 447, 1987.

104. Spaulding, S. W., Age and the thyroid. *Endocrinol. Metab. Clin.*, 16, 1013, 1987.

105. Simpkins, J. W. and Millard, W. J., Influence of age on neurotransmitter function, *Endocrinol. Metab. Clin. North. Am.*, 16, 893, 1987.

106. Bouras, C., Magistretti, J., Morrison, H., and Constantinidis, J., An immunohistochemical study of pro-somatostatin-derived peptides in the human brain, *Neuroscience*, 22, 781, 1987.

107. Najimi, M., Chigr, F., Jordan, D., Leduque, P., Block, B., Tommasi, M., Rebaud, P., and Kopp, N., Anatomical distribution of LHRH-immunoreactive neurons in the human infant hypothalamus and extrahypothalamic regions, *Brain Res.*, 516, 280, 1990.

108. Mezey, E. and Kiss, J. Z., Vasoactive intestinal peptide-containing neurons in the paraventricular nucleus may participate in regulating prolactin secretion, *Proc. Natl. Acad. Sci. U.S.A.*, 82, 245, 1985.

109. Anthony, E. L., King, J. C., and Stopa, E. G., Immunocytochemical localization of LHRH in the median eminence, infundibular stalk, and neurohypophysis. Evidence for multiple sites of releasing hormone secretion in human and other mammals, *Cell Tissue Res.*, 236, 5, 1984.

110. Barry, J., Characterization and topography of LHRH neurons in the human brain, *Neurosci. Lett.*, 3, 287, 1976.

111. Stopa, E. G., Koh, E. T., Svendsen, C. N., Rogers, W. T., Schwaber, J. S., and King, J. C., Computer-assisted mapping of immunoreactive mammalian gonadotropin-releasing hormone in adult human basal forebrain and amygdala, *Endocrinology*, 128, 3199, 1991.

112. Rance, N.E., Young, S., III, and McMullen, N., Topography of neurons expressing luteinizing hormone-releasing hormone gene transcripts in the human hypothalamus and basal forebrain, *J. Comp. Neurol.*, 339, 573, 1994.

113. Vallet, P. G., Charnay, Y., and Bouras, C., Distribution and colocalization of delta sleep-inducing peptide and luteinizing hormone-releasing hormone in the aged human brain: an immunohistochemical study, *J. Chem. Neuroanat.*, 3, 207, 1990.

114. Rance, N. E., Hormonal influence on morphology and neuropeptide gene expression in the infundibular nucleus of postmenopausal women, in *Progress in Brain Research*, Swaab, D. F., Hofman, M. A., Mirmiran, M., Ravid, R., and Van Leeuwen, F. W., Eds., Elsevier, Amsterdam, 1992.

115. Rance, N. E., Uswandi, S. V., and McMullen, N. T., Neuronal hypertrophy in the older men, *Neurobiol. Aging*, 14, 337, 1993.

116. Rance, N. E., McMullen, N. T., Smialek, J. E., Price, D. L., and Young, W. S., III, Postmenopausal hypertrophy of neurons expressing the estrogen receptor gene in the human hypothalamus, *J. Clin. Endocrinol. Metab.*, 71, 79, 1990.

117. Rance, N. E. and Young, W. S., III, Hypertrophy and increased gene expression of neurons containing neurokinin B and substance P messenger RNAS in the hypothalami of postmenopausal women, *Endocrinology*, 128, 2239, 1991.

118. Giusti, M., Marini, G., Traverso, L., Cavagnaro, P., Granziera, L., and Giordano, G., Effect of pulsatile luteinizing hormone-releasing hormone administration on pituitary-gonadal function in elderly man, *J. Endocrinol. Invest.*, 13, 127, 1990.

119. Kaufman, J. M., Deslypere, J. P., Giri, M., and Vermeulen, A., Neuroendocrine regulation of pulsatile luteinizing hormone secretion in elderly men, *J. Steroid Biochem. Mol. Biol.*, 37, 421, 1990.

120. Kaufman, J. M., Giri, M., Deslypere, J. M., Thomas, G., and Vermeulen, A., Influence of age on the responsiveness of the gonadotrophs to luteinizing hormone-releasing hormone in males, *J. Clin. Endocrinol. Metab.*, 72, 1255, 1991.

121. Rossmanith, W., Reichelt, C., and Scherbaum, W., Neuroendocrinology of aging in humans: attenuateal sensitivity to sex steroid feedback in elderly postmenopausal women, *Neuroendocrinology*, 59, 355, 1994.

122. Bloch, B., Ling, N., Benoit, R., Wehernberg, W. B., and Guillemin, R., Specific depletion of immunoreactive growth hormone releasing factor by monosodium glutamate in rat median eminence, *Nature*, 307, 272, 1984.

123. Liposits, Z., Hrabovszky, E., and Paull, W. K., Catecholaminergic afferents to growth hormone-releasing hormone (GHRH)-synthesizing neurons of the arcuate nucleus in the rat, *Biomed. Res.*, 40 (Suppl. 3), 1950, 1989.

124. Van de Nes, J. A. P., Sluiter A.A., Pool, C. W., Kamphorst, W., Ravid, R., and Swaab, D. F., The monoclonal antibody Alz-50, which reveals cytoskeletal changes in Alzheimer's disease, cross-reacts with somatostatinergic neurons in the human hypothalamus of control subjects, *Brain Res.*, 655, 97, 1994.

125. Christiansen, J. S., Jorgensen, J. O., Pedersen, S.A., Moller, J., Jorgensen, J., and Kakkebaek, N. E., Effects of growth hormone on body composition in adults, *Horm. Res.*, 33 (Suppl. 4), 61, 1990.

126. Rudman, D., Kutner, M. H., Rogers, C. M., Lubin, M. F., Fleming, G. H., and Bain, R. P., Impaired growth hormone secretion in the adult population, *J. Clin. Invest.*, 67, 1361, 1981.

127. Rudman, D., Feller, A. G., Nagraj, H. S., Gergans, G. A., Lalitha, P. Y., Goldberg A. F., Schlenker, R. A., Cohn, L., Rudman, I., and Mattson, D. E., Effect of human growth hormone in men over 60 years old, *New Engl. J. Med.*, 323, 1, 1990.

128. Morimoto, N., Kawakami, F., Makino, S., Chihara, K., Hasegawa, M., and Ibata, Y., Age-related changes in growth hormone releasing factor and somatostatin in the rat hypothalamus, *Neuroendocrinology*, 47, 459, 1988.

129. De Gennaro Colonna, V., Fidone, F., Cocchi, D., and Müller, E. E., Feedback effects of growth hormone to growth hormone-releasing hormone and somatostatin are not evident in aged rats, *Neurobiol. Aging*, 14, 503, 1993.

130. Sonntag, W. E., Boyd, R. L., and Booze, R. M., Somatostatin gene expression in hypothalamus and cortex of aging male rats, *Neurobiol. Aging*, 11, 409, 1990.

131. Martinoli, M. C., Ouellet, J., Rhèaume, E., and Pelletier, G., Growth hormone and somatostatin gene expression as measured by quantitative in situ hybridization, *Neuroendocrinology*, 54, 607, 1991.

132. Ferrara, C., Ceresoli, G., Marcezzi, C., and Cocchi, D., Hypothalamic-pituitary somatostatinergic system in middle-aged female rats, *Hormone Metab. Res.*, 23, 243, 1991.

133. Coiro, V., Volpi, R., Cavazzini, U., Bertoni, P., Corradi, A., Bianconi, L., Davoli, C., Rossi, G., and Chiodera, P., Restoration of normal growth hormone responsiveness to GHRH in normal aged men by infusion of low amounts of theophylline [published erratum appears in *J. Gerontol.*, 47(2), M34, 1992], *J. Gerontol.*, 46, M155, 1991.

134. Coiro, V., Volpi, R., Bertoni, P., Finzi, G., Marcato, A., Caiazza, A., Colla, R., Giacalone, G., Rossi, G., and Chiodera, P., Effect of potentiation of cholinergic tone by pyridostigmine on the GH response to GHRH in elderly men, *Gerontology*, 38, 217, 1992.

135. Finkelstein, J. W., Rottwarg, H. P., Boyar, R. M., Kream, J., and Hellman, L. Age-related changes in 24-hour spontaneous secretion of growth hormone, *J. Clin. Endocrinol.*, 35, 665, 1972.

136. Carlson, H. E., Gillan, J. C., Gordon, P., and Snyder, F., Absence of sleep-related growth peaks in aged normal subjects and acromegaly, *J. Clin. Endocrinol.*, 34, 1102, 1972.

137. Iranmanesh, A., Lizarralde, G., and Veldhuis, J. D., Age and relative adiposity are specific negative determinants of the frequency and amplitude of growth hormone (GH) secretory bursts and the half-life of endogenous GH in healthy men, *J. Clin. Endocrinol. Metab.*, 73, 1081, 1991.

138. Müller, E. E., Cella, S. G., de Gennaro Colonna, V., Parenti, M., Cocchi, D., and Locatelli, V., Aspects of the neuroendocrine control of growth hormone secretion in aging mammals, *J. Reprod. Fertil. Suppl.*, 46, 99, 1993.

139. Kremer, H. P., The hypothalamic lateral tuberal nucleus: normal anatomy and changes in neurological diseases, *Prog. Brain Res.*, 93, 249, 1992.

140. Swaab, D. F., Roozendaal, B., Ravid, R., Velis, D. N., Gooren, L., and Williams, R. S., Suprachiasmatic nucleus in aging, Alzheimer's disease, transsexuality and Prader-Willi syndrome, in neuropeptides and brain function, *Progress in Brain Research*, Vol. 72, De Kloet, R. et al., Eds., Elsevier, Amsterdam, 1987, 301.

INDEX

D

U

V

W

X

Z